Moroney's
SURGERY
FOR NURSES

James Moroney, who from 1949—1981 edited fifteen editions of this book, held the following posts: Honorary Consultant Surgeon for the Liverpool Health Authority; Consultant Surgeon, Broadgreen Hospital, Liverpool and Clatterbridge Hospital, Wirral, Merseyside; Clinical Lecturer in Surgery, Clinical Sub Dean and Chairman, Board of the Faculty of Medicine, University of Liverpool; Examiner in Surgery, General Nursing Council for England and Wales; and Hunterian Professor, Royal College of Surgeons of England. He died in 1981.

Moroney's
SURGERY
FOR
NURSES

Edited by

Malcolm R. Colmer MA MB MChir FRCS JP

Consultant General Surgeon and Postgraduate Clinical
Tutor, St Helen's and Knowsley Health Authority,
Merseyside

SIXTEENTH EDITION

Churchill Livingstone

EDINBURGH LONDON MELBOURNE AND NEW YORK 1986

CHURCHILL LIVINGSTONE
Medical Division of Longman Group UK Limited

Distributed in the United States of America by Churchill
Livingstone Inc., 1560 Broadway, New York, N.Y. 10036
and by associated companies, branches and representatives
throughout the world.

First Edition 1950   Eleventh Edition 1967
Second Edition 1952   Twelfth Edition 1971
Third Edition 1955   Thirteenth Edition 1975
Fourth Edition 1956   Fourteenth Edition 1978
Fifth Edition 1958   Fifteenth Edition 1982
Sixth Edition 1959   Sixteenth Edition 1986
Seventh Edition 1961   Reprinted 1990
Eighth Edition 1962
Ninth Edition 1964
Tenth Edition 1966

ISBN   0 443 03355 2

British Library Cataloguing in Publication Data
Moroney, James
    Moroney's surgery for nurses.—16th ed.
    1. Surgical nursing
    I. Title II. Colmer, Malcom R. III. Moroney,
    James. Surgery for nurses
    610.73'677   RD99

Library of Congress Cataloguing-in-Publication Data
Moroney, James.
    Moroney's Surgery for nurses.
    Rev. ed. of: Surgery for nurses. 15th ed. 1982.
    Includes bibliographies and index.
    1. Surgical nursing. 2. Operations, Surgical.
I. Colmer, Malcolm R.   II. Title: Surgery
for nurses. [DNLM: 1. Surgery, Operative—nurses'
instruction. 2. Surgical nursing. WY 161 M868s]
RD99.M73   1986   610.73'677   85-26938

Produced by Longman Group (FE) Ltd
Printed in Hong Kong

Preface to the Sixteenth Edition

It has been the aim throughout, in the preparation of the present edition of this book, to ensure that it is factually correct and up to date. Nevertheless, those concerned have sought to maintain the essential character of a much respected book which, over many years, has stood the test of time. Some chapters, for example those on perioperative care, microbiology, infection, oncology, burns and scalds and cardiac surgery, have been radically revised in an attempt to reflect contemporary knowledge and treatment. Changes have been made in many other chapters with the same end in view.

I wish to express my gratitude to all those who have been so generous with their help in the preparation of the text—the many who have typed the manuscript, provided illustrations and performed many other practical tasks. The publishers have been a constant source of encouragement and support, a role they have fulfilled with considerable patience. Their help and advice have been invaluable.

The overall aim of the book is maintained—that is to provide a straightforward, comprehensive surgical text for the student nurse and a reference book for those who are trained. It does not aim primarily to be a textbook of surgical nursing.

Merseyside, 1986   MRC

Contributors

The editor gratefully acknowledges his indebtedness to all who have contributed so willingly to the preparation of the present editon of this book.

Nursing contributors

Miss M.R. Balmer SRN
Clinical Nursing Officer, Operating Theatre, Whiston Hospital, Merseyside

Mrs P. Comerford SRN RFN DN JBCNS in Stoma Care
Stoma Therapist, St Helen's & Knowsley Health Authority, Merseyside

Mrs M. Crowther RGN DN RCNT RNT
Nurse Tutor, School of Nursing, Whiston Hospital, Merseyside

Mrs E.J. Flinn SRN
Theatre Sister, Whiston Hospital, Merseyside

Mrs S. Goodlad RGN SCM RCNT
Clinical Teacher, School of Nursing, Whiston Hospital, Merseyside

Medical contributors

S.T. Atherton MRCP
Consultant Physician and Director of Intensive Care Unit, St Helen's & Knowsley Health Authority, Merseyside

P.K. Basu FRCS (Ed) FRCS
Senior Surgical Registrar, Whiston Hospital, Merseyside

Jill E.S. Brock MA BCh BM FRCR DMRT
Consultant in Radiotherapy and Oncology, Clatterbridge Hospital, Merseyside

R.J. Donnelly MB FRCS(Ed)
Consultant Cardiothoracic Surgeon, Regional Cardiothoracic Unit, Liverpool; Clinical Lecturer in Cardiothoracic Surgery, University of Liverpool

A.F. Evans FFR, FRCR
Consultant Radiologist, St Helen's & Knowsley Health Authority, Merseyside

Angela Galloway BSc MB BS
Consultant Microbiologist, St Helen's & Knowsley Health Authority, Merseyside

L.A. Holbrook FRCS
Consultant Plastic Surgeon, Regional Burns and Plastic Unit, Whiston Hospital, Merseyside

D. Leighton MD FRCS
Consultant Ophthalmic Surgeon, St Helen's & Knowsley Health Authority, Merseyside

R. Macmillan MB ChB FFARCS
Consultant Anaesthetist, St Helen's & Knowsley Health Authority, Merseyside

J.B. Meade MCh BAO FRCS(I)
Consultant Cardiac Surgeon, Regional Cardiothoracic Unit, Liverpool; Director of Cardiothoracic Studies, University of Liverpool

Janine M. Miller FRCOG
Consultant Obstetrician & Gynaecologist, St Helen's & Knowsley Health Authority, Merseyside

P.K.M. Rostron MCh(Orth) FRCS(Ed)
Consultant Orthopaedic Surgeon, St Helen's & Knowsley Health Authority, Merseyside

J.A. Tappin MD MRCP
Consultant Haematologist, St Helen's & Knowsley Health Authority, Merseyside

Charles West MA BChir FRCS
Consultant Neurosurgeon, Hope Hospital, Salford and Royal Manchester Children's Hospital

Norton E. Williams FFARCS
Consultant Anaesthetist, St Helen's & Knowsley Health Authority, Merseyside

Photography

Mrs D.M. Dean LBIPP
Department of Photography, St Helen's & Knowsley Health Authority, Merseyside

Contents

1

Surgery, the nurse and the patient

HISTORICAL INTRODUCTION

Surgery is one of the most ancient arts in the world. Its oldest branch, obstetric surgery, is almost as old as the world itself. The daring and manual dexterity of the barber-surgeon were surpassed only by the courage and forbearance of his conscious patient. Survival of such an ordeal was followed by many months in bed, during which time 'laudable' pus drained from the wound. A century ago the surgeon of that day operated without even washing his hands, and was clad in a top hat and a frock coat well stained with blood and pus. For convenience, he carried his ligature and suture materials in the buttonhole of his lapel!

The discovery of anaesthetics and the appreciation of the importance of eliminating infection in the patient's wound have transformed the surgical art. Each year adds much to the vast store of knowledge, even to the knowledge of such fundamentals as the sciences of anaesthetics and asepsis. The comparatively recent advances of blood transfusion and chemotherapy are examples of some of the outstanding achievements of contemporary scientists.

A century ago there were few skilled nurses as we know them today. The nurse's predecessor was often an illiterate, rough, dirty handywoman. In many institutions a patient was in great measure dependent on what help he could secure from the patient in the adjoining bed.

Surgery, surgeons, and nurses have changed considerably in a century, but the plea for relief from suffering has remained essentially the same. Every patient is a man, woman, or child living and working in different surroundings and in different spheres of activity. They are all different— different in outlook, different in character, different in their reaction to the same disease. Appreciation of the importance of this individual variation is a fundamental principle of good nursing.

Surgical treatment is usually undertaken away from the patient's own home. The advantages are overwhelming, but there is one serious disadvantage, however, in that hospital staff have few opportunities of visiting ill patients in their own homes. It is surprising at times to see what 'home' means. The advice given to a patient on leaving hospital must be considered against this background. The current trend of nursing education aims at a 'wider basic training' including secondment of the student to the community. The District Nurse Liaison Officer works with other members of the Care Team to ensure a smooth return for the patient to his home environment.

The patient's mental outlook, his fears, his hopes, and his will, may play a part equal in importance to the purely physical treatment of his disease. To ignore, to be unaware of, or to neglect these factors may make a patient prefer death to a struggle, and then no amount of effort may be able to regain the valuable ground which has been lost or opportunities which have been cast away.

As medicine, of which surgery is a branch, becomes more specialised and complex, certain procedures are undertaken in specially equipped centres. Some of these may be comparatively large, such as those for cardiothoracic or neurosurgery, while others may be very small. Where patients suffering from identical or similar diseases meet in the ward or at repeated attendances at a clinic, their conversation inevitably turns to an evaluation of their progress and treatment. Not surprisingly most patients at an artificial limb centre have a very poor opinion of the results of arterial surgery! Nor can one expect a patient who has undergone surgery and perhaps radiotherapy to be enthusiastic about repeated courses of cytotoxic therapy for malignancy.

In other circumstances, a patient of suitable disposition may be most helpful to another sufferer who has undergone, or is about to undergo, a procedure like a colostomy or ileostomy. The nurse has to exercise considerable judgment in all these situations—aware at one moment of the conflicts and despair in the patient's mind, at another of the opportunity where one patient can help another.

THE PATIENT'S CONCEPT OF DISEASE

The term disease has a wider connotation to the nurse and the doctor than it has to the public, many of whom conceive the term as restricted to an infection or, even more narrowly, an infectious disease. Most patients have little appreciation of the nature of their illness and still less of what its cure or control may entail.

As far as possible, making due allowance for intelligence and language difficulties, the patient should be encouraged to take an interest in everything that is happening to him so that the reason for every procedure is understood.

On admission, the patient's condition is assessed by observation and discussion with the patient and his family. From information received his needs are identified and care planned according to the activities of daily living. Throughout his stay the plan is constantly evaluated and up-dated. At each stage he is encouraged to take an active interest in his condition and care. The care of the patient is paramount. In this way the relationship between the patient, his family and the caring team is immediately established.

The patient should be given an explanation of the need for and nature of any investigation or procedure, such as preoperative shaving of the skin, preoperative medication or intravenous infusion. This not only makes the procedure all the more acceptable but encourages the patient to ask questions and perhaps reveal his anxieties. The nature of the operation and its effects should be explained by the surgeon, but a nurse who knows the patient's response to procedures already undertaken by her can brief the surgeon concerning the patient before he explains the operation he advises.

The nurse can do much to allay and alleviate the inevitable anxieties of the surgical patient both on his arrival and throughout his stay in the ward.

FACTORS AFFECTING THE SUCCESS OF SURGICAL CARE

The health care team

Many people from different disciplines are usually involved in the delivery of care and treatment to any particular patient. It is important that such people act as a co-ordinated team, that they communicate together concerning patients' needs and that they value the contribution of each other to the total care of the patient. Such a team includes doctors, nurses, physiotherapists, radiographers, dieticians, occupational therapists, social workers, ministers of religion.

The recognition of specific needs experienced by some groups of patients has led to the development of particular expertise in members of the team e.g. nurses are trained in the fields of stomatherapy, care of the terminally ill and the control of infection.

The application of professional knowledge

There can be no substitute for knowledge gained by study and experience. Since its projection is ultimately on human beings, its first impact is on the patient's mind.

It is obvious that the patient's confidence will only be gained and maintained as he becomes aware of the knowledge, expertise, and understanding of those who care for him.

Appreciation of the aims of modern surgical treatment

Without a high order of technical competence and anatomical knowledge, in surgeon and nurse alike, no operation could be a success. The operation, however, is only a part, albeit an important part, of treatment. To the patient it is dominant and likely to be most feared. While a scar may be the only visible anatomical distortion, physiological and psychological changes may be profound, and with the passage of time, cause increasing disability. To diminish or alleviate these disabilities requires the exercise of sympathy and judgment at least equal to the operative skill.

An operation is not an inevitable sequel of admission to a surgical ward, because many conditions subside without operative treatment. An operation may be:

1. An emergency. This is performed only when there is an immediate threat to life from haemorrhage, respiratory or intestinal obstruction, or a spreading infection not likely to be controlled by conservative measures alone.

2. Planned (elective). Strategically this is the most desirable, because it can be undertaken when the patient's general and local conditions are controlled to the maximal degree.

3. Multistaged. This may be necessary because:

(a) The patient's condition is not good enough to do all that is necessary at once, or

(b) The first operation may be designed to rest or drain an organ or cavity, so that subsequent curative measures can be safely undertaken, or

(c) There is a need for reoperation due to a complication. This is particularly distressing to the patient and disappointing to the surgeon and nurse.

The aim of surgery is to assist and not to usurp the place of natural healing. For this reason timing may be as important as the nature and extent of the operation.

Human sympathy and understanding

It is a fair presumption that one becomes a nurse because one is activated by a desire to help others in distress. In addition, one must have an imaginative mind, considerable tact and patience. Good powers of observation and an ability to listen are essential. Only by imagining oneself in the patient's position can it be realised how he is feeling and how one can help. The background of professional knowledge and detailed care is discussed in Chapter 4. The following aspects of some of these subjects are discussed from the point of view of the nurse–patient relationship.

Reception

The relationship must be established at once—it is that of the good hostess and the welcome guest—natural, kind, and cheerful. Questions should be answered simply. There is no place for dramatisation. Many questions can be answered only by the sister of the ward who will refer all questions on diagnosis and prognosis to the medical staff.

Once settled into the ward environment the patient should be allowed to see his relatives. Prior to leaving the ward the relatives should be given details of the patient's condition, visiting times and ward phone number.

In order to help him settle peacefully, any specific requests by the patient should be met as soon as possible. For example, he may wish to see a Social Worker, regarding home commitments, or a Minister of Religion for his spiritual needs.

Preparation of the patient

The patient may be admitted for an emergency operation, or for one where time is a less urgent factor. Where there are several days in hand, the nurse can get to know the patient as an individual, consider how he will react to the various preparations, and how they can be best undertaken. It is now customary to admit a patient the evening before or even on the day of operation. Many preliminary preparations are undertaken as an outpatient.

1. Consent form. This has to be signed by the patient before any operative procedure can be undertaken. It is a medical responsibility to see that this is done.

2. Collection of specimens. Blood may have to be taken by the doctor or by the phlebotomist for examination or for cross-matching. This is often the first experience of a hospital procedure.

The reason given for the procedure as well as how it is performed may well determine the patient's future attitude. An efficient vein tourniquet and sharp needles, with an adequate choice to ensure that the smallest possible needle is used, are important in fulfilling the promise that it is really 'only a little prick'. A specimen of urine is collected and ward test performed to establish any abnormalities. The patient should be told the result.

3. Dental hygiene may have been poor and require correction. When referring the patient for dental advice the doctor and nurse should remember that they are not qualified to express an opinion. A remark to the patient that he should have his teeth extracted may be as erroneous as it is unprofessional.

4. Physiotherapy may be necessary to improve pulmonary function and prevent postoperative complications.

5. Skin preparation. Specific preparation, discussed fully in Chapter 4, includes shaving of the area followed by a general bath. A quiet unhurried preparation with the patient engaged in conversation may well increase his confidence.

6. Bowel. In the few cases where an enema or washout is necessary the patient will require reassurance. A simple explanation makes the nurse's task easier.

Special points to bear in mind in the postoperative period

The nurse must always look beyond the operation to the postoperative period and anticipate how her own difficulties may be diminished by a judicious word beforehand. The patient is made to feel that everything will be done to minimise the discomfort.

Pain and sleep. The patient quite rightly desires reassurance that he will not be kept awake by pain.

Diet. While everyone may appear very satisfied with the patient, he may be wondering how he will recover on a diet of fluids alone. A simple reassurance of the importance of a fluid diet at this stage can often allay these fears.

Blood transfusion. If a postoperative blood transfusion is likely to be in progress it is as well to say beforehand that this is usual. The patient will feel that he is being well cared for and not that some unexpected complication has arisen.

Oxygen therapy may be particularly alarming, as many patients consider it to be a last desperate measure. If it is to be used postoperatively he should be accustomed to it before operation.

Breathing exercises are important but may be painful. Special care must be taken if the best result is to be achieved. Arrangements should be made for him to see the physiotherapist preoperatively.

Fear of bursting a wound. This is a point on which all patients desire reassurance, because this is exactly the sensation that arises from distension of viscera beneath an abdominal wound. The patient should be shown how to support his wound while coughing.

Drainage tubes. Their removal causes some discomfort. An analgesic one or two hours beforehand may be given but is not usually necessary.

Care of wound. A clean wound maybe kept covered. No special treatment is necessary unless there is reason to suspect that it has become infected. Drainage tubes are usually sited away from the main wound. Daily dressing of the drainage tube site and cleansing should be performed. Not unnaturally, the patient, who is encouraged to move his legs and his chest, may think that his wound has been forgotten and a word of explanation is necessary to ease what may be a suppressed anxiety on this account.

Removal of stitches. Anticipation always worries the patient. It can be quietly explained that it is only the stitch that is cut.

Early mobilisation avoids pressure sores and as muscular strength is not lost, weary legs and painful feet are avoided. The risk of venous thrombosis is diminished, chest movement is improved and bowel action facilitated. The slight change of scene and wider contact, even in the ward, provides relief from the monotony of the patient's bed and improves sleep.

Any other postoperative procedure which may worry the patient should be anticipated in advance. The patient should be encouraged to discuss his anxieties with the nurse in the preoperative period. A full explanation of his expected postoperative condition is given.

Mutilating surgery. The patient for major surgery which will result in altered body image requires much sympathy and understanding. The operation will be fully explained to him by the surgeon, with further discussion by the nursing staff, appropriate specialist nurse and in many instances an ex-patient who has fully recovered from the same type of surgery.

The patient, when he leaves hospital, should feel that, in his misfortune, be it minor or serious, everything possible was done to rehabilitate him. At least he should have no reason to feel that they—'they' in this case being the hospital staff—never realised what they had done to him.

Relationship of disease to emotion and of emotion to disease

With experience, these relationships become well known to the nurse, but there is always the danger that if they are taken too much for granted the patient's complaint may be neglected.

Certain lesions, such as thyrotoxicosis, peptic ulcer, and ulcerative colitis, are conditions where stress seems to play a part in their aetiology or their aggravation. All patients suffering from these conditions are anxious but, of course, there are other causes of anxiety.

The overanxious patient is liable to a higher incidence of complications which a more phlegmatic character may avoid. They include:

1. *Retention of urine.* In many cases, where there is no mechanical obstruction, retention may be purely nervous in origin, particularly following operations on the perineum and anus or when the recumbent position has to be assumed postoperatively.

2. *Air swallowing.* Air swallowing (aerophagy) sometimes results in dilatation of the stomach and again is a nervous reaction.

3. *Deep venous thrombosis.* This is more liable to occur in the patient who lies stiff and immobile in bed. Movement must be encouraged.

4. *Tachycardia.* Many patients develop postoperative tachycardia in the absence of haemorrhage or toxaemia, and it can in itself be very wearisome. Sedation is usually indicated.

5. *General exhaustion* from:
  (a) Lack of rest and inadequate sleep;
  (b) Failure to take adequate nourishment because of nervous upset of digestion;
  (c) Persistent hiccough which is particularly difficult to control.

The mind and body are an integrated whole, and any attempt to manage them in isolation from one another is doomed to failure. The patient may be shy, reserved, taciturn and resent loss of dignity—he may be worried about his job or his family.

In addition to some of the detailed points which have been discussed above, the following are of considerable importance to the patients:

The pattern of his day. The more normal this can be the more normally we can expect the patient to react. Most patients are not accustomed to being awakened in the early hours of the morning, and if this can be avoided it is a great advantage.

The elimination of noise. It is unfortunately true that the hospital environment is often noisy and disturbed rather than quiet and peaceful.

Explanation. A simple explanation of what is happening is too often avoided.

THE ECONOMICS OF MEDICAL CARE

The demand for health care is far in excess of the resources from which it can be provided. The cost may be defrayed by:

1. *The patient.* The majority of the world's population is extremely poor and even in the more prosperous countries the number who can bear the full cost of treatment, directly or indirectly, through insurance provision is negligible.

2. *The state,* which has no money except what can be raised by taxation and borrowing. In spending this money health services are in competition with facilities for education, housing and the many complex services which a modern state has to try to provide.

3. Voluntary contributions and voluntary service is the oldest, and for so long in the United Kingdom, the only provision for the sick, and in many parts of the world is still the only source. Even where the state bears almost all the cost, there will always be ample scope for voluntary effort. The donation of sophisticated equipment from the efforts of charitably disposed contributors may be welcome, but the cost of operating it with the constant attendance of skilled nurses or technicians may be prohibitive.

The task of all engaged in health care is to stretch the available resources to get the maximal value by the elimination of waste and good management. The patient under treatment must not suffer but waste prevents or delays other patients being treated. While the cost of drugs and dressings requires no stressing other sources of misuse are easily overlooked. Excessive investigation, the necessity to repeat investigations because of inadequate preparation or failure to plan investigations in good time are all a cause of waste. Equipment, whether simple or sophisticated, demands instruction in its use. At all stages in caring for a patient the cost of energy is in itself a constricting factor on a hospital's expenditure. Conservation on this as on so many other items used in patient care enables more patients to be treated from a limited budget.

BIBLIOGRAPHY

Campbell E J, Scadding J G, Roberts R S 1979 British Medical Journal 2: 757
Scadding J G 1967 Lancet 2: 877

2

Surgical diagnosis and the nurse

Accurate diagnosis is the corner-stone of treatment. It is the doctor who makes the diagnosis after he has elucidated all the facts. The nurse's observation may be most important, particularly over a period when the patient's condition is changing.

HISTORY

A careful history is the most important single part of diagnosis. What the patient has observed is nearly always significant. The patient's complaints are known as symptoms. He should have the opportunity of giving his account unhurriedly and without interruption in a room or examination bay. His family history, previous medical history, occupation, and the like are sometimes valuable. For example some diseases tend to have a hereditary incidence—carcinoma of the colon is a very striking instance in families suffering from familial polyposis, and haemophilia in males is a well-known example. It is not the nurse's duty to obtain a detailed history as a routine, but patients will often mention to a nurse some fact of great importance which they thought was too trivial to mention to the surgeon. When the nurse is attending to the patient, however, she should always obtain a clear history if the patient complains of a new symptom; for example, if it is pain, its nature, site, radiation, aggravating and relieving factors, should be obtained at once. Sometimes before the doctor arrives the patient's condition may become such that he is unable to give a clear account, and in rare cases he may be unconscious.

CLINICAL EXAMINATION

Facts discovered by examination are known as signs, and for their orderly elucidation the following plan is advisable.

Inspection

Inspection reveals what can be observed by looking. It is surprising how much can be missed by impatience or too cursory a glance. For example, in a patient's face may be seen:

Anxiety or distress	Jaundice
Fright	Oedema
Depression	Partial paralysis
Indifference	A swelling
Stupor	A rash
A flush	Exophthalmos
Pallor	Sweat
Cyanosis	

Any of these observations may be informative. The pallor and sweat may be the result of haemorrhage, and cyanosis may signify increasing respiratory obstruction. Jaundice may be due to obstruction of the bile duct or haemolysis from a recent blood transfusion. Facial paralysis may be caused by a draught from lack of care in the ward, an extending intracranial condition, or the spread of middle-ear disease to the brain or mastoid antrum.

Elsewhere similar careful observation should be made. In all sites previous scars, dilated veins, or the presence of a swelling are important. Anything abnormal should be reported by the nurse, however trivial it may appear.

Palpation

Palpation or examination by feeling with the hands is next performed. To be of value the palpation must always be gentle and the hands must be warm. Tenderness, guarding (stiffness or spasm of the underlying muscles), or a swelling may be discovered. It is well to remember that patients who are in hospital for some other condition are not immune to acute abdominal conditions. Hernias still strangulate and peptic ulcers may still perforate. It has been said with no little truth that the most dangerous place for a patient suffering from a peptic ulcer to perforate is in a hospital!

Percussion

Percussion consists of setting up artificial vibrations in the tissues by means of a sharp tap, usually with the fingers. Considerable experience is required in its interpretation. It is a sign by which a distended bladder gives rise to a dull note on percussion, thus differentiating it from a distended intestine which on percussion is described as being tympanitic (resonant).

Auscultation

Auscultation is particularly valuable to the nurse in the diagnosis and control of atrial fibrillation. It is impossible to control digitalis therapy unless the heart apex rate as well as the pulse rate are counted and charted separately.

The presence of the increased peristaltic sounds of intestinal obstruction may be heard with the stethoscope, but of greater interest is the reappearance of normal peristaltic sounds which signifies that oral feeding can usually be recommenced.

SPECIAL INVESTIGATIONS

Special tests may be necessary to confirm or aid diagnosis, and in carrying out investigations it is important that the regime of preparation is carefully followed.

RADIOLOGICAL INVESTIGATION

Today there are a large range of imaging modalities available for the investigation of the patient within the radiology department. These are:

1. Plain radiographs ⎱ Conventional imaging
2. Contrast studies ⎰
3. Ultrasound*
4. Isotope imaging
5. CT scanning
6. Magnetic resonance*

The primary role of the radiology department is to use the most appropriate technique available to obtain the maximum diagnostic information. Certain of the above imaging modalities can be used in such a way as to prevent excessive and expensive investigation being undertaken.

Recent developments within radiology have extended the role of the radiologist from the pure diagnostician into the realms of therapeutics, i.e. 'interventional radiology'.

1. Plain radiographs

Conventional X-rays have now been available for nearly 90 years. The X-ray image (radiograph) is obtained by passing a beam of X-rays through the patient on to a photographic film. X-rays are selectively absorbed by the different anatomical structures depending on the atomic weight of the molecules which make up the organs through which the beam passes. Hence bones which contain calcium (high atomic weight) appear white whilst air in the lungs or bowel appears black (low atomic weight).

Plain radiographs remain the most widely available method of producing diagnostic images. Despite major advances in imaging they still have a very important role in the initial investigation of the patient. Plain X-rays form the basis of rational radiological investigation in the majority of clinical situations.

A brief outline of the commonly used views follows.

The chest radiograph obtained on inspiration demonstrates the position of the diaphragm, size and contour of the heart and mediastinum, degree of inflation of the lungs, and the bony thorax. A chest radiograph

*These do not utilise ionising radiation.

should include the upper abdomen to demonstrate the normal gastric air bubble and right subphrenic area. Changes in mediastinal and cardiac size, position and contour may reflect cardiac disease and/or the position and size of mediastinal masses, e.g. retrosternal goitre, enlarged hilar nodes in malignant disease, or displacement of the cardiac shadow due to areas of collapse in the lungs.

Masses can be identified on plain chest X-rays within the lung fields, and tomography may aid in identifying the aetiology. Tomography is a geometric method of focusing the X-ray beam within the body, giving clearer focused images within selected slices of the patient. Areas of collapse and/or consolidation due to infection can be identified. The normal lung containing air clearly delineates the de-aerated segments. Lesions of the bony thorax such as fractures or metastases can be seen in the ribs, clavicles and dorsal spine.

Inspiration and expiration chest radiographs clearly delineate pneumothoraces. On the expiration film, denser lung fields contrast well with the air-filled pleural space. An erect film of the chest is the method of choice in visualising a pneumoperitoneum caused by the perforation of a hollow abdominal viscus, for example a perforated duodenal ulcer. Pleural fluid is clearly delineated on the chest X-ray and may reflect intra-thoracic or intra-abdominal pathology.

Plain films of the abdomen demonstrate the intestinal gas pattern and the size and contour of the liver and spleen. The position and size of the kidneys is outlined due to the lucency of the perinephric fat surrounding them. The presence of calcified opacities such as biliary or renal tract calculi can be determined. (90 per cent of renal stones are calcified and visible on plain films, whilst 10 per cent of gall-stones are dense enough and calcified enough to be seen on plain films.) Areas of abnormal calcification can be seen in the pancreas due to chronic pancreatitis or in the liver secondary to parasitic disease, e.g. hydatid cyst. Calcification in the renal tract can be due to tumours, and in the major blood vessels due to atheroma.

Obstruction of the lumen of the bowel is reflected on the erect and supine film of the abdomen by the presence of abnormal air fluid levels on the erect film with distended bowel loops proximal to the obstruction on the supine view. Perforation can be recognised due to the presence of gas outside the bowel wall. (The majority of perforations are most clearly defined on the chest X-ray film.)

Soft tissue radiography can be well appreciated by the technique of mammography. Using a lower powered X-ray beam it is possible to define the internal structures of the breast and detect the presence of both benign (e.g. fibroadenosis, simple cysts) and malignant disease, such as carcinoma.

Peripheral radiographs of the limbs are widely used to detect fractures both traumatic and pathological. Osteomyelitis and bone tumours are often well seen on plain films. The commonest bone tumours are metastatic deposits from primary tumours in the bronchus, breast or renal tract. Primary bone tumours such as osteogenic sarcoma are quite rare. The availability of isotope imaging has meant that bone disease can now be visualised earlier than on plain conventional radiographs of the bones.

Radiographs of the skull are extensively utilised in the casualty department to detect the presence of fractures. Very rarely certain intra-cranial lesions can also be demonstrated. However, the advent of CT imaging of the intra-cranial structures has revolutionised the investigation of the contents of the bony calvarium.

2. Contrast studies

Contrast agents are substances with a very different atomic weight from the organ which the radiologist is visualising. Ideally they should be non-toxic and rapidly excreted from the human body. To be of any use they must be easily visualised on radiographs. By introducing contrast agents into body cavities it is possible to visualise much more anatomical detail and obtain an idea of the function of the organ under investigation. Examples of widely used contrast agents are barium sulphate in the investigation of the gastrointestinal tract and the iodine-containing solutions used in urography, angiography, cholangiography, hysterosalpingography etc. Double contrast examinations of the bowel are obtained by first coating the bowel wall with barium and distending the bowel with a gas; CO_2 in a barium meal for the stomach or air in a barium enema in investigating the colon. Barium meals are performed on the starving patient by paralysing the stomach with a muscle relaxant, distending the stomach with carbondioxide and coating the mucosa of the stomach with an oral ingested barium sulphate suspension. Alteration of the mucosa of the oesophagus, stomach and duodenum are seen in diseases such as carcinoma, when a large filling defect may be visualised. Peptic ulcers cause craters in the stomach and duodenum. Endoscopy is now frequently used in conjunction with barium meals to assess lesions in the upper intestinal tract. Endoscopy has the advantage of allowing biopsy at the time of the examination. The rapidly changing face of radiology has seen a decline in the number of barium meals requested. The ready availability of endoscopy does enable the gastroenterologist to rapidly evaluate the gastrointestinal tract in cases of haematemesis which were at one time primarily investigated by barium meals. Barium enemas are used to assess the colon for the presence of carcinomas, diverticular disease and to assess the extent of inflammatory bowel disease. For a diagnostic study to be obtained the colon must be emptied prior to the examination by adequate bowel preparation. The colon is paralysed with a muscle relaxant, barium is run in, followed by air to distend the colon. The result is a double contrast barium enema which allows adequate visualisation of the mucosa of the large bowel.

Urography is performed using iodine-containing contrast medium. New non-ionic contrast media which have very low toxicity are replacing the previously used ionic contrast agents. Haematuria, dysuria and loin pain (suspected renal pathology) remain the important indications for intravenous urography. In renal trauma an IVU will demonstrate the function of the contra-lateral kidney. This is most important prior to any contemplated surgery on the affected kidney.

Angiography utilises the same contrast agents in visualising the lumina of blood vessels. Complicated radiographic apparatus is necessary to obtain flow studies through the large vessels of the body. The most important indication for angiography is to assess the extent of atheroma in blood vessels prior to contemplated surgery. Angiography is performed by the placement of a catheter within an artery and injecting contrast agents. A new form of angiography has been developed in recent years. This is digitalised vascular imaging. By the use of a computer it is possible to visualise arteries after the injection of contrast media into veins. This technique is not as yet widely available, but undoubtedly, because of the safety factor, will gain widespread acceptance.

Other contrast studies allow visualisation of suspected diseased organs. The gall-bladder is visualised by oral cholecystography. However, the investigation of the biliary system has now largely, although not completely, been superseded by ultrasound investigation.

3. Ultrasound investigation

Ultrasound is increasingly used in the investigation of surgical patients. The principle of medical ultrasound imaging lies in the passing of a beam of high frequency sound into the patient and detecting the returning echoes. These are electronically converted into anatomical images. Since no ionising rays are used in this method of investigation it is extremely safe and can be repeated frequently. Sound waves passed through gas, solid and fluid filled structures travel at different rates with differing degrees of reflection. Gas and bone are not suitable for ultrasound investigation. Gas filled structures such as the lung and bowel are impossible, or at best, very difficult to visualise.

Ultrasound is very useful in assessing the nature of masses either in the abdomen or soft tissues. It is possible to differentiate between solid and fluid-filled masses. For example a mass in the kidney, first seen on a conventional intravenous urogram, can be more accurately assessed with ultrasound. If solid it is likely to represent a tumour, if cystic it would probably be a simple cyst.

Ultrasound is widely used in visualising fluid filled structures such as the gall-bladder, urinary bladder or the blood filled abdominal aorta. It is now the primary means of investigating suspected gall-bladder disease since the radiologist can look at the liver, kidneys and pancreas at the same time. Pathology in these closely related anatomical organs, which may mimic biliary pathology, can be detected.

The majority of ultrasound departments in the U.K. now use real time apparatus. Moving real images of the patient are obtained. Excellent anatomical and pathological detail can be demonstrated. Ultrasound is increasingly used in the investigation of abdominal disease particularly in the solid organs of the abdomen. It is now the primary means of investigating jaundice, demonstrating the presence of liver metastases, or an obstructed biliary system due to calculi or neoplasia of the pancreas. Imaging of soft tissue structures such as breasts and thyroid are now widely available. The intracranial contents of the infant can be assessed by imaging through the anterior fontanelle.

Doppler images are currently being evaluated in assessing blood flow in the major vessels. As yet this technique is not widely available.

4. Isotope imaging

Isotope imaging is based on the principle that certain isotopes emit gamma radiation. By introducing isotopes into the body it is possible to visualise specific regions of interest. Gamma radiation is detected by a gamma camera which contains a large sensitive crystal capable of detecting the emitted gamma radiation and converting this into anatomical images. The isotope image obtained is very non-specific. Many disease processes can give very similar isotope images. However, using chemical compounds labelled with a radio-isotope, it is possible to visualise many organs within the body. Examples of commonly used isotopes include technetium and radio-iodine. Commonly used isotope studies are those where the lungs, brain, thyroid, liver, biliary system, renal tract, bones and blood vessels are visualised. Using organ-specific radiopharmaceuticals it is possible to obtain images of all the above organs. Areas which take up excessive amounts of the radiopharmaceutical appear 'hot', those which take up less than would normally be expected appear 'cold'. Looking at images which have either 'hot' spots or 'cold' spots it is possible to visualise areas of active pathology. Good examples of isotope imaging are those obtained in lung scans where it is possible to define areas of decreased perfusion due to pulmonary emboli. Conventional plain films of the chest show no evidence of pulmonary emboli in the majority of cases. The bone scan is much more sensitive in detecting pathological processes within the skeleton than plain films. For example, isotope images of bones are very much more sensitive in detecting the presence of metastatic disease than plain X-rays of the bones.

Ideal isotopes have been developed in the last decade. They are similar to the iodine containing contrast media in that they are rapidly excreted from the body, non-toxic and readily available on a day-to-day basis.

5. CT scanning

This method of investigation was invented by Houndsfield in the U.K. in the early 1970s. The principle involved is the combination of a rotating X-ray tube moving around the patient together with a series of X-ray detectors which move in a circular fashion completely around the patient. The images obtained from this moving X-ray tube and its detectors are fed into a computer and cross-sectional slices of the patient built up electronically. It is now accepted that all intracranial pathology is probably best demonstrated by CT scanning.

It is possible to demonstrate all the regions of the body. The chest, abdomen, pelvis, neck are all now very often demonstrated by CT scanning.

Originally used without contrast agents it is now common to enhance CT scans with an iodine-containing contrast medium. Because very good anatomical images are obtained by this technique it is extremely useful in demonstrating structures which are otherwise very difficult to visualise. The lungs, heart, major blood vessels, solid organs of the abdomen and pelvis and those which contain fluid are very readily assessed by CT scanning.

6. Magnetic resonance

This is a new imaging modality based on the use of high powered magnets. It is a method of visualising physiological distribution of protons within the body, enabling very high quality anatomical images to be obtained. This has rapidly caught the imagination of the radiological community throughout the world. Unlike CT it is capable of producing images within any plane. The modality has benefited from the previous technological innovations developed for CT computerisation. The NMR signal can be altered by the introduction of new 'contrast' agents. These are paramagnetic substances which interfere with the signal generated by the radio waves within the atom. Recent work has been very promising. Using these new enhanced images very small lesions have been demonstrated within the brain, so small in fact that they were not detectable by any other means.

INTERVENTIONAL RADIOLOGY

Recent advances in the development of needles, catheters and guide wires have led to their increasing therapeutic use. This new field of 'interventional' radiology involves percutaneous biopsy, drainage of obstructed viscera and abscesses, dilatation of vascular and other stenoses and re-canalisation or occlusion of blood vessels. Percutaneous biopsy of lesions demonstrated by the imaging modalities mentioned above is now widely practised. Fine needles can be passed through the body wall into the cavities within the body under fluoroscopic or ultrasound control. These cutting needles can then be used to obtain aspiration specimens from the lesion within the body. Specific pathological diagnosis can then be made from biopsy specimens obtained.

Embolisation and infusion of drugs. Development of angiography has allowed various materials to be injected into specific vessels producing permanent or temporary occlusion. Embolic materials for this purpose include metallic wires, gelatin foam, alcohol and many other agents. Embolisation is used in the control of haemorrhage, for example in the gastrointestinal tract, and in the embolisation of tumours, for example renal tumours or endocrine-producing metastatic lesions in the liver. Preoperative embolisation of tumours is used in an attempt to reduce tumour bulk and haemorrhage prior to surgery.

Percutaneous drainage of the obstructed biliary and upper renal tracts, and of abscesses, can be obtained by modified angiography catheters. Visualisation of the obstructed system or abscess is usually performed using ultrasound or CT. Definitive drainage of subphrenic abscesses can be performed in this manner. In the obstructed biliary or urinary tract percutaneous access for the removal of calculi is possible.

Angioplasty. This is the technique of dilatation and re-canalisation of arteries using catheters which have inflatable balloons built into them. This technique is successful in dilatation of iliac and lower limb vessels. It is now used in aortic and renal obstructions. Currently, coronary angioplasty is gaining widespread use. All of the techniques in interventional radiology are still in their infancy and many exciting developments are expected within the next few years.

Radiology is rapidly changing. The response of the radiographic world to new high technological developments has been very rapid. The widespread acceptance of digitalisation and subsequent computerisation pioneered in CT is now making an impact on conventional radiographs. The drawback in their widespread availability is their high cost. Despite the ever increasing pace of change it is important to remember that the majority of investigations performed within the X-ray department rely on the use of X-rays and will continue to do so in the foreseeable future.

Radiological examination of women of reproductive age. It has become vitally necessary, in the light of present knowledge, to reduce the possibility of performing a radiological examination on any female patient between the ages of 15 and 50 who might be pregnant. It is, therefore, necessary to restrict certain X-rays in these patients to a time when it should not be possible for them to be pregnant, i.e. in that period of the menstrual cycle prior to ovulation. It is necessary to enter the date of the last menstrual period on all X-ray request forms in patients who are menstruating. It may also be necessary to indicate, for the benefit of a clerk, that the examination should be carried out only between certain dates. These would normally be the ten days commencing with the first day of the period or the first day of the next expected period.

The examinations in question are:

- Straight abdomen
- Intravenous and retrograde pyelogram, and cystogram
- Cholecystogram
- Barium meal and enema
- Lumbar spine, sacroiliac joints, sacrum and pelvis
- Hips

ENDOSCOPY

Visual inspection of the interior of many organs is possible either directly or by indirect means, and these procedures are known as endoscopic inspections. They include cystoscopy, laryngoscopy, bronchoscopy, oesophagoscopy, gastroscopy, duodenoscopy, sigmoidoscopy, colonoscopy, and peritoneoscopy. With all these procedures a biopsy may be taken.

LABORATORY INVESTIGATIONS

Any specimens collected must be accurately labelled by the nurse and be sent to the laboratory without delay.

THE NURSE'S SPECIAL CONTRIBUTION TO DIAGNOSIS

Careful observation, accurately recorded, is of great value. The patient in hospital, particularly in a surgical ward, is in highly artificial surroundings. This is greatly exaggerated as treatment progresses, whether by the administration of drugs, artificial feeding, or operation. The patient's physical condition, too, is often quite unstable during the 21 days following an uneventful operation, even though he may have resumed work. He is more liable to sudden complications—for example, pulmonary embolism. The following examples serve as general illustrations of the care which is necessary:

1. Haemorrhage. An increasing pulse rate, a falling blood pressure and a subnormal temperature together with cold and clammy peripheries are characteristic of haemorrhage. For this reason it is important to chart all observations carefully. Increasing pallor is characteristic, but in jaundiced patients it is unobservable, so particular attention to the pulse is essential.

After many operations—for example, mastectomy or cholecystectomy—a drainage tube is inserted. There is always some bloodstained discharge, which should be measured.

Following prostatectomy, if the drainage is light pink in colour haemorrhage is not excessive.

2. Abnormal discharges. The presence of bile from a gall-bladder wound when the common bile duct has not been opened, or of a faecal discharge from an abdominal wound, should be reported at once.

3. Continuous suction and irrigation apparatus can be very treacherous, The danger if the tube blocks is that the cavity is thought to be dry while in fact fluid is welling up and may be causing damage. This is why intermittent suction of the stomach is usually preferable.

Continuous irrigation is sometimes used after bladder operations and a complete suppression of urine may pass unobserved for days unless a strict check of the volume of fluid run in and the volume recovered has been kept.

4. Analgesics and other measures of symptomatic relief. The patient in severe pain cries out for relief but analgesics should be given only in a dosage to control the pain but of an insufficient dosage to produce narcosis. Following the temporary relief of overwhelming pain, the patient is enabled to co-operate by giving a coherent history and being responsive on clinical examination so that a diagnosis can be made.

5. Patients admitted in coma. These patients present special difficulties because a clear history is not always available, but in all cases the nurse should be alert to the possibility of the presence of associated injuries. Fractures without deformity can easily pass unnoticed in the comatose patient and delayed signs of internal injuries may appear some hours or days after admission. The level of consciousness is noted and assessed regularly.

The size of the pupils, whether they are equal or not, whether they are contracted or dilated, and their reaction to light, are essential observations, and any changes which occur should be written down.

The onset of a fit, its type, spread, duration and other features are frequently seen only by the nurse. Her report of the fit may be decisive in some cases. The appearance of slight weakness (paresis) in any muscles, as well as complete paralysis, is important to note.

6. Enemas. Enemas may be prescribed for diagnostic purposes. Occasionally an incomplete intestinal obstruction may be temporarily relieved following an enema, allowing further investigation and planned treatment.

The passage of flatus by a rectal tube when the patient is suffering from an acute abdominal condition or paralytic ileus may be a sign that the condition is responding to treatment.

7. General observation when the patient is washed may be very important. A swelling, an ulcer, a rash, oedema, or distension may be noticed. Such an observation may be the final clue to the solution of the pathology in an otherwise obscure case.

8. Changes in personality and behaviour should be watched very carefully. The effect of the mind on a patient's bodily ills can be profound, and in a surgical ward it is no less disastrous than elsewhere. Patients with a poor psychological background may break down completely before or, what is worse, after an operation. Chronic alcoholics are bad operative subjects and require special care. Not all mental manifestations have their origin in diseases of the mind and the following are examples of gross organic disease which may be present or appearing:

(a) *Slight confusion* is common preceding cerebral thrombosis.

(b) *Confusion, drowsiness and incoherent speech* may indicate the presence of a cerebral tumour which may be primary or secondary. A considerable amount of major surgery is 'cancer' surgery, and secondary deposits are characteristic of a cancer. The brain is one of the sites where a secondary deposit may lodge, and early recognition is important so that the attempt to remove the primary growth is abandoned, as it would now prove fruitless.

(c) *Polydipsia.* Excessive thirst and polyuria (excessive urinary output) are characteristic of diabetes insipidus. This condition is due to disease or injury of the pituitary body situated in the sella turcica in the middle fossa of the skull. Occasionally the condition is caused by a fracture in this area, with consequent damage to the pituitary gland.

9. Deep venous thrombosis complicated by pulmonary embolism is a condition of which every nurse in every surgical ward in every hospital must be aware. It is the one condition which will kill a fit patient with dramatic suddenness.

THE NURSE AND THE RECOGNITION OF DISEASE

There are times when the gravity of a situation is not recognised. The apparent well-being of the patient may be deceptive and yet it is in such situations that it is vital to act almost reflexly correctly. Problems may arise from the following:

1. Organisational failure. The failure to communicate the results of routine laboratory tests used to monitor the dosage of certain drugs in outpatients constitutes a problem. The failure to act correctly is responsible for a number of deaths each year. The two main categories are:

(a) *The anticoagulant drugs* which are extremely dangerous unless controlled by laboratory tests. Any change in dosage should be communicated quickly to the patient and his doctor.

The patient is given a card and the dosage indicated immediately after the test—both in amount and the colour of the tablet.

(b) *Cytotoxic drugs* require monitoring of the white cell count in the blood. Severe white cell depletion necessitates admission to hospital isolation and the administration of penicillin without delay—both difficult steps to take if the patient has been allowed to leave hospital before the results are to hand! With no resistance to infection a journey home in a public service conveyance exposes him to the very hazards he has no resistance to combat.

2. Adverse drug reactions. An adverse drug reaction has been defined by the WHO as 'one which is noxious, unintended and occurs at doses used in man for prophylaxis, diagnosis or therapy' (WHO 1969). New drugs are released for general use only after clinical trials and after ward controlled trials have been undertaken. Nonetheless, spontaneous reporting by individual clinics of any adverse reaction has been a great help in the central registry issuing an early warning. When a new drug is used, a nurse should be specially observant to listen to and report any unusual symptoms of which the patient may complain and to note any unusual signs.

3. Quiet onset. The failure to pass urine is almost always due to urinary retention, usually a painful condition. Anuria (the failure of the kidneys to secrete urine) is usually painless and the patient may initially look and fell very well. The result is that recognition is delayed 24 hours or longer. Only lynx-eyed observation by a nurse will diagnose the condition earlier, and once suspected all treatment should be stopped until a regime which takes account of the new situation has been designed. Drugs which are excreted in the urine can no longer be eliminated from the body and dangerous concentration may occur in the blood. The whole pattern of drug therapy has to be represcribed. Similarly all fluids are stopped and again the whole situation of fluid balance reconsidered (Ch. 42).

4. Omissions. A notable example of this is a full stomach before the induction of anaesthesia. Of course no one would give an anaesthetic to a patient with a full stomach. There is, however, one situation in which this is liable to occur and every year fatalities are recorded. The fit multiparous woman who has had a good meal may go into labour which may be very short indeed. In the rush to deal with her pressing obstetric problem she is given an anaesthetic in a hurry in unfavourable conditions and no one has remembered to pass a nasogastric tube. It is in just such a situation that a thoughtful nurse has so much to contribute.

In summary, careful observation by an alert nurse is always necessary. It may, at times, contribute greatly to the elucidation or prevention of a clinical problem.

3

Identification of the patient

The complexity of modern medical practice arises partly from the rapid increase in scientific knowledge and partly from the fact that the application of this knowledge for the patient's benefit demands that a greater and greater number of people are directly or indirectly concerned in his treatment. The amount of scientific equipment and the range of chemical reagents used in the treatment of a single patient can hardly be realised. Well-equipped operating theatres, laboratories and other departments of investigation and treatment are expensive to build and to staff. For this reason alone, the type of work which the acute general hospital undertakes becomes even more complex.

The result is that the treatment of a particular patient has become and will become more specific. That is to say that the treatment will be so well designed for him and his condition that the first essential is that he must be identifiable with certainty. There is greater liability to mistake or to human error today than ever before. The consequences are liable to be more crippling and more lethal than in the past because many drugs and fluids have narrower margins of safety and are more potent in their effects.

For this reason, the nurse must always ask herself two questions:

1. Is this patient William Smith (or whatever his name may be) who was born on 7.10.27?
2. Is this the correct injection, tablet or blood for William Smith?

She must also be able to ask herself these questions in reverse, namely:

1. Is the next patient for the removal of his appendix William Smith?
2. Is this William Smith now being lifted on to the trolley whom I am taking to the theatre for the removal of his appendix?

Certain well-known facts emerge about patients' behaviour in the stress and strain of going to the operating theatre, receiving injections or even in going from the waiting room to the consulting room of a clinic. For example, a patient sometimes thinks that he has been called when in fact another patient's name has been called. Some patients, hard of hearing, do not like to admit it and even though addressed by another patient's name, keep on saying 'yes' to everything!

This is now the paradoxical situation, that as care and treatment become more specific, more effective and more carefully planned (more personal, in fact), the risk that the plan may misfire through misidentification is greater and more serious.

Many patients have similar names and their place in the ward may be changed, so that identification such as 'third bed from the end on the left' is quite unreliable. A bed card on the wall or locker is certainly useful, but the patient may be moved in the ward and his bed card left, so that this method is not entirely foolproof. The patient's case sheet and records are not suitably kept at the end of the bed so they are not a method of identification.

The only safe method of identification is for every patient to have a name label attached to their person on admission to hospital. This is most commonly in the form of a plastic bracelet, which cannot be easily removed, attached around the wrist (Fig. 3.1). Such a label should contain

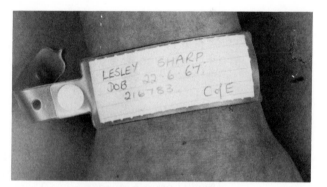

Fig. 3.1 Bracelet label attached to patient's wrist for identification.

the patient's name, date of birth, and hospital registration number. Such identification is particularly important in patients who are seriously ill, going to the operating theatre or unconscious. The latter may, for example require an injection such as insulin, or a transfusion of blood.

A card containing the patient's personal details should be prepared, to attach to his bed.

A sheet of addressograph labels for use on all prescriptions, request forms and specimens should be provided by the records department.

IDENTIFICATION OF THE PATIENT'S SPECIMENS

Every specimen for examination taken from a patient either in the ward or operating theatre should be carefully labelled. In the ward there are certain cardinal points to avoid mishap:

1. Everything necessary to collect the specimen should be taken to the bedside.
2. An addressograph label should be attached by the person taking the specimen in the presence of the patient and at the bedside.
3. Specimens should never be collected from two patients and then two labels attached together.

Blood specimens from patients suspected of suffering from serum viral hepatitis should carry a warning label and should be transferred to the laboratory according to hospital policy for collection of infected specimens.

In the theatre, specimens removed at operations are labelled and sealed after each operation.

THERAPEUTIC FLUIDS, TABLETS, AND OTHER AGENTS

Of all the therapeutic fluids, the one most liable to cause sudden and irreparable damage is incompatible blood. This will be stressed again in the chapter on blood transfusion. The following elementary precautions are essential:

1. The patient must be identified with certainty.
2. The label indicating the cross-match against the patient's blood must be checked against the patient and the bag of blood and also the blood group.

The maze inside a blood refrigerator illustrates how easy it is to pick up the wrong bag.

Other substances particularly liable to cause harm are the anticoagulants, insulin, radium and sedatives. The tragedy of a mistake in the identification of a patient requires no emphasis and in the rush of a busy day it is more likely to occur. Even the coincidence of an identical name, occupation, and disease may play a part, so that the sole identifiable mark may be the patient's home address and his date of birth. If a nurse is in doubt she should never hesitate to share her doubt at once with a more senior member of the staff. No drug or therapeutic substance should be given orally or otherwise without using the correct checking procedure—two persons must always be involved.

The nurse should be able to identify the contents of a medical gas cylinder by its colour. Gas cylinders are now pin indexed—that is, the attachment is so contrived that coupling can be effected only to the correct point on a machine for that particular gas.

4

Perioperative care

The preoperative preparation and after-care of the patient is a subject to which an increasing amount of attention has been devoted in recent years. Complications once believed to be unavoidable have been reduced considerably, mortality and morbidity have diminished and the convalescence of a larger number of patients has been made more comfortable.

The principles of pre- and postoperative care can be readily understood by a moment's reflection on what an operation really means to a patient. In his mind arise thoughts of a wound, loss of blood, an anaesthetic, a period of incapacity in bed, weakness when he gets up, pain and fear of the end result—perhaps of death, perhaps of some incapacity which may prevent him from carrying on his normal life.

The aims of treatment are:

1. To reassure and prepare the patient for operation.
2. To provide safe anaesthesia and to ensure that the patient recovers consciousness without mishap.
3. To prevent or treat shock.
4. To achieve healing of the wound as rapidly as possible.
5. To prevent or treat complications which may arise as a result of recumbency in bed.
6. To restore rapidly the function in all the organs of the body as well as in the mind.

Operations can be broadly divided into two main groups

(a) *Elective procedures.* 'Cold' or non-urgent operations can be planned to take place when the patient is in the optimal condition. Ideally, all patients listed for surgery should have a haemoglobin estimation and urinalysis done in outpatients; the blood pressure should also be recorded at this time. In some hospitals, patients with underlying medical problems may be referred to a pre-anaesthetic clinic for assessment; alternatively the advice of a physician may be sought. Previously undiagnosed conditions (e.g. anaemia, diabetes, hypertension) may be revealed and appropriate treatment instituted. Patients of West African and Indian origins should be screened for sickle cell disease. In this condition aggregation of red cells may result should hypoxia occur during anaesthesia.

If the patient suffers from chronic bronchitis the operation may be scheduled for the summer months. All patients should be encouraged to stop smoking. Perioperative complications are much more prevalent in obese patients; they should be encouraged to lose weight and a diet sheet may be provided. Oestrogens are contained in some contraceptive pills and may increase the likelihood of post-operative thrombosis; alternative contraceptive measures for a few weeks prior to surgery are usually recommended.

(b) Emergency procedures. In these situations the severity of a patient's condition may be life-threatening (e.g. perforated viscus, gastrointestinal haemorrhage), or disabling (e.g. unstable fractures, trauma to limbs). Operation may then be necessary within hours or at the most 1–2 days. In such conditions, thorough preoperative screening may not be possible.

PREOPERATIVE MANAGEMENT

Admission

Patients for elective surgery are usually admitted a day or two before operation. On admission, temperature, pulse and respiratory rates are recorded by the nurse and a sample of urine should be tested. Any abnormality should be recorded and reported. If a patient has a cough or cold or an unexplained pyrexia the operation may be postponed. A note should be made of any known allergies (e.g. skin preparations, dressings and drugs).

The house officer will take a full history and carry out a clinical examination on every patient. Details of existing and previous drug therapy (both prescribed and 'over the counter' remedies) must be obtained and any adverse responses to previous anaesthetics noted.

Patients receiving steroid therapy will require increased dosage in the perioperative period to counteract the stress responses which occur following surgery. Diabetic patients may need further stabilisation prior to surgery and special regimes (e.g. infusions of insulin, glucose and potassium) may be instituted to cover major procedures.

The doctor will request preoperative investigation as required. A chest X-ray and ECG will be required for those scheduled for major surgery and for elderly patients or those with symptomatic disease. Where appropriate, blood will be sent for grouping and cross-matching and other laboratory investigations.

The physiotherapist may visit preoperatively to instruct in deep breathing exercises and expectoration in those patients at risk of postoperative pulmonary complications.

Dehydrated patients (e.g. those with intestinal obstruction) will need replacement of fluids and electrolytes. Where there is a severe blood volume deficit following haemorrhage or shock the infusion of blood and plasma or colloid substitutes may be indicated. In these cases careful monitoring of fluid balance and serial pulse and blood pressure recordings will be necessary.

The risks of inhalation of gastric contents during the induction of anaesthesia are very serious. It must be impressed upon the patient that oral intake is forbidden for 6 hours prior to surgery. However, in emergencies the stomach can never be assumed to be empty; gastric emptying may be delayed considerably by disease or trauma. No method of emptying the stomach is completely reliable although a Ryle's tube will be useful in removing liquid contents, as when obstruction is suspected; the amount and colour of the aspirate should be charted. Patients who are to undergo caesarean section are especially at risk as their gastric juice is often highly acidic. If this is allowed to contaminate the trachea and bronchi irreversible damage (Mendelson's syndrome) and death may ensue. Preoperative administration of antacids such as magnesium trisilicate or sodium citrate will afford some protection in such cases.

Premedication

Morphine in combination with atropine and given by intramuscular injection has traditionally been used as premedication. Morphine will sedate the patient and may reduce anaesthetic requirements; atropine will reduce secretions and inhibit unwanted reflexes which may occur during induction of anaesthesia. Difficulty may be experienced in timing the injection to suit the requirements of a busy surgical list. Furthermore, undesirable side effects such as nausea, dry mouth and palpitations may result from this regime. Modern practice tends toward the oral administration of minor tranquillisers such as diazepam (or dichlorphenazone for the elderly) may also be given in the evening to ensure a good night's sleep.

Perhaps of greater import than the use of premedicant drugs is careful explanation and reassurance by medical and nursing staff. A preoperative visit by the anaesthetist or a member of the theatre team concerned can be of immense value.

Prior to transfer to theatre

The nurse who is to accompany the patient to theatre must ensure that:
- (i)   The patient is correctly identified, by verbal communication, by checking the arm band and by confirming the nature and site of operation.
- (ii) The consent form has been signed (in the case of children under 16 years by the parent or guardian) and is taken to theatre with the case-notes and X-rays.
- (iii) In elective cases that the patient has not had anything to eat or drink in the previous 6 hours, and that the bladder has been voided.

(iv) False teeth and other prostheses are removed; make-up, including nail varnish, should not be worn as colour changes which occur during anaesthesia could be masked. Hair clips, rings and other jewelry are removed (wedding rings may be covered with 'micropore' tape) to avoid the risk of burns if diathermy is used. In extremely deaf patients, the hearing aid may be worn until anaesthesia is induced.

(v) The patient is correctly attired, appropriate skin preparation has been carried out if and when necessary, and warm blankets are available for transport.

(vi) The theatre check-list is completed according to hospital policy.

CONDUCT OF ANAESTHESIA

On arrival in the theatre complex, the nurse may, depending on hospital practice, accompany the patient to the anaesthetic room. At this stage further identification checks should be carried out before induction of anaesthesia.

General anaesthetic techniques

In the majority of cases operations are performed under general anaesthesia which can be described as a state of controlled unconsciousness. A general anaesthetic is usually considered to have three components:

1. Hypnosis or induction of sleep.
2. Maintenance of anaesthesia to prevent awareness, provide analgesia and suppress undesirable reflexes during surgical manipulations.
3. Muscular relaxation which is particularly important when endotracheal intubation is performed and to prevent muscle rigidity during abdominal surgery.

1. Induction of anaesthesia

General anaesthesia is usually induced by the intravenous injection of a rapidly acting barbiturate such as thiopentone or methohexitone. Sleep will ensue within 15 seconds in patients with a normal circulation time; a deep plane of anaesthesia will be achieved, but other agents (gases and volatile liquids) are then introduced from the anaesthetic machine via a face mask in order to maintain anaesthesia, as the patient will waken within 5-10 minutes if the intravenous agent alone is used.

However, it may also be necessary for the anaesthetist to administer a muscle relaxant with the barbiturate in order to intubate the trachea. This is especially important:

(a) When the respiratory tract must be protected from the effects of possible aspiration. In such situations an assistant applies pressure to the cricoid cartilage. By this procedure, not only is the larynx more easily visualised but the muscles at the upper end of the oesophagus are compressed and this prevents egress of the stomach contents.

(b) To prevent aspiration of blood and mucus from the upper airway during intranasal and oral surgery such as tonsillectomy, cleft palate repair, submucus resection. In addition a gauze pack may be inserted into the pharynx to absorb blood and mucus. The pack (and any swabs used by the anaesthetist) must be coloured so that they cannot be confused with those used by the surgeon.

(c) When artificial ventilation is to be continued.

When veins are not easily accessible or in very ill patients where a more 'gentle' induction is desirable anaesthesia may be induced by inhalation methods. These may be accomplished by:

(i) An open mask, e.g. dripping ether onto a gauze pad.

(ii) A face mask connected to an anaesthetic machine using a closed or semiclosed circuit.

2. Maintenance of anaesthesia

This is achieved by continuing administration of inhalation agents. Nitrous oxide and oxygen are delivered from cylinders or a piped supply via a rotameter block where the flow rates can be adjusted to provide a mixture of 30 per cent oxygen and 70 per cent nitrous oxide. This gas mixture may then pass over the surface of a volatile anaesthetic contained in a specially designed chamber (vaporiser) in order to deepen the level of unconsciousness. Such agents include halothane, enflurane and trichlorethylene. Narcotic analgesics such as morphine and phenoperidene may be administered intravenously to enhance the depth of anaesthesia and contribute to analgesia during the recovery period.

Fig. 4.1   The jaw of the unconscious patient is held forward to prevent his tongue falling back.

The maintenance of a free airway is essential. If an endoctracheal tube has been passed there is usually no problem, although malposition or kinking of the tube may occasionally occur. However, if the anaesthetic is to be administered via a face mask, the jaw of the unconscious patient must be held forward to prevent the tongue falling back (Fig. 4.1); alternatively, an oropharyngeal airway is inserted to prevent apposition of the tongue to the posterior pharyngeal wall.

3. Muscle relaxation

Muscle relaxants act by paralysing voluntary muscles including the diaphragm. The short-acting drug suxamethonium is usually administered when rapid intubation of the trachea is desired. The onset of paralysis is preceded by coarse muscle fasciculations which may be evident as twitching. The drug normally acts for 3–5 minutes and is then destroyed by liver enzymes. Longer acting drugs such as tubocurarine, pancuronium and alcuronium are required to produce relaxation during surgical procedures. The effects of such drugs will not have completely worn off by the end of the operation and their action must be reversed by an antagonist, usually neostigmine. This is accompanied by the injection of atropine which prevents the undesirable effects of neostigmine, particularly on the heart.

Artificial ventilation may be accomplished by the anaesthetist 'squeezing the reservoir bag' in the anaesthetic circuit, but more commonly by the use of a ventilator which is connected to the anaesthetic machine and adjusted to provide the required minute volume.

Hypotension and hypothermia

The anaesthetist may deliberately lower the blood pressure during the course of anaesthesia in order to reduce the bleeding which may occur in highly vascular procedures. This is accomplished by the use of hypotensive agents given by intravenous injection or alternatively by producing very deep levels of anaesthesia with, for example, halothane.

Hypothermia may be required for certain cardiac or neurosurgical procedures; lowering the body temperature will reduce the oxygen requirement and thus be protective when vital organs undergo periods of ischaemia. Hypothermia may be achieved by external cooling using ice bags or, in the case of cardiac surgery, by cooling the blood in the cardiac bypass machine.

Spinal and regional anaesthesia

The general condition or personal preference of the patient may preclude the use of a general anaesthetic. Spinal anaesthesia is especially valuable for operations below the umbilicus, e.g. prostatic surgery, amputation of lower limbs, in patients with poor respiratory reserve. Local anaesthetic agents are injected into the cerebrospinal fluid (CSF). The appropriate nerves are blocked as they emerge from the spinal cord.

Motor paralysis usually accompanies sensory loss, and the blood pressure may fall because of paralysis of sympathetic nerves supplying blood vessels.

Epidural anaesthesia is attained by injecting the local anaesthetic into the spinal canal exterior to the meninges. This method has proved very popular as a way of providing analgesia during labour and can be extended to provide anaesthesia for caesarean section.

Regional anaesthesia is particularly useful for hand surgery, e.g. Dupuytren's contracture. The brachial plexus may be blocked either above the clavicle or in the axilla. Blocks of the femoral and sciatic nerves are sometimes valuable for operations on the feet.

If these techniques are used, the operation site must be screened from the patient's view and his attention diverted by engaging him in conversation. Local infiltration of the operation site with an anaesthetic solution containing a vasoconstrictor (adrenaline) may be performed by the surgeon, during a general anaesthetic, in order to reduce bleeding.

Monitoring during anaesthesia

Extreme vigilance on the part of the anaesthetist is essential throughout surgical procedures. Colour, respiration and pulse rate must be carefully observed and particular attention paid to the possibility of leaks in the anaesthetic circuit or failure of the oxygen supply. It may also be necessary to set up an intravenous infusion and to monitor the following:

(i) The blood pressure continuously.
(ii) The ECG using an oscilloscope.
(iii) Blood loss.
(iv) Central venous pressure.
(v) Temperature.
(vi) The composition of inspired and expired gasses particularly O_2 and CO_2.

Positioning of the patient during surgery is also important. At all times special care should be taken to avoid pressure on nerves otherwise paralysis is liable to occur. There is a particular danger of radial paralysis if the arm is allowed to hang over the edge of the table. Arms should not be extended over boards whilst the patient is in the head-down position with shoulder supports because of the risk of damage to the brachial plexus. Elastic stockings reduce the risk of venous thrombosis. If the patient is placed in the lateral position, e.g. for nephrectomy, the underlying arm must remain free from compression. In the prone position, special care must be taken of the eyes.

Recovery from anaesthesia

At the end of the operation the patient should be transferred to a trolley or bed and placed in the lateral position. At this stage a pharyngeal pack (if inserted) will be removed and the trachea extubated. Nursing the patient on his side will facilitate management of the airway and allow pharyngeal secretions to be removed. It is important that the trolley can be tilted rapidly to the head down position. This will promote venous return if the blood pressure is unstable and reduce the likelihood of aspiration of stomach contents. Children are nursed in the tonsil position preferably, i.e. semi-prone with a supporting pillow under the chest.

If the pharyngeal muscle tone is deficient, the patient is at risk from obstruction by the tongue, therefore the jaw must be held forward and the oropharyngeal airway may be retained. Further observation of the patient should take place in the recovery room which must be adjacent to the theatre and be supervised by a trained and experienced nurse. Facilities for suction, delivery of oxygen and blood pressure monitoring should be available. When handing the patient over to the nursing staff the anaesthetist should give written and, if needed, verbal instructions regarding the airway, fluid replacement and pain relief. He may prescribe controlled oxygen therapy administered via a Ventimask or similar device for the postoperative period (28–35 per cent O_2).

The patient should only be allowed to return to the ward when he is able to respond to command. No patient should be permitted to leave the theatre without permission of the anaesthetist. If muscle relaxants have been used during the anaesthetic the patient must also be able to take a deep breath, cough vigorously and lift his head and hold it up for at least 5 seconds.

POSTOPERATIVE MANAGEMENT

Transfer to the ward

A nurse must always accompany the patient back to the ward. The patient should be transferred on a trolley which has oxygen equipment attached, facilities for tilt and cot sides. He must be warmly clad during transport. A pharyngeal airway, mouth gag and tongue depressor should be available should any problems supervene.

On return to bed, patients should continue to be nursed on their side without a pillow. A nurse must stay with them until they are fully conscious. When fully conscious they may assume the most comfortable position. The wound should be inspected regularly for bleeding.

Airway problems which occur at this stage are usually due to inadequate reversal of muscle relaxants. In such instances, respiratory movements are noted to be inadequate and cyanosis may develop. Cyanosis may be difficult to detect in jaundiced patients or in members of coloured races. Oxygen should be administered and the duty anaesthetist called. If the patient becomes pink, but is sweating and has a full bounding pulse, carbon dioxide retention may have occurred because of inefficient ventilation. Assisted respiration and the further administration of drug antagonists may be necessary.

Postoperative pain

Pain after surgery is usually only severe for the first 48 hours. The degree of pain which occurs cannot necessarily be equated with the nature of the operation although pain seems to be most intense after surgery which involves opening the thoracic and upper abdominal cavities. Patients who undergo similar procedures may show a wide variation in their experience of pain. Nevertheless, the control of postoperative pain is most effectively achieved by intramuscular administration of fixed doses of analgesics at intervals frequent enough to prevent the return of severe pain. The timing of the initial dose may be determined by whether the patient has received an intraoperative analgesic or if a local anaesthetic block has been employed in theatre (intercostal nerve blocks or epidural anaesthesia are sometimes used as a supplement to general anaesthesia). In some cases it may be necessary to time a subsequent dose of analgesic so that it will be effective during a potentially painful procedure, e.g. removal of a pack or drain, physiotherapy.

The nurse should be trained to identify postoperative pain; she may be able to make her own assessment of its severity from prior observation and her knowledge of the patient preoperatively. Furthermore, before administering a dose of analgesic drug she should ensure that the pain relates to the surgical procedure. Discomfort can arise from other causes, such as a full bladder, a sore back or from a tight bandage or plaster; excessive restlessness may be due to hypoxia or undiagnosed haemorrhage.

Morphine and its analogue omnipon (Ch. 5) are the most commonly prescribed drugs. Morphine combines good analgesic qualities with a comparable degree of sedation and a sense of well-being. After minor procedures, the oral administration of dihydrocodeine or paracetamol may provide sufficient pain relief.

All analgesics have limitations or side effects when given in sufficient dosage and the nurse should be familiar with the disadvantages of any drug prescribed on her unit.

The control of postoperative pain by intermittent injections is perhaps not ideal. Medical journals have reported on an attitude of 'tight-fisted analgesia' in UK hospitals. Devices have been developed for 'on demand' self-administration of analgesic agents by the intravenous route, but these are too expensive for routine use. The use of equal volumes of premixed nitrous oxide and oxygen (delivered by Entonox apparatus) can provide excellent analgesia but this should be used only for brief periods. The more generalised use of regional blocks with long-acting local anaesthetic agents to 'tide the patient over' the period when pain is likely to be at its worst, probably holds the greatest hope for future management.

Postoperative vomiting

Vomiting, if excessive, leads to rapid salt and water depletion. In most cases vomiting ceases very quickly; if it does not metoclopramide (Maxolon) 10 mg or chlorpromazine (Largactil) 25 mg is usually effective. If the vomiting persists the stomach should be aspirated via a Ryle's tube. The patient is given fluids only at first until the bowel sounds have returned, after which a normal diet is gradually resumed. If vomiting persists or commences 24 hours postoperatively, the possibility of intestinal obstruction must be considered. Persistant hiccough is sometimes a distressing complication of an operation. The treatment is to administer carbon dioxide 5 per cent–10 per cent. If this does not provide relief chlorpromazine 25 mg is sometimes of value. In intractable cases an injection of hyoscine 0.4 mg or blocking the left phrenic nerve in the neck with a local anaesthetic may be necessary.

After gastrointestinal operations fluids by mouth are usually withheld for 24 hours and restricted for the following 24 hours. During this period careful attention to mouth hygiene and frequent mouthwashes will improve the patient's morale. If vomiting is not a problem, dentures may be worn. In ill patients or those incapacitated by intravenous drips, the nurse must carry out routine oral care.

The care of the mouth

If a patient who is confined to bed can clean his own teeth, he is given a beaker of water or mouth wash, and a bowl into which to spit.

When a patient is unable to use his hands but is otherwise well, the nurse can clean his teeth for him, using the patient's own toothbrush, and toothpaste, and allow him to rinse his own mouth, spitting into a bowl held by the nurse.

When the patient cannot co-operate in caring for his mouth, a special technique is carried out according to the acceptable hospital procedure.

Any unusual condition of the mouth is reported to the Sister or Charge Nurse, who will order any special treatment.

Care of dentures

When a patient can clean his own dentures, he is given a bowl of cold water in which to do so, and also a beaker of water or mouthwash with which to rinse his mouth.

When it is necessary for a nurse to clean the patient's dentures, they are removed and placed into a denture container. Taking the dentures and the patient's toothbrush to the bathroom, she cleans the dentures over a sink using *cold* running water. It is most important for modern dentures that the water used should be cold. They are returned to the patient, who is allowed to rinse his mouth before replacing them.

When a patient does not wish to retain his dentures, or in the case of a very weak or unconscious patient, the dentures are first cleaned and then placed in a denture container labelled with the patient's name, and stored in his locker. Before replacing the dentures which have been stored, they should be rinsed in cold water.

Maintenance of nutrition

If the operation is a short one, such as uncomplicated appendicectomy, no special difficulty arises in feeding. The patient takes fluids shortly after recovering consciousness and soon resumes a normal diet. Following a long period of anaesthesia or major surgery the maintenance of nutrition is essential. Of all the constituents of diet, fluid is the most important. Until the patient is able to drink, the fluid balance is maintained by the administration of fluid by other routes.

In severely ill patients or following extensive resections of the intestinal tract where it is clear that there is no likelihood of maintaining nutrition by eating within a couple of days, nitrogen imbalance (Ch. 14) has to be restored. An elemental diet may be given through a nasogastric tube or if this is not possible, feeding by the intravenous route is established (Ch. 14).

Deep-breathing exercises

Deep-breathing exercises, particularly in the 48 hours following the operation, do much to eliminate pulmonary complications. These should be taught by the physiotherapist in the preoperative waiting period if possible.

The wound

The diminution or elimination of infection at the site of the disease

A wound will heal rapidly only if it is non-infected. The wound includes not only the incision in the skin, fascia and muscles, but in all the deeper organs which have been opened. If infection is present in the organ to be operated on it should, if possible, be controlled before the operation takes place. Not only is the operation easier and safer, but the patient's convalescence is smoother.

In some cases several weeks' preparation may be necessary before the operation is undertaken. To illustrate this principle, operations at the following sites may be taken as examples:

1. The lungs. In Chapter 30 this problem is considered in detail. In the condition known as bronchiectasis, for which a lobe of the lung is removed, every effort is made to empty the cavities of pus and render their walls as clean as possible. Expectorant mixtures, antibiotics, postural drainage, breathing exercises, and physiotherapy are all prescribed for this purpose.

2. The stomach and duodenum. Operation is commonly undertaken for chronic gastric and duodenal ulceration which has failed to respond to medical treatment, or because the ulcer has produced an obstruction to the outlet of the stomach (pyloric stenosis). If the emptying of the stomach is defective, gross infection results in the stagnant food. The stomach must be washed out repeatedly.

3. The intestine. It is impossible to sterilise the intestinal contents, but the degree of infectivity can be reduced considerably. The incision and suture of a septic swollen intestine are fraught with considerable danger. The stitches may cut out, resulting in leakage of the intestinal contents. Before an operation on the intestine, the diet should consist of food which leaves no residue, so that faecal accumulation is diminished. Antibacterial drugs are administered systemically with the premedication or in the anaesthetic room. Attempts to sterilise the bowel by oral administration have been less effective.

4. The urinary tract. A wound communicating with the urinary tract will be very slow to heal in the presence of grossly infected urine. The consumption of about 3000 ml of fluid daily is adequate to ensure elimination of waste products and not too excessive to dilute the concentration of antibacterial drugs in the kidneys.

The same principle applies to all sites where an operation may be performed, whether it be the mouth, the eye, the ear, or the joints. The methods of controlling infection will be discussed in detail (p. 65). Some surgeons like to operate under an 'antibiotic umbrella' if there is a risk of infection, but experience has shown that this is not as effective as one may think.

The preparation of the skin

The preparation of the skin is a procedure common to almost all operations. The skin should be shaved, and if the patient is fit a bath or better a shower is given to remove loose hairs. The skin is then washed with soap and water and dried on a clean towel. The nails, the hair and the umbilicus should be clean. After this preparation the patient is put into a theatre gown and goes to bed in freshly laundered sheets. No antiseptic, towelling or dressings are applied in the ward.

The skin of the thighs of a patient who is incontinent of faeces requires special preparation if anaerobic infections are to be avoided after operations such as amputation or nailing operations for fracture of the femoral neck.

The importance of adequate vitamin C in the body

If vitamin C is deficient the healing of the wound may be delayed or fail to occur, but in the United Kingdom vitamin C deficiency is now uncommon except in the elderly who live alone.

The care of the wound

This is considered in Chapter 11.

Prevention and treatment of shock

This subject is considered in detail in Chapter 13.

Usually until 4 hours before the operation the patient may drink freely. If drinking is difficult or the patient is vomiting, fluids must be administered by the intravenous route. In pyloric stenosis, or intestinal obstruction, as fluid cannot leave the stomach, fluid by mouth is prohibited for hours or even days preoperatively. A patient depleted of salt and water becomes collapsed very rapidly. Severe purgation, once thought to be a good preoperative measure, is now known to be harmful since it produces severe dehydration and loss of electrolytes. In most cases a reduction of diet is all that is necessary.

An anaemic patient collapses very easily, and slight haemorrhage increases this tendency. A preliminary blood transfusion is given and may be continued during the operation. Fear predisposes to shock and sedatives and hypnotics may be useful. The relief of pain and the promotion of sleep are important. Analgesic and hypnotic drugs are administered, but an uncomfortable bandage or an awkward position in bed should be corrected. The patient must be returned to a warm bed, but excessive warming only increases the degree of shock.

After operation the nurse should note carefully the patient's colour and the state of his skin, any increase in the rate of the pulse, its quality, and any irregularity, and a strict check on the blood pressure is also indicated. In more serious cases a half-hourly check is recorded or the heart rate is monitored. Basically the treatment of shock is relief of pain, fluid or blood transfusion and elevation of the foot of the bed as a temporary short-term measure.

The prevention and treatment of complications which arise as a result of recumbency in bed

With very few exceptions no patient should be confined to bed before operation. The principal exception is a patient suffering from thyrotoxicosis and even in this condition confinement to bed to secure complete rest to the heart is now rarely necessary as modern antithyroid drugs control the toxicity so effectively.

The complications which may arise are:

1. Difficulty with micturition. Many patients find it difficult to pass urine while lying flat in bed and the difficulty is increased if there is an abdominal wound. The patient may sit or stand up or use a commode. Relaxation is necessary and the relief of pain essential. The treatment of this condition is discussed in Chapter 43. Catheterisation is not resorted to until all other measures have failed. A patient suffering from a minor degree of prostatic obstruction should have a catheter passed in the theatre after any operation which may precipitate retention. It can be removed in a day or two when he is up and about and pain has diminished.

2. Difficulty with defaecation. Difficulty in defaecation arises from conditions similar to those which interfere with micturition. The main factor in this condition, however, is intestinal distension with gas causing pain, and in all cases it should be relieved at regular intervals by the passage of a flatus tube—otherwise the heart and lungs may be embarrassed and the onset of the condition known as paralytic ileus may be encouraged.

Distension may be induced by an unsuitable diet during the two days before operation. Foods likely to cause residue and flatulence, such as vegetables, pastries, and large quantities of milk, should be avoided. The immediate preoperative care of the bowel has been discussed, but if the bowel is the site of the operation, as in removal of a portion of the colon, extra precautions are necessary (Ch. 39).

3. Respiratory complications. Respiratory complications are very com-

Fig. 4.2 Pitting oedema and swelling of the leg due to thrombosis.

mon. Many anaesthetic mixtures are irritant and produce excessive secretion. This may result in bronchitis, retained secretions or massive lobar collapse of the lungs. Pneumonia is an occasional complication. Many patients are afraid to take deep breaths because of fear of damage to their wounds. Lack of movement and shallow breathing increase the liability to pulmonary complications. The patient needs help and supervision. He is encouraged to use his hands to support the abdominal wound.

Inhalations, of which steam is the most important, are sometimes of value. Alternatively an ultrasonic nebuliser producing 'cold steam' or an electric nebuliser may be used. Nebulisers may be fitted to the oxygen supply. The moisture produced by either method reaches the smaller bronchioles and liquifies the mucus.

Pulmonary complications following operation are much commoner after interference in the upper abdomen and in all operations are more closely related to pre-existing bronchitis rather than the type of anaesthetic. Preoperative assessment and treatment with bronchial dilators, breathing exercises and, if necessary, antibiotics and steroids, diminish the risk. In addition the patient should stop smoking. Good postoperative physiotherapy is essential.

4. Thrombosis. Inactivity from rest in bed and an increase in the number of platelets in the blood as the result of a wound are conditions which favour the occurrence of a blood clot (or thrombus) in the veins of the legs (Fig. 4.2). Movement of the clot into the general circulation (embolism) may give rise to sudden death. Measures to diminish thromboembolism are discussed in Chapter 18. Preoperative oestrogens have already been mentioned as likely to increase thrombosis. Operating on the patient with the heels slightly elevated off the table diminishes the risk of thrombosis by taking pressure off the calves and aiding venous return. Continued slight bed elevation postoperatively also helps. In high-risk patients prophylactic heparin therapy may be prescribed (Ch. 18).

5. Pressure. Great care should be taken to prevent pressure sores after operations and in any severe illness. Their treatment is described in Chapter 22.

6. Muscular disuse and deformity. Muscular disuse and deformity have to be carefully guarded against, especially in orthopaedic conditions where they are most likely to occur, but they are none the less important in all conditions where the patient has been confined to bed for a considerable period.

7. Mental inactivity. Many patients tend to deteriorate mentally during a long stay in bed, and occupational therapy has a useful part to play.

Postoperative mania may occur in unstable subjects after operation. Old people are liable to develop mental changes. This is also liable to occur in toxic conditions. A suitable tranquilliser is usually prescribed if the patient is otherwise uncontrollable.

Delirium tremens may occur in chronic alcoholics.

8. Diminution in circulating blood volume. This occurs with bed rest and increases the risk of circulatory collapse (shock) during operation. It may be further aggravated by the vasodilatation produced by many anaesthetic agents in current use.

9. Postoperative pyrexia. Following operation many patients develop a rise in temperature which usually subsides after 24 hours. If it persists the following steps are advisable:

(a) The wound should be inspected for swelling or tenderness, which may be due to haematoma formation or infection.

(b) The urine is examined for pus and organisms.

(c) The legs are inspected for signs of thrombosis (Ch. 18).

(d) The chest is examined and a radiograph may show a segment of collapse.

(e) After an abdominal operation a residual abscess in the pelvis (detectable by rectal examination) or a subphrenic abscess should be suspected (Ch. 34).

(f) A white blood count is examined for leucocytosis.

Restoration of function

The restoration of function in the organs of the body by rehabilitation, re-education, exercises, and an adequate convalescence are most important.

The advice given to a patient on leaving hospital on such special points as diet, care of his wound, fitness for work, and other activities will do much to ensure a good result. Such advice must however be given against the knowledge of the patient's social background, his psychological attitude, education and personal character.

DAY SURGERY

Day surgery requires the cooperation of the general practitioner, the community nurse and the hospital. It increases the work of the hospital and good organisation is essential to its smooth running. There is a danger that as the patient has such a short time in contact with the staff he may feel that he has received treatment which was technically competent but that there was no personal concern. A word to show that the nurse who receives and sees him on discharge fully realises this possibility is most welcome. Another difficulty nurses experience in day wards is finding medical staff to come to discharge the patient.

Preoperatively the suitability of the patient's home is assessed, a note is sent to the hospital of any drugs which the patient may be taking, X-rays, blood and urine examination are undertaken before the day of admission but urine must always be examined again on the day of operation. Before the patient is discharged following day surgery he should be:

(i) seen by the doctor at the hospital and kept in if there is any doubt about his fitness;

(ii) given analgesics or a note of what treatment is necessary;

(iii) warned about bleeding;

(iv) told to report back to the hospital if necessary.

The patient's general practitioner, together with the community nurse, will be able to continue treatment at home. In some cases where equipment or home help facilities are necessary the social services of the district authority may be used.

5
Pain

Pain is one of the commonest presenting and continuing symptoms of organic and psychiatric disease. The mechanism of its production and perception are ill understood. It is rarely felt as an isolated sensation—a pin-prick is a mixture of touch and pain. The simple conception of pain receptors conveying impulses along a sensory nerve to a tract in the spinal cord and then to the cerebral cortex which localises the site of the pain is not confirmed by modern physiological research.

Pain arising in the skin can be localised accurately but pain of visceral origin is usually felt in the skin or muscular wall far distant from the organ involved. Conversely, it has been shown that vascular changes and alterations in the tone of a viscus can be produced by stimulating a localised area of skin. Such changes may provide a rational explanation for the use of counter-irritant measures and for acupuncture.

GATE CONTROL THEORY OF PAIN

Melzack and Wall in 1965 postulated the theory of a 'gate control' of pain within the spinal cord. The large 'A' fibres which conduct generalised sensation tend to close this gate while the small 'C' fibres tend to open it. If the 'A' fibres are damaged as in herpes zoster the smaller fibres are uninhibited and the gate is opened giving rise to pain. Electrical stimulation of the large nerve fibres, either at peripheral sites (transcutaneous nerve stimulation) or within the spinal cord (dorsal column stimulation), is effective in the control of some types of pain.

Pain is subjective and cannot easily be measured or monitored like the temperature or the pulse rate. A nurse will confirm from her own experience on the wards the apparently enormous variation in the degree of pain felt by two different patients from what appears to be an identical clinical lesion. In making this assessment the family doctor with intimate knowledge of a patient and his background has a great advantage over hospital staff. Anxiety and depression are important factors in the causation and escalation of pain. All pain is real to the patient and it may well be that pain of psychological origin is even more severe. To doubt this is to place oneself at a great disadvantage in the management of the patient. The only pain which is not genuine is one 'produced' for malingering or fraudulent purposes. Pain may be caused by tissue destruction with the release of chemical substances locally as well as by hypoxia. Lack of oxygen is a well-recognised cause of myocardial pain, as it is of intermittent claudication in peripheral arterial disease. The products of the inflammatory reaction are well-recognised sources of the origin of pain although the exact nature of the substances and the mode of action are open to more doubt. That cancer causes so little pain in the earlier stages is an important cause of delay in diagnosis. Pressure on nerve roots is believed to be a cause of pain and in prolapsed interverte-bral disc this is undoubtedly true because removal of the disc cures the pain. It is also believed that collapse of a vertebral body from secondary carcinoma causes pain by compressing the nerve root below, but the fact that removal of even one adrenal gland in a responsive case of breast cancer will relieve the pain immediately provides a nice enigma which baffles explanation on present knowledge. A single dose of oestrogens for a similar pain arising from cancer of the prostate may have the same dramatic effect.

The administration of steroids is effective in relieving susceptible pain but there is a danger that they may mask, exacerbate or reactivate a lesion which in their absence the body would overcome uneventfully. A healed peptic ulcer or a healed focus of pulmonary tuberculosis may become very active.

The endogenous opiates are substances of different structure to the opiates but with apparently similar function. They latch on to the same receptors as morphine and their effects like morphine are reversed by the narcotic antagonist drug naloxone. There are two groups, the encephalins and the beta-endorphins. Electrode percutaneous stimula-tion or acupuncture techniques take about twenty minutes before the patient feels any effects, presumably because it requires this time for sufficient quantities of the substances to be released. Beta-endorphin is a neurohormone secreted into the pituitary and Bowsher suggests that its release at the same time as ACTH in stress may explain why soldiers on the battlefield or sportsmen may feel no pain and be unaware at the time that they have been injured.

The prostaglandin PGE$_2$ secreted locally in inflammatory conditions dilates the blood vessels and increases capillary permeability. It is believed that this mechanism is blocked by cortisone or aspirin, with the result that the symptoms may be relieved.

CLINICAL MANAGEMENT

The significance of pain as a symptom of disease has to be evaluated by a full examination of the patient so that a diagnosis can be made. Analges-ics are restricted in patients suffering from acute abdominal pain until a diagnosis is made. Even in these conditions a sensible explanation will do much to relieve pain by allaying anxiety. In some acute situations an analgesic may have to be administered before transport of the patient to hospital, but the amount should be kept to the minimum and a note made of what has been administered. The dosage and the time of administration should accompany the patient. Obviously the sooner the diagnosis is established and a plan of treatment instituted the better.

The converse situation also holds great danger for the patient. The diagnosis has been clearly established—the patient either complains of repeated pain or the pain suddenly becomes more severe. The alert nurse should ask herself two questions before repeating analgesics—'Is this the same situation?' or 'Has a complication arisen?' Two examples are:

1. The patient under medical treatment for a peptic ulcer may have repeated pain—one danger is perforation, and it is a regrettable truth that the mortality is higher if the patient perforates in hospital rather than at home or even on the street! Only awareness of the hazard and re-examination of the patient complaining of repeated or severe pain will enable the diagnosis of perforation to be made when it occurs and prolonged delay by giving analgesics is avoided.

2. Most patients with gall stone colic are treated conservatively. Occasionally a gall stone will obstruct the small intestine—a condition which requires an urgent operation for its relief.

The ultimate relief of pain in acute organic disease is cure of the disease. As this will usually be of short duration the problem of the relief of pain is not a difficult one. Appropriate analgesics are prescribed and the danger of addiction is negligible. None the less, the drugs are chosen after assessment of the pain arising from the local condition, the degree of anxiety or fear and the stability or otherwise of the psychological background. Above all else it must never be suggested to a patient that he or she is too intolerant of pain—pain is never to be equated with an endurance test. In practice the total amount of analgesics can be considerably reduced if they are given in small frequent doses before the pain recurs rather than after the patient has been in pain for some time.

DRUGS

There is an endless variety and combination of drugs but in practice an individual unit will usually use a small number which have been found to be adequate. Rapid and effective absorption is essential for their action. If the patient is unable to eat or drink a parenteral route is essential for their action. The only parenteral route which is effective in the shocked patient is the intravenous one. Subcutaneous or intramuscular injections are not absorbed when the patient is shocked and an undesirable cumulative dosage may arise as recovery occurs.

Analgesic drugs may cause respiratory depression, nausea, constipation or hypotension.

Narcotic analgesics

Narcotic analgesics are indicated in the treatment of severe pain, especially that arising from deep (e.g. visceral) structures.

Morphine (10-15 mg) is an excellent analgesic but decreases respiration and should be used with care in bronchitic or asthmatic patients. Many patients complain of nausea and the drug tends to cause constipation. The action of morphine can be reversed by the administration of naloxone.

Omnopon (papaveretum) (15-20 mg) is a semisynthetic mixture of narcotic drugs extracted from opium, and contains about 50 per cent morphine. It is commonly used as a postoperative analgesic.

Pethidine (50-100 mg) is an effective analgesic but is less powerful than morphine. It is less likely to cause respiratory depression but may lower the blood pressure.

Diamorphine (heroin) (5-10 mg) is a powerful analgesic. The use of heroin is usually restricted to the management of intractable pain associated with incurable malignant disease and in the relief of pain for patients on coronary care units.

Dihydrocodeine (DF118) (30-60 mg) is suitable for moderate pain.

Pentazocine (Fortral) (30-60 mg) is an intermediate between morphine and codeine. It has a low risk of dependence but can cause hallucinations.

Buprenorphine (Temgesic) (0.3-0.6 mg) is a similar drug which can also be administered by the sublingual route. Unlike the other drugs previously mentioned, parenteral preparations of pentazocine and buprenorphine are not subject to Controlled Drug Regulations.

Non-narcotic analgesics

Non-narcotic analgesics are useful in the treatment of milder forms of pain which are usually of superficial origin.

Aspirin (300-600 mg) is a widely used and highly effective analgesic. Its use is sometimes limited because of the risk of gastric bleeding in susceptible patients; it may also interfere with blood coagulation by increasing the prothrombin time. The use of other non-steroidal anti-inflammatory drugs (NSAIDs) such as ibuprofen and naproxen may lessen but not abolish the risk of gastrointestinal haemorrhage.

Paracetamol (0.5-1g) does not have anti-inflammatory effects and does not cause gastric bleeding. It is a useful alternative to aspirin. Some advantage may be conferred by using these drugs in combination or in compound preparations containing less powerful narcotic analgesics (e.g. Paracodol, Solpadeine).

CHRONIC PERSISTENT OR RECURRENT PAIN

Acute pain is fairly easily relieved by analgesics while measures are taken to cure its cause. The pain is protective. In many cases of persistent or recurrent pain the pain is in itself the dominant feature. Such patients may be divided into two categories:

1. Those in whom the expectation of life is short, usually a patient with advanced malignant disease.
2. Sufferers who have a normal life expectancy but persistent pain which is overwhelming. These include arthritics, post-herpetic neuralgia and many other conditions.

The patient with malignant disease can be treated with analgesics and anxiolytic drugs and in severe pain there is a variety of methods listed below which may be effective in a particular case. The patients in the second group present a much more difficult problem. In all it is essential to be certain that pain is the symptom complained of and not just itching or numbness. A careful clinical examination and investigation is indicated to exclude any obvious remedial cause. Special pain clinics have been established to aid in the management of such problems.

Methods of treatment

1. Analgesics similar to those administered for acute pain are used— the danger of drug dependence in patients with benign disease is an overriding consideration and should intensify the efforts to use other methods of control. For patients with malignant disease a slow release preparation of morphine (MST) may provide more sustained pain relief. Sublingual and rectal preparations of narcotic analgesics may produce a more rapid or additive effect. Continuous administration of powerful analgesics into subcutaneous sites via infusion pumps is of value in refractory cases: heroin, by virtue of its high aqueous solubility, is very useful in this context.

2. Other drugs may also be valuable. Anticonvulsants can diminish the transmission of pain within the CNS. Tranquillisers and antidepressants will be useful if there is underlying depression or anxiety associated with the pain.

3. Local injection of nerves or ganglia. Repeated injections of long-acting local anaesthetics into pain pathways can break the 'vicious circle' of pain.

4. Destruction of nerve routes or tracts by:
   (a) Injection of phenol or alcohol.
   (b) Surgical section.
   (c) Electric coagulation.
   (d) Cryoprobe therapy.

Despite such radical measures, in time the pain recurs in many patients. Trigeminal neuralgia (Ch.45) which does not respond to carbamazepine (Tegretol) is treated by injection of the ganglion or nerve section.

5. Radiotherapy is often effective for the relief of pain from secondary malignant deposits in the spine.

6. Hormonal methods including oophorectomy, adrenalectomy or hypophysectomy (Ch. 28).

7. Sympathectomy is indicated for true causalgia—a burning pain which occurs after injury to a peripheral nerve.

8. Electrical stimulation. This may be achieved by the use of surface electrodes placed over the painful area. In special circumstances, an

electrode can be implanted into the dura mater adjacent to the dorsal columns of the spinal cord. This is connected by a subcutaneous lead to a receiver implanted in the groin. An external stimulator and transmitter are provided to allow stimulation whenever required.

The control of intractable pain is far from easy and with further understanding of its physiology better methods of control will be discovered.

BIBLIOGRAPHY

Bowsher D 1978 Pain topics. In: Academy News Bulletins Inc, p 3
Melzack R, Walls P D 1965 Science 150: 971
Scottish Health Service Library Bibliography No 14

6

Microbiology

All infections are caused by micro-organisms. These are broadly divided into four categories—bacteria, viruses, fungi and protozoa. Bacteria are approximately 1μ in diameter ($1\mu=0.001$ mm) and can be seen with the aid of a laboratory microscope; viruses are very much smaller and can only be seen with the aid of an electron microscope. Micro-organisms may be classified as 'pathogens', capable of causing disease, or 'commensals', which are found in the normal body flora. However, it has been recognised more recently that the pathogenicity of a microbe depends on the host as much as the microbe and 'commensals' may act as pathogens in a susceptible patient. Pyogenic organisms are those capable of producing pus.

BACTERIA

Classification

Bacteria are described according to their shape, as seen under the microscope, and their staining characteristics. There are three main groups of bacteria—those that are readily Gram stained, acid-fast bacilli (AFB) and spirochaetes (Table 6.1). Organisms which hold the Gram stain are known as Gram-positive. Those in which it disappears after washing with acetone are known as Gram-negative and need to be counter-stained to be visible under the microscope. Acid-fast bacilli need strong stains to be visible e.g. Ziehl-Neelson stain.

Bacilli are rod-shaped.

Cocci are rounded.

Spirochaetes are corkscrew-shaped in appearance, but do not take up the Gram stain.

Physiology

Effect of atmosphere

1. **Aerobic** bacteria are organisms which need oxygen to grow.

Table 6.1 Classification of bacteria

A. Bacteria that are readily Gram stained

	Gram positive	*Gram negative*
Cocci	Staphylococci	Neisseria
	Streptococci	e.g. *N. meningitidis*
	e.g. *Strep. pneumoniae*	*N. gonorrhoeae*
	Strep. pyogenes	
	Strep. faecalis	
Bacilli	Bacillus	Escherichia ⎤
	e.g. *B. anthrax*	e.g. *E. coli* │
	B. cereus	Klebsiella │ Coliforms
	Corynebacteria	Proteus ├─
	e.g. *C. diptheriae*	Salmonella │
	Listeria	Shigella ⎦
	Clostridia	Pseudomonas
	e.g. *Cl. perfringens (welchii)*	Haemophilus
	Cl. tetani	Yersinia
	Actinomyces	Vibrio
		e.g. *V. cholerae*
		Campylobacter
		Bacteroides

B. Acid-fast bacilli

Mycobacteria
e.g. *M. tuberculosis*
M. leprae

C. Spirochaetes

Treponema
e.g. *T. pallidum*
Leprospira
Borrelia

2. **Anaerobic** organisms can survive only when oxygen is absent or present in very low concentrations. In the body anaerobic conditions are, in practice, only created when the blood supply has been cut off so that no oxygen reaches the part, for example, in dead muscle.

Artificial growth of organisms

This is known as culturing. Various substances known as media are used to grow organisms artificially; that most commonly used is agar. Pus-containing organisms, swabbed onto an agar plate and kept at body temperature (37°C) overnight, will produce a growth varying in appearance with the strain of the organism.

Effect of temperature

Conditions favourable to a growth of micro-organisms are warmth, moisture and an adequate supply of nutrients. Cold inhibits the growth of most bacteria. It interferes with their ability to divide and multiply, but it never kills them. Some organisms provide for their survival by the formation of spores. A spore is a bacterium in a modified form, modified to protect itself in unfavourable surroundings. As soon as the conditions are most favourable it develops into a normal organism. While moist heat at 100°C kills all organisms, spores require a temperature of 116°C to 127°C for their destruction.

Sensitivity testing

This is determined by adding a particular antibiotic to the culture media and if growth is prevented the organism is described as sensitive.

Virulence factors

Bacteria may produce enzymes which aid their pathogenic effect, for example *Staph. aureus* produces coagulase which acts on plasma components at the site of infection and leads to a deep deposit of fibrin around the bacteria and so protects it from the host immune defences. *Strep. pyogenes* produces several enzymes or 'toxins', including haemolysin, streptokinase and hyaluronidase, which cause tissue damage. Other bacteria, for example *Haemophilus influenzae*, *Strep. pneumonia*, produce capsules which make them relatively resistant to phagocytosis by white cells.

COMMON PYOGENIC ORGANISMS

1. Gram positive

The commonest organism is *Staphylococcus aureus*—**Staphylococci** are rounded bacteria and under the microscope appear in clusters like bunches of grapes (Fig. 6.1). Boils, carbuncles, and many abscesses in the skin and subcutaneous tissues are due to staphylococci. They are the most common cause of bone infection. Less frequently they cause infection elsewhere, for example, a perinephric abscess or pneumonia.

Streptococci viewed microscopically usually appear in chains (Fig. 6.1). Some strains haemolyse blood on a blood agar plate and they are known as the haemolytic variety; the remainder are non-haemolytic. The haemolytic streptococci can be divided into a number of broad groups determined by the chemical nature of the carbohydrate contained in the cell wall of the organism. Group A haemolytic streptococci *(Strep. pyogenes)* cause an acute sore throat. Local extensions from a throat infection may cause peritonsillar abscess (quinsy), sinusitis, otitis media, mastoiditis or meningitis. It also may cause severe spreading skin infections (cellulitis), erysipelas and impetigo. Healthy individuals may carry *Strep. pyogenes* in the throat without causing them harm. There is, however, risk to patients from infection by this organism.

Pneumococci *(Strep. pneumoniae)* are always in pairs (diplococci) (Fig. 6.1). They are the usual cause of lobar pneumonia and occasionally are responsible for meningitis and septicaemia.

2. Gram negative

Gonococci are also diplococci and are the causal organism of gonorrhoea.

Escherichia coli (Fig. 6.1) is a rod-shaped organism whose natural habitat is the intestine where it is non-pathogenic. Like most Gram-negative organisms it produces a powerful endotoxin and may be the

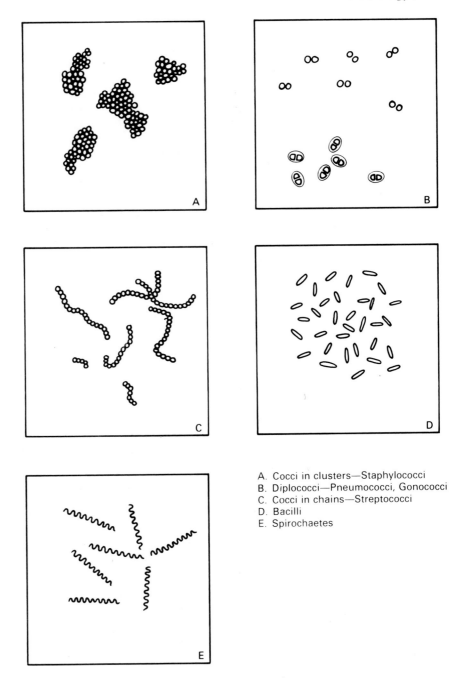

A. Cocci in clusters—Staphylococci
B. Diplococci—Pneumococci, Gonococci
C. Cocci in chains—Streptococci
D. Bacilli
E. Spirochaetes

Fig. 6.1 Microscopic appearance of some micro-organisms.

cause of septicaemic shock. Perforation of the intestine enables the organism to gain access to the peritoneal cavity, where it is pathogenic (disease causing). Hence it is found in peritonitis secondary to appendicitis and diverticulitis, but is greatly outnumbered by anaerobic organisms of the bacteroides group. Urinary infections such as cystitis and pyelonephritis are frequently due to E. coli.

The Proteus group of organisms are well recognised urinary tract pathogens where they cause pyelonephritis as well as infection of the lower urinary tract. They can also contaminate and infect wounds and burns.

Salmonella may cause typhoid fever (due to *Salmonella typhi* or *paratyphi*) in travellers from abroad but in the UK other salmonella strains (e.g. *Salmonella typhimurium, hadar, virchow*) are more common and usually cause gastro-enteritis. Septicaemia, however, may occur with any of these strains particularly in the very young, the old and the debilitated.

Shigella are Gram-negative bacteria which cause bacillary dysentry. *Shigella sonnei* is commonly seen in Britain among small children where it may cause outbreaks of diarrhoea.

Escherichia coli, Proteus, Klebsiella, Salmonella and *Shigella* are known as coliforms.

Pseudomonas aeruginosa can infect almost any external site or organ in the body especially in hospital inpatients. It may cause persistent urinary tract infections as well as infections in ventilated patients. The great danger of Pseudomonas is that it develops in wounds when the competition from more sensitive bacteria has been removed. The young, the old, the burnt and patients receiving wide spectrum antibiotics or on steroid treatment are liable to develop this infection.

Yersinia are small Gram-negative rods. Examples are *Y. enterocolitica* and *Y. pseudotuberulosis*, which may cause mesenteric adenitis and mimic acute appendicitis.

Campylobacter is a comma-shaped Gram-negative bacteria which commonly causes gastro-enteritis.

The bacteroides are another prominent group of non-spore bearing anaerobes which commonly cause infection and peritonitis. They are the predominant organisms in the large intestine where they outnumber *E. coli*. The bacteroides predominate the bacterial picture in peritonitis, caused by perforation of the intestinal tract, and in abdominal wound infection.

Anaerobic infections in man are most commonly caused by these non-clostridial anaerobes (Willis). They are part of a normal bacterial flora of the alimentary canal and the lower female genital tract. From their normal habitat they invade tissues debilitated by diabetes, trauma or other pathological conditions. The pus produced is particularly foul smelling and copious. While surgical drainage is of the first importance, metronidazole is highly effective in treatment.

ORGANISMS WHICH CAUSE SPECIFIC INFECTIONS

Clostridium tetani is an anaerobic spore-bearing organism which is very resistant to ordinary methods of disinfection. It is present in soil and dust and the large intestine of several animals, including sheep. Catgut (made from sheep's intestine) has been the source of infection in some postoperative cases of tetanus. The sterility of surgical catgut is now rigorously controlled in Britain.

It elaborates a powerful toxin which poisons the motor nerve cells with the result that spasm occurs in the muscles supplied by the corresponding nerves. The disease is known as **tetanus.**

Clostridium perfringens *(Cl.welchii)* and its associated organisms is also an anaerobic inhabitant of the intestine and proliferates in damaged muscle, producing gas and toxins, causing **gas gangrene.** It is a complication of wounding. Contaminated clothing embedded at the time of the accident is commoner than soil as the source of the organism. It is penicillin-sensitive but surgical measures are also essential in its treatment (Ch. 9).

Mycobacterium tuberculosis is an aerobic rod-shaped organism, which causes **tuberculosis.** It does not stain readily with the Gram stain but retains hot carbol fuchsin which resists decolorisation by acid. It is therefore referred to as acid-fast.

Treponema pallidum is a spirochaete (Fig. 6.1) and is the cause of **syphilis.**

VIRUSES

While immunisation for the prevention of viral disease is highly effective, chemotherapy for established infection is limited to the treatment of herpes infection. In addition to causing infection, there is a suspicion that viruses may be the cause of some forms of malignant disease.

Many infectious diseases such as measles, smallpox, mumps, influenza and the common cold are due to a virus. Of special interest to the surgical nurse are:

1 Poliomyelitis (infantile paralysis).
2 Hepatitis B (Ch. 36) from blood products.
3 Herpes (zoster and simplex)—the cause of shingles and cold sores respectively.
4 Rubella (German measles) in the pregnant woman on account of the risk of congenital deformities to the fetus.

Before a virus can cause disease it has to enter and multiply inside the body of a living cell. Similarly, viruses will only grow in living cells in the laboratory. Tissue culture is therefore used in specialised laboratories to grow viruses. More commonly, the diagnosis of a viral infection depends on the demonstration of antibodies to the virus in the patient's serum.

FUNGI

Fungi are large branched or budding organisms. Three groups are of surgical interest.

1. **Tinea pedis** (athlete's foot) causes infection in the web of the toes and *Tinea cruris* infects folds of skin in the thigh and groin.

2. **Candida albicans** (causing moniliasis) is a fungus which is normally suppressed by harmless bacteria but may cause a virulent infection following the administration of broad range antibiotics. It is a common cause of infection in the mouth (thrush) or in the vagina.

3. **Actinomyces** may cause infection arising in the floor of the mouth and neck, in the lungs, or the ileo-caecal region of the intestine. It also may cause pelvic sepsis in a patient fitted with an intrauterine device. The organism *Actinomyces israelii* is too large to invade the lymphatic system, but causes destruction of tissue producing typical 'sulphur granules' pus. Actinomyces are truly bacteria but closely resemble fungi.

THE PROTOZOA

The protozoa are the cause of a wide spectrum of diseases in the world. The surgical complications of amoebiasis and hydatid disease are the only ones the nurse is likely to encounter in the British Isles and then only very occasionally.

Entamoeba histolytica is the parasite responsible for **amoebiasis.** While dysentry is the commonest manifestation, surgical complications such as perforation of the intestine, abscess and stricture formation may occur. A liver abscess is a well-recognised complication. Metronidazole is the most effective drug.

Echinococcus granulosa causes **hydatid disease** which may affect many parts of the body but 80 per cent of lesions occur in the liver as a hydatid cyst. Surgical treatment is necessary when there are complications, e.g. obstruction, abscess formation.

ANTIBACTERIAL THERAPY

Antibiotics have made surgical procedures safer, increased the scope of surgery, and reduced the incidence of postoperative wound infection in contaminated surgery. They have not, however, diminished the need for supportive measures, such as good hygiene in the wards, or the need for an incision to evacuate pus. Antibiotics may be bactericidal—that is they destroy the organism, for example, penicillin and the aminoglycoside group (gentamicin and tobramycin). Others such as tetracycline and chloramphenicol which prevent propagation are known as bacteriostatic.

Before discussing the more important agents briefly, some general principles should be considered:

Choice of agent

Modern chemotherapy has taught us to think not so much in terms of disease but in terms of sensitive organisms. If the organism is known and is sensitive to an antibiotic, cure is certain. This presupposes that the facilities for identification and tests for sensitivity are universally available. It also assumes that the organism can be readily isolated from the patient. Isolation, culture, assessment of sensitivity by the bacteriologist and the administration of the appropriate antibiotic is ideal. Unfortunately this is only possible in certain types of infection and in many cases it has to be assumed that the organism is the one commonly responsible for the condition and the antibiotic to which it is usually sensitive is chosen. The patient's response is used as an indication to sensitivity. If, after 72 hours, there is no response the antibiotic is changed or if, before this period has elapsed, the organism can be isolated and sensitivity tests show that a different antibiotic is indicated, therapy is changed.

When an antibiotic is prescribed it should be:

1. Administered by the *correct route* which may be orally, intramuscularly, intravenously, intrathecally or by local instillation.

2. Given at the stated intervals in the dose prescribed, so that its concentration in the bloodstream is maintained.

3. Continued over a sufficient period of days to cure the infection.

A sufficient quantity of fluid has to be taken so that the antibiotic can be excreted by the kidney if this is its route of elimination, and if used for treatment of urinary infection the fluid intake should not be so great that the concentration of the antibiotic in the urine is so low as to be ineffective. An intake of 3 litres per day is probably the optimum.

It is inadvisable to prescribe antibacterial therapy for mild self-limiting infections. These substances are expensive, not without complications and may produce resistant organisms. It used to be thought that antibiotics given prophylactically would prevent postoperative infection, but experience has shown that this is not so and careful aseptic technique is the best safeguard.

Prophylactic antibiotics are used when either the risk of infection postoperatively is high or the risk of infection is low but there would be serious consequences of any infection. Prophylaxis is therefore used for:

(a) Amputation for gangrene (p. 244).

(b) Abdominal surgery—particularly on the large bowel or for peritonitis.

(c) Operations on patients with congenital or rheumatic heart disease who are at risk of developing endocarditis.

(d) Hip replacement.

(e) Open heart surgery.

Complications of antibiotic therapy

1. Resistant organisms

Penicillin was introduced to widespread use in the 1940s. At that time almost all staphylococci were penicillin-sensitive. 1965 saw the emergence of penicillin resistance. Flucloxacillin or cloxacillin became then the antibiotic of choice for staphylococcal infection. However, more recently flucloxacillin (methicillin) resistant staphylococci have emerged as a problem in several hospitals. These resistant organisms have been difficult to eradicate and do not have a predictable sensitivity pattern.

Gram-negative bacilli resistant to the aminoglycosides have caused similar problems. Numerous outbreaks of such resistance have been described. These organisms carry a resistant plasmid which can be transferred to other bacteria (not necessarily of the same species) and this causes the organism to become resistant. The emergence of Gram-negative organisms resistant to many antibiotics and the increase in this type of infection in hospital is probably due to the widespread use of broad spectrum antibiotics as well as the increased use of catheters and tubes in the:

(i) Urinary bladder for drainage.
(ii) Veins for infusions.
(iii) Respiratory tract for suction.
(iv) Stomach.

Any patient who is infected or colonised by a multiply resistant organism should be nursed in isolation so that it is not propagated in the ward and spread to other patients. Antibiotic therapy should cease when the period for which it has been prescribed has elapsed. Inappropriate antibiotics should be stopped immediately.

2. Sensitisation

Sensitisation of the patient or staff may occur with any antibiotic. For this reason antibiotics are not prescribed for trivial infections. Sensitivity reactions take the form of a skin rash or even, in some cases, severe anaphylactic shock may result.

The following precautions are of value in protecting the nurse from sensitivity:

(a) The same needle can be put into the bottle of solution and also used for injection into the patient.
(b) Air in the syringe should be expelled with the needle in the bottle. Spraying it into the atmosphere causes skin reaction on the face and arms.
(c) The overall precaution, of course, is for the nurse to wear gloves.
(d) Hermetically sealed or orally administered capsules of antibiotics prevent skin contact with the antibiotic. Disposable syringes and hand washing to remove any particles after handling antibiotics are probably as important in preventing reactions in the nurse.

3. Toxic reactions

Toxic reactions are almost unknown with penicillin, but damage to the 8th nerve may occur with the aminoglycoside antibiotics. Streptomycin and gentamicin affect particularly the vestibular branch while neomycin and kanamycin affect the auditory branch and both are more likely to occur in the presence of poor renal function. With local or topical use, neomycin, in addition to damage to the auditory division of the 8th nerve, is dangerous in the presence of hepatic failure as well as when renal function is impaired.

Another well-known toxic reaction is the danger of aplastic anaemia from chloramphenicol. This antibiotic is therefore reserved for use in life-threatening conditions, for example, meningitis, typhoid fever.

4. Super infection

Suppression of the normal flora by antibiotics may unleash the activities of organisms which are normally held in check. Examples are pseudomonas infection, moniliasis and staphylococcal enterocolitis. Antibiotics may also promote *Clostridium difficile* colonisation in the gut. This may lead to the development of pseudo-membranous colitis.

ANTIBACTERIAL AGENTS

A. PENICILLINS

Benzyl penicillin (Penicillin G)

Penicillin was the first and is still the safest of the antibiotics. It is destroyed in the stomach by the action of gastric acid and must therefore be given by intravenous or intramuscular injection (see below). It is active against most *streptococci, gonococci, meningococci, Clostridium perfringens* and *Clostridium tetani,* but has no activity against *coliforms, Mycobacterium tuberculosis* or *Pseudomonas aeruginosa.* It is destroyed by penicillinase produced, for example, by most strains of *Staph. aureus.*

Intramuscular injection

An injection into the muscle tissue which has a good blood supply enabling drugs to be readily absorbed. Large amounts of drug may be injected in this way (1 ml to 5 ml)

    Requirements:
      Receiver
      2 or 5 ml syringe
      Needle—size 23G 1¼ (1) or 21G 1½ (1)
      Needle—19G (2)—for drawing up if required
      2 Mediswabs
      Prescription and recording sheet

Disposable gloves should be worn when potentially sensitising drugs are to be injected.

The injection is prepared in the treatment room. Using the aseptic technique the guarded needle and syringe are assembled and placed in the receiver. The drug is checked by two nurses (one of whom is qualified), the ampoule opened, or the cap of a multidose bottle wiped with a mediswab. The needle guard is removed. The drug is drawn up into the syringe, the amount being regulated according to the prescription. The drug is again double checked with the prescription sheet. Air bubbles are expelled, the needle guard is secured, and the syringe and needle are replaced in the receiver together with a Mediswab.

The patient is advised of what is to happen. Privacy is ensured and the patient placed in a suitable position. The clothing is arranged so as to expose the site. The site chosen is the lateral aspect of the thigh (Fig. 6.2). If this cannot be used, the ward sister or the unit officer is informed and they may give it into the buttock (Fig. 6.3). The nurse and witness check with the prescription sheet. The nurse cleans the skin with the Mediswab.

Fig. 6.2   The safest site for intramuscular injection.

Fig. 6.3   If the buttock is used the upper and outer quadrant is the only safe area.

The needle is inserted at an angle of 90°, care being taken to avoid touching the bone. The plunger is withdrawn slightly to ensure a blood vessel has not been punctured. If blood is seen entering the syringe, the needle is withdrawn, and firm pressure applied to the puncture site for 10 seconds. An adjacent site is then chosen for the injection. If no blood is seen, the fluid is instilled gently. The Mediswab is placed over the needle track and the needle withdrawn smoothly. The underlying tissues are massaged, and/or the patient is instructed to carry out 'quadriceps' exercises to aid absorption of the drug and to reduce discomfort. The patient is made comfortable and the recording sheet initialled by the nurse giving the injection. Used equipment is discarded, and the nurse washes and dries her hands.

Subcutaneous or hypodermic injections. Although not used for anti-biotics they are necessary for the administration of many drugs. The sites used are, the upper outer surface of the arm, the front of the thigh or the abdomen.

Requirements are:
   Receiver
   2 ml syringe
   Needle—size 25G 1 (1)
   Needle—21G 1½ (1)—for drawing up if required
   2 Mediswabs
   Prescription and recording sheet

The needle is inserted at an angle of 45°, care being taken not to insert it right up to the hub. The plunger is withdrawn slightly to ensure a vein has not been punctured, depressed gently and the fluid instilled. The Mediswab is placed over the needle track and the needle withdrawn smoothly. The skin is massaged gently to aid dispersion of the fluid.

The patient is made comfortable, and the recording sheet initialled by the nurse giving the injection. In the case of a controlled drug, the nurse and the witness sign the register. Used equipment is discarded, and the nurse washes and dries her hands.

Apart from a mild skin rash no toxic reactions from systemic penicillin have been reported but as with any drug an acute sensitivity reaction may occur. A few reports of fatal collapse following intrathecal penicillin have been reported. It is advisable to enquire if the patient is known to be sensitive to penicillin and to ensure that any allergy is clearly recorded on the patient's case-sheet.

Phenoxymethyl penicillin (Penicillin V)

This is not destroyed in the stomach and can therefore be given by mouth. It has the same spectrum of activity as benzyl penicillin and is also destroyed by penicillinase.

Penicillinase-resistant penicillins

These include methicillin, cloxacillin, oxacillin and flucloxacillin. Infection due to *Staph. aureus* is usually treated using one of these antibiotics. However, resistant staphylococci are emerging and may be difficult to treat.

Broad spectrum penicillins

1. Ampicillin has activity against the organisms sensitive to benzyl penicillin and in addition is active against *Streptococcus faecalis* (a penicillin-resistant streptococcus) and *some coliforms* but *not pseudomonas*. Resistance among the coliforms has increased over the last few years but ampicillin may be used for urinary tract infections if the infecting organism is known to be sensitive. It is useful for the treatment of chest infections as the common infecting bacteria are usually ampicillin sensitive (*Haemophilus influenzae* and *Strep. pneumoniae*). Amoxycillin is a derivative of ampicillin which is better absorbed orally but has the same spectrum of activity.
2. Antipseudomonal penicillins. Ticarcillin, piperacillin, azlocillin and mezlocillin are all broad spectrum penicillins which must be given by injection. They have similar activity to ampicillin but are more active against *coliforms* and *Pseudomonas aeruginosa*. They are used usually in conjunction with an aminoglycoside and metronidazole for the treatment of serious infection.

B. AMINOGLYCOSIDES

Gentamicin, tobramycin

These are the two aminoglycosides commonly used in the UK. They are powerful broad spectrum antibiotics with high activity against *coliforms, pseudomonas* and *staphylococci*. They are not active against streptococci or anaerobic bacteria. They must be given by injection and blood levels must be monitored to avoid toxic levels. Toxicity is associated with damage to the inner ear leading to deafness and vertigo. Renal failure may also occur. Coliforms resistant to gentamicin and tobramycin have caused outbreaks especially in catheterised patients. Infections caused by these multiply-resistant organisms may be difficult to treat and cause mortality due to inappropriate therapy.

Netilmicin

This is similar to gentamicin and tobramycin but may be active against some multiply-resistant coliforms.

Amikacin

This has an increased spectrum of activity and is usually active against multiply-resistant coliforms. It is, however, not as active as gentamicin or tobramycin against sensitive coliforms. Amikacin should therefore be reserved for the use of resistant infections only.

Streptomycin

This was the first aminoglycoside to be used but is now reserved for the treatment of tuberculosis. Like the other aminoglycosides it needs to be given by injection and is therefore a second line antituberculous drug.

Neomycin, kanamycin, framycetin

These are used for topical treatment of minor infection or orally in regimes for bowel decontamination prior to colonic surgery or in the immunosuppressed patient.

C. CEPHALOSPORINS

This group of drugs now consists of more than 15 different agents. They include cephalexin, cephradine and cefaclor which can be given orally, and cefoxitin, cefuroxine, cefotaxine, ceftazidime which need to be given parenterally. They have activity against *staphylococci, streptococci* (excluding *Strep. faecalis*) and *many coliforms*. Most have little or no activity against pseudomonas. There is a cross-hypersensitivity between penicillin and cephalosporins which may occur in up to 10 per cent of patients with penicillin allergy.

D. METRONIDAZOLE

Metronidazole may be given orally, as a suppository or intravenously, and is important in the treatment of anaerobic organisms, for example in faecal peritonitis, pelvic sepsis and as a prophylactic agent in colo-rectal surgery. It is often used in combination with an aminoglycoside for the treatment of serious sepsis. It is also used in the treatment of protozoal infection, for example trichomoniasis, amoebiasis and giardiasis.

E. OTHER ANTIBACTERIAL DRUGS

Sulphonamides, trimethoprim and co-trimoxazole

There are many sulphonamides available but the development of resistance by many bacteria has reduced the usefulness of these agents as single drugs. They do however penetrate well into the cerebrospinal fluid and are useful for prophylaxis following fractures of the skull. Non-absorbable sulphonamides may be used for bowel decontamination prior to surgery, e.g. colectomy. Trimethoprim is usually used in combination with sulphamethoxazole as co-trimoxazole and this greatly potentiates its effective range of activity. Co-trimoxazole is used for the treatment of urinary tract infections and chest infections.

Tetracyclines

The tetracyclines include oxytetracycline, tetracycline, doxycycline and minocycline. They are broad spectrum bacteriostatic agents and are useful for treating some infections due to intracellular organisms such as brucella and chlamydia and for treating infective exacerbations of bronchitis.

Erythromycin

Erythromycin has a similar range of activity to penicillin. It is useful for the treatment of staphylococcal sepsis and other conditions when penicillin might be used, if the patient is allergic to penicillin.

Fucidin

Fucidin is an antistaphylococcal antibiotic of narrow spectrum. It is administered orally or intravenously but resistance rapidly develops if used alone.

Chloramphenicol

This is a broad spectrum antibiotic with good penetration into tissue. Potentially fatal bone marrow toxicity restricts its systemic use to treating life-threatening infections, for example meningitis, typhoid fever. Topically it is commonly used for the treatment of superficial eye infections.

Lincomycin, clindamycin

These antibiotics have activity against staphylococci and clindamycin has been used for treating anaerobic infections. Both these antibiotics are not used routinely due to the potential toxicity associated with pseudo-membranous colitis.

Vancomycin

Vancomycin is a potentially toxic drug when administered intravenously. It is used for treating selected patients with endocarditis or septicaemia due to antibiotic-resistant strains of *Staph. aureus*, *Staph. albus* or for patients with penicillin allergy. Orally it is used for the treatment of pseudo-membranous colitis as it is poorly absorbed.

Nalidixic acid, nitrofurantoin

These are antibiotics used for the treatment of cystitis.

Noxythiolin, chlorhexidine

These are antiseptics commonly used for the local treatment of wounds or in the bladder for instillation.

Clavulonic acid

This is not active alone as an antibiotic but is a very powerful inhibitor of penicillinase and is used in combination with, for example amoxycillin, to increase its activity against staphylococci and coliforms.

BIBLIOGRAPHY

Bint A J, Reeves D S 1978 British Journal of Hospital Medicine 19: 335
Shanson D C 1982 Microbiology in Clinical Practice, 1st edn. Wright, Bristol
Willis A T 1977 Anaerobic bacteriology. In: Clinical and laboratory practice, 3rd edn.
    Butterworths, London
Willis A T 1978 British Journal of Hospital Medicine 20: 579

7

Infection

Infection is the successful invasion and growth of micro-organisms in a body tissue. The severity or mildness of the resulting disease depends upon:

The dosage and virulence of the organisms.

The resistance of the patient.

THE DOSAGE AND VIRULENCE OF ORGANISMS

By dosage we mean number of organisms. Obviously a more severe infection is produced by 10 000 000 organisms than by 1 000 000 of the same strain.

Different strains of the same organism vary in their inherent power to attack the body, and this property is known as virulence; organisms of the same strain vary in virulence under different conditions. The virulence is sometimes a property of the body of the organism when the toxin is known as an endotoxin; and sometimes it is due to a toxin or poison which the organism produces called an exotoxin. In clinical practice the sensitivity or response of an organism to antibacterial drugs may well be decisive in determining the severity of the clinical infection.

THE RESISTANCE OF THE PATIENT TO INFECTION

This depends on the following:
1. The skin and mucous membranes, by providing a protective cover, deny organisms access and are the first line of defence.
2. Antibodies if present in the blood stream and the tissue fluids will prevent the disease developing.
3. The third and final defence is the development of inflammation.

The skin and mucous membranes

Of all the protective coverings, the skin is structurally the best equipped

Keratin

Stratified squamous
epithelial membrane
with keratin

Simple columnar
epithelial membrane

Fig. 7.1 The skin with its many layers of cells (*top*) is more resistant to infection and injury than the more delicate single layer of cells (*bottom*) lining most glands and viscera.

because it has a thick layer of squamous epithelium, and organisms on its surface (normal skin flora) are denied access to the body. In most surgical procedures the skin is incised, the underlying tissues are exposed to the air and the skin adjoining the wound, so that the risk of bacterial invasion is immediate. Single layered mucous membranes are easily damaged and have less strength in combating assault from bacteria (Fig. 7.1).

Types of immune response

When an antigen, which may be a micro-organism or a microbial product, enters the body, two different types of immunological reaction may occur.

1. Humoral immunity

This is the synthesis and release of free antibody into the body and other body fluids. This antibody acts, for example, by coating bacteria to enhance their killing and by combination with and neutralisation of bacterial toxins. Antibodies may arise in the body actively as a response to the presence of an antigen or they may be passively acquired by the administration of gammaglobulin or by transfer from a mother to her baby in utero. Active immunity may be produced by previous infection with the microbe or it may be artificially induced by the administration of a dead or weakened organism. This type of active immunity gives more prolonged and better immunity than passive immunisation.

Antibodies are produced by certain lymphocytes which transform into plasma cells and form the group of substances known as immunoglobulins.

2. Cell-mediated immunity

This involves the production of 'sensitised' lymphocytes which are themselves the effectors of cell-mediated immunity. These lymphocytes are distinct from those which produce antibodies. This type of immunity confers protection against organisms such as the tubercle bacillus and viruses. In individuals immune to tuberculosis, the 'sensitised' lymphocytes interact with the injected tuberculin antigen to produce a skin response—this is known as the Mantoux reaction. Sensitised lymphocytes are also responsible for the rejection of skin grafts and transplanted organs.

The degree of immunity

This varies from patient to patient and with different types of organisms.

The following factors may alter, usually unfavourably, the degree of immunity:

1. Age. In infancy antibody production has not developed because the infant has not been exposed to latent infection. In extreme old age it may be depressed like all the other vital functions.

2. Race. The introduction of a new infection to a native race is usually catastrophic. The inhabitants have no natural immunity to a new disease. For instance, tuberculosis has almost wiped out the Red Indians in North America.

3. The following conditions diminish resistance to infection with a resultant lowering of the degree of immunity:

(a) Metabolic diseases, e.g. diabetes mellitus.

(b) Severe anaemias, hypoproteinaemia and blood diseases.

(c) Uraemia.

(d) Cold, exposure, starvation, haemorrhage, and metallic poisoning.

(e) Radioactivity.

(f) A poor blood supply or a wound filled with serum or a haematoma.

Susceptibility to surgical infection

The susceptibility of a patient to infection depends upon the freedom of access of organisms to his body and the degree of immunity which he possesses to the particular organism once it is implanted on his tissues.

Access of organisms. An intact healthy skin or mucosa is the greatest barrier against infection. Organisms may gain access from a wound, or may be inhaled or swallowed.

Great stress has rightly been laid on protecting the patient from infection arising from outside sources (exogenous infection) but insufficient attention has been paid to infection arising from the patient himself (endogenous infection). The importance of eliminating endogenous sources efficiently, particularly in intestinal surgery, is now more widely recognised (Ch. 39).

The whole complex organisation of surgical technique is designed with the sole object of preventing the access of organisms to wounds. This is known as asepsis—literally, no infection.

CLINICAL APPLICATION OF IMMUNITY

Diagnostic

The estimation of the presence of antibodies in the blood may be of value in diagnosis. The test is usually performed on the blood serum. The specimen of blood should be collected with no anticoagulant in the specimen tube, so that the serum can separate from the clot. The Widal test for the diagnosis of typhoid fever and the Wassermann reaction for the diagnosis of syphilis are examples of its use.

Prophylactic and therapeutic

Tetanus toxoid is administered if the patient has been recently exposed to tetanus. Human antitetanus immunoglobulin is used in treatment of the disease.

Active immunisation is effected to prevent several diseases, for example, tetanus, diphtheria, poliomyelitis, whooping cough, measles, rubella and tuberculosis.

Active immunisation is undertaken for tetanus, and anyone liable to be at risk, such as agricultural workers, children and members of the services, are included. The following schedule of active immunisation is advised in children. At twelve weeks the first injection of diphtheria, pertussis and tetanus (triple vaccine) is given, and then the second and third injections are given at 5 months and 11 months respectively. Poliomyelitis vaccine (Sabin type) is given orally at 5 months. After the first year the child is inoculated against measles. A booster dose of diphtheria and tetanus antigen is given when the child starts school and again at the age of 10 years.

BCG (Bacille Calmette-Guerin) immunisation is offered to school children found to be Mantoux negative at the age of 13 years.

Immunisation in older children or adults can, of course, be given by an injection of tetanus toxoid on its own. This is usually given as two injections at four-weekly intervals. For complete protection booster doses should be given. There is a tendency to forget or neglect the every 5 years necessity for immunisation when the disease is rarely seen.

Rubella vaccine is offered to school girls between 11 and 14 years of age for protection against the risk of congenital foetal malformations in pregnancy. The vaccine can also be given to older women who have been tested and found to have rubella antibodies absent from their blood. The patient of child bearing age should ensure she does not become pregnant for 2 months after rubella vaccination because the vaccine contains a living virus.

Smallpox, as a human disease, has been successfully eradicated from the world due to the use of vaccination.

Hypersensitivity reactions

When an individual has been exposed to an antigen, further contact with the antigen leads to secondary boosting of the immune response which normally protects against infection. However, the reaction may be excessive and lead to tissue damage (hypersensitivity) if the antigen is present in large quantities or if the humoral or cellular immune defences have already been stimulated. These excessive reactions are not normally employed by the body in combating infection and are rarely seen. However, their importance lies in the severity of the reaction and this may result in the death of the patient.

There are four types of hypersensitivity reaction:

1. *Anaphylaxis.* This does not occur when an injection is given for the first time but develops on subsequent exposure to the antigen to which the patient is allergic. For this reason, careful inquiry should always be made to elicit whether the patient has had a previous injection of serum or is allergic to foreign protein. Anaphylaxis is a frightening condition— the most severe cases collapse and die almost at once in a state of shock and respiratory embarrassment. Intramuscular or subcutaneous adrenaline is administered to counteract the reaction.

2. *Cytotoxic hypersensitivity.* An example of this is the transfusion of an incompatible unit of blood to a patient. Antibodies in the patient's serum react with the transfused red cells and cause them to lyse.

3. *Complex-mediated hypersensitivity.* In this case the combination of soluble antigens and antibodies in the body causes the formation of complexes which stimulate an acute inflammatory reaction. Circulating complexes give rise to serum sickness. This may occur after the first injection of a foreign protein and may produce rash, albuminuria, headache, nausea, vomiting and joint pains. This reaction occurs 7–10 days after the first injection.

4. *Cell-mediated (delayed type) hypersensitivity.* This is encountered in many allergic reactions to bacteria, viruses, fungi, in the contact dermatitis due to sensitisation with certain chemicals and the rejection of transplanted tissues. The reaction forms the basis of the Mantoux test.

THE PREVENTION AND CONTROL OF INFECTION

Infection is always inimical to the interest of the surgical patient. It adds to his suffering, delays his recovery, and may cause such destruction to his tissues that his last state is worse than his first. If it is severe enough it may cause death.

Many surgical conditions are primarily infective and the prevention of the spread of infecting organisms to other patients is a cause of constant anxiety. In subsequent chapters considerable attention is paid to the practical details of this problem, but certain general principles are worthy of special notice.

1. General measures of hygiene are of the first importance for the patient and the nurse. Cleanliness of the ward, the handling of food, crockery, and personal cleanliness are of the greatest importance. An individual thermometer for each patient commonly stored dry after wiping with a Mediswab is an example of the type of measure which it is necessary to take.

2. Control of special local conditions in a surgical wound. Injury or bruising of a wound increases the risk of infection. The patient is instructed not to touch dressings or his skin which may have been contaminated by pus. Hand washing should be frequent and an anti-bacterial soap is used. Masks should not be touched with the fingers, changed frequently and as soon as a dressing has been finished discarded so that the nurse is able to breathe freely and diminish the risk of infection into her own nose.

3. Special methods of protection such as immunisation and antibiotic prophylaxis.

4. Recognition. Because some degree of infection is inevitable, it is easy to fail to recognise the outbreak until it has reached serious proportions. Routine recordings of the temperature and pulse rate are invaluable and inspection of the wounds is undertaken. A separate register of any infection which arises in a wound should be kept in each ward. A control of infection officer (often a nursing sister) is invaluable to a hospital.

5. Prevention. The following measures are important:

(a) Bed spacing should be as generous as possible. A minimum of 2.4 metres is essential.

(b) Staff with minor septic lesions should not be on duty in a surgical ward.

(c) Contaminated dressings and instruments are treated as appropriate by disinfection or incineration.

(d) Sterilisation must be effective and recontamination prevented (Chapter 10).

(e) Bed clothes should be handled gently to reduce the risk of dissemination of infection.

(f) Flies should be denied access and destroyed without delay if they do break bounds.

(g) Flower vases are a further source of contamination and require disinfection.

(h) Antibiotics should be used with care and not indiscriminately (Ch.6).

(i) The dressing of surgical wounds requires special care (Ch. 11). The patient should be instructed not to interfere with the dressing and to report if he requires attention for oozing of serum, pus or blood (Ch. 12).

(j) Nothing that is to be put into the bed should be placed on the floor —back rests, bed cradles and bedpans.

(k) Screen covers and curtains around the bed require regular laundering.

(l) Isolation. Where facilities are available, patients with infections due to organisms known to give rise to epidemics, e.g. certain staphylococcal infections, are barrier nursed in a separate cubicle.

(m) Indwelling tubes and catheters are a constant hazard. It has been suggested that 1 in 10 000 patients admitted to hospital dies of septicaemia due to catheterisation of the urinary tract. That would account for 500 deaths in Great Britain yearly (Strong 1980).

6. Control. Patients with an infected wound should, if possible, be isolated. If this is impossible barrier nursing has to be instituted at once. Infection spreads on the hands of the staff, fomites or clothes and through the air or by droplets. Hands should be washed inside the cubicle and *dried outside* to obviate contamination from paper cloths or paper towels stored in the cubicle. Unless gowns are used intelligently they are better not used at all. A surgeon dons a sterile gown before beginning an operation and discards it at the end. The same practice must be adopted in barrier nursing—such a practice need not add unduly to the laundry problem since the used gown usually need be only autoclaved and not laundered. Many modern gowns are disposable.

It may be desirable to close the ward to further admissions if the sepsis rate is rising or to empty the ward for cleaning and disinfection if there is a severe outbreak of infection.

Investigations should include bacteriological examination of:
(a) the wound.
(b) the mouth, hands, throat and skin of the staff and careful clinical examination to discover any infective lesions in other patients.

BIBLIOGRAPHY

Roitt I 1980 Essential immunology, 4th edn. Blackwell Scientific Publications.
Strong J 1980 Surgical News 9

8

Inflammation

Inflammation is the response of the body to an irritant. The irritant may be a burn, a chemical, a wound, or a micro-organism. It is usually painful. Pain warns the patient that the enemy has arrived and is an indication that his body has risen to the attack.

It is only the body tissues which can overcome the irritant. By treatment we can, at best, only aid this struggle. If necessary, the body will sacrifice much of tissue to survive, and when its superiority has been established it will cleanse and repair its wound.

STAGES OF INFLAMMATION

The modern conception of inflammation recognises four stages as illustrated in wound healing. Wound healing always follows a regular pattern:

Stage 1. Traumatic inflammation. During this phase the edges of the wound become oedematous and matted together with fibrin. Within a few hours of injury the capillaries dilate and fluid leaks through the damaged endothelium and accumulates in the interstitial space. The body temperature may rise as in acute inflammation elsewhere. Lymphangitis and lymphadenitis occur at this stage.

Stage 2. Destruction, in which necrotic material is removed. It is characterised by the migration of leucocytes and macrophages into the wound. These cells engulf and destroy dead or dying tissue. It is terminated by the formation of pus. If the destructive stage is very severe the process goes on to necrosis, which is death of a small area of tissue as opposed to gangrene, which may also occur and means gross death.

Stage 3. Proliferation. When epithelium and connective tissue develop, new capillaries sprout off the sides of existing wounds. Fibroblasts appear alongside the capillaries. These two together constitute granulation tissue. Fine fibrils soon form in the ground substance and then gradually aggregate into typical collagen fibres. The stage of proliferation starts from the 4th to 14th day. During this phase all the cells forming the surface epithelium undergo rapid division and migrate as a thin film

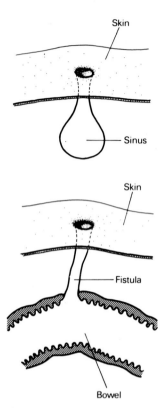

Fig. 8.1 A sinus ends blindly — a fistula connects two epithelial surfaces — in this case the skin and the intestine.

covering the wound. They also grow down as several sprouts into the depth of the wound. It is thought by some pathologists that these tiny growths of epithelial cells stimulate the formation of granulation tissue.

Stage 4. Maturation. During this phase the blood vessels gradually disappear and the number of fibroblasts in relation to fibres diminish. The red elevated recent scar is gradually changed into a thin white line.

Healing by first intention (primary healing) and *healing by second intention* (healing by granulation) were in the past considered to be distinct processes. Healing by granulation is essentially the same as primary healing, the only difference being that usually, as a result of infection, the stage of destruction is greatly prolonged and results in a deep cavity which is filled gradually from the bottom by granulation tissue.

Tissue repair

Repair is the process by which tissue is replaced — the simpler the tissue the more effective repair can be. As tissue, i.e. cells, become highly specialised repair becomes more difficult. Epithelial surfaces and fibrous tissue will regenerate without too much difficulty, but most other cells, and in particular nerve cells and structures like the glomerulus in the kidney, are not replaced but the space they occupy is filled with fibrous tissue. Some apparently highly specialised epithelial tissue is capable of regeneration. This is particularly true of the liver following destruction by disease.

If granulation tissue is excessive it is raised above the level of the approaching epithelium and forms an insurmountable barrier to the spread of epithelium. This is corrected by cauterising the granulation tissue to the level of the epithelium with silver nitrate (Fig. 11.7).

A blind track which may persist following inflammation or infection is known as a sinus. It is usually due to the presence of a foreign body such as a knot of unabsorbed catgut or deficient drainage of a cavity. If the track to the skin surface communicates with another epithelial surface through the granulation tissue the condition is known as a fistula (Fig. 8.1).

THE SPREAD OF INFECTION IN THE TISSUES

According to the form of spread which occurs, special terms are used to describe the process.

1. Cellulitis. It is the direct spread of infection in the tissues, or more strictly, in the extracellular spaces.

2. Lymphangitis (Fig. 8.2). The lymphatic vessels between the site of infection and the regional lymphatic glands may be inflamed. Classically they are best seen as red lines on the arm of a patient suffering from a septic finger. This is called lymphangitis.

3. Lymphadenitis. The lymphatic glands (syn. nodes) are invaded by organisms carried by the lymph stream in the lymphatic vessels (Fig. 8.2).

The lymphatic glands, which become swollen and tender, are structurally well equipped to deal with infection by their complex network, which filters the organisms.

The common sites for lymphadenitis and the areas from which they are infected are:

Glands enlarged and tender

Lymphangitis

Septic finger

Fig. 8.2 Spread of infection in the lymphatic system.

Glands	*Area of infection*
(a) The neck	Face, mouth, tongue and scalp
(b) The axilla	Breast and upper limb
(c) The groin	Lower limb, groin and perineum

4. Bacteraemia. Bacteraemia is the spread of organisms into the bloodstream. They are usually destroyed spontaneously.

5. Septicaemia. Septicaemia is the invasion and multiplication of bacteria in the bloodstream. The onset is usually heralded by a single rigor followed by persistent pyrexia.

6. Other forms of spread. In the body cavities and the lumen of tubed viscera, infection can spread very rapidly.

Two other terms must be mentioned: *toxaemia*, which is the spread of the toxic products of inflammation from the site of infection into the blood stream; and *suppuration*, which is the process of pus formation (an abscess, see Fig. 8.3).

FAILURE OF THE INFLAMMATORY REACTION

In severe infection the inflammatory reaction may fail to develop and the patient succumbs rapidly. More commonly the failure is partial and it is important to recognise at once the factors which may be preventing its full development. They are:

1. Poor arterial blood supply

(a) Age—arteriosclerosis.
(b) Site—the lower third of the leg—gross scarring.
(c) Tight dressings. Tourniquets.
(d) Arterial thrombosis or embolism.
(e) Shock—a poor blood supply diminishes the supply of leucocytes and allows bacteria to multiply.
(f) Gas pressure—gas gangrene.

2. Deficient venous drainage

(a) Venous thrombosis.
(b) Varicose veins.

Fig. 8.3 An acute abscess of the arm.

3. Depression or deficiency of the quality of the blood

    (a) Anaemia—nutritional.
                     haemorrhage.
    (b) Leucopenia. Steroids suppress the action of the leucocytes.
    (c) Hypoproteinaemia. Plasma protein levels below 5 g per 100 ml are insufficient for a skin graft to take.

4. Malnutrition and dehydration

    (a) General.
    (b) Vitamin deficiency.
    (c) Zinc deficiency.

5. Excess of fluid in the tissues

    Oedema—cardiac.
              nephritic.
              lymphatic obstruction.
              venous obstruction.

6. Metabolic

    (a) Diabetes.
    (b) Nephritis.
    (c) Uraemia.
    (d) Portal cirrhosis.
    (e) Jaundice.

7. Drugs

    (a) ACTH.
    (b) Corticosteroids.
    (c) Metallic poison.
    (d) Cytotoxic drugs.

PATHOPHYSIOLOGICAL CHANGES IN INFLAMMATION

The blood

The normal count of white blood cells (leucocytes) ranges between 4000 to 10 000/mm³ in the adult and 10 000 to 25 000/mm³ in the infant and consists of:

    Granulocytes (polymorphonuclear leucocytes)
        Neutrophils   40-75 per cent
        Eosinophils   1-6 per cent
        Basophils   1 per cent
    Lymphocytes   20 to 50 per cent
    Monocytes   1 to 6 per cent

The increase in the number of neutrophils in acute infections is rapid and they may account for 95 per cent of the total white cell count. If for any reason this increase fails to occur, the disease takes a more severe course than would otherwise have been expected. If the production of granulocytes is markedly depressed for any reason—e.g. in leukaemia, after treatment with cytotoxic drugs or radiotherapy, the patient is unable to combat even the mildest infection and death results. Clinically the most obvious feature of granulocytopenia is a destructive condition in the tissues of the mouth and throat because the patient has no resistance to the vast number of organisms he normally inhales and ingests without ill effect each day. The most valuable drugs for this condition are the antibiotics which help to combat infection.

Almost all acute infections result in an increase in the white cells, but there are important exceptions. For example, in typhoid fever, the white cell count is below normal, of the order of 2000 to 3000 mm³. The term leucopenia is applied to those states in which the *white cells* are fewer than normal.

Pyrexia

The body temperature is usually raised in response to infection or inflammation.

Pyrogens act by the release of a prostaglandin in the temperature regulating centre in the brain. The antipyretic effect of aspirin is due to blocking of the formation of the prostaglandin.

If the infection is mild, the rise in temperature is slight. However, in severe infection and as a result of infection in organs like the kidney or liver where the vascular mass is considerably higher than most, a persistent high temperature may cause dehydration and electrolyte imbalance.

Sometimes the temperature may be the presenting sign and, in the absence of an immediately obvious cause, a diagnosis of 'pyrexia of unknown origin' is made. Painstaking investigation and observation will be required to reveal the cause. Occasionally a pelvic infection may present with pyrexia without any local symptoms and of course deep seated infection elsewhere in the body may be very difficult to locate.

The rise in temperature increases metabolism and increases the demand for oxygen. A notable exception to a rise in temperature from infection is where the body is flooded rapidly with endotoxins. The temperature is subnormal and the patient in a condition of shock (endotoxic shock).

Metabolism

This is increased and in prolonged suppuration, protein loss is considerable.

Oliguria

The amount of urine secreted is diminished to preserve fluid in the body and it is highly concentrated.

INVESTIGATIONS

In the vast majority of infections no investigation is necessary because, if the infection is mild, the inflammatory response can be seen or detected on clinical examination. The nature of the infection can be determined and the site localised.

In more severe infections or in conditions where the nature of the disease is obscure investigation will be necessary and include the following:

1. *White blood cell count* which in acute infection will reveal a leucocytosis.

2. *Bacteriological examination* of material recovered from the site of infection—for example the throat, the urine or a wound as appropriate. The nature and antibiotic sensitivity of organisms discovered is determined. If septicaemia is suspected blood is taken for blood culture. The culture medium should be at hand so that blood is withdrawn when the patient's temperature, if swinging, is at its height or, if rigors are a feature, as soon as the next rigor occurs.

3. *Serum tests for the presence of antibodies* may occasionally be valuable in the diagnosis or exclusion of certain infections like syphilis or typhoid fever.

4. *The urine* is tested for sugar to exclude diabetes. Proteinuria commonly occurs in any febrile illness.

THE SYMPTOMS AND SIGNS OF INFLAMMATION

The constitutional symptoms include malaise, loss of appetite, fatigue and sleeplessness. The temperature is elevated and the pulse rate is increased. All these symptoms are due to the toxins which are liberated by the invading organism into the blood stream. In overwhelming infection the patient may be in septicaemic shock.

Local symptoms and signs

1. Redness is caused by dilatation of capillaries in the inflamed area.
2. Heat is due to the increased blood flow.
3. Swelling occurs because plasma is poured into the surrounding tissues. The degree of swelling is dependent to some extent on the natural laxity or otherwise of the tissues. For example, inflammation below the eyes causes an extreme degree of swelling at a very early stage.
4. Pain is due to the accumulation of toxins which irritate the nerve endings and hormones released locally from stretching of the tiny nerve twigs caused by the excess of fluid in the tissues, which increases as tension becomes greater.
5. Loss of function occurs as a result of pain, swelling and the toxic effect on the tissue itself. The patient's natural desire is to rest and to avoid using any painful part.

THE TERMINATION OF INFLAMMATION

This may be by:
  (a) Resolution
  (b) Suppuration
  (c) Ulceration
  (d) Gangrene
  (e) Fibrosis

MANAGEMENT AND NURSING CARE

General management

Most infections are mild and the patient's resistance is high so that resolution is rapid and only the simplest measures are required. These include rest, a liberal fluid intake, and the avoidance of cold, physical exertion or mental anxiety all of which depress resistance. Antibiotics which are expensive and not without risk are unnecessary in most cases.

The necessary measures and the vigour with which they are pursued depends on the severity, course and site of the disease. They include:

1. Assessment of the patient's resistance. All the factors which may cause the inflammatory reaction to be limited (p. 69) are assessed and as far as possible appropriate action taken. This will include bringing a diabetic condition under control, increasing the dosage of steroids if the patient is on steroid therapy, remedial vitamin therapy if necessary and reviewing the administration of cytotoxic drugs which the patient may be receiving. The presenting picture in leukaemia may be an infection and in a known leukaemic patient infection is a constant hazard.

2. Rest is a fundamental principle.

General rest to the body increases resistance, diminishes strain on the heart which may be poisoned by circulating toxins, and ensures conditions in which sleep can be promoted.

Local rest in addition to diminishing pain relieves the part or organ from the stress and strain of its normal function. It has to be interpreted in relation to the part affected. It consists of a darkened room for an inflamed eye, a bland diet for a gastrointestinal infection or a sling to rest an infected arm.

3. Relief of pain by analgesics enables the patient to sleep.

4. Diet. If the condition is severe or prolonged there is loss of fluid from sweating resulting in dehydration and electrolyte imbalance. A fluid balance chart and electrolyte estimations are necessary so that corrective measures can be taken. The increased metabolism from pyrexia and the breakdown of body protein requires a high protein and high calorie diet. In addition, vitamin supplements are necessary. Vitamin A is anti-infective, vitamin B is necessary when administering many antibiotics and vitamin C is required for healing.

5. Antitoxins and antibacterial substances are prescribed as appropriate and have revolutionised the management of infective disease.

6. Pyrexia. Rigors are particularly unpleasant for the patient. A temperature of 39.5°C or over is in itself dangerous and described as hyperpyrexia so that every effort is made to prevent it rising further. Frequent tepid sponges, fans, and in severe cases even ice packs, may be advisable.

7. Prevention of further contamination. The nurse should explain to the patient that the skin around a suppurating wound is highly infected and warn him that he can, with his fingers, spread the infection to his eye or ear. The surgical conversion of an open wound into a closed wound, or the deviation of normally infected bowel contents by a colostomy in acute diverticular disease of the colon, are examples of the same principle.

Local measures

1. Rest has already been mentioned and is the most effective non-operative measure.

2. Increasing the blood supply. The only measure to increase the blood supply which may be undertaken occasionally for a chronic ulcer of the leg is sympathectomy. In such patients the arterial supply of blood to the limb is already deficient.

Surgical measures

Excision of an infected focus is an ideal method of treatment but it is rarely possible—a notable and very effective example being appendicectomy for an acute appendicitis.

Incision and drainage is necessary once an abscess has formed. The incision has to be sufficiently large to allow free drainage. A tube stitched to the skin is usually inserted and the surgeon will give instructions when it has to be shortened or removed. Its removal should be recorded in the patient's notes. If pressure has to be applied to the sides of a wound to express pus, drainage is inadequate and further incision is necessary. The skin surrounding the draining wound is cleansed with an antiseptic when the wound is dressed. A sinus or fistula which persists has to be laid open and dressed as an open wound—a corner of a gauze pack is tucked very lightly into the wound to keep the skin edges apart while healing proceeds from the depths. Tight plugging with gauze is not only painful but also prevents free drainage by acting as a plug.

Failure to heal may be due to the presence of a foreign body including a lost drainage tube. Other causes include all the conditions, mentioned on page 69, causing a failure of the inflammatory reaction. The patient's condition is reviewed with all these in mind and corrective measures undertaken.

A sinus from a wound can discharge for years or a chronic skin ulcer may eventually undergo malignant change.

A persistent sinus or fistula has to be laid open in order for it to heal.

RESTORATION OF FUNCTION

From the beginning the restoration of full function should be the aim of the nurse and the surgeon and if this is unlikely to be achieved as much function as possible must be preserved. The cooperation of the patient in movement of joints in an affected limb or exercise of muscles liable to waste can be encouraged with sympathy and firmness. A skin graft may be necessary to accelerate healing and diminish scarring. The objective is explained to the patient. The physiotherapist has often an important role. The Social Worker, the patient's family and in some cases the Psychiatrist may have parts to play in the restoration of full function and health.

9

The specific surgical infections

A specific surgical infection is a disease which can be caused only by a particular strain of organism.

TETANUS (LOCK-JAW)

Tetanus is commonly known as lock-jaw, because the muscular spasms which characterise it frequently attack the muscles of the jaw. The discovery of an antitoxin and methods of active immunisation as well as control of the preparation of catgut have made tetanus a rare disease in the West. In the developing countries it is responsible for 500 000 deaths each year.

The organism, the *Clostridium tetani* (Ch.6), usually gains access through a deep punctured wound but all contaminated wounds are dangerous.

The organism elaborates a powerful toxin which poisons the motor nerve cells, with the result that spasm occurs in the muscles supplied by the corresponding nerves.

Symptoms and signs

The first symptom is slight stiffness of the muscles, particularly those of the jaw. The patient is anxious, but mentally clear. As the disease progresses the classical picture of tetanus appears.

The back is arched and the head may be thrown back (opisthotonos). The facial muscles are in spasm, the mouth can be opened only with difficulty (trismus). Drawing up of the angle of the mouth gives rise to the characteristic smile (risus sardonicus).

Spasms may affect every muscle in the body, and in severe cases the muscles rupture. Spasm of the sphincter muscles of the body render swallowing, defaecation, and micturition very difficult. Spasm of the respiratory muscles causes long periods of anoxia until death ensues. The temperature is elevated and the pulse rate is increased.

Prognosis. The longer the incubation period the more hopeful the outlook.

Treatment and nursing care

Prophylactic. Careful surgical toilet and a prophylactic dose of penicillin is the best prevention. If the patient has not been immunised human anti-tetanus immunoglobulin is the ideal.

If an old accidental wound has to be reopened (perhaps years later) tetanus spores may be lying dormant in its substance. Their reactivation may give rise to tetanus. This danger is described as latent tetanus. The best prophylatic treatment is active immunisation against tetanus.

If one can be certain of the patient's immunity status, a patient who has been actively immunised should be given a booster dose of tetanus toxoid, but within three years of immunisation it can be omitted.

Therapeutic—specific treatment. Penicillin is bactericidal and is administered in all cases of tetanus. Human antiserum is given.

The wound must be excised and irrigated with hydrogen peroxide, because the tetanus bacillus will not grow in the presence of oxygen. The wound is not sutured.

General treatment. Absolute rest and isolation are important, since the slightest noise or flicker increases the spasms. The patient is nursed in a quiet dark room which must be draught-free. The door should be fitted with suitable closing springs to prevent slamming. The nurse should warm her hands before touching the patient to avoid stimulating further spasms.

Most deaths are due to lack of oxygen and pulmonary infection. The toxin infects the bulbar nuclei so that the muscles of the pharynx and larynx are affected; the larynx is no longer the watch-dog for the lungs. Coughing is ineffective and anything that the patient swallows or regurgitates from the stomach is liable to infect the lungs. The important points in treatment are:

1. A nasogastric tube is passed in all but the mildest cases and the stomach is aspirated before each feed if nasogastric feeding is permitted.
2. A tracheostomy is performed and suction applied at regular intervals. Controlled respiration using a mechanical respirator should be used as soon as possible. Regular suction produces sympathetic overactivity with a resultant fall in blood pressure and tachycardia. The pulse should therefore be checked and any alteration reported.
3. Muscle relaxants relieve most of the symptoms. The eyes are protected if curare is used, otherwise conjunctivitis develops.
4. The maintenance of fluid balance by intravenous fluids. The relaxant is injected into the infusion by the anaesthetist.
5. Sedatives are used very sparingly and are almost unnecessary if relaxants are used correctly.

GAS GANGRENE

Wounds which contain lacerated or crushed tissue are those most likely to develop gas gangrene. The organism may be present in a wound but the anaerobic conditions in which a tissue has lost all or most of its blood supply are essential for its proliferation. The organism is *Clostridium perfringens (Cl. welchii).* See Chapter 6.

Sources in hospital

The organism arises from the patient's own intestinal flora. It is particularly important that, if gas gangrene is to be avoided following amputations or operations on the hip in these patients, the skin should be treated with extra care and care should be taken to exclude faecal matter from the wound. Additionally, penicillin is administered intramuscularly at the beginning of the operation.

Symptoms and signs

Pain in the wound is extremely severe. It is important to remember that the disease may develop in a wound under plaster. Never neglect the pain of a patient in a plaster—it may only indicate a pressure sore but it may also be a symptom of gas gangrene.

The wound, which may be green or black, has a strong 'mouselike' odour. Small bubbles of gas may be seen escaping and the surrounding tissues are swollen and crackle when touched (crepitus). Untreated, deterioration is rapid.

In early cases, radiographic examination may reveal the presence of gas in the tissues.

Treatment

The patient is resuscitated with blood, and penicillin is administered. Anti-gas gangrene serum may be prescribed.

Wide excision of all infected tissue must be performed and the wound left open. The wound is irrigated with hydrogen peroxide and eusol, and the danger has passed only when granulations appear.

Hyperbaric (i.e. at a pressure greater than the atmosphere) oxygen therapy may save the limb but is of no value until after wound excision has been performed.

SURGICAL TUBERCULOSIS

Tuberculosis is still a prevalent infectious disease in many countries and amongst immigrants from Asia and Africa in the United Kingdom. In one London borough 250 out of 290 notifications were immigrants and many lesions were extrapulmonary.

Not common enough to be a major health concern yet not rare enough to be ignored, tuberculosis is still a fatal disease if not diagnosed and managed effectively (Grange 1979).

The organism may be ingested, inhaled or inoculated through the skin. The pathological reaction of tissues to the bacillus is known as a tubercle which consists of a central necrotic mass of caseous or cheese-like material containing giant cells surrounded by a layer of lymphocytes. It may liquefy to form what is known as a cold or tuberculous abscess which may point on the surface and become infected with organisms on the skin. The result is that chronic infection with pyogenic organisms results in a persistent discharge. At any stage of the disease healing may occur by fibrosis of the tubercle, and this is sometimes consolidated further by calcification of its substance.

Cold abscess (Fig. 9.1). The tuberculous abscess is described as cold because the skin temperature is not raised. Erythema of the skin and pointing of the abscess develop slowly. Frequently these changes never appear, because resolution occurs and the pus is absorbed.

If pointing is threatened, aspiration is performed through an area of relatively healthy skin. The greatest care is taken to prevent secondary infection. Very rarely are tuberculous abscesses incised, and then only if it is possible to eradicate the underlying focus.

Treatment

1. Specific treatment. The oral administration of rifampicin and isoniazid for 9 months with the addition of ethambutol for the first two months is recommended by the British Thoracic and Tuberculous Association. This regime is more acceptable than streptomycin which has to be injected and combined with PAS (para-aminosalicylic acid) which causes nausea.

In almost all cases the patient is cured.

2. Surgical treatment. The scope of surgical treatment has greatly diminished since the advent of chemotherapy, but it still has a place in the excision or partial excision of an organ infected with tuberculosis, and the management of a cold abscess is still an important surgical condition.

THE VENEREAL DISEASES

Those most commonly seen in Britain today are gonorrhoea and non-specific urethritis. Over 70 000 new cases of each are seen in England and Wales each year and the incidence is rising.

Genital herpes has become increasingly recognised and is now a common sexually transmitted disease among young adults.

Syphilis is now uncommon in Britain but may cause widespread lesions which may also be evident years after the initial infection.

Chancroid or soft sore is rarely seen in Britain and is mainly a disease of the tropics.

SYPHILIS

Congenital syphilis

The mother may infect her unborn child in utero, and this may result in

Fig. 9.1 Cold abscess (collar stud type) in the neck.

Breaking down of tuberculous lymph gland

Collar-stud tract

Cold abscess

Deep fascia

Skin

abortion, stillbirth or the birth of a child which may show the signs of syphilis or subsequently develop them. Early signs of syphilis include rash, rhinitis, poor feeding. Hepatosplenomegaly, meningeal involvement and periostitis may occur. Late syphilis is characterised by interstitial keratitis, Hutchinson's teeth (abnormal upper incisors) and deafness.

Acquired syphilis

The primary lesion of syphilis is the chancre, or septic sore at the site of infection—in men usually on the penis and in women either on the vulva or the cervix of the uterus. Occasionally chancres are found elsewhere, for example, on the lips, or on the nurse's finger from contact with a syphilitic lesion while in attendance on the patient. The primary lesion has an incubation period of 1 to 3 weeks and is painless; it is highly infectious, and must never be touched with the naked finger. Untreated, it rapidly heals and gives rise later to almost any symptoms in any part of the body. After its disappearance the patient may have no further clinical evidence of syphilis until he develops lesions many years later, or he may pass into the secondary stage 2 to 6 months later.

Secondary syphilis. An extensive rash is the characteristic symptom. It is usually a dull copper-coloured eruption, particularly on the back and face.

A similar lesion occurs in the throat, and the moisture of that area produces what is known as a snail-track ulcer. The presence of secondary syphilitic lesions in the anal region produces large soggy thicknesses known as condylomata.

All the lymphatic glands are very much enlarged. They are rubbery to the touch and are not tender.

Tertiary stage. This may occur years after the primary or secondary lesion. The characteristic lesion is known as a gumma, and may occur in any organ of the body. The tibia and skin overlying it, as well as the palate, are favourite sites. It takes the form of a hard mass which gradually breaks down to form an ulcer, which has a typical punched-out appearance.

Parasyphilitic lesions. These are the most dreaded of all manifestations of syphilis, and include tabes dorsalis, general paralysis of the insane, and lesions of the heart and circulatory system, such as aortic regurgitation and aneurysm of the thoracic aorta.

The diagnosis of syphilis

The finding of the *Treponema pallidum* in the primary lesion is the most certain method of diagnosis. A specimen is taken by the doctor by means of a capillary tube and then examined unstained immediately under a microscope by darkground illumination.

The Kahn or Wassermann reaction is positive on examination of the blood 2 to 3 weeks after the appearance of the primary lesion. More specific tests are used to confirm the diagnosis, e.g. *Treponema pallidum* haemagglutination test (TPHA) and the fluorescent treponemal antibody test (FTA).

Treatment

Penicillin is now the drug of choice but penicillin sensitive patients must be treated with tetracycline or erythromycin.

GONORRHOEA

Gonorrhoea is due to a diplococcus known as the *Gonococcus*. It is an aerobic organism and extremely delicate. The acute symptoms appear after about 3 days from the time of infection. They consist of irritation of the urethra in the male, followed by a copious, yellow, purulent discharge. The patient is toxic, complains of malaise, and has a high temperature. There is frequency of micturition and the patient finds walking uncomfortable. In the female, Bartholin's glands may be swollen and a local abscess or cyst may form.

In pregnant women there is sometimes surprisingly little evidence of infection.

Gonorrhoea may spread through the whole of the genital tract. In the female, infection of the cervix uteri and of the Fallopian tubes (salpingitis) is not uncommon. In the male, the Cowper's glands, the prostate, and sometimes the epididymis may be affected.

Chronic lesions of gonorrhoea

Any of the acute lesions in the urinary tract may become chronic, but, in addition, infection may spread to other regions of the body. Arthritis, particularly of the ankles, is not uncommon. In babies, conjunctivitis and keratitis may be acquired during birth. The treatment of ophthalmia neonatorum is described in Chapter 49. Rarely gonorrhoea is responsible for infective endocarditis.

The outstanding chronic surgical lesion resulting from gonococcal infection is stricture of the male urethra.

Treatment

The most useful drug in the treatment of gonorrhoea is penicillin. If resistant strains have developed, spectinomycin or cefuroxime may be prescribed. Patients allergic to penicillin can be treated by co-trimoxazole or spectinomycin.

Repeated examinations by direct smears and cultures are essential before declaring the patient cured.

It is not very uncommon for a patient to be suffering from both gonorrhoea and syphilis. It is important that this should be discovered by the appropriate serological tests as short term penicillin therapy will cure gonorrhoea but only mask syphilis.

NON-SPECIFIC URETHRITIS

This condition is becoming increasingly prevalent and is now commoner than gonorrhoea in the male. The commonest cause of non-specific urethritis (NSU) is *Chlamydia trachomatis.* Symptoms in the male are similar to those of gonorrhoea and include a purulent urethral discharge and dysuria. Female patients with NSU usually have no symptoms but may have cervicitis and some urethritis.

Treatment consists of tetracyclines for three weeks. Erythromycin may be used for pregnant women or chlamydial infection in neonates (neonatal eye infection or pneumonia).

SOCIAL ASPECTS OF VENEROLOGY

Follow-up contact tracing and publicity campaigns are important in limiting the spread and prevention of disease. The patient is more likely to continue treatment until a cure is effected and to cooperate in tracing contacts if the doctors and nurses treat him with human understanding, tact and compassion.

BIBLIOGRAPHY

British Thoracic and Tuberculous Association 1976 Lancet ii: 1102
Grange J M 1979 British Journal of Hospital Medicine 22:540
Shanson D C 1982 Microbiology in clinical practice, 1st edn. Wright, Bristol

10

The operating theatre

The operating theatre should provide a place in which surgical procedures can be undertaken with maximal safety to the patient. It is a complex of engineering to provide power for lighting, ventilation and the working of machines as well as to meet many demands which are essential for the care of the patient. The prevention of infection which is the most demanding of his requirements is the most difficult to satisfy.

Infection prolongs convalescence, increases morbidity and, if sufficiently severe, will start a chain of events which ultimately may result in death of the patient. Sterilisation and the use of disinfectants will destroy micro-organisms but unfortunately many objects which come in contact with the patient cannot be sterilised. The only course available is to deny the micro-organisms access—a technique called asepsis of which sterilisation is a component. This forms the basis of all theatre procedures and has a discipline all of its own demanding constant vigilance.

STERILISATION

Sterilisation is the destruction of all micro-organisms and spores. Most equipment including linen and instruments are supplied already sterilised either from a central sterile supply department or from commercial sources. This saves the nurse's time and permits the use of the most efficient methods of sterilisation. The nurse's task is to select the correct pack, open it without contamination and dispose of the contents after use so that there is no spread of infection or wastage of recoverable objects. If the container is made of glass or plastic it is examined for cracks or damage and if these are discovered the pack is discarded. Similarly, packages of dressings, operating gowns or instruments wrapped in paper are rejected if tears or dampness are discovered. The high pressure autoclave tape is inspected and any discrepancy in the black lines on the tape indicates that the pack is unsafe to use.

A few objects such as endoscopic instruments may be sterilised in a chemical solution chosen by the theatre team of the nurse's own hospital. The instrument should be fully immersed in the solution for the correct time and rinsed before use with sterile water to remove all trace of chemicals which may be irritant to the body tissues. Sterile water is produced by some form of steam distillation, bottled and sterilised in the autoclave (steam under pressure).

Sterilisation undertaken commercially is effected by the use of irradiation, ethylene oxide, or ultraviolet light while central sterile supply departments use an autoclave.

The provision of materials, already sterile, in a smooth continuous flow is ideal. However, as in all commercial operations, the supply may suddenly cease from a shortage of materials, lack of fuel, transport or industrial disruption and a hospital will then have to rely on its own limited resources and expertise. The least fortunate hospital will be the one where modernisation has removed not only all the water sterilisers but also the autoclave outside its curtilage to a central sterile supply department which may have ceased to function.

Boiling and chemical methods of sterilisation fall short because they do not destroy spores or viruses, but the risk of such infection is smaller than doing nothing for a patient suffering from general peritonitis or from an accidental wound.

The discussion which follows is a bare outline of those methods. Before sterilisation is undertaken by nursing staff whose normal duties do not encompass the mechanisms of sterilisation procedures, they should consult the excellent publications listed at the end of this chapter for detailed information. If an autoclave is available some instruction from an expert will be essential.

Chemical sterilisation

Chemical sterilisation and the methods which are used commercially have been mentioned above.

Heat sterilisation

The possible methods likely to be available in hospital all utilise heat.

1. Dry heat

Dry heat is one of the most efficient methods of sterilisation. The object to be sterilised is sealed in a container and placed in a hot air oven at a temperature of 160°C. This is maintained for 1 hour. The destruction of spores is complete. It is suitable only for glassware, all glass syringes, metal instruments and ointments and powders. In order to prevent reinfection the materials must be sealed in a container. Nowadays, most syringes are disposable.

2. Moist heat

Moist heat is one of the most important and most universally applicable methods of sterilisation. Autoclaving uses steam under pressure.

Steam-pressure autoclaves

The sterilising times and the temperature of steam-pressure autoclaves are determined by the following:
    Size of autoclave
    Amount of load
    Type of material for sterilisation.
    Autoclaves are of different types depending on the method of removing air.

Downward displacement autoclave (DDA)

The DDA can be controlled manually or automatically with a timed cycle. It is run on gas, electricity or from a mains supply. It may be used with or without a drying process, depending on requirements. The downward displacement autoclave destroys bacteria and spores by coagulation. The modern high-vacuum high-pressure steriliser will, after 3 minutes at 143°C, 10 minutes at 126°C and 15 minutes at 121°C and a pressure of 2 kg per cm², sterilise its contents. Less modern autoclaves require a longer period.

The following points, are important:

The containers must be such that adequate penetration by the steam is possible. Suitable material must:
1. Allow steam to penetrate it to sterilise its contents.
2. Afford adequate protection against bacterial contamination and infestation.
3. Be light to transport.
4. Be inexpensive.
5. Have a long shelf life.
Paper, metal, balloon cloth, linen and calico are all used. Packs must be stored on slotted shelves, kept free from dust, and dated.

Moist textiles. If dressings or gowns are damp then they should be regarded as unsuitable for use. Gloves should be sterilised at the same pressure, temperature, and time as dressings and textiles. It has been shown that it is quite unsafe to accept a lower standard. In modern rapid autoclaving at high temperature the gloves are not damaged. Most disposable gloves are now sterilised by gamma radiation.
    Objects may be unsterile because of:
    (a) Incorrect packing.
    (b) Incorrect loading of the autoclave.
    (c) Mechanical defects such as a blocked air ejector.
    Daily testing of the autoclave should eliminate objects being unsterile. The thermocouple is an indicator proving that the correct temperature has been reached and held for the correct time. The thermocouple is inserted into the centre of a load for sterilisation and viewed at the completion of the process.

Autoclaving record chart. This is a permanent record of the temperature reached and time held during the cycle of sterilisation.

Sterilisation checks.

1. **The Bowie-Dick test** is a method for testing complete penetration of heat to whole areas of a load and is designed for use in high vacuum high pressure autoclaves. The principle is that high pressure autoclave tape is placed in the centre of a pile of 30 towels (made of Huckaback). The pile is placed in the centre of the autoclave for the first process of the day. On completion of the cycle the autoclave tape is inspected. Any discrepancy in the black lines on the autoclave tape indicates a faulty cycle.

2. **Bacteriological.** Spore-bearing organisms are put in the centre of a pack of dressings and the bacteriologist determines if the destruction has been complete.

3. Boiling

Boiling used to be the method in common use but should only be used for surgical procedures when no other means are available. This method destroys bacteria only and not spores. However, it may be the only method available. It is important to ensure:

1. That all instruments are opened before immersing them completely;
2. That the time taken for boiling should commence after the cold instruments have been immersed and the water has started to boil again, the time being 5 minutes or over at a temperature of 100°C.

ASEPSIS AND THEATRE TECHNIQUE

ASEPSIS

Asepsis is the underlying principle of surgery by which organisms are denied access to the patient. Asepsis has a discipline all its own. From the commencement of her career the nurse must train herself to recognise at once conditions which are at variance with an aseptic technique.

Micro-organisms are to be found everywhere. Objects which can be sterilised and wrapped in sterile containers present the least difficulty provided sterilisation has been adequate, but many objects which come into contact with the patient are either impossible to sterilise or are easily recontaminated.

Practical points of importance

1. There are particles in the air, i.e. dust and droplets, which are the ideal vehicle for the dissemination of airborne organisms. To lower the bacterial count of the air the following precautions are essential:

   (a) *Ventilation*. Ideally air should be filtered, moistened, and warmed or cooled to the regular temperature. An air-conditioning plant should be capable of changing the air in the theatre suite 15 or 20 times in each hour. When a wound is exposed movement is kept at a minimum. Doors and windows are kept closed. (If the room is air conditioned windows will always be kept closed.)

   (b) *Speech* should be limited to the minimum and masks worn for the elimination of droplets.

(c) *Bodily movement* should be gentle and unhurried because in so doing the dust particles are kept to the minimum.

(d) *Movement of the patient* within the theatre suite should be kept to the minimum.

(e) *Cleaning procedures* should be completed 1 or 2 hours prior to use of the theatre with a recommended disinfectant.

(f) *The patient is transferred* from the trolley to the table in the anaesthetic room or at interchange areas and vice versa at the end of the operation. Patient trolleys and ward blankets should not enter the theatre.

2. Many objects cannot be sterilised

(a) The patient's skin.

(b) The hands of the surgeon or nurse. It has been shown, however, that routine baths before operation tend to increase and not diminish infectivity.

(c) The throat, nose and mouth of the staff.

3. The operating table and floor are easily contaminated from infected material during the operation.

4. Blood stains and pus are excellent media for the propagation of organisms, especially as the temperature (68°–72°F) is usually fairly high and the atmosphere humid. Cross-infection can occur from anaesthetic apparatus, which should be pasteurised. Theatre staff, as all nursing staff, should be very careful in handling blood and its products since pricking of the skin or abrasions of the finger may be an entry for viruses which are sometimes present not only in stored blood but also in the patient's blood.

5. Recontamination of sterile objects may occur because of:

(a) Inefficient sterilisers or condensation of steam.

(b) Inefficient air conditioning.

(c) Poor technique in the handling of sterilised instruments and materials. This may cause infection in a patient.

6. Faulty packaging of disposable articles and faulty storage may result in infection.

7. Theatre clothing should be laundered daily and footwear cleaned daily.

8. Rings and jewellery should not be worn.

9. Blankets are a source of infection and should be changed after each patient.

Theatre design

Because of the importance of maintaining asepsis, operating theatres should be designed so that they have:

(a) Air-conditioned ventilation.

(b) A Charnley enclosure for orthopaedic work, especially joint re-placement.

(c) Easily cleanable fabric.

(d) A one-way traffic circulation from 'clean' area to 'dirty' area.

(e) Adequate shower facilities for medical and nursing personnel after they have finished a day's operating.

THEATRE TECHNIQUE

The theatre nurse is a member of a team, and unless she and all the theatre staff carefully observe all the principles and techniques of asepsis, infection in the patient's wound is an inevitable result of the operation.

Theatre dress

The nurse should be clean in her person, her hands kept free from cracks and abrasions, and the fingernails kept short, rounded and unvarnished. In the theatre she should wear the special uniform provided, which usually consists of an overall-type dress with short sleeves, or trousers and top. The material has a smooth surface and is boilable, so that all germs are destroyed in the laundering process. Mitchell et al have shown

---

CONSENT BY PATIENT

I, ...

of ....

hereby consent to undergo the operation of ....

....

the nature and effect of which have been explained to me by

Dr./Mr. ....

   I also consent to such further or alternative operative measures as may be found to be necessary during the course of the operation and to the administration of a general, local or other anaesthetic for any of these purposes.

   No assurance has been given to me that the operation will be performed by any particular surgeon.

Date .... (Signed) ....
(Patient)

   I confirm that I have explained to the patient the nature and effect of this operation.

Date .... (Signed) ....
(Physician/Surgeon)

CONSENT BY RELATIVES

I, ...

of ....

the *husband/wife/parent of the above-named ....

hereby consent to my *wife/husband/child undergoing the operation indicated above.

*delete as necessary.

(Signed) ....

Fig. 10.1 Example of a consent form for operation.

that when all theatre staff, scrubbed as well as unscrubbed, wear suits or dresses made of a non-woven fabric, air bacterial counts during an operating session are reduced by 50 per cent. All hair should be concealed under a special cap. Footwear with antistatic and impervious soles should be kept in the theatre cloakroom and never worn outside the theatre. It is possible to carry micro-organisms into the theatre from outside. The nose and mouth are covered with a mask whilst the operation is in progress and whilst the theatre is being prepared. Nurses from the ward must change into theatre clothing like the theatre staff, if they enter the operating theatre.

Theatre bedding

Blankets or blanket substitutes from the ward are not taken into the theatre because they are a source of infection. The patient's blanket should be removed on entering the theatre and the patient covered with a clean cotton blanket. Ideally the patient should be visited the night before surgery by the theatre nurse and she should explain what he is to expect when entering the theatre suite.

The ward nurse and the theatre

The ward nurse accompanying the patient to the theatre entrance must comfort and inspire confidence.

At the theatre entrance the patient is received by the theatre nurse, who accepts the patient from the ward nurse, ensuring that she has the

---

Patient's
Surname ....

Forenames ....   D.O.B. ....

Ward ....)
Operation ....)   *To be completed by*
Date ....)   *Theatre Sister*

                                           Tick   *Tick*

Premedication given ....

Dentures removed ....

Urine tested and recorded ....

Signed Consent Form enclosed ....

Signature of   *Signature of*
Ward Sister or   *Anaesthetist*
Staff Nurse

....

Fig. 10.2 Example of a final check form before anaesthesia.

right patient and all documentation is complete, together with any relevant information, e.g. if the patient is deaf, the patient has a stiff hip, etc. The consent form (Fig. 10.1) is checked by the theatre nurse. If it is not signed then the operation must not commence. The theatre nurse accompanies the patient into the anaesthetic room and stays with the patient during induction of anaesthesia. It is most important never to leave the patient prior to induction. The patient may be confused due to drugs or very apprehensive. Each patient should have a label attached to his wrist which is checked by the theatre nurse, the anaesthetist and the surgeon. The final check form (Fig. 10.2) is signed by the anaesthetist. Some of these duties may be undertaken by an operating department assistant (ODA).

The patient is positioned on the theatre table with the aid of the operating department assistant, and the theatre nurse. The position for an abdominal operation is shown in Figure 10.3 and for other regions in the relevant chapters in this book.

After the operation the patient remains in the theatre suite or recovery area until conscious and until the anaesthetist considers him fit to return to the ward.

Fig. 10.3 Usual position for abdominal operation. Note elevation of the calves by pads under the heels.

The ward nurse returns to the theatre to collect her patient, ensuring that she is aware of the nature of the anaesthetic, the diagnosis at the operation, the nature of the operation which has been performed, the number of tubes and drains inserted and any special instructions from the surgeon or anaesthetist about postoperative care.

The ward nurse is entirely responsible for the patient during transit from the theatre to the ward. She must above all keep the airway clear and have with her a receiver with an airway, tongue depressor and gauze swabs. Care must be taken with the intravenous line, and the patient should be kept warm during transit.

The duties of the theatre nurse

It is the scrub nurse who is responsible for the instruments. She wears a

Fig. 10.4 The tapes of a backwrap gown are held by 'scrubbed' member of the staff and one tape is passed to the sister's left hand so that she can tie it in front.

theatre cap which conceals her hair and a mask. The hands and arms are soaped and the nails are scrubbed for 5 minutes with an antiseptic soap. There are many antibacterial agents on the market which may be used for hand washing. The hands and arms are then dried with a sterile towel. The hands are inserted through the armhole of the sterile gown. It is pulled on by the circulating nurse and the back tapes tied. A back wrap gown (Fig. 10.4) has two tapes on the front one of which is handed to another scrubbed nurse or the surgeon who encircles the gown and hands it to the wearer to tie in front. This is done after putting on gloves. The outside of the gloves and gown must not be touched by the ungloved hand. The hands are powdered and the first glove put on, touching the inside of the cuff only with the bare hand. The second glove is put on, touching the outside of the glove only with the other gloved hand. (Fig. 10.5).

When both gloves are on, the cuffs are pulled over the gown at the wrist. Back wraps on the gown are then tied with the help of another gowned and gloved member of the theatre team. Once scrubbed, hands should be held in front and above waist level. The nurse who has scrubbed up now handles only sterilised materials. Should she inadvertently touch something which is non-sterile she must change her gloves, and gown. She supervises the instruments, prepares ligatures and sutures, and keeps the surgeon supplied with swabs (which are wrapped in bundles of five), tubes, or anything else which is needed during the operation. She must be quick to respond to the whispered word or gesture, for unnecessary speech is out of place in the theatre.

The instrument nurse takes the soiled swabs from the surgeon and disposes of them into a bucket or container for the circulating nurse to hang on the swab rack (Fig. 10.6).

Fig. 10.5 Correct method of putting on gloves. A. Picking up the first glove. B. Putting on the first glove. C. Picking up the second glove. D. Both gloves drawn over the cuffs. The outside surface of the glove is never touched by the skin of the hand.

It is the responsibility of the scrubbed nurse, at the end of the operation, to account for all instruments and materials used.

Duties of the circulating nurse

The circulating nurse is responsible for supplying all additional equipment for the surgical team and for assisting in swab check procedures. She retrieves all the used swabs from the bucket and hangs them in fives on the swab racks to be checked by the scrub nurse. All swabs contain a radio-opaque thread for ease of identification (Figs. 10.7 and 10.8). All materials used in the operation are counted and checked by the two nurses and the Record Book completed and signed by the scrub nurse.

Specimens in a swab tube or test tube for bacteriological examination or in a specimen pot containing the correct fluid, for histological examination are sealed and labelled so that the patient's identity is unmistakable. The container is then placed in a paper bag for transport to the laboratory after the surgeon has completed the request form indicating the examination he requires.

Other duties may include checking on pharmacy supplies and the ordering of packs and trays. Each theatre nurse must be aware of the importance of working as a team. She must always maintain a high standard, behave quietly and decorously and never discuss anything which she may see or hear during her theatre duties.

Fig. 10.6 Swab rack on which *all* swabs should be hung and counted.

Fig. 10.7 Swabs contain a radio-opaque thread.

Fig. 10.8 Radiograph of a swab in the abdomen which cannot be closed until it is recovered.

Prevention of infection

Because skin cannot be sterilised this remains one of the most important sources of infection in the theatre. The patient's skin is cleaned with an antiseptic solution, those most commonly used being povidone iodine or chlorhexidine in spirit. The skin adjoining the wound may be covered so that it is isolated. There is considerable difference of opinion as to the best method of doing this. The choice is:

1. Muslin towelling.
2. Semitransparent sheeting.
3. Adhesive surgical film.
4. Ventile water-repellent material.

An additional precaution is to use a separate sterile needle for every skin stitch, but in practice this is rarely done.

Septic case—clearance of the theatre

The main aim is to confine the infected materials to the one operating room by restricting movement of contaminated staff. All equipment and materials used should be kept to the minimum. Precautions should be taken from the start of the operation contaminated with pathogenic bacteria. Any staff entering the contaminated theatre should be warned of infection, taking the necessary precautions.

1. A towel soaked in a suitable disinfectant is placed on the floor of the theatre entrance as a mat.
2. Any equipment that will not be in use during the operation is removed.
3. Personnel involved should remain in the theatre during the procedure.
4. A runner should be stationed outside the door to provide any anaesthetic or surgical requirements.
5. Swabs and towels should not be dropped on the floor but put in a plastic bag.
6. The circulating nurse should wear rubber gloves for picking up swabs.
7. At the end of the operation the linen is placed in a plastic bag and sent to the laundry immediately, the laundry having been informed that the linen is infected.
8. Instruments should be returned to the Tray Service Supply Unit immediately, the Tray Service Supply Unit having also been informed that they are infected. If there is no Tray Service Supply Unit, instruments should be left to soak in a bowl filled with strong disinfectant for at least 2 hours. Any adhesive strapping that has come in close proximity with the patient should be discarded. Swabs should be placed in a plastic bag and burnt in the incinerator immediately. Theatre staff then discard their theatre clothing and gloves, and the theatre is thoroughly cleaned with a disinfectant before further use. This is often achieved by the use of a machine which emits a vaporised antiseptic (called 'fogging'). All staff should change into clean theatre clothing afterwards. Shoes should be disinfected for the recommended period.

Prevention of burns and explosion in the operating theatre

In the operating theatre the patient is vulnerable to burns and explosions which can be avoided by remembering the following:

Anaesthetic explosions. When inflammable agents are used for anaesthetising a patient the presence of a naked flame or sparks from faulty switches can induce violent explosions, extensive burns and death to the patient and theatre staff.

Static electricity. Theatre staff should be aware of static electricity and its dangers. Static electricity is generated when two materials are separated. It may not cause friction. The surface of one material or object becomes positively charged and the other negatively charged, and when these two are separated the static electricity disperses and may produce a spark. Wool and nylon together will build up static electricity.

The following precautions are important:

1. All metal apparatus should be fitted with antistatic rubber wheels.
2. Good earthing of all apparatus.
3. Theatre shoes should be made of a conductive rubber.
4. Theatre staff should wear cotton clothes.
5. Mattresses should be of sorbo and covered with antistatic rubber.
6. All rubber parts of the anaesthetic apparatus should be antistatic type.
7. Floors throughout the suite should have metal strips let in at regular intervals to earth any static electricity. This is not required with some newer types of flooring.
8. Cotton or flannel sheets should be used on the patients' trolleys.
9. The humidity of the theatre should be checked regularly. The higher the humidity in the theatre the less likely is static electricity to build up. Safe humidity should be 60 per cent.

Surgical diathermy. Surgical diathermy is a very high frequency electric current produced by a diathermy machine. The machine consists of a mains switch, foot pedal, active electrode, indifferent electrode, coagulating and cutting dials.

The active electrode is used by the surgeon, the indifferent electrode is a disposable metal plate which is fixed onto the patient's thigh and bandaged (Fig. 10.9).

Electrode

Lead to machine

Fig. 10.9 Passive diathermy electrode on the thigh.

The active electrode can coagulate bleeding points or cut through tissue.

To make a complete electrical circuit through the patient the surgeon uses the active electrode and the current passes to the tissues, where heat is generated and the tissues are coagulated.

If the patient is lying on the operating table touching metal, the patient will be burnt at the point of contact if he is not earthed.

Diathermy disposable plates (Fig. 10.9) should be only used once and care should be taken that the whole of the plate is touching skin.

Electrical equipment. All electrical equipment used in the operating theatre should be checked regularly for faults and repaired by a qualified engineer or electrician. Any equipment that is not in good working order should immediately be removed from the theatre and checked.

All the threatre staff must make themselves conversant with an electrical failure in the theatre suite as the patient's life will be at risk.

ELECTRICITY FAILURE IN HOSPITAL

Sudden failure of electric power becomes increasingly significant as the patient's needs become more dependent on its use. Most people think at once of the theatre lighting and the danger which may ensue for a patient undergoing an operation. In practice, this is usually very well taken care of by the theatre emergency lighting, provided from a 12-volt wet battery. The danger to the patient arises from:

1. Mechanical ventilators (artificial respirators)

This transcends in importance everything in the hospital. The patient whose life is dependent on an artificial mechanical respirator which is powered by electricity is saved by the fact that all machines can be operated manually, and the nurse needs to know how to use those in her own hospital.

2. Blood transfusion

The blood in the refrigerator will usually be safe for some hours but the advice of the blood transfusion officer must be sought. The nurse should consult the medical officer about securing further blood for patients under-going transfusion or already suffering from haemorrhage.

3. Suction apparatus

For operations such as tonsillectomy, alternative suction should be available in every theatre. This can be provided very simply by syphonage from a water tap or by a foot pump.

Other effects on the hospital are:
(a) Theatre—sterilisation, diathermy cautery, endoscopic lights, pump for open heart surgery, heating, and even the water supply may be threatened.

(b) In the laboratory there are no lights, the incubator may be out of action, and microscope lights may be ineffective.

(c) In the maternity department incubators for premature babies are affected.

(d) General—X-ray department, kitchen, dispensary, general heating, lighting, laundry, and physiotherapy departments are all affected.

Modern units tend to have a self-starting diesel alternator as an alternative in case of power failure.

BIBLIOGRAPHY

Brigden R J 1980 Operating theatre technique, 4th edn. Churchill Livingstone. Edinburgh
Cranfield A B 1972 Theatre nurses handbook. Butterworth, London
Dixon E P 1976 An Introduction to the operating theatre, Churchill Livingstone, Edinburgh
Mitchell N J, Evans D S, Kerr A 1978 British Medical Journal 1: 696

11

Surgical ward dressings

MAINTAINING ASEPSIS IN THE WARD

The provision of a bacteriologically clean atmosphere is one of the greatest of surgical problems. In operating theatres this is attempted at great expense. In the hospital of the future a similar but smaller scale provision will be built on every ward. This would consist of a dressing room which is air conditioned with a 'clean' and 'dirty' room on either side of it. All dressings would be performed in the dressing room, the only exception being infected cases which would be nursed and dressed in their own isolation ward. In the meantime, however, the vast majority of patients will be nursed in large wards and the problems which arise will have to be dealt with as they occur.

It is inevitable that the more patients there are in a ward the greater is the risk of infection, whilst an ideal number of patients from this point of view is one that is economically impossible. However, the situation can be controlled by the separation of clean from infected cases in the ward. A small isolation ward attached to the main ward is a great advantage and glass partitions in the ward diminish cross-infection.

Patients particularly liable to infection are diabetics, amputees and patients on steroid or immunosuppressive drugs.

Where wounds become infected this is most likely to have occurred in the theatre. *Other sources of wound infection are:*

(a) Dust in the air of the ward
(b) Poor hygiene in nurses or patient
(c) Lack of cleanliness of the ward environment
(d) Infected droplets from mouths and noses
(e) The hands of the dresser or contamination of instruments during procedure
(f) Cross-infection from other infected wounds.

Dressings should ideally be carried out in a room or cubicle specially designed for the purpose. Where this is not practicable the following points should be observed.

1. The air in the ward. The bacterial content of the air in the ward rises to a maximum in the early morning owing, among other factors, to the domestic activities in the ward, including the cleaning of floors, dusting, bed-making, etc. Bacteria are less likely to be scattered if the precautions mentioned on page 65 are observed with the following additional measures:

  (a) When making beds the clothes are handled slowly and gently.
  (b) Bed-making, floor-cleaning and dusting cease at least 1 hour before the first dressing is uncovered.

When dressings begin the ward is closed to all visitors and all unnecessary personnel. Windows and doors are shut.

2. Droplet infection. To prevent the spread of infection, surgeons, nurses, students, orderlies and domestic workers with respiratory infections or septic lesions should not be on duty in a surgical ward.

3. Hands. Hands cannot be properly sterilised, though thorough washing can remove recent contamination. It is essential, therefore, that during a dressing the hands should not come in contact either with the wound itself or with any material in the vicinity of the wound. The hands should be thoroughly washed, using plenty of soap and water, paying particular attention to the nails, which should be cut short and free of varnish. A Towelmaster or disposable paper towels are used to dry them and the dressing is performed, using sterile forceps.

4. Masks should always be worn during dressings. Efficient masks made of paper are now in use. They should be changed hourly, since after that period they only present a further source of infection, and should not be touched with the fingers during use. As soon as the need has passed, the mask should be removed. To go around all day with a mask covering the nose is to increase the chance of infection because of lack of proper ventilation to the nose.

Nonetheless there are some who advise that masks are unnecessary.

Protective dressings for the wound

Dressings for a wound may consist of one or more of the following: gauze, lint, cotton-wool, gamgee, cotton or crepe bandage, various prepared adhesive dressings, Elastoplast, elasticated tube bandage or net of various shapes, adhesive tape.

The advantages of protective dressings for wounds are many, but one disadvantage is that evaporation from the skin surface is hindered. This may be overcome by:

1. No dressing. A little gauze is strapped on the wound for 6 hours until the edges have become sealed off with exudate. After this all dressings are abandoned.

2. A plastic skin dressing. Such dressings consist of an acrylic resin dissolved in a mixture of acetic esters. When applied to the skin the solvent evaporates, leaving a transparent, adherent, and elastic film. This film is impervious to bacteria but pervious to evaporation from the skin surface. It must not be used unless haemostasis is perfect. It may be sprayed or spread with a glass rod. A thick layer may be peeled off; a thin layer may be dissolved with ether or acetone.

The advantages of a plastic skin dressing are that:

(a) the wound is sealed and cannot be infected; this is particularly important if a colostomy or ileostomy is functioning near a fresh wound.

(b) the progress of the wound can be seen without disturbing the dressing.

(c) the patient can take a bath as the dressing is impervious to water.

Clean wounds which have been closed without drainage and have a dressing need not be uncovered until it is time to remove the stitches.

Infected discharging wounds require regular dressing.

Changing a simple dressing—one nurse

A basic trolley is prepared. The nurse washes and dries her hands, and puts on a mask.

Using Jontex cloth the whole trolley is washed with soap and water and dried. It is then swabbed with a disposable swab soaked in 70 per cent spirit—in some hospitals a similar antiseptic is sprayed over the trolley and allowed to dry.

A basic dressing pack (containing woollen balls, gauze swabs), adhesive tape, recommended antiseptic and any other necessary equipment are placed on the bottom shelf. A 'used instrument bag' is attached to one end of the trolley with a strip of adhesive tape. Two strips of adhesive tape are attached to the rail at the other end for the soiled dressing bag.

The procedure is explained to the patient. Privacy is ensured and nearby windows are closed as necessary. The trolley is then taken to the bedside.

Using her scissors the nurse cuts the sealed end of the pack and tips the inner pack on to the top of the trolley. She attaches the outer pack to the other end of the trolley, for receiving soiled dressings. The patient is placed into an appropriate position and made comfortable. The bedclothes and personal clothing are adjusted as necessary. The nurse loosens the bandage or adhesive holding the dressing. She then thoroughly washes and dries her hands. The inner wrapping is then opened and partially spread by pulling on the first three corners. The fourth corner is lifted carefully with one hand and the nurse picks up the first pair of forceps with the other and continues to spread the final corner. Using the pair of forceps she arranges the sterile field and tray, placing the instruments on the side of the tray. The forceps are then placed at the side of the trolley with the points only on the sterile field. She opens any supplementary packs. She pours out the antiseptic. Using the first pair of forceps she removes the soiled dressing, discarding it into the appropriate bag. The soiled forceps are placed into the used instrument bag. She picks up two pairs of forceps. If towels are necessary, they are arranged around the wound.

With the forceps in her left hand she picks up a swab, dips it into the antiseptic and transfers it to the forceps in her right hand. The wound is cleaned and the swab discarded. As many swabs as necessary are used, each swab being used once only. She discards the forceps in her right hand, and transfers those in her left hand to the right hand. In her left hand she picks up the remaining forceps. Using the two forceps the dressing is applied. Both forceps are discarded. The dressing is secured, using adhesive or bandage as indicated. The patient is made comfortable.

Any unused wool or gauze is saved for suitable unsterile procedures. The tray is then placed into the used instrument bag which is disconnected from the side of the trolley. The sterile field, used towels, and the nurse's mask are placed in the soiled bag, which is also disconnected from the side of the trolley and closed tightly by squeezing the top. The bag containing used instruments is taken to the sluice (or dirty room) and thence to the Central Sterile Supply Department (CSSD). The soiled dressings are also taken in the sealed bag to the sluice and sent for incineration. The trolley is removed and cleaned. The nurse washes and dries her hands. She reports to Sister or Charge Nurse as necessary.

THE STITCHES

The skin edges of a wound must be approximated and held together until the wound has healed. This is usually achieved with skin stitches of non-absorbable material, e.g. nylon or silk. They are removed at times varying from the 3rd to 10th postoperative day. The timing depends on such things as the site of the wound (skin crease incisions with no tension heal quickly), the general state of health of the patient, the nature of the disease, the presence of obesity, complications in the wound. If deep tension sutures have been used they are removed on the 10th to 14th postoperative day. When removing skin stitches the cut stitch must be extracted from the skin towards the wound—pulling it away from the wound may disrupt its edges. Some types of skin stitches are illustrated in Figure 11.1.

Fig. 11.1 Types of skin sutures.

Metal clips or staples are increasingly being used instead of stitches, mainly in skin crease incisions with little tension across them. They are removed from the 2nd to 5th postoperative day.

Butterfly plasters or adhesive tape strips are also sometimes used instead of stitches.

A stitch which is cutting through the skin may give rise to considerable pain. The surgeon's attention should be drawn to this to see if the stitch can be removed earlier than usual. Swelling in the wound because of inflammation, usually due to infection, is the common cause of such a problem.

A stitch abscess may develop if infection is present. The stitch concerned should be removed to provide free drainage. One or more stitches may need to be removed, when a wound infection develops, to allow free drainage of pus.

DRAINS

Drains are used:
1. to drain fluid which has collected or is expected to collect, e.g. blood, serum, pus, bile.
2. as a safety valve to an anastomosis or suture line, e.g. the duodenal stump after gastrectomy or the ureter after removal of a stone.

In the first case the drain is removed when drainage has become negligible or has ceased. This is often within 1 to 3 days.

In the second case the drain is removed once the danger of leakage has passed. This is usually 4 to 5 days.

The drain is usually brought out through a small incision separate from the main wound, to avoid both interference with healing and contamina-

Fig. 11.2 Some types of drains—rubber and plastic tubes, corrugated and Penrose.

Fig. 11.3 *Above*: Wrong. Gauze plugs the wound, obstructs drainage and is painful.
    Below: Correct. Tube allows free drainage.

tion of the wound. Sometimes it is brought out through the wound, while in certain circumstances the wound itself requires drainage.

Wherever a drain is inserted it should be covered with a sterile dressing or, if a tube, its exit from the skin surrounded with such a dressing.

Types of drain

1. Tubing—fenestrated or split
    plastic, latex or rubber
2. Corrugated—plastic or rubber sheeting
3. Penrose tubing—soft, thin, flat latex tubing
4. Shaped drains for specific purposes, e.g. catheters for certain cavities, T-tubes for the common bile duct.

Some varieties of drain are illustrated in Figure 11.2.

Gauze is not a drain. As figure 11.3 shows, its misuse prevents drainage.

The drain is stitched to the skin. A safety pin should be put into a corrugated drain to prevent it slipping deep to the skin.

Drainage

Drainage may be:

1. *Open*
    (a) Directly on to dressings.
    (b) Into an adhesive plastic bag stuck to the skin around the drain.
2. *Closed*
    (a) Tube or catheter into a sealed sterile disposable bag.
    (b) Chest tube to an under fluid seal (p. 321).
    (c) Suction-tube attached to a low grade suction machine or to a sealed vacuum apparatus (e.g. Redivac drain illustrated in Fig. 11.4). The practical details of the management of such drains vary with the make of drain used.

In closed drainage, organisms from the air are excluded, the discharge can be measured and the main wound can be kept dry.

Management of drain

The nature and quantity of drainage should be carefully noted. The quantity of fluid draining can be measured accurately if it is collected into a bag or suction apparatus. This should be recorded every 24 hours, or more frequently if there is a large quantity.

Some surgeons advocate that drains should be shortened gradually by pulling them out a little and cutting off the excess, so that the drainage track can heal from the bottom, and that tube drains should be rotated so that they do not adhere to the tissues. However, many simply remove the drain when it has ceased to fulfil a useful function.

The following complications may arise if a tube is left in situ for too long a period:

Fig. 11.4 Redivac drain.

Infection
Intestinal obstruction
Erosion of a blood vessel causing a secondary haemorrhage
Perforation of an organ causing a fistula
Adhesions
Incisional hernia.

HEALING OF WOUNDS

Healing by *first intention* is the aim in all wounds. The raw edges of the wound are approximated with stitches or other materials (see above) and the wound heals unhindered. If the wound edges overlap, are indrawn, or sucked under due to loss of tissue beneath, delay in healing will result. Wounds heal best when immobilised and, if covered, left untouched. Daily dressings are not necessary.

Sometimes a wound is left open to heal by *second intention*. This is usually because of infection or loss of tissue. Examples of this are following excision of a pilonidal sinus (Fig. 11.5), incision and drainage of a perianal abscess, excision of dead tissue due to trauma. Such a wound should be narrow at the bottom and wide at the top, in general terms conical in shape. The base and sides become lined by granulation tissue.

Fig. 11.5 Open wound following excision of infected pilonidal sinus.

The wound fills in from the bottom and becomes gradually covered with skin. An open wound should be kept clean. This is achieved by daily dressings and the use, if necessary, of saline soaks, irrigation with hydrogen peroxide or saline baths. In the early stages analgesics may be necessary about half an hour prior to the dressing to control pain. Damage to the granulation tissue by the dressing should be avoided but the wide top of the wound should be kept open so that it heals last.

Fig. 11.6 (a) Silastic foam mould, seen from deep surface. (b) Silastic foam mould in position in wound (same patient as in Fig. 11.5).

Various dressings can be used including petroleum jelly gauze, gauze soaked in eusol and paraffin or flavine emulsion, or a silastic foam moulded bung. The latter is mixed according to the manufacturer's instructions and poured into the wound as a liquid. It sets solid, with a sponge-like consistency, as a mould in the shape of the wound (Fig. 11.6). It is washed daily in antiseptic and replaced in the wound. A new mould is made once a week to allow for shrinkage of the wound. Such a dressing is good for outpatient use.

COMPLICATIONS OF WOUNDS

The nurse must know when to suspect complications which necessitate inspection of the wound. The following are a guide that all may not be well:
1. the continued presence of pain.
2. swelling and/or redness around the wound.
3. persistent rise of temperature and/or an increasing pulse rate.
4. presence of toxaemia, indicated by the onset of vomiting, diarrhoea, loss of appetite and increasing pallor.
5. discharge from the wound.
6. any symptoms of tetanus—very rare nowadays.
7. any symptoms of too tight a plaster or dressing e.g. pain, tingling or cyanosis of the tips of the fingers or toes.

The following complications can occur in a wound

Infection

This may vary from redness around the wound (erythema) to abscess formation. The patient complains of pain. The temperature and pulse are raised. The wound is usually red, swollen and tender. Pus, if present, will discharge. Some stitches may have to be removed and the skin edges separated with sinus forceps to allow free drainage. Wound swabs are taken to isolate the causative organism and enable appropriate antibiotic treatment to be given if indicated. If the wound is draining freely, antibiotics are unnecessary. In the presence of spreading cellulitis, toxaemia and some specific infections they should be given. However, there are differing opinions concerning the use of antibiotics in wound infection.

Regular dressings, often several times a day, are required for infected discharging wounds. Gauze packing of a subcutaneous collection of pus delays healing and blocks drainage. It should not be used. A small drain inserted into the wound may be helpful. Irrigation with antiseptic lotions such as eusol or hydrogen peroxide will help clean the wound. An apparatus is available which can be stuck over an infected wound to allow continuous irrigation.

If granulation tissue becomes excessive (proud flesh) and grows above the level of the skin, the exuberant patches should be burnt down by the careful application of a silver nitrate stick (Fig. 11.7). The nurse must take

Fig. 11.7   Cauterisation of excessive granulation tissue.

care not to damage any portion of the patient's skin or her own hands. When an infected wound has become clean, secondary suture of the skin may be performed or a skin graft may be possible.

Antibiotics are used prophylactically in some circumstances to try to prevent wound infection, e.g. in operations on the large bowel.

Prolonged discharge from wounds and consequent loss of protein is liable to give rise to hypoproteinaemia. Patients with such wounds should have a diet rich in protein and vitamin C.

Haemorrhage (see also Ch. 12)

Primary haemorrhage. This is bleeding from the wound immediately following surgery. Re-stitching of the wound, additional stitching or local pressure dressings can be used to stop it. Occasionally the patient has to be taken back to the theatre for the bleeding to be controlled surgically.

Secondary haemorrhage (p. 112). The commonest cause of this is wound infection. It occurs around the 7th to 10th postoperative day. Treatment is that of the infection, and blood transfusion if necessary.

Haematoma formation (p. 128). When the sutures are about to be removed it may be noticed that there is some tension in or swelling of the wound, due to a haematoma. If this is the case the edges should be separated gently with sinus forceps, the haematoma expressed if possible, and a small strip of plastic or rubber drain inserted for 48 hours.

Failure to heal

This may vary from a little gaping of part of the skin wound on removal of the sutures to complete dehiscence (falling apart) of the wound, e.g. 'burst abdomen'. The treatment varies from that of an open wound to partial or complete resuturing, depending on the size and depth of the defect.

Local causes of failure to heal are:
(a) infection
(b) haematoma
(c) tension in wound e.g.—abdominal distension or bad cough causing tension in abdominal wound; skin stitched under tension
(d) poor blood supply e.g.—in lower third of leg; limb wounds in peripheral arterial disease; at edges of large skin flaps

General causes of failure to heal are:
(a) diabetes
(b) malnutrition—hypoproteinaemia; vitamin deficiency, especially vitamin C; shortage of trace elements, especially zinc
Such problems usually arise from prolonged or severe illness.
(c) anaemia
(d) steroids—given as treatment for the disease in question or for something else
(e) carcinoma—especially abdominal carcinomatosis
(f) old age.

Sloughing

This is when part or all of the skin adjacent to a wound becomes dead (necrotic). The causes are poor blood supply, tension or sometimes infection. The skin first becomes a dusky blue colour and later turns black. The necrotic tissue either separates spontaneously in due course leaving the wound to heal by second intention (granulation) or it has to be removed surgically.

Sinus or fistula formation

A discharging sinus (blind ending track) may persist in a wound following infection. This is either because there is an infected cavity beneath the skin with only a small opening on the surface or a 'foreign body' in the wound, commonly non-absorbable suture material. In the first case the cavity may have to be laid open, while in the second the suture material may have to be removed.

Less commonly, a discharging wound may communicate with the epithelial lining of another organ, forming a fistula. Thus, following surgery on the gastrointestinal tract, a fistula may in some circumstances form discharging intestinal contents on to the surface. The management of a fistula depends on its site and its cause. The discharge is often irritant to the skin, which should be protected by barrier paste or adhesive waterproof material. The discharge should preferably be collected in an adhesive bag or via a tube inserted into the fistula. This also permits measurement of the quantity of discharge.

Contracture

Scar tissue contracts. This may give rise to problems in some wounds, especially those across joints, in the hands and following extensive tissue

Fig. 11.8   Keloid in abdominal scar.

damage or loss (e.g. burns). Proper splinting in the early stages and later active movement help to minimise the problem. The physiotherapist normally supervises the movement and rehabilitation of the patient but the nurse may have to assist with this.

Keloid formation

A keloid (Fig. 11.8) is a condition of excessive thickening of a scar. The cause is unknown. It can occur at any site in the body but is particularly liable to occur around the shoulders and in the upper half of the trunk, especially in the midline anteriorly. It is also liable to develop after operations on tuberculous foci and following wounds in members of the coloured races.

Treatment is difficult. The keloid may soften and fade with time. Masking it with make-up may be required. Excision is of no value for it recurs. Other treatments that are sometimes tried are local application of steroid-impregnated tape or injection of steroids, local application of pressure by a tailor-made pressure garment and shaving flat followed by skin grafting.

12

Haemorrhage

Haemorrhage is the loss of blood from a blood vessel. The blood lost is described as extravasated (outside the vessels). It may lie on the surface of the body, on the patient's clothing or on the floor. Blood which is extravasated into the tissues, a body cavity or the lumen of a hollow organ may in itself be very significant quite apart from any effect which may ensue from loss to the circulation. This problem is considered at the end of this chapter.

Clotting is the circulatory system's defence mechanism to leakage. Clot formation may be deficient from disease, the absence of essential clotting factors or the use of anticoagulant drugs. To be effective in sealing the leakage the clot has to be inside the lumen of the vessel (intravascular)—clot formation inside a viscus but outside the blood vessels increases the bleeding for reasons given in Figure 12.1. When bleeding occurs and blood is spilt into a receiver or shed on to the floor it is always worth noting whether clots are forming since in conditions of

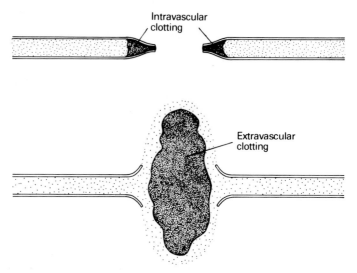

Fig. 12.1 Haemorrhage is arrested by clotting *inside* the vessel but aggravated by clots outside which prevent the severed ends from retracting.

defective clotting or active fibrinolysis the patient bleeds but clots either do not form or are quickly lysed. Replacement of the missing clotting factors, e.g. by fresh frozen plasma, may be necessary when there is defective clotting. In conditions of fibrinolysis it may be necessary to give an antifibrinolytic agent such as tranexamic acid, with or without replacement of any clotting factors which may have been depleted by the lysis.

Blood may be lost from all three types of vessel, the arteries, the veins, or the capillaries. The type of haemorrhage is named accordingly. Bleeding which occurs as soon as the vessel is divided is known as primary haemorrhage. If the patient is collapsed the vessel may not bleed immediately, but as recovery takes place the blood pressure rises and bleeding occurs—this is known as reactionary or intermediate haemorrhage. If infection is present, the walls of the blood vessels may be eroded and may burst, causing what is known as secondary haemorrhage.

TYPES OF HAEMORRHAGE

1. Arterial.
2. Capillary.
3. Venous.

Arterial haemorrhage. The blood is bright red and spurts with the heart beat. The escape is from both ends of the vessel not only from that nearer to the heart. Blood loss is more rapid than from a vein of corresponding size.

Capillary haemorrhage. The blood oozes over the surface and is darkish red in colour. Oozing over several hours can result in considerable blood loss.

Venous haemorrhage. The blood is dark in colour, there is no spurting and the rate of loss is much less severe than arterial haemorrhage. Since the large veins are big cave-like structures, injury to them is a serious matter. A further danger is that air may be sucked into the damaged veins, giving rise to fatal air embolism in which the blood and air may form 'foam'.

Increased intravenous pressure with even greater blood loss occurs in rupture of a varicose vein, in portal hypertension and in asphyxia. Blood loss from the pulmonary artery is dark unoxygenated blood while that from the pulmonary vein is fully saturated with oxygen and is, therefore, bright red.

TIME OF HAEMORRHAGE (in relation to time of wound)

1. Primary.
2. Reactionary or intermediate.
3. Secondary.

Primary haemorrhage is immediate, e.g. a cut finger or an operative incision.

Reactionary haemorrhage occurs in the first 24 hours after operation. The more severe the operation the more likely it is to occur, especially after the patient has recovered from circulatory collapse. Operations on the kidney, the thyroid and the breast as well as total hysterectomy are particularly liable to be followed by reactionary haemorrhage.

Coughing or vomiting, by increasing the pressure in the veins, are contributory factors.

Secondary haemorrhage is due to sloughing of the wall of a blood vessel. The commonest cause is bacterial infection, but in the absence of infection it may be caused by the action of an enzyme, for example acid pepsin on a peptic ulcer. The pressure of a drainage tube, a bone fragment or the presence of carcinoma may also be factors. The vessels are eroded. The thinnest walled vessels, the capillaries, burst first and a few specks of blood are found on the dressing. This should be immediately reported. It is a warning that the larger vessels are also being eroded, and in another few days, commonly the 10th after operation, a main artery may burst, giving rise to a torrential, fatal haemorrhage.

Most symptoms of blood loss complained of by patients at diagnostic clinics are in fact small secondary haemorrhages.

THE SEVERITY OF HAEMORRHAGE

In the body of a healthy adult there are approximately 5.8 l of blood with a haemoglobin concentration of 14.6 g per dl. If 1.8 l of blood are lost very rapidly—for example in half an hour—death usually results. However should loss occur at the rate of 1 litre over the whole day for several days there would still be very little less than 5.8 l of fluid in the circulation: the haemoglobin concentration, however, might be only 2.9 g per dl. The fluid lost from the circulation is replaced by fluid from the tissues, so that the volume of blood is restored, but since vast numbers of red blood cells have been shed, the oxygen carrying power is depleted.

It is always a matter of great surprise to junior nurses to learn that the blood volume of a new born baby is about 350 ml, i.e. less than one pint, and consequently a loss of 100 ml is a very serious haemorrhage.

An estimation of the extent of the blood loss is made by clinical observation of the patient (p. 116), records of the pulse, temperature and blood pressure (Figs. 12.2 & 12.3) and the central venous pressure. Blood haemoglobin and packed cell volume (PCV) estimations are essential. In the theatre the weighing of swabs is undertaken and the volume of blood in any suction apparatus is measured. In the ward the quantity of blood vomited or aspirated from the stomach or lost in a bed pan is also measured.

THE NATURAL ARREST OF HAEMORRHAGE (Fig. 12.4)

Adequate amounts of calcium and all the clotting factors are essential for the natural arrest of haemorrhage. The blood in circulation is kept fluid by a fine balance between clotting and fibrinolysis. As a result of a complex series of reactions starting when tissue is damaged, prothrombin is converted to its active form thrombin in the presence of calcium.

Fig. 12.2   The rising pulse and falling temperature of haemorrhage.

Fibrinogen is then transformed by thrombin to fibrin, which forms a mesh in which platelets and other blood cells become entangled to form a clot. Alterations of these factors by drugs form the basis of anticoagulant and fibrinolytic therapy.

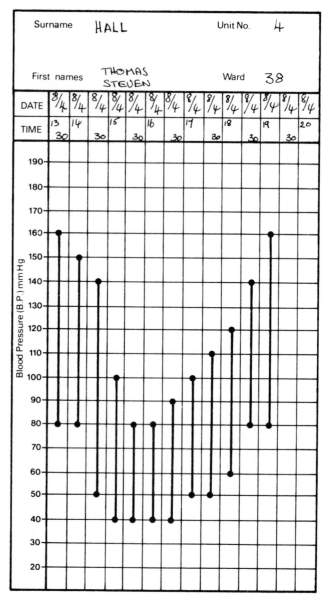

Fig. 12.3 The systolic and diastolic blood pressure is recorded, showing a fall due to haemorrhage.

Factors affecting clotting

1. Calcium may be displaced from blood by:
(a) A 3.8 per cent solution of sodium citrate.
(b) Acid citrate dextrose solution.
(c) Citrate phosphate dextrose solution.
(d) Oxalate.
(e) Ethylenediamine tetra-acetic acid (EDTA).
Clinically sodium citrate prevents the formation of clots in the bladder; acid citrate dextrose and acid citrate phosphate solutions are used to

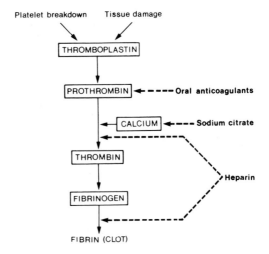

Fig. 12.4 Mechanism of clot formation and the site of action of anticoagulants.

prevent clotting of stored blood. Because stored blood has had its calcium displaced, a patient receiving blood requires 10 ml of a 10 per cent solution of calcium chloride for every four units of blood transfused.

Oxalate or EDTA is used in pathological specimen tubes when it is desired to prevent clotting of the blood sample.

2. Prothrombin is formed from vitamin K, a fat-soluble vitamin absorbed from the small intestine. A patient suffering from obstructive jaundice will not absorb vitamin K and therefore is liable to bleed if operated upon. For this reason vitamin K is given by injection until the prothrombin level of the blood has been restored. Oral anticoagulants like warfarin act by preventing the liver utilising vitamin K, thus reducing the formation of prothrombin. The dosage is controlled by the prothrombin time. If it is necessary to reverse the process, vitamin K is given, but it may be too slow to act and a transfusion of fresh frozen plasma may be necessary.

A more immediately acting anticoagulant is heparin given intravenously by continuous infusion. Its action can be rapidly reversed with protamine sulphate, if necessary.

3. Fibrinogen is the precursor of fibrin. In the absence of fibrinogen severe bleeding may occur. Fibrinolysins are substances which dissolve fibrin by a phenomenon known as fibrinolysis. The fibrinolytic activity of the blood may be increased:

(a) In complicated obstetric cases associated with haemorrhage.

(b) After strenuous exercise.

(c) In the presence of some malignant growths.

(d) Occasionally after operations such as prostatectomy, the fibrinolysin known as urokinase being the cause.

(e) In certain streptococcal infections—streptokinase releases an endogenous activator or fibrinolysin.

Patients suffering from increased fibrinolysis will show reduced evidence of clotting. They may be treated by neutralisation of the fibrinolysins by the administration of tranexamic acid or the administration of fibrinogen. Fibrinolysins such as streptokinase may be used in the dissolution of thrombi in cases of deep venous thrombosis and pulmonary embolism.

Fibrinogen is also consumed in the condition known as disseminated intravascular coagulation (DIC). In this condition very small clots are formed inside the blood vessels. This leads to a haemostatic defect caused by consumption of clotting factors and platelets in the clotting process. There may be secondary activation of the fibrinolytic system in an attempt to keep the vessels patent. Disseminated intravascular coagulation is more common than primary fibrinolysis and may complicate the following conditions:

(a) Obstetric accidents e.g. placenta abruptia.

(b) Surgery, especially that involving the heart and lungs.

(c) Gram negative and meningococcal septicaemia.

(d) Haemolytic transfusion reactions.

(e) Widespread carcinoma.

(f) Acute leukaemia.

Patients with DIC must never be given tranexamic acid or the protective fibrinolysis may be inhibited, giving rise to widespread and possibly fatal thrombosis. The cause must be treated and the consumed clotting factors replaced.

THE SYMPTOMS AND SIGNS OF HAEMORRHAGE

Clinically, haemorrhage may be of two types:

1. Revealed or external, i.e. the bleeding can be seen.

2. Concealed or internal, i.e. the bleeding cannot be seen. The bleeding occurs into one of the body cavities, such as the abdomen, into the lumen of a hollow organ, such as the intestine, or into the tissues. It may later become obvious, e.g. by being vomited or passed per rectum, or by formation of bruising and swelling on the surface of the body. Since it is concealed it must be diagnosed on the presence of symptoms and signs alone. These do not develop until a moderate sized bleed has occurred.

When the loss of blood is rapid the symptoms and signs are those of acute circulatory collapse. When the loss of blood is slow the symptoms and signs are those of a progressive anaemia as well as water and salt depletion.

Early symptoms and signs

1. *Restlessness and anxiety.* The patient is conscious that all is not well and feels faint.

2. *Coldness.* The temperature is slightly subnormal, 36.9°C (98°F).

3. The *pulse rate* is slightly increased.

4. The *blood pressure* is lowered.

5. *Pallor* increases.

6. The patient is *thirsty*.

Symptoms and signs after severe haemorrhage

1. *Extreme pallor.* The face may be ashen white, and clammy with cold sweat. The colour as well as the temperature (as palpated with the hand) of the nose and digits are very significant.

2. *Coldness* is profound. The temperature is of the order of 36°C (97°F) or lower (Fig. 12.2).

3. *Air hunger.* The patient literally gasps for breath. The respirations are rapid and sighing.

4. *The pulse* is very rapid in rate, thready in volume and frequently is irregular in rhythm.

5. *The blood pressure* is extremely low (Fig. 12.3).

6. *Thirst* is extreme.

7. *The volume of urine* secreted is diminished—acute renal failure may occur.

8. *The central venous* pressure is low and often negative (Fig. 13.2).

9. *Blindness, tinnitus (buzzing in the ears) and coma* occur in this order prior to death.

Diminution of the volume of blood in the circulation with depletion of the supply of oxygen to the tissues is the first and most important result of haemorrhage.

THE TREATMENT OF HAEMORRHAGE

This may be summarised under three headings:

1. The arrest of haemorrhage, i.e. its control.

2. Restoration of the blood volume.

3. The fate of the extravasated blood.

1. THE ARREST OF THE HAEMORRHAGE

External haemorrhage

Pressure will control all forms of external haemorrhage. According to its severity there is a choice of methods.

1. Pad and bandage. This simple method of applying direct pressure to a bleeding wound is applicable to the vast majority of cases. It is effective and causes no damage.

2. Digital pressure, applied over the pressure point of the artery supplying the area of the wound, will control haemorrhage temporarily. This is called indirect pressure. It is particularly valuable in the neck, where other methods are inapplicable.

3. Elevation of the limb will control venous haemorrhage. This is the classical method of dealing with a sudden haemorrhage from a ruptured varicose vein of the leg.

4. Application of a tourniquet. This is rarely required except for the control of a torrential haemorrhage from a limb. *It is not without danger.* A temporary tourniquet may have to be devised in a sudden emergency. A pad, e.g. a handkerchief, is placed over the line of the vessel and a tourniquet—which may be a scarf, a tie, or whatever is available—is bound around the limb and tightened if necessary with a small piece of wood. More usually, in hospital, three types of tourniquet are used:

    The Samway anchor tourniquet

    Esmarch's elastic bandage

    Inflatable cuff tourniquet.

The great danger of a tourniquet, if left on for more than 30 minutes, is that gangrene of the limb may occur. Damage to the nerves is not infrequent, especially if the skin has not been protected before its application. It is essential, therefore, to slacken the tourniquet intermittently and tighten it again if bleeding persists.

The time of application and removal of a tourniquet should be recorded on the theatre blackboard. Some theatres have a stop clock with an alarm which can be set. The limb on which a tourniquet has been used should be kept elevated afterwards to control oedema which may result from venous congestion.

5. Surgical ligation is necessary if the bleeding is persistent.

6. Coagulation of the bleeding point with electrocautery or diathermy may be required.

7. Therapeutic embolisation means the deliberate occulsion of blood vessels by means of emboli introduced through an angiographic catheter in a clinical situation where it is necessary to obliterate local blood flow. The material used ranges from Sterispon (Gelfoam) to lyophilised human dura mater (Lyodura). Haemorrhage from oesophageal varices and gastric ulcers has been controlled by this method (Allison 1978).

8. A pack will temporarily control very severe haemorrhage. This method is used in the theatre to control temporarily a sudden haemorrhage. The theatre nurse should always have a pack readily available for this emergency.

9. Styptics, such as snake venom or adrenaline (1: 1000), may be used locally in certain cases. Thrombin and Gelfoam have their uses in appropriate cases such as low pressure bleeding from venules and capillaries.

Internal or concealed haemorrhage

Pressure cannot be employed internally except by surgical ligature or packing. Many internal haemorrhages are secondary in nature, and will cease if the infection can be controlled and the vessels encouraged to contract. The following methods are involved in its control:

1. The organ is emptied of blood clot if possible. In a case of severe bleeding from the bladder a catheter is passed and the bladder emptied. The blood vessels in a dilated paralysed organ are unable to contract.

2. The vessels are encouraged to contract. A lotion of saline or sodium bicarbonate, to which a few drops of adrenaline solution (1: 1000) have been added, is of great value in washing out the organ. This can be repeated every two hours. The use of ergometrine after the birth of the placenta is an example of stimulating the vessels to contract.

Pitressin intravenously may be effective in the control of bleeding from oesophageal varices (p. 418).

3. The coagulability of the blood is increased. This is not very valuable unless the mechanism of clotting is deficient, due to the absence of an essential constituent of the blood. The parenteral administration of vitamin K is important to a jaundiced patient who is bleeding, because its absorption from the intestine is deficient. In haemophilia, the administration of factor VIII concentrate or cryoprecipitate is indicated and increases coagulability.

4. Packing with gauze soaked in adrenaline is effective at certain sites, and Oxycel, which is absorbable gauze impregnated with fibrin, is used extensively. A piece of the patient's own muscle, crushed, can be used in the same way.

5. Surgical ligature e.g. in the case of a ruptured spleen.

6. Antibiotics. A secondary haemorrhage, whether internal or external because it is infective in origin, requires the systemic administration of antibiotics in addition to measures to control the bleeding and restore the blood volume.

7. Internal pressure. This may be applied by the balloon of a triluminal tube in bleeding oesophageal varices or by the balloon of a Foley catheter in a prostatectomy cavity.

8. Antifibrinolytic therapy such as tranexamic acid (p. 115).

2. RESTORATION OF THE BLOOD VOLUME

BLOOD TRANSFUSION

Indications

1. To counteract the effects of severe haemorrhage and replace the blood lost.

2. To prevent shock in operations where blood loss is considerable, such as rectal resection, hysterectomy and arterial surgery.

3. In severe burns to make up for blood lost by burning but only after plasma and electrolytes have been replaced.

4. To correct severe anaemia from cancer, marrow aplasia and similar conditions, and from slow continuous haemorrhage.

The blood volume can be fairly accurately estimated by a machine using a radio-iodine technique to determine plasma volume and micro-haematocrit to estimate red cell volume.

As described earlier, in slow haemorrhage the blood volume is restored by fluid from the tissues. In cases of severe haemorrhage, where large volumes of blood are lost rapidly, the blood volume must be restored by blood transfusion or, if not immediately available, by plasma substitutes.

Blood used

Blood is collected from healthy donors, 420 ml being collected on each occasion. Blood which is administered in the same form as it is collected, apart from the addition of an anticoagulant, is described as whole blood.

In some cases 'packed red cells' are given. This consists of the cellular elements left after siphoning off the supernatant plasma from whole blood. It is used in cases of chronic anaemia where the volume of blood is not substantially diminished and a large volume may induce cardiac failure.

Selection of donors

They should be in good general health. The blood tests for syphilis and serum hepatitis must be negative, and they must not have had infective hepatitis or malaria.

Collection of blood

Blood is collected into a plastic bag containing either 75 ml acid citrate dextrose (A.C.D.) solution or 63 ml citrate phosphate dextrose (C.P.D.) solution. A needle is inserted into a vein at the elbow after the application of a sphygmomanometer cuff to the arm and 420 ml blood are withdrawn to make a total unit of 495 ml if A.C.D. solution has been used or 483 ml if C.P.D. solution has been used. If the blood is not required for immediate use it is stored in a special refrigerator at a temperature from 4° to 6°C.

Blood grouping

All human beings have one of four main blood groups—A, B, AB or O—according to the nature of the blood group antigen which is carried on the red cells. Thus group A persons have A antigen on their red cells, group B have B antigens, group AB have both A and B antigens and group O have neither A nor B antigens.

A and B antigens have natural antibodies carried in the plasma known as anti-A and anti-B. Anti-A antibody will clump A red cells (and AB) causing a transfusion reaction. Similarly anti-B will clump B cells (and AB). Thus the main groups are made up as follows:

Group	Red cells (antigen)	Plasma (antibodies)
A	A	Anti-B
B	B	Anti-A
AB	A + B	O
O	O	Anti-A and Anti-B

The percentage of the population in the various blood groups is:

Group A	42.0 per cent	Group AB	3.0 per cent
Group B	8.5 per cent	Group O	46.5 per cent

The Rh system

There are six antigens involved in the rhesus blood group. The antigen most frequently involved in incompatibility and haemolysis is D, which is present in 85 per cent of the population. These people are known as rhesus-positive. The 15 per cent of people whose blood does not contain

D antigen are known as rhesus-negative. The main problem is the Rh-negative person who if given Rh-positive blood will come to no harm on the first occasion but will produce antibodies against antigen D, and further transfusion with Rh-positive blood will cause haemolysis.

Clarke and others have shown that the production of Rh antibodies in Rh-negative mothers by Rh-positive babies may be prevented by the injection, after the baby is born, of gammaglobulin containing high titres of antibodies active against the Rh-positive antigen of the foetus.

In addition to the main blood groups there are many rare sub-groups which because of their rarity may present great difficulties when blood has to be obtained for transfusion.

The patient's blood group is determined by reacting his red cells with a number of different sera, each containing a known antibody. If the red cells clump, or agglutinate, with a particular serum, then they contain the antigen corresponding with the antibody in that serum and vice versa. It can thus be concluded whether the patient's blood group is A, B, AB or O and whether it is Rh-positive or Rh-negative.

Cross matching of blood

It is important that the transfused blood (i.e. the donor blood) should be compatible with the recipient's blood (i.e. the patient's blood). The antibodies in the patient's plasma should not react with the antigens of the donor red cells, thus avoiding clumping or agglutination of the latter.

Cross-matching of blood is carried out to determine compatibility (i.e. to avoid incompatibility). The serum of the recipient is reacted in tubes against the red cells of the donor and the presence or absence of agglutination is noted. Agglutination must be absent for the bloods to be compatible.

To achieve the high degree of safety necessary in cross matching blood this test is checked under the microscope after 2 hours incubation in tubes.

In an emergency, where there is doubt as to a patient's blood group, it is necessary to cross match a unit of group O Rh-negative blood.

On the bag containing the blood is marked the group and the latest date for use. It is important that the blood should not be 'outdated' or haemolysed when given. Another important point is that the blood should not be taken out of the refrigerator more than half an hour before use and not over-heated.

Large transfusions of blood may cause citrate intoxication and after every 4 units (2 l) 10 ml 10 per cent calcium chloride should be injected intravenously. When blood is stored potassium leaks from the red blood cells into the anticoagulant. High levels of potassium may be present in older blood, thus making it unsuitable for transfusion into infants or babies.

Transfusion into the patient

Closed infusion is the usual method of transfusion (Fig. 12.5 and 12.6). The blood is given into the vein of the arm or, very rarely, into a vein of

Fig. 12.5 Blood transfusion using the standard gravity drip-giving set, with fine screen filter in use.

Fig. 12.6 Teflon cannula in the vein.

the leg. The arm is the more usual site because there are many more suitable veins and the patient's mobility is less inhibited.

Scalp vein drips. This is often the site used for transfusion in infants. An area of the scalp selected by the medical officer is shaved and a special fine scalp vein needle inserted into the vein. The needle with attached polythene tube is held in position with plaster of Paris.

In young children and babies a special drip set with a graduated burette is used to facilitate the accurate administration of small volumes of blood or other fluids.

The most important precaution to take in preparation for blood transfusion is to check that each bag of blood to be given to the patient is: (a) of the correct group for that patient; (b) that the cross-matching label on each bag bears the full name, date of birth and ward of the patient to whom it is to be given as well as his unit number; (c) that the expiry date on the bag has not been reached; (d) and that the cross-matching label attached to the bag matches the label on the bag. These checks should be done by two persons, one being a qualified nurse or a doctor.

Blood, like plasma, is not normally heated before use but when rapid transfusions are undertaken it is necessary to take measures to warm the blood. This is done by using some form of heating coil which is connected somewhere between the drip set and the patient. Suitable drip heaters set at body temperature are available for this purpose. Blood must never be heated in any other way.

The rate of blood flow is carefully regulated on the doctor's instructions by the clip on the delivering tube. The limb is lightly splinted. If the cannula slips out of the vein, blood escapes into the tissues and the patient complains of pain. The tube should be clipped off and the doctor summoned.

In blood transfusion, as in all intravenous injections, the tubing and other portions of the delivery apparatus must be free of air. Air embolism is the danger.

The drip may fail to run because:

(a) The vein is obstructed by too tight a bandage.
(b) The outlet of the cannula is against the wall of the vein. This is corrected by adjusting the position of the cannula and fixing it with adhesive strapping to the skin.
(c) The head of pressure is too low (corrected by elevating the container).
(d) The delivery tube is blocked. This can be tested by disconnecting the tube from the shaft of the cannula.
(e) Venospasm has occurred. This may be lessened by:
    (i) the injection by the doctor of 2 per cent procaine around the vein.
    (ii) keeping the patient's arm warm. Warmth dilates the vein and is permissible in this strictly localised area.

The drip that is running satisfactorily may stop because:

(a) The cannula has come out of the vein.
(b) The bag of blood was allowed to empty before it was changed.
(c) Blood has clotted in the cannula. The blood running into the patient will not clot because it contains an anticoagulant. The clotting occurs because the patient's blood has been allowed to be siphoned back into the cannula. This can be avoided when changing the bag by:
    (i) Clamping off the delivery tube as gently as possible.
    (ii) Turning off the drip set when changing units of blood.

Other difficulties which may arise are:

(a) *An airlock* which can be cleared by disconnecting the delivery tube from the cannula and running the blood through.
(b) *The drip-chamber becoming too full.* This difficulty can be overcome by turning off the drip and holding the bag upright, i.e. with the neck upwards. Gentle pressure on the drip chamber will cause air to re-enter this chamber.

Fine screen filters

It is now well established that microaggregates in stored blood contribute significantly to many cases of pulmonary insufficiency by blocking the pulmonary capillaries. These aggregates are not removed by the 170 micron filter supplied with standard blood administration sets. A fine screen filter e.g. 20 microns will remove the aggregates and should be used in the following situations:-

(a) Patients who are likely to require a transfusion of three or more units of blood.
(b) Major trauma, including chest trauma and multiple fractures.
(c) Major surgery.
(d) Major obstetric bleeding and surgery.

(e) Gastro-intestinal bleeding.
(f) Vascular surgery.
(g) Previous pulmonary disease.
(h) Patients who have had a febrile reaction during a previous blood transfusion.

Transfusion of blood under increased pressure

In some circumstances, usually of large rapid blood loss, it may be necessary to transfuse blood more quickly than is possible by the simple gravity drip method outlined above. This is achieved by increasing the pressure at which the blood is transfused. This should only be done by medical staff or under their direct supervision.

The following methods are available:

Pressure cuff. This is an inflatable cuff placed around the bag of blood. When inflated, by means of the attached bellows, it exerts external pressure on the bag of blood, thus increasing the flow of blood into the patient (Fig. 12.7).

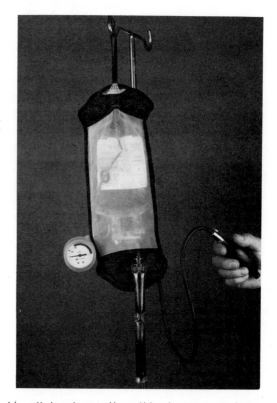

Fig. 12.7 Inflatable cuff placed around bag of blood to increase infusion pressure.

Pressure pump administration. Some transfusion giving sets permit either a gravity or pressure pump administration of blood (Fig. 12.8).

The inbuilt blood pump permits the rapid administration of blood. It is always there and obviates the necessity to set up ancillary pumping

Fig. 12.8 Baxter pressure transfusion set. Note self-sealing rubber (third left) to enable intravenous drugs to be given rapidly into the set.

equipment in an emergency. It eliminates the hazards of positive air pressure systems. It cannot pump air.

When pressure transfusion is required, the regulating clamp is closed and the lower (pump) chamber squeezed and then released so that it fills completely and so that the float occludes the inlet. The regulating clamp is opened and the pump chamber alternately squeezed and released, allowing it to fill completely between each action. Pumping action should be discontinued as soon as the container is empty. To return to gravity transfusion the bag is removed from the stand to the upright position and, by squeezing the pump chamber with tubing clamped off, the excess fluid is discharged back into the container. The bag is resuspended and the set tapped briskly to disperse any froth.

The Martin's pump (Fig. 12.9) is another type of pressure pump available in many hospitals for use when rapid transfusion is required. The pump is clamped to the drip-stand and the drip tubing is inserted into a grooved channel. Manual turning of the handle moves rollers against the tubing producing pressure to force blood into the vein.

Precautions during transfusion

Patients and transfusion apparatus must be kept under constant supervision during the entire period of the transfusion.

The medical officer must inform the nurse of the rate at which the transfusion is to be maintained. Forty drops per minute is the usual rate of transfusion, which means that a bag is transfused in four hours. Patients suffering from haemorrhage may need to be given transfusion at a much greater rate.

Sufferers from cardiac or pulmonary disease, and severely anaemic patients, must be transfused at a slow rate, sometimes as slow as 12 drops per minute. Packed cells may be used because of their smaller volume.

Fig. 12.9 Martin's pump.

When a transfusion is in progress half-hourly pulse and hourly temperature records are kept. If the transfusion is for shock the blood pressure and the pulse are recorded after each unit of blood.

Because stored blood contains large amounts of particulate debris, which if infused may cause pulmonary complications by collecting in the lungs, it is wise to insert a special filter into the transfusion system if large quantities of blood are likely to be used.

All patients should be watched for the symptoms of transfusion reactions (see below) after the first few millilitres of blood from each unit of blood. Immediate treatment should be given and the medical officer informed without delay.

Measurement of the central venous pressure may be of assistance in assessing the amount of blood required.

Procedure after transfusion

The details of the transfusion, with serial numbers of bags given and the time taken for the transfusion, must be entered in the case records. A note should be made of any untoward reactions.

The used blood bags, containing their residues of blood, should be kept in the ward (preferably in a refrigerator) for 24 hours. The small amount of blood remaining in each bag may be required in the investigation of transfusion reactions.

When 24 hours have elapsed after transfusion, the used bags should be disposed of by incineration. Any unused or partly used bags of blood which have been left at room temperature for one hour or more should be labelled 'dangerous for patients' and returned to the laboratory.

Complications of blood transfusion

1. *Allergic reactions* may occur in patients with a previous history of allergic reactions to transfusion or who have a history of asthma or similar allergic conditions. The reaction tends to occur after about 300 ml of blood have been given. There is no need to stop the transfusion. It is characterised by itching and urticaria. Intravenous antihistamine preparations will usually control it.

2. *Pyrexia* from pyrogens in the blood may occur. It is usually due to dirty apparatus and is very much rarer since fresh disposable apparatus has been used. Infected blood is another rare cause of pyrexia.

3. *Haemolysis* gives rise to rigors at an early stage. The transfusion should be stopped and Mannitol infused.

4. *Citrate intoxication* may manifest itself by an irregular slow pulse. After every fourth unit of blood 10 ml of 10 per cent calcium chloride is injected intravenously.

5. *Overloading* gives rise to signs of right heart failure. It is very rare if the transfusion is controlled by measurement of the central venous pressure.

6. *Transmission of infection* may occur of which the most important is serum hepatitis.

7. *Air embolism* is avoided by keeping air away from the lower portion of the drip chamber and beyond.

8. *Thrombophlebitis* is an occasional complication usually at or near the transfusion site.

9. *Renal failure* is usually caused by mismatched blood.

10. *Pulmonary complications* may arise (particularly after large amounts of unfiltered blood—see above).

After blood transfusion it is advisable to check the haemoglobin to ensure that the patient has received some benefit. Normally a unit of blood should raise the haemoglobin 1 g per dl. In some cases blood is rapidly destroyed and the patient receives little or no benefit from the transfusion.

Special problems of massive transfusions

The administration of large quantities of blood in a short period gives rise to two special types of problems—haemorrhagic manifestations and metabolic effects.

1. Haemorrhage. Bank blood stored for more than 24 hours contains no functioning platelets and almost no factor VIII (antihaemophilic) factor. A transfusion equal to the blood volume of the patient dilutes the number of circulating platelets and the amount of clotting factor. These are corrected if necessary by infusion of concentrated platelets and fresh frozen plasma.

2. Transfusion haemosiderosis. Patients receiving regular blood transfusions for chronic anaemia become iron-overloaded. A litre of blood contains 350 mg of iron while the normal excretion of iron is only 1 mg per day. Weatherall et al (1977) have shown that the amount of iron excreted can be increased to 70 to 120 mg by continuous infusion of desferrioxamine using a small portable pump over 12 hourly periods each week.

Clinical use of blood and blood products

Whole blood or some specially prepared constituent of blood may be used in clinical practice.

1. Whole blood is used for replacement in haemorrhage. The usual anticoagulant is citrate phosphate dextrose.

2. Concentrated red cells (packed cells) replace haemoglobin in anaemia without greatly increasing the circulatory volume.

3. Platelets prepared by concentrating the plasma after removal of the red cells may be used in thrombocytopenia.

4. Plasma replaces protein lost in burns and large wounds. Dried pooled plasma has been replaced by plasma protein fraction (PPF) which is supplied as a solution. Whereas dried plasma may transmit the virus of serum hepatitis, plasma protein fraction is heated to inactivate the virus.

5. Fresh frozen plasma (FFP) contains all the clotting factors and is invaluable in bleeding states with loss of coagulation factors.

6. Cryoprecipitate contains a high concentration of factor VIII. It is

used for treating patients with haemophilia. Freeze-dried factor VIII is given as soon as possible after bleeding. It arrests haemorrhage which relieves pain. If the patient is unable to give it intravenously himself a competent relative may be taught to administer it.

7. Fibrinogen is used in conditions of hypofibrinogenaemia such as occur in the defibrination syndrome.

8. Gammaglobulin is used for immunisation against such conditions as hepatitis.

3. FATE OF THE BLOOD LOST IN HAEMORRHAGE

At the beginning of this chapter it was noted that all the patient's problems may not be resolved when the bleeding ceases or the blood volume has been restored. In some haemorrhages the amount of blood loss is insignificant, but the actual blood lost is highly destructive in specialised tissues such as those of the eye or small but important areas of the brain or spinal cord. In body cavities such as the skull, the brain may be compressed by extravasated blood lying between the bone and the meninges or between the meninges and the brain. In the chest a large effusion of blood and blood clot may interfere with the action of the heart or lungs. In the pharynx, larynx or trachea, blood may seriously obstruct respiration and give rise to a lung infection including an abscess. In more disastrous circumstances the patient may die from flooding of the whole lung with inhaled blood.

Terms to describe extravasated collections of blood are:

1. *Petechiae* or purpura—tiny pinpoint haemorrhages from capillary damage.
2. *An ecchymosis*—a small area of skin bruising.
3. *Haematoma*—a sealed collection of blood and clot. It may be sealed beneath:
    (a) a wound.
    (b) a tissue such as the periosteum (subperiosteal) or beneath the capsule of an organ (subcapsular).
    (c) a tear of a soft organ such as the spleen or liver.

Complications of a haematoma are:

(a) infection—'stale blood' is an ideal medium for the growth of organisms.
(b) rupture—in large haematomas profuse internal 'delayed' haemorrhage may result.

HAEMORRHAGE FROM SPECIAL SITES

The occurrence of haemorrhage from special sites is designated by special terms.

Epistaxis—bleeding from the nose.
Haemoptysis—the expectoration of blood from the lungs.
Haematemesis—vomiting of blood.

Melaena—the passage of dark blood per rectum from a site high in the intestinal tract.

Haematuria—blood in the urine.

Haemothorax—bleeding into the chest.

Haemoperitoneum—bleeding into the peritoneum.

Haemarthrosis—bleeding into a joint.

Menorrhagia—excessive menstruation at normal intervals.

Metrostaxis—(metrorrhagia)—excessive, irregular or continuous bleeding per vaginam between the periods.

Haemopericardium—bleeding into the pericardium. This may cause cardiac tamponade.

Haematomyelia—bleeding into the spinal cord.

BIBLIOGRAPHY

Allison D J 1978 British Journal of Hospital Medicine 20: 707.
Machin A 1979 British Journal of Hospital Medicine 21: 294.
Weatherall D J, Pippard M J, Callender S T 1977 New England Journal of Medicine 297: 445 (Editorial).

13

Shock

DEFINITION

The supply of oxygen to the tissues is the first essential in the maintenance of life, and this can only be ensured when the circulatory system is functioning normally. Shock is defined as a failure of the circulation to adequately supply the tissues with oxygen.

CAUSES

The circulation may fail from:

1. Sudden malfunction of the heart. This may occur as a result of:
(a) *Coronary arterial occlusion* with acute myocardial ischaemia.
(b) *Trauma* with structural damage to the heart.
(c) *Toxaemia*—bacterial or viral.
(d) *Effect* of drugs.

Complete cardiac arrest is the most urgent of all conditions, and death is an inevitable sequel unless the heart can be restored within three minutes. External cardiac massage (ECM) may be the only hope, and is discussed in detail at the end of this chapter. In certain arrhythmias such as ventricular fibrillation, a defibrillator is required.

2. Deficient oxygenation of the blood in the lungs. Amongst the many causes the following are the most important surgically:
(a) *Postoperative atelectasis* (collapse of a large segment of lung) and pneumonia.
(b) *Thoracic injuries,* particularly 'stove in' chest, tension pneumothorax, bruising and laceration of the lungs (Ch. 30).
(c) *Obstruction of the pulmonary artery by an embolus.* If it is complete sudden death occurs.
(d) *Disturbances of lung function* following surgery and anaesthesia.

The complicated issues involved in this form are discussed in the chapters on Respiratory Failure and Diseases of the Lungs and Chest Wall.

3. Reduction in the blood volume (oligaemia or hypovolaemia). This may occur from loss of:
(a) *Whole blood*—haemorrhage (external or internal).
(b) *Plasma.* This is particularly significant in burns.

(c) *Water and electrolytes*, which occurs in (i) peritonitis, (ii) intestinal obstruction and paralytic ileus, (iii) acute dilatation of the stomach, and (iv) severe diarrhoea and vomiting.

4. Septic shock. This is a complex process involving both depression of the heart and loss of fluid from the circulation into body tissues. The fluid loss is due to capillary leakage and may give rise to oedema.

5. Miscellaneous. There are a number of other conditions that may lead to a shocked state with low blood pressure.

(a) *The common faint.* The arterioles in the muscles relax.

(b) *Acute anaphylaxis (p. 64).*

(c) *Acute adrenal deficiency (Addison's disease)* due in part to salt and water loss.

(d) *Overdosage of drugs, for example, analgesics like pethidine.*

(e) *Following therapy with beta-blocking agents (for angina, hypertension, etc.).*

(f) *Noxious stimuli* such as pain will, if sufficiently severe, cause vasodilatation, particularly of the splanchnic vessels with 'pooling' of blood in the area. This is the mechanism of primary or neurogenic shock. It is a condition of short duration because either the patient dies immediately or recovers spontaneously if the causal stimulus is removed or severe pain is relieved; otherwise it passes into 'secondary' oligaemic shock.

Clinical causes

A. *Hypovolaemia*

(a) Haemorrhage—internal e.g. multiple fractures
ruptured spleen or liver
bleeding peptic ulcer
—external e.g. large scalp wounds
compound fractures
lacerated artery

(b) Severe burns

(c) Peritonitis from perforated viscus.

B. *Cardiogenic*

(d) Myocardial infarction

(e) Pulmonary embolism

C. *Mixed type*

(f) Septicaemia

(g) Adrenal failure

(h) Severe pain

COMPENSATORY MECHANISMS

Whatever the cause of sudden collapse there are certain compensatory physiological mechanisms which occur.

1. Posture. A patient in acute circulatory failure falls down. He should be left flat or, better, kept in the head-down position to an angle of 5°. This helps to supply more blood to the brain but an angle of more than 5° is harmful because it causes venous congestion. The best position is with the head flat and the legs raised.

2. Contraction of the skin vessels. Contraction of the arterioles and venules of the skin is usual so as to conserve the blood supply to the more vital centres. The application of heat dilates the skin vessels, thereby aggravating the condition, and should not be used.

3. Insensitivity. A very collapsed patient usually has little pain. Large quantities of pain-relieving drugs are unnecessary and, in any case, are ineffective because they cannot be absorbed unless given by the intravenous route. Administered subcutaneously they may result in cumulative overdosage as the circulation recovers. Because the shocked patient is insensitive his skin is more easily damaged, so he has to be handled very gently.

4. Urinary secretion is diminished to conserve fluid in the body, but it is also a sign that tissue perfusion (the circulation of blood through the kidney and other tissues) is inadequate.

5. The heart rate accelerates in most forms of circulatory failure with the important exception of the common faint. It is an attempt to ensure that the remaining fluid is circulated as rapidly as possible, thereby providing sufficient oxygen to the tissues.

6. The temperature is subnormal. This reduces the requirements of the tissues for the diminishing amount of oxygen available. The core temperature may actually be raised. The difference between the two is a measure of the degree of shock.

All these compensatory factors are temporary in their beneficial effects and, if the condition of the circulation is not restored to normal without delay, irreversible changes set in.

CLINICAL ASPECTS OF SHOCK

Clinical appearance of patient

The face is ashen pale and expressionless. The eyes are still and the patient takes little or no interest in his surroundings, although he may answer, slowly, questions which are asked. He may make no complaint of pain.

The skin is cold, white, and clammy.

Respiration is rapid and shallow.

The pulse is usually rapid and weak, although sometimes it is below normal in rate.

The most constant and important finding is a *low systolic and diastolic blood pressure.*

If septicaemia is suspected, a blood culture is performed.

Clinical management

The **aim of treatment** is to restore normal tissue perfusion. Of the many disturbances which occur in shock, oligaemia is the one best understood and most easily remedied. Its control requires observation of:

1. The blood pressure. The reversal of hypotension is in itself an unreliable sign unless accompanied by reversal of the other signs of oligaemia.

Taking the blood pressure. The patient should be at rest lying in bed. The sleeve of the gown/jacket is rolled back or removed as necessary. The arm is extended and supported. The cuff of the sphygmomanometer is wrapped firmly and smoothly round the upper arm well above the elbow flexure. The manometer is placed level with the patient's arm, the scale being visible to the nurse. It is connected to the cuff. The nurse palpates the radial/brachial pulse, she inflates the cuff and notes the point on the manometer at which the pulse disappears. (N.B. Care should be taken to avoid discomfort to the patient by the cuff being overinflated or inflated for too long a time.) The cuff is deflated. She adjusts the ear pieces of the stethoscope, and places the other end over the brachial pulse (artery). The cuff is reinflated to above the previously noted point on the manometer. It is slowly deflated. When a tapping sound is heard, the nurse notes the point on the manometer—this gives the systolic pressure. As the cuff is deflated further, the sounds become louder, suddenly they change to a muffled sound, and then cease altogether. The point at which the sound changes from loud to muffled is noted—this gives the diastolic pressure. The manometer is disconnected. The cuff is removed and folded away into the manometer box. The patient is made comfortable.

The result is charted immediately, e.g.

BP $\dfrac{120}{80}$ or filled in on a chart (Fig. 13.1)

Any significant change from previous recordings is reported to the nurse in charge. When there is difficulty in hearing the sounds or in obtaining the readings the nurse in charge should be asked to help.

2. The heart rate is rapid in shock. The pulse is felt first at the wrist (radial). If this is poorly felt, as may occur in shock, then the carotid or femoral pulse should be felt. In hypovolaemic shock, when the circulating volume is restored, the pulse becomes stronger and less rapid (Fig. 13.1).

3. Urinary output. The production of urine reflects the flow of blood through the kidney. In shock or hypovolaemia the kidney will produce only small volumes of concentrated urine and, if prolonged, may fail to produce any urine at all. In severe cases the assessment of urine production will require an indwelling catheter and hourly measurement of urine volume. Urine flow should be maintained at about 50 ml/hour or above. The measurement of specific gravity of the urine will assess the ability to concentrate, which is an important function of the kidney.

Urine output is an indirect guide to the adequacy of perfusion of other organs.

4. The central venous pressure. This is a useful guide to the effective

| Surname | ATKINSON | | | | | | | | | | | | | | | | | | | | | | Unit No. | 7 |

| First names | JAMES ROBERT | | | | | | | | | | | | | | | | | | | | | Ward | 29 |

Fig. 13.1 Pulse, blood pressure and central venous pressure chart. The arterial blood pressure is measured in mm. Hg., the C.V.P. in cms. of water.

circulating volume. It may be measured by inserting a cannula into one of the great veins—preferably the superior vena cava. This is normally done via the veins at the elbow, the neck veins (internal jugular) or the subclavian veins at the root of the neck. When correctly sited there is free rise and fall, of fluid in the attached manometer, with respiration. Before using the line to administer any fluids a chest X-ray should be taken to confirm the site of the cannula and exclude complications. The greatest complication is collapse of the lung due to pneumothorax. The cannula must be fixed when measurements are not being made and continuous infusion should be maintained to keep it patent.

The cannula is connected to a special venous pressure measuring drip set (Fig. 13.2).

This is distinguished by having a long side-arm. It is provided with a centimetre scale. In use, the side-arm is filled with fluid and is then connected to the patient's venous system. The level above the manubri-

Solution bottle

Cotton air filter

Self-adhesive monometer tape
(centimetre scale)

Tape

Stopcock

FLO-TROL clamp

Fig. 13.2 The estimation of central venous pressure using a special Baxter drip set.

um sternum at which the fluid in the side-arm comes to rest is a measure of the central venous pressure. In the normal subject the value will be from 0 to 2 or 3 cm of water.

In the shocked or hypovolaemic patient it will be negative while in patients who are in heart failure or who have been overtransfused it may be very high (10 to 25 cm of water).

5. Temperature and temperature gradient. Observations of differences between the peripheral skin temperature and the rectal temperature (measured by electrical thermometers) are helpful in estimating the peripheral circulation. If the temperature in the rectum and on the surface of the big toe are recorded and it is found that the big toe temperature drops or fails to rise, then all is not well. It is an even finer guide than urinary excretion to the state of tissue perfusion.

6. Expansion of the circulatory volume until it is adequate as shown by reversal of the signs of failure. This remains the most hopeful method of treatment whatever the metabolic disturbance, since restoration of normal tissue perfusion is essential.

Drugs and other specific treatment

1. *Fluids* must be administered intravenously to restore the circulating volume.
2. *Electrolyte imbalance* must be corrected.
3. *Oxygen lack* is corrected by administration with nasal spectacles or mask.
4. *Correction of acidosis.* A solution of 8.4 per cent sodium bicarbonate may be advisable and arterial blood-gas estimations are of value in making this decision.
5. *Vasodilators* may be of value after the blood volume has been restored

on the basis that prolonged splanchnic vasoconstriction (constriction of the arteries to the stomach and intestine) causes irreversible changes. Phenoxybenzamine has been reported to be of value as has isoprenaline which has a direct inotropic effect as well as being a vasodilator.

6. *Diuretics.* Mannitol (a 6-carbon sugar) is an osmotic diuretic which is neither absorbed in the renal tubules nor metabolised. It may be given when acidosis and oligaemia have been corrected but if oliguria persists frusemide may also be given. If diuresis does not occur within half an hour of 40 mg of frusemide being given severe renal damage has occurred and the intake of fluid may have to be restricted on this account.

7. *Dopamine* by low dose infusion is sometimes used to improve the blood pressure.

8. *Antibiotics* are essential if a bacterial element is present.

9. *Anticoagulants* may occasionally be indicated if microcirculatory thrombosis is suspected.

10. *Hydrocortisone* 100 mg or more in the infusion may be effective. It probably acts by stabilisation of the cell membranes.

11. *Analgesics* are rarely necessary until the patient's condition has been restored.

Internal haemorrhage from a ruptured organ may occur so rapidly that the risk of operating on a patient suffering from shock has to be accepted. Rapid transfusion should be performed until the haemorrhage has been controlled surgically and continued until the blood volume has been restored. The shorter the period the patient is collapsed, with a low blood pressure, anoxia and loss of tissue perfusion, the better, otherwise there is a risk of irreversible damage to the kidneys, the liver, and the brain, especially in the elderly.

Whatever the cause of circulatory collapse the following general principles evolve:

1. Treatment must be instituted without delay and continued until the condition has been reversed.

2. In difficult cases, where the response is slow or inadequate, the diagnosis of the cause may have to be revised.

3. Once the patient's condition has improved every precaution must be taken to see that shock does not recur. Observations on the pulse, temperature, the colour and state of the skin, and urinary output are important. Examination of the blood and urine should be continued and the return to a sitting-up position should be instituted gradually and observantly.

THE PREVENTION OF SHOCK

Preoperative measures

Circulatory collapse should be avoided by strenuous measures if at all possible. Preoperatively the patient should be as fit as possible, and from the point of view of the circulatory system:

Fig. 13.3 Trendelenburg position.

1. His blood should be adequate in quality and in volume.
2. His tissues should be adequately hydrated.
3. He should be mobile so that there is no stagnation in the circulatory system.

Perioperative measures

Every operation is an injury, but operative trauma differs from all other injuries in that the surgeon and nursing staff know its nature in advance. Further, we know the early signs of circulatory collapse.

1. The patient is kept warm on his journey from the ward to the theatre and back. Blankets should be warmed. Fear is allayed and tranquillising drugs are commonly used preoperatively.

2. The blood pressure is recorded, and in serious cases monitored continuously. Blood and fluid replacement should be commenced in good time. Major operations are commenced only after satisfactory infusions have been established.

3. The head of the table is lowered if the blood pressure falls (the Trendelenburg position), shown in Figure 13.3.

4. The anaesthetist induces and maintains an adequate level of anaesthesia ensuring good oxygenation and tissue perfusion.

The blood pressure and pulse rate are recorded regularly, together with drugs and fluids administered.

Postoperative measures

1. Postoperatively, fluid and electrolyte replacement (saline, 5 per cent, dextrose, Hartman's solution, plasma or blood as indicated), rest and relief from pain are continued.

2. Gentle handling of the patient by the nursing staff is very important in the prevention of shock.

There are few conditions in which a patient can improve or deteriorate so rapidly as in circulatory failure. Its treatment calls for the best organisation of the resources of a hospital and the most painstaking care from the nursing staff.

CARDIAC ARREST

The signs of cardiac arrest are:
1. Sudden collapse and the onset of unconsciousness.
2. Cessation of the heart beat—no palpable pulses.
3. Cessation of breathing—severe cyanosis.
4. Dilated pupils.

Fig. 13.4   External cardiac compression.

Fig. 13.5   Electrocardiograph. Normal tracing showing P Q R S and T waves.

Fig.13.6   Sinus rhythm going into ventricular fibrillation.

The interval between 'clinical death' which occurs with cessation of the heart beat and respiration and biological death is 3 to 5 minutes. This may be prolonged by:

1. Cardiac massage (external cardiac compression).
2. Hypothermia.
3. Extracorporeal circulation with artificial oxygenator.

Sudden stoppage of the heart requires immediate action on the part of the nursing staff, because after three minutes of cessation of blood flow to the cerebrum, cerebral damage is permanent and irreversible.

The alarm should be raised and the cardiac arrest team summoned. Ventilation of the lungs should be established at once. An unobstructed airway is essential. Teeth, vomitus and debris should be cleared, the neck extended and the jaw pulled forward. In the absence of equipment expired air ventilation using the mouth to mouth or mouth to nose method should be employed. If available a bag and mask may be used to ventilate with air or oxygen. The lungs should be inflated 3 to 5 times and then, if no pulses are felt, external cardiac massage started.

This may be performed by the nurse while another nurse continues mouth to mouth breathing simultaneously. The patient is laid flat on a firm surface (a mattress is too soft), a fracture board on a bed will do, and regular manual compression is exerted against the lower sternum at a rate of 60 times per minute (Fig. 13.4). Properly performed it can be a very exhausting procedure. The rib cage may be damaged. A machine has been designed for the purpose but it is not generally available. The patient's legs should be slightly elevated to aid venous return. As soon as medical assistance arrives an endotracheal tube is passed to ensure and maintain an unobstructed airway.

As soon as possible an ECG machine should be attached to the patient in order to establish which type of heart rhythm is present (Figs. 13.5 and 13.6). An intravenous infusion should be set up and a sample of heparinised arterial blood is sent for blood gas analysis. 100 mmol sodium bicarbonate should be infused.

Solutions of 1 in 10 000 adrenaline and 10 per cent calcium chloride should be immediately available for intravascular injection.

Cardiac arrest produces a severe metabolic acidosis and solutions of sodium bicarbonate will need to be infused before satisfactory cardiac action can be restored.

The provision of a cardiac arrest resuscitation trolley is now a regular feature in many blocks of wards. In addition to an oxygen cylinder with a regulator it should be furnished as follows:

Top shelf—

Ambu foot sucker
Suction catheters size 16
Suction catheters size 14
Ambu-type bag with oxygen line
Airway no. 3
Airway no. 2
7 mm endotracheal tube
8 mm endotracheal tube
9 mm endotracheal tube
20 ml syringe

Catheter mount
Ryle's tube
Laryngoscope
Tube KY jelly
Spencer Wells
Brook airway
Roll of Blenderm
3 in. No. 9 drain

Lower shelf—

Baxter intravenous set + meal hook
200 ml polyfusor sodium bic. 8.4%
500 ml dextrose 5%
Cut down set
Medicut cannulae 18g
Medicut cannulae 16g
12 cm 14 or 16g cannulae
(for internal jugular line)
Three-way taps
20 ml syringe
5 ml syringes
23 g needles
21 g needles
19 g needles

21 g butterfly
19 g butterfly
Mediswabs
Greengauze swabs
Ethilon 320
Plain 439
Ethilon 795
22 g surgical blade
15 g surgical blade
Roll of Blenderm
5 in. filling tubes

Fig. 13.7   Tray of drugs ready for rapid use in cardiac arrest.

Because every second is vital a 'cardiac arrest drug tray' (Fig. 13.7) should be in readiness and each compartment *boldly* labelled so that no time is wasted.

If ventricular fibrillation is present an electrical defibrillator will be required to administer an electric shock to restore normal rhythm.

Observations which should be made whilst the patient is receiving treatment are:

1. Feel for the pulse in the groin. If the circulation is maintained the pulse will be palpable.
2. Note if the pupils constrict. The pupils always dilate with circulatory arrest.
3. ECG will show activity.
4. Arterial blood gas analysis.

Aftercare. If normal cardiac function is restored these patients should be treated in an intensive care unit and be carefully monitored.

ECG control for 24 to 48 hours is desirable. Occasionally measures to reduce cerebral oedema are necessary. Renal failure may follow a period of hypotension.

A useful aid to memory in the sudden emergency of the management of cardiac arrest is:

A Airway
B Breathing
C Cardiac compression
D Drugs and drip
E Electricity—ECG machine and a defibrillator.

14

Fluid, electrolyte balance and surgical nutrition

The method and forms of administration of fluid together with its complications are discussed in Chapter 15. Since fluid and electrolyte balance is a subject of great complexity and much still requires to be known, this separation is deliberate. The present discussion is a subject for the senior student.

Before abnormal states are considered an outline of the normal processes is essential.

THE FLUID

Water is the basis of all body fluids. The total quantity of body water is approximately 42 litres. This represents about 60 per cent of body weight and varies with build (a lower percentage in the obese) and age. It is divided into (Fig. 14.1):

1. Water inside the cells (intracellular water), 30 litres
2. Extracellular water, 12 litres.
   of which:
   (a) the plasma constitutes 3 litres (intravascular)
   (b) the water in the tissue spaces 9 litres (interstitial).

The intracellular water is the fluid in which the essentials of nourishment are consumed and metabolites accumulate. The water in the tissue spaces is outside the blood stream and outside the cells. Its electrolyte composition is almost identical with that of blood plasma.

Examination of the various substances in the plasma will provide information about the composition of the fluid in the tissue spaces, but it will not tell us what the position is inside the cells.

THE ELECTROLYTES

An electrolyte is a substance which when dissolved in water splits (dissociates or ionises is the correct expression) into electrically charged particles known as ions (ion, Greek = wanderer). Each electrolyte splits

Fig. 14.1 Composition of the body.

into an equal number of positively (+) charged ions (known as cations) and negatively (−) charged ions (known as anions).

In food an electrolyte is consumed as an independent substance, for example, common salt. To be an independent substance, which can be seen and handled, it must exist in molecular form as NaCl (its chemical formula) but in the body it exists as Na^+ (sodium ions) and Cl^- (chloride ions). Because electrolytes exist as particles, they used to be measured in terms which expressed their biological activity, namely milliequivalents per litre (mEq/l) but in the international system (SI) are now expressed in terms of their molecular weight as millimoles per litre (mmol/l).

The principal electrolytes are sodium (Na^+), potassium (K^+), chloride (Cl^-) and bicarbonate (HCO_3^-). There are many others like calcium, magnesium, phosphate, and sulphate.

Distribution of electrolytes

The extracellular and intracellular fluids show a marked difference in concentration of electrolytes. The most striking are:

1. Potassium (K^+) is the dominant cation inside the cell. Its concentration is about 144 mmol per litre against 8 mmol per litre for intracellular sodium (Na^+).

2. Sodium (Na^+) is largely concentrated in the extracellular fluid and plasma with a concentration of 140 mmol per litre against 5 mmol per litre for that of potassium (K^+).

Normal metabolism tends to a production of an excess of anions over cations in the blood with the result that there is a tendency to acidosis. This state of affairs is corrected in health by the production of an acid urine. The glomeruli of the kidneys filter 170 l of fluid from the blood in 24 hours, but 168.5 l are reabsorbed by the tubules allowing 1.5 l to be passed as urine.

NORMAL CONTROL OF WATER AND ELECTROLYTES

The facts described below are illustrated in Figure 14.2.

Intake or gain is by mouth, followed by absorption from the gut.
Excretion or loss is from:

1. *Extrarenal sources*—the skin, respiration, and faeces. This amounts to about 1 l per day.
2. *The kidneys.* Five hundred millilitres of water is the minimum in which a healthy kidney can excrete the body's metabolites. The daily amount is, therefore, this quantity in addition to fluids consumed in excess of 1.5 l.

Renal control

For the kidney to function adequately it must have:

1. An intact blood supply and the blood must be supplied at adequate pressure. Its blood vessels must be intact to filter the enormous quantity of 170 l per day. In any condition of *hypotension* the mechanism fails. In acute nephritis the glomeruli are swollen and diseased so that they allow blood to pass into the urine. In chronic nephritic conditions the glomeruli are inadequate in number and structure.

2. **Normal acting tubules.** To function normally and concentrate the

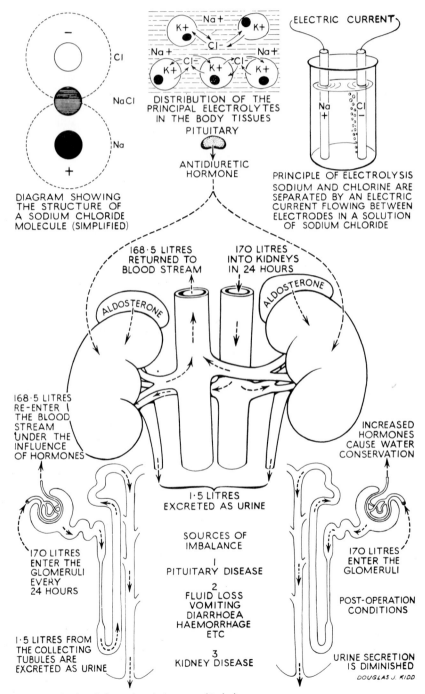

Fig. 14.2 Fluid and electrolyte balance and imbalance.

glomerular filtrate from 170 to 1.5 l the tubules must be intact. More than this, they are under the control of hormones, viz:

(a) *The antidiuretic hormone of the pituitary.* If this is inadequate in amount the glomerular fluid is not concentrated and large quantities of water are lost. The condition known as diabetes insipidus in which a vast quantity of pale urine is passed is an extreme example of this failure. Pitressin by injection or by 'snuff' controls the condition.

(b) *Aldosterone.* This is a hormone which is secreted in the adrenal cortex and increases the reabsorption of sodium (Na^+) from the filtrate. This is present in large quantities in the blood and hence also in the glomerular filtrate.

Estimation of electrolytes

Electrolyte estimations are determined by the laboratory on specimens of plasma from blood which has been collected in tubes containing lithium heparin. Care must be taken not to haemolyse the specimen by using a wet syringe, spirit, shaking the blood or squirting it through a fine needle. If the red cells rupture (haemolysis) they liberate enormous amounts of potassium into the plasma and render this determination valueless.

THE METABOLIC RESPONSE TO INJURY

When a patient is injured, using injury in the widest sense and including bacterial infection and surgical operation, the two hormones acting on the renal tubules are excreted in excess. This is a physiological protective mechanism. The result is:
1. Water is conserved in the body. It is an everyday observation that in the first 24 to 48 hours postoperatively there is oliguria.
2. Sodium (Na^+) and chloride (Cl^-) are conserved in the body and not excreted in the urine.
3. Potassium (K^+) is lost in the urine. Potassium increases in the blood from the breakdown of cells, which is just what occurs in trauma.

The kidney allows potassium (K^+) to pass more freely, since potassium in excess is lethal, but gross lack, too, can be serious.

Once the blood volume has been restored, that is, once circulatory failure has been adequately treated, further fluid in the 24 hours postoperatively is unnecessary and may be harmful.

PATHOLOGICAL STATES

Depletions of fluid and electrolytes rarely occur in 'pure' forms. Sodium and water depletions, except in conditions like miner's cramp (where water has been taken without salt), usually occur together.

Sodium

Depletion occurs in:
1. Vomiting.
2. Gastric aspiration.
3. Intestinal obstruction.
4. Addison's disease.

The clinical features are those of 'dehydration', namely a dry tongue, dry wrinkled skin, sunken eyes, and a rapid, weak pulse.

It is corrected by adequate quantities of isotonic saline.

Retention is due to deficiency in the mechanism of elimination and is common in oedematous conditions. In addition, drugs such as cortisone, testosterone and stilboestrol tend to cause retention. The treatment is restriction of salt and fluid intake and the use of diuretics.

Potassium

Depletion occurs in any illness in which there has been prolonged discharge like a fistula, paralytic ileus, or severe diarrhoea.

The clinical picture is one of apathy, drowsiness, loss of muscle power. The electrocardiogram shows characteristic changes.

The treatment is the administration of potassium salts.

They must always be given with caution and, if by the intravenous route, very slowly. There must be an adequate urinary output (at least 500 ml) before they are given at all.

Excess is particularly dangerous and is usually due to failure of elimination by the kidney. It occurs in conditions of:

Uraemia

Acidosis

The treatment is that of anuria (Ch. 42).

Fluid requirements

The amount of fluid the patient requires is:

Extrarenal loss	1000 ml
Add urinary loss	
Add pathological loss:	
1. Aspiration	
2. Fistula	
3. Drainage	
4. Diarrhoea	

Total fluid required in 24 hours

Fluid balance charts may be quite simple and all fluid must be measured in millilitres and totalled every 12 hours. The precise type of fluid to be given is determined by the clinical condition and the nature of the fluid lost. The state of the blood chemistry is only a rough guide in treatment and by no means helpful as a constant check. The more important normal levels are:

Serum	mmol/l
Na^+	136–144
K^+	3.4–5.0
Cl^-	95–105

Solutions

The more important solutions used in maintaining or correcting fluid and electrolyte balance are:

1. *Sodium chloride* (0.9 per cent)—Isotonic saline. Replaces Na^+ and Cl^-.
   154 mmol Na^+ and 154 mmol Cl^- in a litre.
2. *Glucose* (5 per cent)—Isotonic.
   Replaces water.
3. *Hypertonic saline*
   Replaces Na^+ and Cl^- without water.
   Hypertonic saline (1.8 per cent) contains
   154 mmol Na^+
   154 mmol Cl^- } in 500ml.
4. *Potassium*—5 ml 20 per cent pot. chloride w/v (13.5 mmol of K^+). Added to 500 ml glucose (5 per cent).
   Replaces K^+.
5. *Compound sodium lactate solution injection BP* (formerly known as Hartman's solution)—Na^+ 131 mmol/l, Cl^- 111 mmol/l, K^+ 5 mmol/l and calcium lactate.
   Replaces Na^+, K^+, Cl^-, and corrects acidosis.

THE MAINTENANCE OF NUTRITION

The maintenance of a good nutritional state presents a problem in patients who are unable to take ordinary diets by mouth. For short periods in patients who start off fit the problem is not important, as long as fluid and electrolyte balance is attended to, but the longer the inability to eat continues the more important it becomes. The patients particularly affected are long term respiratory cases, head injuries, laryngopharyngeal operations and cases of major abdominal surgery complicated by ileus, fistulae or sepsis.

The daily dietary requirements of the normal adult are:

Protein	80–100g (provides 13–16.25g of nitrogen)
Carbohydrates	400–500g
Fats	80g
Sodium	2–5g
Potassium	2–5g
Calcium	1g

Trace elements—iodine, copper, manganese, zinc, phosphorus and fluoride.

Calorie requirements 2500–3000 per day.

Nitrogen balance. A minimum of 40g of protein (6.59 g of nitrogen) is necessary to repair the normal breakdown of protein tissues in health. If the intake is below this level the individual is said to be in negative nitrogen balance and protein is mobilised from the body tissues which become wasted. A negative balance of 62.59 g of protein (equal to 10 g of nitrogen) causes a loss of 300 g of muscle. The estimation of the urinary nitrogen is a guide to the patient's requirements but if he has a fistula a further allowance is added for this source of protein loss.

Many diseases, including burns and septic states, produce a hypercatabolic state with increased energy and protein requirements. To ensure that protein is used to rebuild the tissues and not wasted as an energy source the ratio of calories to protein should be about 200 calories per gram of nitrogen, e.g. 20 g of nitrogen to 400 calories.

Folic acid and phosphate are vital ingredients in the catabolic patient and in addition trace elements may be added when intravenous feeding is prolonged. Magnesium, which is necessary for enzyme formation, may have to be given but most trace element deficiencies can be corrected by blood transfusions.

Methods of feeding

Two methods of feeding other than by mouth are available:

1. Intravenous

Solutions of 50 per cent, 20 per cent and 10 per cent dextrose are available as are aminoacid solutions and fat emulsions. These, together with vitamins and trace elements, enable a diet of carbohydrate, protein and fat to be administered. A wide variety of solutions, excepting the fat emulsions, are available, and there are arguments about which solution is likely to be of the greatest benefit, dependent upon its aminoacid formulation. The use of a carbohydrate source other than dextrose has been discarded.

The precise structure of an intravenous feeding regime will depend upon many factors but should include adequate sources of dextrose, protein and fat. Vitamins, folic acid, trace elements and electrolytes will need to be added. These solutions (except the fat emulsion) are hyperosmolar and irritant to small veins. Therefore their use necessitates central venous cannulation.

Finally the use of blood plasma as a means of restoring plasma proteins should not be forgotten. It may be used in above normal concentrations for this purpose.

Indwelling venous cannulae are an important cause of hospital acquired septicaemia which is frequent after cannulation of the large veins when this route is used for feeding. Sepsis is more frequent if blood is withdrawn through the cannula. If infection is to be kept to a minimum it must be used for no purpose other than to administer parenteral nutrition (Ryan 1974).

2. By gastric tube

While the recent innovations in intravenous feeding have produced satisfactory methods they still involve intravenous infusions which have many hazards (upsets of fluid balance—infection—thrombosis of vessels). They are also extremely expensive. Therefore intragastric feeding has become popular for any patient who is unable to take oral food, but who has an intact and functioning gut. In this form of feeding a tube is passed via the oesophagus into the stomach and 60 ml of water are put down it hourly until it is established that the stomach is emptying normally. Then fluid diet is passed into the stomach at appropriate intervals—usually 2, 3 or 4 hourly or by a continuous drip.

Diets may be made up of eggs, milk, protein, hydrolysates and sugar, but unless great care is taken these tend to cause intractable diarrhoea.

A satisfactory method is to take the ordinary ward meals, complete with bread, butter and fish and chips not forgetting the salt and the sugar in the tea, and put it all into a liquidiser together with an appropriate amount of water. The resultant thin gruel is then passed down the intragastric tube using a funnel. Three main feeds a day (or more if required) may be given. Volumes of 300 ml per feed are acceptable to most patients. Additional in-between feeds of fluids will bring the total fluid intake up to 2.5 to 3 litres. Following severe trauma this method may fail to supply the very high calorie requirements of such patients. If this is so, intravenous feeding will have to be used.

Tube feeding should proceed very cautiously until it is established that it is well tolerated. Unless the mixture is maintained at an osmolarity of 300 ml/l severe diarrhoea may result. In all forms of artificial feeding a fluid balance chart is kept and daily serum electrolyte estimation undertaken.

Alternatively the longer arm of a double barrelled nasogastric tube can be threaded into the small intestine at operation and the patient fed from the first postoperation day.

Preformulated liquid diets

Powders made up with water or liquids, containing protein, fat, carbohydrate, vitamins and trace elements which are administered orally or via a nasogastric tube are available. They supply all the daily nutritional requirements and are easily absorbed. They are particularly useful in patients with intestinal fistulae who need nutrition with no residue.

BIBLIOGRAPHY

Ryan J A et al 1974 New England Journal of Medicine 290: 757

15
Fluid administration

The administration of fluids is amongst the most arduous tasks the nurse can undertake. The safest and simplest route of all is by drinking. This requires:

A cooperative conscious patient

A normal alimentary tract

Adequate renal function.

In these circumstances no real problem arises although occasionally gentle persuasion is required. Fluids consumed by drinking are absorbed in the lower small intestine and proximal colon, and normal excretion occurs from the kidney.

There are two main routes by which fluids may be given:

1. Enteral (by the gut). This includes:

(a) Drinking.

(b) By nasogastric tube; the lower end of the tube is in the body of the stomach.

(c) By gastrostomy or jejunostomy.

2. Parenteral (by the side of the gut—which means that the fluid does not traverse the intestinal mucous membrane to reach the circulation). The fluids are administered intravenously.

ENTERAL ADMINISTRATION

Drinking

Provided the patient is conscious the nurse can do much to increase the intake if this is desirable, but she must never attempt to pour fluid into the mouth of a patient whose cough reflex is absent. It will flow into the lungs with disastrous effects.

Nasogastric tube

This may be used for a patient who has difficulty in co-operating but it is essential to ensure that the tube is in the stomach (and not coiled in the mouth or trachea) prior to feeding. This is done by aspirating a small amount before the feed and testing it with litmus paper which will turn red to indicate the presence of acid.

Gastrostomy and jejunostomy

Gastrostomy is performed in the management of infants with oesophageal atresia. A temporary jejunostomy is a little commoner. The advantage is that a wider variety of nourishment may be given than is possible by parenteral routes.

The jejunum will absorb large quantities of fluid which have been withdrawn by gastric or duodenal suction, but the extra volume of fluid which can be given should be limited to 1500 ml in 24 hours. The best method of feeding is by a continuous intrajejunal drip. Aspirated fluid should be filtered before being replaced and additional fluid which is given should be rich in carbohydrate, contain fat emulsion of small particle size, and ordinary salt is best avoided. Considerable trial and error has to be undertaken with the exact mixture of the food if severe diarrhoea, which is one of the great troubles of this type of feeding, is to be avoided.

PARENTERAL ROUTES

The intravenous route is the usual one for parenteral administration.

Blood, plasma, plasma substitute, and a wide variety of fluids for artificial feeding and the correction of electrolyte imbalance are administered by an intravenous cannula.

The type and amount of fluid required is discussed in detail in Chapter 14. This is a complex and comparatively advanced study but in this section discussion is confined to the care necessary during administration and the complications which may arise. It should be read in conjunction with the section on blood transfusion in Chapter 12.

The infusion is usually given into a vein in the forearm or hand by using the standard blood transfusion gravity set. If intravenous therapy is to be prolonged, or highly irritant solutions have to be used, a Teflon or silicone catheter is passed into one of the vena cavae. This may necessitate open insertion but more often percutaneous puncture is used.

The veins of choice are those in the lower half of the forearm. This has the following advantages:

(a) The patient's joints, particularly the elbow, are not immobilised.
(b) The more proximal veins are intact should further infusion be necessary.

All containers for use should be sealed and labelled with the nature and strength of the solution. If full volume is not present, then a crack must be suspected and this, as well as debris or solid matter in the flask, is an indication to abandon it. Modern practice tends to rely more on fluids supplied in flexible plastic containers. The batch and the container number should be noted in the case sheet.

The danger of plasma—that hepatitis due to a virus may be transmitted to the patient—has now been overcome by using plasma protein fraction (PPF) (Ch. 12).

To overcome the disadvantage of the danger of hepatitis from plasma, many plasma substitutes have been developed. They include:

(a) Dextran, a polysaccharide of high molecular weight.
(b) Rheomacrodex, which has the property of preventing 'sludging' of red cells and increases blood flow through the capillaries. It is a dextran of medium molecular weight.
(c) Haemacel, a 3.5 per cent colloidal infusion solution containing gelatin.

Dextran maintains blood pressure if blood is not available, and the number of patients surviving when it is given instead of plasma closely approximates. The amount should be limited to three bags or bottles (540 ml each). Because of its anticoagulant effect, it is liable to cause some aggregation of the red cells and 10 ml of blood should be withdrawn and kept from every patient about to receive dextran. This enables blood grouping and cross-matching to be carried out with the usual technical ease should blood transfusion be called for in the next few days.

If the cause of shock is blood loss, blood has to be administered instead of plasma.

Intravenous infusion

Equipment required:
I.V.-giving set
Mediswabs
Selection of i.v. needles and cannulae
Syringe and needles
Sterile towels
Gauze swabs
Adhesive tape, Elastoplast
Appropriate fluid, e.g. normal saline
Splint
Crepe bandage
Receiver
Fluid balance chart
Local anaesthetic, syringe and needles
Intravenous infusion stand
Tourniquet
Sphygmomanometer
Blood filters if blood transfusion is contemplated.

The patient is informed of the procedure and his co-operation obtained. Privacy is ensured. He is given an opportunity to empty his bladder. The site is shaved if necessary.

The apparatus is taken to the bedside, preferably on a trolley. The site is exposed, usually the arm the patient uses least frequently. The arm is removed from the pyjama/gown sleeve. The patient is made comfortable and kept warm.

The doctor or nurse primes the giving set, fluid being caught in the receiver and air excluded. He applies the tourniquet, perhaps using the sphygmomanometer for this purpose. A bleb of local anaesthetic is injected into the skin at the proposed puncture site. Using the aseptic technique, he introduces the needle and cannula into the vein. The cannula is advanced into the vein and the needle is withdrawn. He attaches the giving set to the cannula and ensures the fluid is flowing. The cannula is secured in position by adhesive tape. The limb may be lightly bandaged to a splint, taking care not to obstruct the flow.

The patient is made comfortable and the used equipment cleared away. The doctor prescribes the fluid to be given and the rate of flow. Whilst the infusion is in progress the nurse observes the rate of flow, the presence of fluid in the drip chamber/airlock, the amount of fluid remaining in the container and the giving set, the position and coverings of the cannula, the patient's arm and his general condition.

When the container is changed, two nurses check the fluid to be given. The guidelines on administration of parenteral infusion fluids are as follows:

The rate of infusion. This is determined by the doctor. The amount is determined by the size of the drops and the nurse should read the graduation of drops per millilitre on the package supplied with the set. In many sets 15 drops make 1 ml. Therefore a rate of 30 drops per minute will infuse just under 3 litres in 24 hours.

Complications

Thrombophlebitis. All solutions are mildly irritant to the wall of the vein. Its incidence is diminished by:
   (a) Atraumatic vein puncture.
   (b) Maintaining asepsis.
   (c) Limiting the time any one vein is used, ideally not more than eight hours but in practice usually 24-48 hours.
   (d) Giving specially irritant solutions by caval catheter.
   (e) Changing the giving set regularly.

Extravasation of fluid into the tissue is due to the point of the cannula slipping out of the vein. The infusion usually stops and some swelling of the tissues occurs. The cannula is removed and the puncture wound dressed. Special care is required if an irritant solution is being infused. Extravasation causes necrosis of the tissues. Some antibiotic solutions such as the tetracyclines and cytotoxic agents may produce this effect.

As soon as possible fluids are taken by mouth, which is the natural and best route of all. If the patient is co-operative he takes just the right quantity. The dangers of the artificial routes are:
   (a) Excess of fluid may be given, resulting in pulmonary oedema.
   (b) Too little fluid is taken, causing water depletion.
   (c) The wrong type of fluid may be given.
   (d) Infection may be introduced or thrombosis may occur in the vein.

Contamination of intravenous fluid was extensively investigated by the Clothier Committee, and the fundamental cause of disease was found to be human failing ranging from simple carelessness to poor management of men and plant. In particular:

1. A bottle or bag which looks suspicious should not be accepted.
2. Defaced labels, loose collars, weeping from the bung, and turbidity or opalescence in the fluid render the contents suspect.

The Control of Infection Officer should be informed and stocks in the pharmacy should be immobilised pending investigation if any of the above defects is discovered in a single container.

Unit of measurement of fluid. This is expressed in the metric system. A one-thousandth part of a litre is a millilitre (ml).

16

Respiratory failure

PHYSIOLOGY

Respiration is the process whereby the tissues are provided with oxygen (O_2) and carbon dioxide (CO_2) is eliminated. There are certain basic requirements.

1. A mechanically efficient bellows consisting of the ribs, and the muscles of respiration (i.e. the intercostals and diaphragm) with an airtight chest wall and a clear passage to the outside air through the trachea, the larynx, the mouth and the nose.

2. Enough sound lung to oxygenate the blood which passes through it and at the same time to eliminate all the carbon dioxide (CO_2) from the blood.

3. An adequate circulation of blood through the lungs and the rest of the body to carry the gases.

4. The central mechanism in the brain which controls respiratory efforts must be working and the nervous pathways from this to the muscles it controls must be intact. This centre initiates rhythmic impulses which drive the muscles of respiration and is situated in the medulla oblongata. It is sensitive to chemical changes in the blood (e.g. excess of carbon dioxide and lack of oxygen) and adjusts the rate and depth of respiration to maintain normal blood levels of those substances.

RESPIRATORY FAILURE

Respiratory failure may occur if any or all of these mechanisms are destroyed or deranged to a sufficient extent to prevent them carrying out their function.

Defects of the bellows mechanism. The bellows mechanism may be put out of action. Causes of this are:

1. Extensive fractures of the bony thoracic cage or trauma to the diaphragm.

2. Tears in the chest wall, allowing the pleural cavity to communicate with the atmosphere and hence preventing the normal lowering of

intrathoracic pressure associated with inspiration which sucks air into the lungs.

3. Paralysis of the muscles of respiration may occur due to overdosage with muscle relaxant drugs (often used in anaesthesia), poisoning with organic phosphorus insecticides.

4. Structural deformities of the chest such as kyphoscoliosis or ankylosing spondylitis.

5. Neurological paralysis of the muscles of respiration including brain damage, spinal cord injury, poliomyelitis and peripheral neuropathies such as lead poisoning, Guillain Barré syndrome and acute porphyria.

6. Muscle disorders such as myasthenia gravis and muscular dystrophy.

7. Obstruction of the airway may prevent the bellows from sucking in air. This is often due to foreign bodies, sputum, secretions or trauma to the air passages or the face.

Inadequacy of lung tissue. An inadequacy of lung tissue is due either to disease e.g. chronic bronchitis and emphysema, pneumonia, pulmonary oedema, pulmonary fibrosis, tuberculosis, carcinoma of the bronchus, pneumoconiosis, etc., or to destruction of lung tissue by surgery, irritant gases or chemicals. An example of the latter is the destruction of lung tissue caused by poisonous gases such as chlorine.

Inadequate circulation of blood. Inadequate circulation of blood may occur from heart failure or sometimes due to vascular accidents such as emboli or thrombosis within the lungs themselves.

CYANOSIS

Cyanosis is a blue or sometimes a greyish colour of the skin produced by abnormally large amounts of reduced haemoglobin or less frequently by abnormal pigments such as methaemoglobin or sulphhaemoglobin.

It may be:

1. Central

(a) Failure of the lungs to adequately oxygenate the blood, due to lung parenchymal disease, obstruction to the air passages or paralysis of the respiratory muscles.

(b) Blood is shunted from the pulmonary artery to the pulmonary vein without exposure to the alveoli.

2. Peripheral. The arterial blood flow in the tissues is slowed by vaso-constriction and cyanosis occurs because of the large amount of time available in the tissues for gaseous interchange. Shock and Raynaud's disease (Chs. 13 and 24) are conditions in which this may occur.

TREATMENT

The principles underlying the treatment of all forms of respiratory failure are the same. The cardinal rule is to ensure that the lungs are ventilated efficiently by whatever means are available.

First in order to ventilate the lungs a clear airway via the mouth or nose and trachea to the lungs must be ensured. Therefore foreign bodies secretions, etc. are removed and the tongue and jaw must be held forward in the unconscious patient. Artificial respiration is commenced. The most efficient and only really satisfactory method of doing this as a first aid measure is by mouth to mouth or mouth to nose respiration. By this method the patient's lungs are inflated by the nurse blowing through his mouth or nostrils—then they are allowed to deflate again by their own elasticity.

Mouth to mouth or mouth to nose breathing

Firstly, the air passages must be cleared of any obstruction. The occiput should rest on a surface in the same plane as the patient's shoulders and buttocks and the patient's neck is extended from the normal lying position so that the tongue does not fall back and close the glottis. A special airway (Brook's), or, alternatively, a handkerchief to fit over the lips can be used if contact with the patient's mouth is undesirable.

Many favour mouth to nose instead of mouth to mouth, but for the less expert it is probably easier to nip the nose than to keep the patient's mouth closed. If a 'bag mask' type of inflating unit is available it can be used only if the operator is quite sure that she has the necessary skill.

As soon as possible this method of maintaining gaseous exchange ought to be replaced by some sort of formal artificial ventilation of the lungs.

Artificial ventilation

This may be accomplished by passing an endotracheal tube into the trachea and inflating the lungs with air or oxygen either manually, using a rubber bag, or, better, by one of the many machines available.

All mechanical lung ventilators work by intermittently blowing respirable gases into the patient's lungs. The lungs deflate by virtue of their own elasticity. Such a machine is the Manley ventilator which is driven by compressed gas. Other varieties are powered by electric motors.

The more sophisticated machines such as the Elema-Servo ventilator, have what is known as a patient-triggering device which enables them to assist the inadequate efforts of a partially paralysed patient without his attempts to breathe conflicting with the work of the machine.

All mechanical ventilators must be equipped with efficient humidifiers so that the inspired gas is saturated with water vapour. These may be devices rather like an electric kettle in which the gas is passed over hot water or may be nebulisers, either mechanical or ultrasonic. Some such as the Bennett cascade may also be heated. If the inspired gases are not rendered wet the patient's tracheal and pulmonary secretions dry up and are difficult to remove and may even crust on the tracheal mucosa.

It is essential that all equipment used in mechanical ventilation should be sterile before use. Accessories such as endotracheal and tracheostomy tubes are sterilised by steam or radiation. (Ethylene oxide should be used with care as it may become trapped between the layers of rubber—only to be liberated later when the tube is in use.)

The ventilator itself should have its working parts sterilised by ultrasonically nebulised alcohol (70 per cent solution), ethylene oxide gas or suitable chemical solutions, or should be autoclaved.

Ventilators should be fitted with bacterial filters on both their inspiratory and expiratory tubes. These should be autoclaved frequently and always before the machine is used on a new patient. It is important to ensure that these filters do not become waterlogged during use as this may give rise to respiratory obstruction. Waterlogging may be avoided by siliconising the filter or by heating it.

If the use of a mechanical ventilator is expected to last for more than 48 hours it is often considered desirable to carry out a tracheostomy and inflate the patient's lungs via this route.

The reasons are:

1. Prolonged presence of an endotracheal tube in the larynx may cause sloughing with subsequent stenosis. An endotracheal Lanz tube with its overpressure safety is mandatory for prolonged use or when a cuffed tracheostomy tube is required.
2. It enables the attendant to remove secretions from the bronchial tree with great ease. This is accomplished with the aid of a suction machine and catheter (Fig.16.1).
3. The patient may in fact find a tracheostomy less distressing.

Fig. 16.1 Suction through the tracheostomy tube. The nasogastric tube is for feeding.

It is important that the nurse should understand the care of a tracheostomy. The tube which will be used for this type of patient is of plastic and has an inflatable cuff which prevents leakage of air from the trachea. The mechanical ventilator is attached to a swivel connection at the end of this tube. Whenever secretions accumulate in the tube or air passages they should be removed at once. After a suction session it is desirable to inflate the patient's lungs using a rubber bag as an inflating device.

It is impossible to overemphasise the importance of two factors in the care of a tracheostomy.

Firstly, every effort should be made to avoid introducing infection into the bronchial tree during the repeated bronchial toilets which must be carried out and, secondly, at all costs the inspired gases must be prevented from drying out the tracheal and pulmonary secretions.

Because the nose, which normally moistens the inspired air, has been bypassed patients breathing through a tracheostomy tube tend to get tenacious and viscous sputum which is hard to remove. This evil can be mitigated by humidifying all gas used in machines. Some rely on heat to saturate the gas with water vapour while others introduce an extremely finely divided spray of water into the gaseous stream. The Radcliffe humidifier is a good example of the first type. A more modern one is the Bennett cascade.

It is important to remember that whilst artificial ventilation by a machine will keep the patient alive almost indefinitely, machine failure which goes unobserved will kill him within minutes. Therefore machines should never be left unattended and manual means of inflation should always be immediately available for use in emergency.

Whilst mechanical ventilation is in progress the cause of the respiratory failure should be treated if this is possible. Infection is treated with antibiotics or the pressure on nerves caused by fractures is relieved.

Where a mechanical ventilator is in use the patient requires feeding. Some are able to take ordinary light diets, others need intragastric feeds. If they are lying very still in bed they ought to be gently rolled from one side to the other every 2 hours to prevent hypostatic pneumonia of the dependent parts of the lungs. Care of the pressure areas is important.

The services of well trained physiotherapists are essential.

TRACHEOSTOMY

Tracheostomy, or an artificial opening in the trachea, is necessary to relieve sudden laryngeal obstruction. In the very young nasotracheal intubation with a plastic Jackson-Rees tube is used rather than tracheostomy.

INDICATIONS FOR TRACHEOSTOMY

Obstructive conditions of the larynx

1. Acute oedema of the glottis. This may occur as a result of Ludwig's angina, carcinoma of the tongue, or as a result of a radium reaction inside the mouth.
2. Carcinoma of the larynx.
3. Foreign bodies impacted in the larynx.
4. Trauma.
5. Burns of the mouth or larynx.
6. Acute laryngitis particularly diphtheria; the diphtheritic membrane may block the airway completely.

Paralysis or spasm of the respiratory muscles and respiratory failure

1 Bulbar paralysis including poliomyelitis.
2. Tetanus and certain stages of coma, including some head injuries.

Some types of inability to maintain satisfactory blood gas levels during prolonged artificial ventilation

Such as reversible respiratory failure due to asthma, adult respiratory distress syndrome and chest wall trauma.

Haemorrhage into a cystadenoma of the thyroid gland is not an indication for tracheostomy, but for laryngeal intubation followed by partial thyroidectomy.

THE TIME FOR OPERATION

The nurse must be familiar with the conditions in which a tracheostomy may be indicated, and once the possibility has arisen the instruments must be at hand and ready sterilised.

In a case of progressive respiratory obstruction a tracheostomy is usually indicated when the accessory muscles of respiration commence to be used, namely, the alae nasi and the sternomastoid. Recession of the epigastrium is also present. The patient is usually cyanosed, and the accompanying mental stress is very considerable.

Artificial respiration will not be of the slightest use should the patient collapse, because he has not a free airway, and collapse due to respiratory obstruction is an indication for lightning speed in effecting an artificial opening.

THE OPERATION

If the patient is collapsed and no instruments are at hand a mini tracheostomy (Portex) should be inserted percutaneously through the cricothyroid membrane. This should always be available for it negates the need to use such things as a penknife in the emergency situation. The patient's head must be kept well extended over a pillow or sandbag.

When making a formal tracheostomy, after the opening has been made in the trachea, a tracheostomy tube, to which two tapes are attached, is inserted. The tapes must be tied immediately at the side of the patient's neck in a knot and bow. If they are tied at the back of the patient's neck they are uncomfortable to lie on, inaccessible and may be untied by mistake if the gown is also fastened by tapes. If a ventilator is to be used a cuffed plastic tube is essential.

POSTOPERATIVE TREATMENT

The patient is exhausted and dozes off to sleep. He should be laid flat in bed, rolled from side to side hourly to promote drainage and exudate should be sucked from the tracheostomy tube. When he awakens he should be propped up and kept in this position for 48 hours. If metal tracheostomy tubes have been used the inner tube will require frequent removal and a supply of autoclaved tubes should be available.

Deep breathing exercises are carried out under the direction of a physiotherapist. A suction machine must be available to enable the nurse to clear secretions from the airway, together with a supply of sterile suction catheters. Personnel should be trained in the methods used to avoid introducing infection into the trachea. Humidified oxygen may be administered via a tracheostomy mask. A pair of tracheal dilators must be always at hand in case the tube is coughed or pulled out, and a pair of scissors to cut the tapes in case the outer tube becomes blocked. A spare correctly fitting tube should be available. Gentle handling is essential as the posterior wall of the trachea is very thin and easily eroded.

All these measures are designed to prevent pneumonia, which is a very likely complication.

Swallowing may be difficult but small amounts of fluid can usually be taken. If the patient is very thirsty fluids may be given parenterally.

If the case is one of carcinoma of the larynx a tracheostomy will be permanent, but in other cases the tube is removed when the cause of the obstruction has subsided. In children, removal of the tube may be followed by considerable fright because the voice is absent *unless the wound is completely covered.*

RULES FOR TRACHEOSTOMY MANAGEMENT

The following rules are essential:
1. Scrub the hands, wear sterile disposable gloves and a mask.
2. Use prepacked sterile disposal catheters.
3. Do not allow the catheter to touch *anything* before aspirating the trachea.
4. Discard the catheter after aspiration.
5. Replace the inner tube as required. A supply of autoclaved inner tubes should be available.
6. Clean the tracheostomy wound and renew the dressing regularly. A keyhole gauze dressing is used.
7. Micro-organisms live everywhere and may kill if introduced into the bronchi. *Escherichia coli, Klebsiella bacilli* and *Pseudomonas aeruginosa* are the most common.
8. Always inflate the lungs after a suction session.
9. The use of a word chart (Fig.16.2) to enable the patient to communicate.

CARE OF A PATIENT WITH A TRACHEOSTOMY

The following articles should be kept at the bedside:
Sterile tracheal dilators
Selection of sterile suction catheters
Sterile disposable gloves

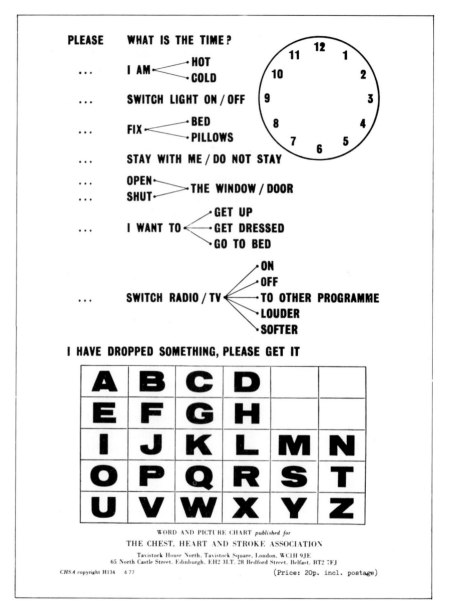

Fig. 16.2 On a table within reach of the patient is a word and picture chart, a bell, a pencil and a writing pad. (Illustration by courtesy of the Chest, Heart and Stroke Association.)

Suction machine with half an inch of Savlon 0.5 per cent in the suction bottle

Bowl of Savlon 0.5 per cent

Brown wax bag

Small gallipot containing small amount of sterile normal saline to act as a lubricant. This sterile normal saline is removed from the container using a sterile syringe and needle.

The tracheostomy tube is held in position by tapes, which are tied at the side of the patient's neck.

The tube is sucked out whenever necessary, but at least at 2-hourly intervals. Disposable gloves are put on. The packet containing the catheter is cut at the wide end of the catheter, which is connected to the pressure tubing of the suction machine. The wrapper is removed. The catheter is nipped in order to prevent suction, and dipped into the normal saline in order to lubricate it.

The tracheostomy tube is steadied and the catheter inserted not more than 4 inches. It is released to allow suction, turned and slowly withdrawn while turning. Should it be necessary, the catheter can be reinserted once only.

When a Y-shaped connection is used, the side-arm can be opened or covered to prevent or allow suction.

After withdrawal the catheter is washed through with Savlon 0.5 per cent. It is disconnected and discarded into the brown wax bag. The pressure tubing is fixed to the handle of the suction machine using a bulldog clip. The gloves are removed and discarded into the brown wax bag.

Ideally the suction session should be attended by an anaesthetist who together with the nurse form a team and engage in what is known as 'bagging and sucking', an exercise designed to remove as much moist secretion as possible and in a way that will reduce the risk of infection and post-suction lung collapse.

Care of the tube

A cuffed tube requires attention at intervals, e.g. 2-hourly or as otherwise instructed. The pharynx is sucked out especially if the patient is not swallowing. The tracheostomy tube is sucked out using another catheter. The cuff is released for 2 minutes and then reinflated (Fig. 16.3).

The inner tube of a metal tube is removed, e.g. 2-hourly and the outer tube sucked out. The inner tube is washed in sodium bicarbonate, and is sterilised in special Savlon or by boiling and reinserted.

The wound is cleaned as required, e.g. 4-hourly, using a suitable antiseptic aseptic technique. A gauze swab may be placed under the tube if necessary.

Emergency. If the tube becomes dislodged and the patient is having difficulty in breathing, the tapes holding the tube are cut, the tracheal dilator inserted and held open to allow entry of air. Assistance is called for. The tracheostomy may require to be sucked out.

OXYGEN THERAPY

Air contains about 20 per cent of oxygen. This is adequate to saturate the haemoglobin of the blood in a patient whose respiratory and circulatory systems are normal. In many surgical conditions the respiratory and cardiovascular systems have suffered from severe interference. The result is that the circulating haemoglobin is reduced in amount or is inadequately saturated with oxygen. For this reason the percentage of oxygen in the inspired air has to be increased.

Fig. 16.3 The cuff of the tube fills the trachea when inflated. Its deflation for two minutes two hourly relieves pressure on the softer posterior wall of the trachea and prevents ulceration. (See also Fig. 28.10)

The indication for use is hypoxia (deficient oxygen in the blood from any cause). The distress of respiratory failure is often really due to CO_2 retention, not to lack of oxygen.

CAUSES OF HYPOXIA

1. Respiratory obstruction. This includes all conditions in which the normal exchange of gases in the lungs is impeded:
  (a) Laryngeal obstruction.
  (b) Laryngeal spasm.
  (c) Pneumonia.
  (d) Collapse of the lungs.
  (e) Pneumothorax.
2. Shock and heart failure. Stagnant anoxia.
3. Diminished oxygen-carrying capacity. Anaemia due to haemorrhage being the most important surgically.
4. Increased oxygen consumption, such as continuous hyperpyrexia.
5. Post-operative causes. It is important to stress that the decreased respiratory movements which occur postoperatively may be due to:
  (a) The effects of the anaesthetic not having worn off.
  (b) Bandages being too tight and impeding respiratory movement. The patient whose chest is 'crushed' should nevertheless be tightly bandaged in order to stabilise the thoracic cage.
  (c) Pain.

Fig. 16.4 Disposable oxygen Ventimask.

These may be indications for assisted respiration or analgesics rather than a supply of oxygen.

ADMINISTRATION OF OXYGEN

Oxygen is supplied in cylinders at a pressure of 13 800 kPa (2000 lb/in²; 6.9 kPa, or kilopascals, = 1 lb/in²) or possibly by a pipeline from a central depot. A reducing valve brings this pressure down to 34.5 kPa and a flowmeter is attached which measures the quantity of oxygen delivered in litres per minute.

Oxygen may be administered by:
1. *A face piece*—(a) the ordinary mask of an anaesthetic machine, (b) the polythene mask (Fig.16.4).
2. *Nasal inhalation*—(a) nasal mask such as a Polymask, (b) nasal tube, nasal spectacles or a nasal catheter.
3. *Oxygen tent*—The oxygen tent has been largely abandoned. It is hot, septic and the concentration of oxygen is frequently inadequate.
4. *Incubator for newborn hypoxic babies.*

Method of administration

Pure oxygen is administered until the patient shows the maximal improvement. The oxygen is then gradually reduced, the patient's condition being satisfactory only when he can inhale air alone without any deterioration. The usual rate of administration is 4 l per minute. All oxygen should be moistened. The nose requires careful toilet if an indwelling catheter is being used and 0.1 per cent Hibitane in Xylocaine jelly is useful.

In patients such as chronic bronchitics who normally have a high blood carbon dioxide (P_{CO_2}) and low blood oxygen (P_{O_2}) care should be taken to limit oxygen flow to 4 litres of 24 per cent oxygen per min to avoid total suppression of respiration, or to use one of the special masks such as the Ventimask which restricts the inspired oxygen content to 24 or 28 per cent.

Special precautions to be taken with oxygen therapy

There are no toxic changes in the fully formed tissues from a concentration of up to 70 per cent oxygen. Retrolental fibroplasia is a danger in premature infants.

The most important danger is that of fire. This is increased by:
1. Greasing the valve.
2. Smoking, the use of a naked light or electric toys.
3. The use of spirit or ether for the treatment of the patient.
4. The production of static electricity—for example by too active bed-making or nylon clothing.

Before connecting up the oxygen supply, grit should be blown out. When the oxygen cylinder is empty it should be removed and marked accordingly. If 'piped' oxygen is used the nurse must know where the cut-off valves are situated outside the room or ward in case of fire.

Details of administration of oxygen

The doctor ordering that oxygen shall be given to a patient, should indicate the means of administration and the rate of flow. Many devices are available for this purpose e.g.:

Nasal spectacles
Ventimask
Edinburgh mask

In emergency, until the arrival of the doctor the nurse may give oxygen using the nasal spectacles with the rate of flow adjusted to 4 litres per minute.

The procedure is explained to the patient, and his co-operation obtained. The nostrils are cleaned using a wool swab held in sinus forceps and moistened in sodium bicarbonate solution. After use the swab is removed with dissecting forceps and discarded.

The nurse checks that oxygen is flowing from the piped supply. She fills the humidifier (nebuliser) with distilled water up to the level of the mark. The apparatus is connected and the flow of oxygen set to the prescribed rate. The spectacles or mask are placed in position. The patient is made comfortable. Observations are made on the effects of the oxygen on the patient's colour, breathing and general condition.

When oxygen is being administered intermittently, on the same patient. the spectacles or mask are stored in a clean paper bag attached to the locker, until next required.

The spectacles or mask and length of tubing are changed after 24 hours or more frequently as necessary. Being disposable they are discarded.

When the administration of oxygen is discontinued, the spectacles, mask and length of tubing are discarded. The humidifier is emptied. washed in Savlon 0.5 per cent, rinsed and dried, and placed back in position near the flow meter until required again.

When an oxygen cylinder is used, it is prepared and turned on outside the ward. The assembled apparatus consists of:

    Cylinder with reducing valve, gauge and flow meter
    Humidifier
    Appropriate tubing
    Appropriate means of administration.

Hyperbaric oxygen therapy

A tiny amount of oxygen is dissolved in the blood plasma. This amount can be considerably increased if the patient is placed in a chamber and oxygen is administered at a pressure of 2 atmospheres. (Oxygen at a greater pressure than that of the atmosphere is described as hyperbaric.) This may be of value in saving a threatened limb. There is a specially devised bed which avoids the necessity of a pressure chamber. It has been used before megavoltage radiotherapy to increase the response to treatment. It is also used for patients in severe shock, for enhancing the chances of 'take' in extensive skin graft, in the treatment of gas gangrene and in combating carbon monoxide poisoning. Paradoxically the development of North Sea gas, which contains no carbon monoxide, has reduced the need for hyperbaric oxygen as a treatment for gas poisoning but increased the demand for hyperbaric facilities in hospitals close to off-shore rigs because of the conditions of pressure in which divers work.

INTENSIVE CARE UNITS

An intensive care unit is one where there is the concentration of skill, equipment and staff required for the treatment or resuscitation of a seriously ill patient. The object is to maintain the highest level of medical and nursing care by day and by night. The essential features are:

1. Structure

Extensive floor space per patient is necessary and easy access all around the patient's bed should be provided. There should be good observation of the patient from a centrally placed panel. Exceptionally extensive electrical provisions are made for portable X-rays as well as for respirators, suction machines and monitoring apparatus. At the nurse's station are telephones and light indicators for night use, switches for the control of lighting and indicators relating to piped oxygen, suction and emergency electricity generation.

2. Equipment

This is necessarily on a lavish scale. The nurse cannot be expected to know how everything works but she should know what she may or may not do with it, whether it is working and what measures to take if it ceases to function. The most efficient suction machine will not function if the top of the reservoir is not fitted in an airtight manner! All the equipment necessary and already discussed in the sections on acute circulatory and respiratory failure must be available. A small laboratory near by is an essential.

Because of the ever-present danger of cross-infection, facilities for the total isolation of 'very clean' from 'very dirty' patients are an essential feature of all modern intensive care units.

3. Staff

To afford complete 24-hour coverage a three-shift system of duty is required with an average of five trained nurses and supporting nursing auxiliaries or ward orderly staff for each patient.

The types of condition for which patients are admitted vary enormously. They may be postoperative conditions, severe road accidents, coal-gas poisoning, frost-bite, myocardial infarction or cerebral thrombosis. Most will have some degree of respiratory, circulatory or metabolic disturbance. In addition to specialised procedures to counteract these conditions all patients require good basic nursing care. Careful records, attention to general and oral hygiene are as important as elsewhere in the hospital.

CONTROL OF RESUSCITATIVE THERAPY

The control of resuscitative therapy, amongst which may be included oxygen, mechanical ventilation and the correction of acid base disturbances, is often achieved by reference to blood gas estimations. These are carried out on arterial blood samples taken into heparinised syringes. Specimens which cannot be examined at once should be refrigerated.

The normal values are:

pH   7.4
Standard bicarbonate 25 mmol per litre
P_{CO_2} 5.4 kPa
P_{O_2} 13.3 kPa

Collection of specimens

Taking blood for estimation of blood gases

On a tray is placed:
A receiver
Heparin 5000 units per ml
Syringe 5 ml
Needle size 21 x 1½

     Wax carton of ice
     Strapping
     Red caps
     Mediswabs
     Packet of gauze swabs

A piece of strapping with the patient's name written on it is attached to the barrel of the syringe.

The doctor takes the blood from the patient's femoral artery. He removes the needle. He fixes a red cap to the nozzle of the syringe. He gently rotates the syringe. It is plunged into the wax carton of ice. It is taken immediately to the unit laboratory. The nurse maintains digital pressure on a gauze swab over the femoral artery puncture for at least 5 minutes and continues observation for several hours for signs of haemorrhage.

17

The nature of disease

In the preceding pages the various processes of disease have been covered. For the remainder of the book, disease as it affects specific systems and organs of the body will be described. This chapter serves as a link between the two sections, and provides an opportunity to take a slightly broader view of the nature of disease before proceeding to a more detailed description of its site.

THE NATURE OF THE CHANGES PRODUCED BY DISEASE

The causes of disease are of fundamental importance. The clinical picture as revealed by symptoms and signs has to be known if it is to be recognised and the correct treatment undertaken. Changes which result from disease have one or more of the following effects:

1. *Tissue destruction.* When it is gross it is known as gangrene or putrefaction; lesser degrees of destruction are termed necrosis.

2. *Obstruction* is a common cause or result of disease. Lesions occur in far dispersed sites in the body which have little or nothing in common aetiologically yet they share an identical, simple mechanical process. It is more likely to occur in the narrowest part of an organ or duct. Some of these sites are illustrated in Figure 17.1.

Loss or diminution of blood supply is due to obstructive changes in the blood vessel walls or the valves of the heart. Solidification of normal contents in other channels results in stone formation in the biliary or urinary tract whilst the same process in the blood is called thrombosis. In addition to disease of the wall and obstruction of the lumen the whole organ may be compressed by pressure from without.

3. *Fluid leakage.* Fluid loss may be in a gross clinically perceptible form such as occurs in haemorrhage, perforation, ascites, burns, diarrhoea, vomiting or only in a more delicate physicochemical sense of change between the extracellular spaces and the blood.

4. *Degeneration.* The tissues wear out.

5. *Hormonal excess or inadequacy.*

ANATOMICAL NARROWS

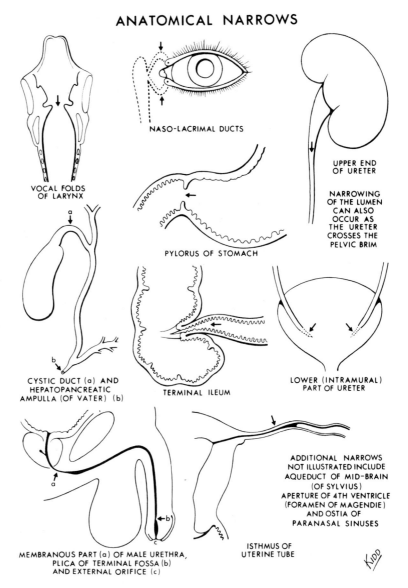

NASO-LACRIMAL DUCTS

VOCAL FOLDS
OF LARYNX

PYLORUS OF STOMACH

UPPER END
OF URETER

NARROWING
OF THE LUMEN
CAN ALSO
OCCUR AS
THE URETER
CROSSES THE
PELVIC BRIM

CYSTIC DUCT (a) AND
HEPATOPANCREATIC
AMPULLA (OF VATER) (b)

TERMINAL ILEUM

LOWER (INTRAMURAL)
PART OF URETER

ADDITIONAL NARROWS
NOT ILLUSTRATED INCLUDE
AQUEDUCT OF MID-BRAIN
(OF SYLVIUS)
APERTURE OF 4TH VENTRICLE
(FORAMEN OF MAGENDIE)
AND OSTIA OF
PARANASAL SINUSES

MEMBRANOUS PART (a) OF MALE URETHRA,
PLICA OF TERMINAL FOSSA (b)
AND EXTERNAL ORIFICE (c)

ISTHMUS OF
UTERINE TUBE

Fig. 17.1 Obstruction is more likely to occur where the lumen is narrowest.

In any illness an assessment has to be made of the nature of the changes produced.

The following are a few examples:
(a) A small wound causes fluid leakage due to haemorrhage and fluid leakage occurs from the inflammatory reaction in healing;
(b) a 30 per cent burn causes fluid leakage and tissue destruction;
(c) in a strangulated hernia containing a loop of small intestine the blood vessels to the bowel are obstructed and the flow of intestinal contents along the lumen of the intestine is prevented.

The degree or severity of the change

Taking the above examples:

(a) is usually completely trivial;

(b) requires immediate and urgent treatment of the extensive fluid loss if the patient is to survive;

(c) unless there is immediate surgical relief the patient will die.

If the normal vital reactions of the body can restore health no special treatment is required. If these reactions are overwhelmed treatment is necessary.

Health is the preservation of a constant internal environment in the body. Small changes in this environment—the 'milieu interieur' of Claude Bernard—produce reactions which restore this state. Living cells apart from those on the surface of the skin are provided with a fluid environment, with a constant hydrogen ion concentration, osmotic pressure and temperature. Oxygen and food are carried to the cells by the arterial blood which is oxygenated in the lungs and waste products including carbon dioxide removed by the venous blood and the lymphatic system to be eliminated by the lungs and the kidneys. The whole process is regulated by the activities of the hormones and the nervous system. Cannon named this restoration of a constant environment 'homeostasis'.

Many diseases produce a state in which these reactions are strained or severely threatened and unless efforts are successful in re-creating conditions in which it is possible for the body to readjust the patient will lose his life. Treatment must be based on measures which logically assist these reactions. It is very easy to aggravate the patient's condition by well meaning but thoughtless action. For example, it is not so very long ago that heat in the form of hot water bottles and radiant heat cradles which appear so comforting in the management of the shocked patient were used routinely. They caused dilatation of the skin vessels which the physiological reaction was trying to constrict to maintain the blood pressure as well as to retain fluid in the body and provide as much blood as possible to the vital centres within the brain.

The measurement of the pulse, temperature and respiration are routine checks on the physiological state of the patient, but in serious conditions many more parameters of the body's activities have to be checked—the arterial blood pressure, the central venous pressure, the blood gases, the serum electrolytes, to mention only a few examples. Since the patient's condition is changing rapidly many tests have to be repeated at frequent intervals. In many cases a continuous check—monitoring—is essential. It is for this reason that a patient who requires such observation is nursed in an intensive care unit.

Man has survived much injury and disease from Adam to the present day without the help of antibiotics, extensive resuscitative measures and all the other facilities of modern medicine, including the social services. It is but a few years ago that the pulse, arterial blood pressure, temperature, blood haemoglobin and the blood urea were the only physical and chemical measurements of his well-being. To understand what we are really trying to do to help the patient it is worth considering very briefly what vital reactions occur in the patient's body, all of which are designed for his survival. It is the study of these in depth that has enabled considerable progress to be made in the care of the patient.

VITAL REACTIONS

1. Haemostasis has been considered in detail in Chapter 12. It is a natural reaction and, however large or small the haemorrhage, it is essential in controlling bleeding. Detailed study of its mechanism has enabled us to make good deficiencies of clotting factors as well as to prevent or disperse undesirable thrombus formation. Blood transfusion has saved lives of patients whose blood loss has been too rapid and too great to be overcome by the body.

2. The reaction to injury explains how the body takes special precautions to conserve vital fluids and electrolytes when it is assaulted by injury, using the term 'injury' in the widest sense of physical trauma or bacterial invasion. The immediate changes are:

(a) *Increased secretion of antidiuretic hormone by the pituitary.* The result is that water is conserved in the body. The kidney secretes a highly concentrated urine of high specific gravity. The volume is small so that what fluid is lost as urine is used to the greatest advantage to remove the maximal quantity of waste products.

(b) *The adrenal glands* secrete large quantities of aldosterone which has the effect of retaining Na^+ in the body; K^+ is increased in quantity from the breakdown of protein tissue and an excess, which is very toxic, is freely excreted by the kidneys in larger quantities than normal. These changes are reversed when the body commences to rebuild—Na^+ is freely excreted and K^+ necessary for the building up of cells is retained.

There are many other reactions but the above are examples of the types of changes which occur.

3. The inflammatory reaction has already been discussed and its failure to occur may be fatal (Ch. 8).

4. Physiological changes in fluid loss whether of whole blood, water, plasma, or electrolytes (Ch. 14).

5. Immunological reactions are generally beneficial but a fuller understanding is necessary to treat and prevent organ rejection.

6. Psychological reactions to disease are important to the surgical nurse and the surgeon in the management of the patient and his disease. The interrelationship between the patient's disease and his hopes and fears, his family, his environment, his work and leisure must be appreciated.

All these vital reactions occur in and around a living cell in a fluid medium. The one essential is an adequate supply of blood and efficient venous drainage. Figure 17.2 illustrates in simplified diagrammatic form how the normal mechanism operates at the level of a single cell. For the purposes of illustration a single cell in the upper part of the small intestine secreting intestinal juice (succus entericus) is taken as an example and for the purposes of illustration only we shall assume that the

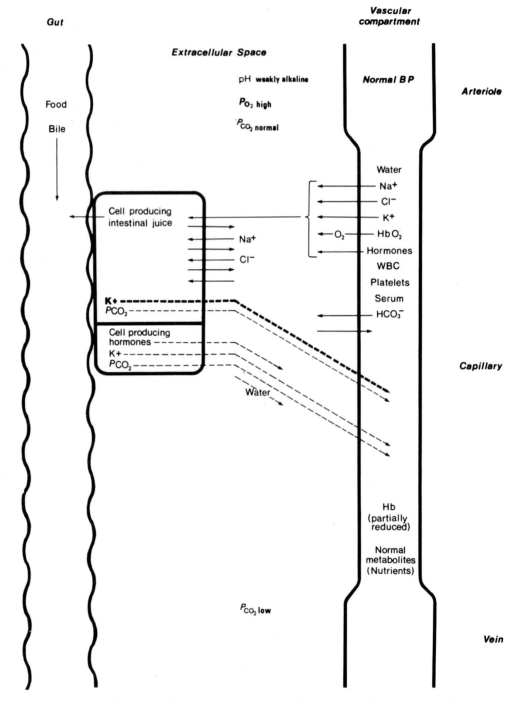

Fig. 17.2 Some of the normal exchanges at cell level in the small intestine in health (see text). K^+ and Na^+ pass freely across the cell membrane, CO_2 is excreted. Intestinal juice is produced and intestinal hormones are secreted and carried away in the venous blood.

adjoining cell secretes the hormone secretin which warns the pancreas that pancreatic juice should be secreted.

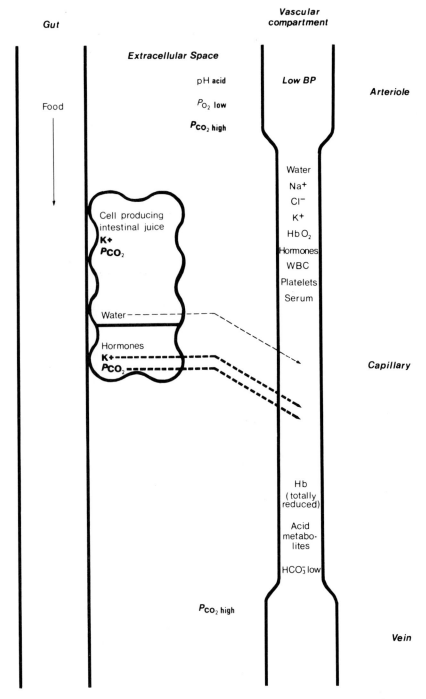

Fig. 17.3 The effect of a severe haemorrhage. The cell is denied oxygen and nourishment. Water is withdrawn from the extracellular space and ultimately from the cell. CO₂ first accumulates in excess in the cell then in the extracellular space and in the venous blood.

Figure 17.3 shows the changes which occur in the cell as a result of depletion of blood volume from haemorrhage anywhere in the body.

Relation of vital reactions to care of patients

The junior nurse may well think—this is all very interesting, but has it any relevance to what she does at the bedside? Indeed it has. For example, it determines many nursing procedures.

1. *The position of the patient.* It explains why pressure sores may develop and are kept active. The blood supply is compressed and the cell dies. If there is an excess of fluid in a limb from deficient venous drainage raising the limb will help increase the flow of fluid from the leg. When the femoral artery is blocked by an embolus the patient is nursed on the opposite side and not resting on his buttock, so compressing the little blood which could flow in from this area to the leg.

2. *The prevention of thrombosis.* It is obvious that the more dehydrated the patient the greater is the viscosity of the blood (Fig. 17.3) and the more likely thrombi are to form. The risk of thrombosis is increased if the patient is immobilised or the blood platelets are increased as after splenectomy.

3. *Corticosteroid therapy* by interfering with fluid exchange and causing water retention interferes with normal reactions. It also prevents the adrenal glands from functioning normally and in stress more corticosteroids have to be supplied or the patient will collapse since he is unable to react to injury.

4. *The poorer reaction of the older patient* is in large measure due to inadequate blood supply because the vessels are arteriosclerotic. Hormones, immune bodies, white blood corpuscles, and antibiotics are not so easily concentrated where they are required as they are in the younger patient with a better cardiovascular system.

5. *Abnormal white cells* are ineffective in infection and the leukaemic patient is unable to deal with invading organisms. Shortage of white cells has a similar effect.

6. *Inadequate renal or pulmonary function* results in a build-up of waste products.

The outstanding lesson that emerges from a study of the changes in disease at the cell level is that the shorter the time that elapses from deprivation of blood and all the bad things it brings the better it is for health.

18

Thrombosis and embolism

THROMBOSIS

Thrombosis is defined as the formation of a solid or semisolid mass from the constituents of the blood within the vascular system. It is not identical with the clotting of shed blood. Although the incidence of disease is higher in the arteries, thrombosis is commoner in veins where the more sluggish blood flow predisposes to its formation.

A thrombus may:

1. Extend and spread while still attached to the vessel wall.
2. Lyse (dissolve) spontaneously without permanent damage.
3. Organise into fibrous tissue so that the lumen of the vessel is permanently obstructed, partially obstructed or its valves (if a vein) damaged.
4. Become detached in whole or in part and be swept away into the blood stream until it lodges and blocks another blood vessel. This process is known as embolism, the detached thrombus being the embolus and the area deprived of blood is known as the infarct.

Thrombi may form in any part of the vascular system. The common sites are:

(a) *The veins of the lower limb and pelvis.* Detachment from this site gives rise to pulmonary embolism.
(b) *The left heart chamber* in valvular disease or myocardial infarction. As the heart recovers and its action improves, an embolus may be expelled. It may lodge in an artery of the leg causing acute gangrene (Ch.23) or in cerebral vessels causing a hemiplegia.
(c) *On an atheromatous patch in an arteriosclerotic artery.* This compromises the blood flow through an already diseased artery, resulting, for example, in threatened gangrene in a limb.

FACTORS WHICH PREDISPOSE TO THROMBOSIS

In general the factors which predispose to thrombosis are changes in the vessel wall, changes in the blood or changes in the blood flow.

1. *The vessel wall* may be damaged by trauma including pressure during operation. Many substances injected or infused intravenously damage the vessel wall predisposing to thrombosis.

2. *Structural changes in the vessel wall.* Arteries already the site of sclerosis may be further obstructed by thrombosis.

Veins with damaged valves are more liable to form thrombi, as are heart valves which have been damaged by disease.

3. *The prostaglandins and thrombosis.* Platelets synthesise the prostaglandin TXA_2 which induces the platelets to stick to each other and to foreign surfaces including the wall of diseased blood vessels. The normal lining endothelium cells secrete a different prostaglandin PGI_2 which counteracts the action of TXA_2 reducing the tendency of the platelets to aggregate. In a diseased blood vessel which cannot make PGI_2 the aggregating action of TXA_2 is unopposed. This is a contributing factor in thrombus formation. The possibility that PGI_2 will be available for therapeutic anticoagulation is very real (Horton 1979).

4. *Changes in the nature of the blood.* Dehydration increases the viscosity of the blood. Other factors which increase its coagulability are leukaemia, splenectomy (because platelet destruction is delayed), drugs such as oestrogens (included in the contraceptive pill), malignant disease, smoking, and other diseases in which plasma viscosity is raised. In many cases there is a combination of factors present. Thrombosis is sometimes the first clinical feature of malignant disease.

5. *Slowing the blood flow* increases the risk of thrombosis. Confinement to bed for any reason, obstruction to the flow of blood by constricting bandages or bad positioning on the operating table may be contributing factors.

6. *Pelvic operations* are more likely to be complicated by thrombosis because of local damage to or pressure on the veins.

7. *Age.* The incidence of thrombosis increases with age.

CLINICAL FEATURES

Arterial thrombosis causes loss of function and usually severe pain. Common examples are coronary thrombosis or thrombosis in the main artery of a leg. In this chapter, however, we are primarily concerned with venous thrombosis. This may be present as:

1. Thrombophlebitis. In this condition there is not only thrombosis in the vein but also concomitant inflammation of the vessel wall. It usually affects superficial veins of the leg which are already varicose. The thrombus is unlikely to become detached. It is painful. The skin over the vein is reddened and the vein itself is usually palpable as a tender, firm cord.

2. Deep vein thrombosis. This refers to thrombosis in the deep venous system of the lower limb.

There is evidence that in some patients this passes undetected with no clinical features to suggest its presence. If the thrombosis is in the soleal venous sinuses or veins below the knee there is some aching pain in the calf of the leg, particularly on walking, pain in the muscles of the calf on

Fig. 18.1 Swelling of left leg due to thrombosis of the left iliofemoral vein.

dorsiflexion of the foot (Homan's sign), tenderness in the calf of the leg, and slight oedema of the foot. There may be a slight rise in the patient's temperature. If there is extensive thrombosis in the common femoral or ileo-femoral veins, rapidly increasing swelling of the limb occurs due to oedema (Fig. 18.1). The limb feels heavy, the unaffected superficial veins may be very prominent, but the limb is often relatively painless. Occasionally the thrombosis is so extensive that the blood flow through the limb is severely compromised. The limb is dusky in colour, tensely swollen throughout, and painful. Venous gangrene, though rare, may ensue.

3. Pulmonary embolism (p.184) may be the first indication that thrombosis has occurred.

INVESTIGATION

Established thrombosis may be obvious clinically or only suspected. In either case further investigations are advisable to confirm the diagnosis and to establish the site and extent of the thrombosis. Such investigations are also sometimes used to gauge the response to treatment.

Radiography

The veins of the leg and pelvis can be visualised following injection of contrast medium. This is usually injected into a dorsal vein of the foot and forced into the deep veins by a tourniquet just above the ankle. The procedure is called phlebography (or venography). By this method the site and extent of thrombosis is determined. It can also be seen whether the thrombosis completely or partially blocks the veins. Occasionally the contrast medium has to be injected directly into the femoral vein or into the greater trochanter of the femur (perosseously) to outline the pelvic veins.

Isotope scanning

^{125}I-labelled fibrinogen, when injected intravenously, becomes incorporated in a thrombus (if present) and may be detected by Geiger-counter scanning of the legs.

The ultrasonic doppler

The flow in blood vessels can be detected with the ultrasonic doppler machine using a simple probe over the vessel at various sites. It can thus be used to detect changes in venous flow due to thrombosis. The ultrasonic response to an increased venous flow against an obstruction has been termed the A-wave. The test can be repeated as frequently as desired to assess progress without any discomfort to the patient and therefore has an advantage over radiographic and isotopic measures, but is not as accurate.

MANAGEMENT OF VENOUS THROMBOSIS

Prevention

Prevention of venous thrombosis in the legs should always be the aim. The principles involved are to maintain a normal or increased venous blood flow, to avoid pressure on or damage to the veins, and to consider altering the coagulability of the blood in those patients particularly at risk.

The practical procedures employed are as follows:

1. Preoperatively.

(a) Physiotherapy. Leg and breathing exercises are taught, to be used pre- and postoperatively.

(b) Elastic stockings. Full length elastic stockings are worn from shortly before operation until the patient is mobile afterwards. They exert a diminishing pressure on the leg from the ankle to the thigh, compressing the superficial veins and encouraging flow in deep veins. Some surgeons advocate their use in all patients, while others reserve them for those at greater risk (e.g. older age group, specific operations, major surgery).

(c) Varicose veins. Patients with varicose veins should wear elastic stockings while in hospital undergoing surgery for other conditions. Sometimes varicose veins are treated surgically before treating other major conditions.

(d) Drugs liable to produce thrombosis such as oestrogens (mainly the contraceptive pill) are stopped four to eight weeks preoperatively in elective procedures.

(e) Smoking. This increases the viscosity of the blood and should therefore be stopped.

(f) Subcutaneous heparin. This is used prophylactically in high-risk patients to reduce coagulability of the blood, thus reducing the incidence of venous thrombosis. Significant reduction of venous thrombosis has been demonstrated in some groups of patients with the use of subcutaneous heparin. High-risk factors are age (over 40 years), obesity, previous venous thrombosis or known venous abnormality, pelvic operations, operations on hips and legs, prolonged major surgery, immobility or prolonged bed-rest postoperatively, malignant disease, emergency surgery on patients taking oestrogens. The risk of haemorrhage is the reason why some surgeons do not use this method. It should not be used in patients with known cardiovascular disease (e.g. hypertension, previous cerebrovascular accident), the very old, in operations where severe haemorrhage is particularly likely (e.g. prostatectomy), or where haemorrhage could be dangerous (e.g. neurosurgery).

Calcium heparin in a dose of 5000 units is injected subcutaneously 2 hours preoperatively and repeated 8 hourly for 3 to 5 days. The skin of the abdominal wall or thigh is marked in squares, a different square being used for each injection to avoid the use of any site more than once. The skin is pinched up and a fine gauge needle (26G⅜) used for the injection.

2. Peroperatively.

(a) Position on the operating table. If possible the foot of the operating table is slightly elevated to encourage venous return from the legs. The heels are supported by padded rings so that the calves are lifted off the table. If the legs are supported in stirrups these should be well cushioned and any local pressure avoided. Pressure on or damage to the veins during surgery is avoided as far as possible.

(b) Pneumatic stockings. These are inflatable below-knee stockings which exert pressure on the leg. They incorporate a 'pulsatile' impulse which increases this pressure, thus actively improving venous flow. Where they are available some surgeons use them on all patients. Others use them only on high-risk patients.

(c) Calf muscle stimulation. By the use of special equipment the calf muscles are stimulated electrically and intermittently. This produces a similar effect to pneumatic stockings.

(d) Adequate fluid intake or replacement should be ensured to avoid dehydration and consequent increased viscosity of the blood.

(e) Low molecular weight dextran. Infusion of this during operation and in the early postoperative period has some effect in reducing the incidence of venous thrombosis.

3. Post-operatively.

(a) Adequate and regular analgesia. Good pain relief makes movement easier.

(b) Early mobilisation after the operation. This means walking if possible, but if the patient is sitting then the legs should be elevated. The nurse should inspect the patient's ankles for swelling when bed-making.

(c) Aspirin. This is thought to reduce platelet stickiness and is therefore used by some people with the object of preventing venous thrombosis. However, such use is not common.

Treatment

The objects of treatment are:
1. To prevent extension of the thrombus.
2. To lyse (dissolve) or remove the thrombus.
3. To prevent detachment with embolus formation.
4. To prevent long-term occlusion of or damage to the vein, including the valves.

The relative importance of these objectives varies depending on the site and size of the thrombus. The methods of treatment available will be described under each of these objectives.

1. Prevention of extension of thrombus. Thrombosis tends to extend proximally in the vein to the next large tributary. It may continue beyond that level. This is prevented by:

(a) Maintaining good flow in vein:
  —elevate foot of bed
  —elastic stocking to compress superficial veins
  —maintain mobility to aid venous return

(b) Administration of anticoagulants. This stops the blood clotting. Heparin 5000 units intravenously is given at once, followed by 12 000–20 000 units 12 hourly by continuous intravenous infusion using a clockwork syringe. This dose is controlled by measurement of the kaolin cephalin clotting time (CCCT). This is continued for 10 days. If at any time it is necessary to reverse the effects of heparin (e.g. because surgery is indicated, unwanted bleeding occurs) this can be achieved by intravenous injection of protamine sulphate; 10 mg will neutralise 1000 units (10 mg) of heparin. After 10 days oral anticoagulants are introduced. They are slower in achieving their effect, usually about 24 hours. The dose is controlled by estimation of the prothrombin time, the aim being to keep this about two and a half times the control (normal) value. When effective, their administration is continued and heparin therapy stopped. The dose varies with the preparation used. Warfarin has an initial dose of 30 to 40 mg on the first day, none on the second day and a maintenance dose of 2 to 20 mg daily, adjusted to keep the prothrombin time at the required level. The prothrombin time should be estimated at midday and the anticoagulant given before midnight each day. Once a stable maintenance dose is achieved, the prothrombin time can be estimated once a week. If the need for rapid reversal of anticoagulation is remote the oral anticoagulant therapy can be instituted at the same time as heparin and the latter stopped once satisfactory anticoagulation is achieved. If necessary warfarin can be neutralised by vitamin K 10 mg intravenously but this may take up to 24 hours to be effective. Transfusion of fresh frozen plasma may be needed in some circumstances. Too high a dose of oral anticoagulant may cause abnormal haemorrhage (e.g. haematuria, purpura, heavy periods, haematemesis). Drug sensitivity may occur and be manifest by delayed haemorrhage, pyrexia, skin rash, albuminuria, jaundice, granulocytopenia or diarrhoea. Steroid therapy may be required to treat this. There are many drugs which increase or decrease the effect of oral anticoagulants. It is the doctor's responsibility to ensure that the patient is aware of this. The patient should not take alcohol.

2. Lysis or removal of thrombus. The natural history of a thrombus is that it becomes organised and the lumen of the vein recanalised. This may result in a fairly normal vein, or, more commonly, one with a narrowed irregular lumen in which valves have been damaged. The following methods are available to aid lysis or removal of thrombus.

(a) Heparin. This increases the lysis (dissolution) of thrombus to some extent but is probably not of great importance in this respect.

(b) Fibrinolytic agents. These may dissolve an established clot. This is more likely to happen if the clot is non-occlusive (i.e. it does not completely block the lumen of the vein). In this case the fibrinolysins are able to circulate around and come into contact with the clot. Streptokinase 600 000 units is given intravenously over 30 minutes, followed by 100 000 units hourly. The exact dose required should be determined in the laboratory by special tests. After 48 to 72 hours repeat venograms are done to check that lysis has occurred. Close observation is required for signs of hypersensitivity to the drug and for signs of haemorrhage.

(c) Surgical removal of thrombus (thrombectomy). A clot can be removed directly from large veins or, more commonly, by use of a Fogarty venous thrombectomy catheter. The operation is similar to removal of an embolus from an artery (p. 237). Anticoagulants are administered per- and postoperatively. The incidence of re-thrombosis is disappointingly high.

3. Prevention of detachment with embolus formation. This is achieved by trying to ensure one or more of the following—that the clot sticks to the vein wall, that it does not become detached, that it is dissolved or removed, that if it becomes detached it cannot get very far.

(a) Bed rest. The rationale of this is that the clot becomes firmly adherent to the vein wall during rest. Also bits are less likely to break off while the patient is at rest. Bed rest with the feet elevated should continue until the temperature subsides and the signs of deep venous thrombosis disappear—usually 5 to 8 days. Anticoagulants should be administered at the same time.

(b) Fibrinolysins (see above). The risk is removed by dissolving the clot. This is particularly important where there is non-occlusive clot in the large veins of the upper thigh or the pelvis.

(c) Surgical removal. The rationale for this is as in (b).

(d) Ligation of veins above clot. In some circumstances, where recurrent pulmonary emboli are occurring or are likely to occur, veins are tied above the clot to prevent the latter travelling far in the circulation. This may be done in the leg (long saphenous, superficial or common femoral vein), in the pelvis (iliac veins) or in the abdomen (inferior vena cava). If the inferior vena cava is selected as the site for surgical attack it is better to plicate it, so that some blood can circulate while clots are held up. Alternatively, a small umbrella-like sieve can be inserted into the inferior vena cava under local anaesthetic via a vein in the neck. The sieve catches the emboli.

4. Prevention of long-term occlusion of or damage to the vein. This can only be achieved if the clot is dissolved or removed and does not recur. As indicated above this is almost impossible to achieve. Some degree of permanent damage in the deep veins of the leg is very common. This may result in symptoms and signs of the post-thrombotic syndrome (Ch. 24).

There is a good deal of controversy as to which is the most appropriate form of treatment in a given situation. The following table summarises this:

Site of clot	Treatment
1. Below knee—patient mobile	elastic stocking elevate foot of bed maintain mobility ±anticoagulants
2. Below knee—patient immobile	elevate foot of bed anticoagulants elastic stocking when up
3. Above knee	bed rest elevate foot of bed anticoagulants
4. Upper thigh and/or pelvis	bed rest elevate foot of bed anticoagulants
—if non-occlusive clot	streptokinase or surgical removal ±ligation of veins or continue as above
—if pulmonary embolus	streptokinase or surgical removal ±ligation of veins or continue as above

Fig. 18.2 Pulmonary embolism. The thrombus has formed in the posterior tibial veins and passes via the femoral, external iliac and common iliac veins to the inferior vena cava and thence to the right atrium of the heart. From the right atrium it passes to the right ventricle which pumps it in this case into the left pulmonary artery with infarction of the left lung.

Most people think that if anticoagulants are used in the treatment of deep venous thrombosis they should be continued for 3 to 6 months. This view is not universally accepted.

EMBOLISM

An embolus is a foreign body momentarily free in the blood stream. The most common variety is a detached thrombus from a vein which gives rise to pulmonary embolism. Detachment of a thrombus from the left side of the heart may cause gangrene of a limb (p. 237). It used to be thought that pulmonary embolus, apart from the immediate postoperative period, was rare, but more careful observation has shown that it is not uncommon at other times. Other forms of embolus are considered and mentioned at the end of this chapter.

PULMONARY EMBOLUS (Fig. 18.2)

Since embolism is a complication of thrombosis, prevention depends on avoiding thrombosis and in detecting established thrombosis as early as possible. The effect of an embolus is entirely dependent on its size. Three syndromes are recognised:

1. A relatively small embolus occludes a peripheral pulmonary artery and produces the classical picture—pleuritic-type pain, haemoptysis and a shadow of infarcted lung on the X-ray.

2. Repeated small or micro-emboli, without pain initially, with gradually increasing breathlessness, fatigue and a feeling of collapse on exertion. An isotope lung scan and phlebography may be necessary to confirm the diagnosis. This syndrome is sometimes associated with the oral contraceptive pill.

3. A massive pulmonary embolus occluding about two-thirds of the circumference of the pulmonary artery. The onset is sudden, there are signs of right heart failure, the patient's skin is clammy and cyanosed and the veins in the neck are distended. The diagnosis from myocardial infarct, though often difficult, is vital since pulmonary embolectomy may be the only hope of survival and such a procedure would be rapidly fatal in a patient with coronary thrombosis. Electrocardiography and lung scanning with radioactive xenon may be needed. Pulmonary angiography may confirm the diagnosis with certainty, but the patient may be too ill for it to be undertaken. Blood gases should be estimated—hypoxia and hypocarbia may be diagnostic of pulmonary embolism.

Treatment

The occurrence of a relatively small pulmonary embolus always gives rise to anxiety since it may be the forerunner of a massive embolus. Movement is reduced to a minimum, anticoagulant treatment instituted and analgesics given. Chest physiotherapy is used cautiously. Some add prophylactic antibiotics. The deep veins of the legs and pelvis are investigated by bilateral ascending phlebography. Any clot detected is treated as indicated above.

Repeated micro-emboli require treatment with anticoagulants, sometimes for several years.

Massive pulmonary embolus presents great difficulties in the choice and timing of treatment. Many patients die rapidly within an hour. The patient is left absolutely still and oxygen administered. If the condition is improving treatment is conservative. Either anticoagulants or fibrinolysins are administered, together with prophylactic antibiotics and analgesics (as necessary). If the patient survives an hour and is not improving pulmonary angiography is considered to accurately assess the embolus with a view to pulmonary embolectomy. The latter requires the facilities of cardio-pulmonary by-pass (although the operation can be done without this). Such a procedure is not often appropriate. The legs and pelvis must be investigated for causative thrombus, this being treated as outlined above.

Most patients suffering a massive pulmonary embolus have already had a small embolus. Such a small warning embolus must therefore be taken very seriously and further emboli prevented as far as possible.

OTHER FORMS OF EMBOLISM

1. Fat embolism. Fat embolism is usually associated with fractures of large long bones. Fat globules escape into the circulation as emboli. In severe cases respiratory distress occurs due, not to the emboli in the lungs, but to their effect on the brain which may cause death. Assisted respiration is advisable.

2. Air embolism. Air embolism is a risk of venous haemorrhage in which air is sucked into an open vein. The air causes frothing of the blood particularly in the heart. This may prove fatal. It is avoided in intravenous injections, including transfusion, by ensuring that only fluid and no air is injected.

3. Bacteria spread by emboli may be recognised by the presence of purpuric spots on the skin, tiny splinter haemorrhages under the nails, retinal haemorrhages, or from the presence of red blood cells in the urine (e.g. in cases of infective endocarditis).

4. Malignant cells. These can spread by the bloodstream as emboli.

5. Foreign bodies. The most important to avoid clinically is a detached portion of an intravenous catheter. This is a rare accidental occurrence associated with the use of central venous catheters.

BIBLIOGRAPHY

Horton E W 1979 British Journal of Hospital Medicine 22:260

19

Burns and scalds

DEFINITION AND CAUSES

A burn or scald implies some destruction of the body surface by an external cause such as:
1. Dry heat—flame or any hot object.
2. Moist heat—hot water or steam. This is what is meant by a scald.
3. Corrosive chemicals—acids or alkalis.
4. Electricity.
5. X-rays or other ionising radiation.
6. Friction.

CLINICAL FEATURES

The two most important factors are the extent of the skin area involved and the depth to which it is damaged.

1. **The area** of skin involved, measured as a proportion of the patients total body surface, determines the immediate risk to the patients life from loss of body fluid. This loss is comparable to severe bleeding and can produce a state of 'shock'. In this sense, the word shock implies a sequence of events in which the amount of circulating blood is reduced, the blood pressure falls and the heart can no longer sustain an adequate circulation. If not treated promptly, this state becomes irreversible and death ensues.

2. **The depth** of the damage determines whether the burn can heal spontaneously. For practical purposes there are two possibilities:

(a) *Partial thickness burn.* This implies that some skin cells remain alive throughout the area and healing will proceed if they are protected from infection or dehydration. The category includes burns ranging from the very superficial ones which heal rapidly without a permanent scar to those where only small remnants of skin survive in the deeper parts of the dermis. These heal slowly with much scar formation.

Because partial thickness burns will include some surviving nerve endings, they are painful and sensitive to any touch.

(b) *Full thickness.* Here the complete thickness of the skin is destroyed and healing can only occur from the edges. In practice, the lost skin must be replaced by some form of graft.

Because the nerve endings have been destroyed, the area will be insensitive and relatively painless.

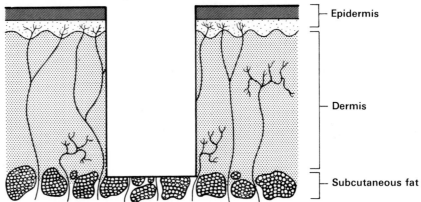

Example of partial thickness (first degree—in the old Dupuytren classification)

Partial thickness there will be epithelium in sweat glands and hair follicles to this depth

Full thickness (Third degree in old Dupuytren classification)

Epidermis

Dermis

Subcutaneous fat

Fig. 19.1   Diagram to illustrate depth of burn.

TREATMENT AND NURSING CARE

The percentage of the body surface involved in the burn is calculated from 'Wallace's Rule of Nine' (Fig. 19.2).

Fluid loss and replacement

If more than 15 per cent of the surface in an adult, or as little as 10 per cent in a small child, is involved, intravenous fluid replacement is needed at once. This need continues from the moment of the burn for a period of at

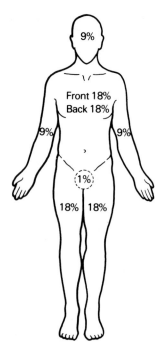

9%

Front 18%
Back 18%

9%   9%

1%

18%   18%

Fig. 19.2 Wallace's 'Rule of Nine' for estimating fluid requirements in the first 48 hours after burns.

least 48 hours, though the actual rate of fluid loss gradually diminishes during this time. The diminishing rate can be expressed by dividing the 48 hours into a series of time periods, during each of which the fluid loss/replacement need will be roughly equal. The time periods are:

4 hours	4 hours	4 hours	6 hours	6 hours	12 hours	12 hours

The fluid loss during each period is estimated thus:

$$\frac{\% \text{ area burned} \times \text{patient's wt in kg}}{2} = \text{ml fluid required}$$

Thus a 70 kg man with 50 per cent burns requires:

$$\frac{50 \times 70}{2} = \frac{3500}{2} = 1750 \text{ ml fluid per period or}$$

8750 ml in the first 24 hours. This is a vast quantity of fluid, far exceeding the normal blood volume.

Ideally, it should be given as plasma or human plasma protein solution, as this is what the patient is losing. Towards the end of the 48 hours, some whole blood may be used if there is a high proportion of full thickness burn which will have destroyed many of the red blood cells. Further amounts of electrolytes such as normal saline will be needed, in addition, to replace normal losses in urine and expired air.

During this resuscitation, the following are monitored:
1. Pulse rate
2. Blood pressure — usually ½ hourly
3. Respiration
4. Temperature
5. Urine output, plus check on specific gravity, blood and protein content. — hourly
6. Haematocrit—after each resuscitation period
7. Blood urea and electrolytes—at least daily

Meticulous fluid balance charts must be kept. If the hourly urine output falls below 20 to 30 ml, Mannitol is given to stimulate a diuresis, though a low urine output and a high haematocrit also imply that in spite of the calculated need, more fluid is required.

An indwelling catheter is essential to ensure that the hourly urine flow can be recorded.

Even after 48 hours, the i.v. infusion is discontinued only if oral intake is adequate. Other factors such as vomiting may greatly prolong the time. At best, when the acute resuscitation phase is over for an extensive burn, oral intake cannot quite keep pace with the patient's metabolic needs and feeding supplements may be given via a fine naso-gastric tube.

Care of the burn itself

During the all-important resuscitation, the highest priority is given to fluid replacement and the burned surface is protected in the simplest practicable manner. Ideally the patient is nursed in a special room and, so far as possible, aseptic techniques are used, similar to those of the operating theatre. The burn itself can then be simply covered by sterile towels. Definitive treatment of the burn must wait until the need for resuscitation has been satisfied though there are a few exceptions. These are:

1. Burns involving the upper respiratory tract may need urgent tracheostomy to maintain an airway.

2. Full thickness burns which completely encircle a limb, the neck or the chest may cause such constriction that circulation and/or breathing cease. This is because the burned skin shrinks in exactly the same way that bacon rind shrinks when it is cooked, the final effect being like a tourniquet. The complete insensitivity of a true full thickness burn can be exploited to release the constriction by incising with a scalpel, no anaesthesia being needed.

3. Only slightly less urgent than the above are full thickness eyelid burns which may need grafting within the first 24 hours to prevent exposure keratitis of the cornea.

Otherwise care of the burn itself can be carried out as follows:

(a) **Partial thickness burn.** Protection is required to expedite the natural healing potential. In addition to aseptic handling techniques, the taking of swabs for culture of bacteria and the use of antibiotics where necessary, various forms of direct protection are used according to the site.

  (i) Sterile occlusive dressings, usually just a non-adherent material such as Vaseline gauze covered by plenty of padding and bandages, changed only when needed as each dressing change increases the risk of introducing outside bacteria and disturbs the healing surface. This is suitable for most areas of the body.

  (ii) Sterile plastic bags applied over some lubricant and usually antiseptic cream such as Hibitane cream or silver sulphadiazine cream; the particular use for these is in treating burned hands, movement being unimpaired by such dressings.

  (iii)Simple exposure, allowing a natural coagulum to form on the surface which then acts as a dressing if left undisturbed. This is particularly useful for the face, but can be employed over much larger areas.

Healing should take place within about three weeks. Beyond that, the partial thickness nature of the burn is called into question and treatment as for full thickness burn becomes more appropriate.

(b) **Full thickness burns.** If of appreciable size, the area will need some form of skin replacement:

  (i) The burned skin may be completely excised immediately, or at some time after any resuscitation is completed, and split-skin grafts applied to the raw surface. Full thickness hand burns, small enough to require no resuscitation, are ideal for immediate excision as the risk of infection and the period of immobilisation are minimised by this technique.

  (ii) The burns may be allowed to deslough themselves over a period of weeks assisted by dressings similar to those used in partial thickness burns, but with greater use of antiseptic creams. Skin grafts are then applied when all the dead tissue has been shed and a clean, vascular raw surface remains. In practice, some combination of the two alternatives may be used, final desloughing of the surface being performed as an operation. This slower method is more appropriate in larger burns where the patient's general condition may have precluded early surgery.

The skin grafts used are most often so-called split skin. The outer layers of the skin are removed from an unburned area using a variety of special knives, leaving some living dermis behind. This donor site heals just like a partial thickness burn. The removed outer layers are applied to the raw surface at the burn site and will unite to it within a few days, given suitable conditions of immobility and freedom from infection.

Sometimes, very deep burns may expose bone or tendon and the above simple graft has no vascular surface to which it can unite. In these cases some form of skin-flap is required, transferring a piece of skin and fat, sometimes with fascia and muscle attached, but always with the retention of a blood supply. This means that either one edge of the flap must remain attached to its original site, or its blood vessels must be re-connected by microvascular anastomosis.

Nursing care of the skin grafts

Once the grafts have been applied, they need to be protected from disturbance, as any movement between graft and the recipient site will prevent union. This is mainly achieved by the dressing or suturing technique of the surgeon, but it is important to leave the dressings intact for at least five days and avoid unnecessary movement of the area during other nursing procedures.

Sometimes, skin grafts are just taken from the donor site and stored for later application on the ward, when it becomes part of the nursing procedure to apply them to the raw surface at the next dressing change. It is also usual to store any surplus graft for later application if some of the original graft should fail. The stored skin is wrapped in gauze moistened with sterile Normal saline and kept in an ordinary refrigerator at 4°C. It will remain usable for up to three weeks.

It must be always remembered that the donor site is very painful (cf. partial thickness burn) and its dressing should not be disturbed for the best part of two weeks.

Use of antibiotics

There is little value in prophylactic antibiotic treatment used as a routine on all burns. It is better to treat any infection which arises, choosing the antibiotic indicated by the culture and sensitivity reports. The antibiotics are given orally or intramuscularly. The use of antibiotic creams and ointments is best avoided as they tend to be ineffective and promote the development of resistant bacteria. If topical ones are ever used, they should not include the antibiotics which one is likely to need to give systemically.

Many bacteria can infect a burn, but two merit particular mention:

1. *Streptococcus*: the particular form of the haemolytic streptococcus known as Lancefield Group A is particularly destructive of skin grafts and can also cause a dangerous spreading cellulitis. The same organism causes acute sore throats, scarlet fever and, more indirectly, acute nephritis and rheumatic fever. It is always sensitive to penicillin, but the co-existence of a resistant staphylococcus may make simple penicillin ineffective in practice.

2. *Pseudomonas pyocyaenia*: this can be a great nuisance in burns and may cause a fatal septicaemia. It resists many antibiotics though gentamycin often succeeds against it. This is why it is important to reserve gentamycin for systemic use and not risk creating resistant pseudomonas by its casual use in ointments.

General nursing care

In addition to the dressings, observations and care of the intravenous infusion, other special points arise in the nursing of burned patients.

1. Burned skin is much more vulnerable to local pressure than is undamaged skin and a partial thickness burn will rapidly become full thickness under the circumstances which will produce pressure sores. Because of the other needs of the patient it may be very difficult to protect pressure areas, but every care must be taken to overcome this. Sometimes special beds are used, e.g. water beds or so-called low air-loss beds where the aim is to 'float' the patient on a cushion of water or air.

2. The use of bedpans calls for great care and patience to overcome the inevitable discomfort. It does not solve the problem to allow the patient to become constipated.

3. Apart from the initial drastic fluid loss, severe burns greatly increase the patient's dietary needs. High protein intake and a high calorie intake in general are needed to replace the tissues destroyed by the burn and the far greater amount of body protein which is broken down by the increased katabolism which occurs. This need coincides with many factors such as pain, general ill-health, discomfort, and the unpleasant sights and smells of the burns which tend to suppress appetite. Many patients need coaxing, hand feeding and even extra supplementary feeding via a naso-gastric tube. Even then, a patient with a severe burn will lose weight.

4. It must never be forgotten that the patient needs as much emotional support as can be given. The horror of the original experience, the pains and discomfort of prolonged treatment, the fear of permanent disability and disfigurement and of death all combine to destroy morale and constant encouragement is a great help.

SPECIAL COMPLICATIONS OF BURNS

1. *Overwhelming infection.* Local infection at the burn site can progress to a septicaemia and secondary infection of any part of the body. In spite of modern antibiotics, the situation can prove rapidly fatal.

2. *Extensive oedema.* There is always oedema at the burn site and this, to some extent, accounts for the loss of fluid from the circulation. It usually begins to re-absorb after about 48 hours. Oedema within the upper respiratory tract, from the mouth and nose to the larynx, can obstruct the airway and demand a tracheostomy. Oedema of the lungs from inhalation of smoke or other hot gases may require artificial ventilation and other urgent measures.

3. *Other respiratory problems.* Any extensive burn can cause changes in the lungs which lead to a serious failure of oxygenation, even where no inhalation burn has occurred.

4. *Renal failure.* This may be due to the failure to give adequate fluid replacement in time to prevent a prolonged fall in blood pressure. The renal circulation is the first to suffer and once urine secretion ceases, the patient will progress rapidly to complete renal failure. This is often irreversible and in spite of renal dialysis, death is the usual result. Renal failure can also occur due to blockage of the renal tubules with haemo-globin released into the circulation from the many red blood cells destroyed by deep burns. The intact cells cannot enter the tubules, but in this situation, the free haemoglobin may.

5. *Gastro-intestinal bleeding.* This occurs quite often as a reaction to extensive burns. Occasionally, a true acute duodenal ulcer develops, known as Curling's ulcer.

6. *Anaemia* can result from a number of factors; initial destruction of red cells, gastro-intestinal bleeding as above and later depression of the bone marrow due to chronic infection.

7. *Scar hypertrophy and contracture.* All scars shrink as they mature and extensive burn scars can cause disabling contractures as they do so, limiting the movement of joints. Burn scars often form excessive masses of scar tissue leading to great disfigurement. These are known as hypertrophic or keloid scars. They are best prevented by expediting healing by early grafting where necessary and by the use of special elastic pressure garments when healing is complete.

SPECIAL BURNS

1. Chemical burns. These are most often due to strong acids and alkalis such as sulphuric acid, widely used in car batteries and in many industrial processes, or caustic soda, used in some paint strippers. Either acid or alkali requires neutralisation to arrest its action. As a first aid measure, copious amounts of water will dilute either and special buffer solutions can be applied when available. These contain mixtures of chemicals which tend to neutralise either acid or alkali, the great advantage being that one does not need to know the exact nature of the burning agent.

One special acid is hydrofluoric acid which is used in the chemical industry and also to etch glass. It causes painful, spreading destruction of tissue by abstracting calcium ions and if at all extensive, can cause a fatal fall in serum calcium level. It is treated by local application of calcium gluconate and, where necessary, by intravenous calcium.

2. Certain other substances cause contact burns, not by corrosive action but by their property of producing great heat in reacting with other materials. For example, metallic sodium or potassium when in contact with water commences a violent chemical reaction, giving off intense heat. In contact with living tissue, the water in the tissue sets this off. Likewise, phosphorus contrives the same effect when in contact with air.

3. Radiation. Any ionising radiation, including X rays, will cause burns if the exposure is sufficient. The effect may be delayed some hours after the exposure.

20
Trauma

Trauma means injury. People may be injured singly or many at a time, e.g. train crashes, multiple pile-ups on the motorways and, regrettably, terrorist activities. When there are many injured patients the accident services of the hospital to which the casualties are taken will be severely tested. Most hospitals will have a published plan to deal with such situations. Nurses should make quite sure that they are familiar with such major disaster plans as the efficient treatment of a large number of casualties presented in a very short time depends to a large extent upon the efficient organisation of the medical and nursing staff and the ancillary staff.

MAJOR DISASTERS: SURGICAL TRIAGE

Triage is a military term used to describe the initial sorting of injured patients. This concept has been adopted to deal with major disasters in civilian hospitals. The method used to sort injured patients is to divide them into three groups. The first group of patients to identify are those whose life-threatening conditions will benefit most rapidly from the provision of basic resuscitative techniques. The second group of patients are those with serious injuries which will need hospital treatment but whose treatment can safely be deferred without threat to life until the first group of patients have been dealt with. The third group are those patients with lesser injuries who do not require urgent medical attention; many of them do not require admission to hospital.

Surgical triage: multiple casualties

Group I	Group II	Group III
Life threatening conditions	Injuries requiring hospital treatment as inpatients, but whose treatment can *safely* be deferred until Group I dealt with	Minor injuries requiring O.P. or G.P. treatment.
Airway obstruction		
Haemorrhage		
Major chest, abdominal or head injuries		

The critically injured patients, in the first group, are those in whom the air-way is at risk, or whose blood volume is seriously diminished, and those with major chest, abdominal or head injuries.

Patients with threats to the airway

Threats to the airway must receive absolute priority in order to re-establish a patent airway. A patient with otherwise minor injuries may very quickly die because the airway is obstructed by vomit, blood or foreign bodies. Once the airway has been re-established by removing any obstruction, by ensuring that the tongue has not fallen back into the pharynx, by endotracheal intubation or by tracheostomy then other serious injuries can be dealt with. Naturally occurring surgical diseases are usually confined to natural anatomical regions, e.g. the stomach, the peritoneum, the lung. This is not so in the case of traumatic lesions which may transgress many anatomical boundaries. Their treatment requires a very sound knowledge of anatomy and a wide experience of surgery.

Blood volume

Serious external blood loss is uncommon and can in most cases be stopped fairly easily by the application of direct pressure. On the other hand blood lost internally, either by bleeding into the abdominal or thoracic cavities or by bleeding into soft tissue planes from such injuries as multiple fractures, is less easy to recognise and is often underestimated. It should be suspected in all patients who have multiple fractures, a history of high speed injury or a penetrating injury. It is rarely necessary to transfuse such patients with uncrossmatched blood as the blood volume can be maintained with various intravenous fluids until adequately crossmatched blood is available.

Chest injuries

All patients with major chest injuries are at risk to their life until the lungs can be re-expanded and kept adequately ventilated. Such patients will usually need to be kept in the resuscitation area until they are stabilised, and may well need chest drains and intermittent positive pressure respiration. See Chapter 30, Figure 30.1.

Abdominal injuries

Major abdominal injury can be life-threatening. This is usually due to severe internal haemorrhage from a ruptured spleen or liver. The diagnosis is often clear on clinical grounds, but in the presence of multiple injuries it may be more difficult. Peritoneal tap or lavage are helpful in detecting free blood. The patient requires urgent blood transfusion and urgent laparotomy to control the haemorrhage.

Head injuries

Patients with severe head injuries often require urgent resuscitation and attention to the airway (see Ch. 44).

The second group of patients should be assessed in the resuscitation reception area but are usually able to be passed through this area fairly quickly and admitted to the ordinary wards for treatment when time becomes available.

The third group of patients will also need assessment in the Casualty reception area but can often be referred for out-patient treatment or treatment by their own doctors after initial assessment.

It is important in the treatment of a large number of casualties that the nursing staff should follow directions of the nursing officers in charge who will in turn be working in close conjunction with the medical staff. The most important member of the medical staff in such a situation is a senior doctor who has been appointed as the triage officer and this will usually be a senior accident surgeon. He will often ask the nursing officers to allocate a nurse to a particular patient as continuous observation and re-assessment of priorities is necessary. It may be necessary to empty a ward of routine patients to use it as a special reception ward for the injured. This will require a high level of nursing staff.

Documentation of the injured patients presents many difficulties as some of the patients may be unconscious and no names may be available. In addition the care of property of the injured patients will also have to be specially organised. Continuous liaison with the police and arrangements to deal with the press and enquiries from patients relatives will have to be planned.

Shock in injured patients

This is considered in detail in Chapter 13. Shock may be caused by severe pain, by emotional factors, or by severe diminution in the blood volume. Pain can of course be relieved. Emotional factors need to be considered and a good nurse will always try and reassure a patient that he or she is in good hands and will be well looked after. The nurse should always have time to answer patients questions and to keep the patient informed as much as possible as to why various procedures are necessary. Loss of blood volume is dealt with by intravenous transfusion of blood, plasma, plasma expanders such as dextran or other intravenous fluids as the doctor directs.

Infection

Patients with open wounds or compound fractures (remember that fractures of the base of the skull into the pharynx, the middle ear or the sinuses; fractures of the jaw into the mouth; fractures of the ribs which may penetrate the lungs; and fractures of the pelvis which may damage the bladder, the rectum or the intestines are technically compound fractures) are at risk of infection and for this reason antibiotics are usually prescribed to cover the first few days of healing. Such wounds are often contaminated with foreign bodies (pieces of clothing, oil, metallic fragments or road debris) and the initial treatment should always include removing all the foreign material that can be identified in the wound. It is quite often necessary to excise the whole wound surgically in order to be sure of obtaining clean surfaces which will heal satisfactorily. In some cases it is advisable not to close the wound immediately but to use the method known as delayed primary repair where the wound is cleaned and dressed and is not sutured for 3 or 4 days. This method is quite commonly used in crush injuries or in missile injuries. Its application in war time or as a result of terrorist activities has saved many lives.

The crush syndrome

After a compressing injury of several hours duration, usually of the limbs, the patient may develop hypotension followed by acute renal failure. This is known as the crush syndrome. It is thought to be due to the release from injured tissues of substances toxic to the renal tubules.

The treatment is both to manage the renal injury by suitable dialysis and intravenous treatment, and to excise or even amputate the crushed tissue, taking special precautions to avoid infection, as this always makes the syndrome more dangerous.

Thrombosis

Thrombosis, or clotting of the blood in the large veins, is a frequent complication of injury especially in older people. Sometimes the clots break away from the walls of the vein and enter the venous circulation, passing through the heart and becoming impacted in the pulmonary arteries—pulmonary embolism. This is a serious and often fatal complication so precautions are often taken to prevent venous thrombosis by the administration of plasma expanders or occasionally by the use of anticoagulant drugs.

Sloughing in wound and adjacent tissues

Tissues in the depth of the wound may be deprived of their blood supply and become necrotic. This is known as sloughing and will often require excision of the dead tissue. It may not be obvious at the time of injury how much tissue has become avascular.

Secondary haemorrhage

This is haemorrhage which presents a week or 10 days after injury and is almost always due to infection which erodes the wall of the small blood vessels in the base of the wound. Such a complication may be dealt with by means of direct pressure but usually requires surgical ligation of the eroded artery and the administration of antibiotics.

Failure to heal

Persistent infection sloughing, haemorrhage or retained foreign body may lead to failure of the wound to heal. This is dealt with in detail in Chapter 11.

Wound healing

Healing of the wound depends not only upon the accurate apposition and repair of wounded tissues but on the general condition of the patient, so it is important to ensure that the patient's nutritional state is good and that there is an adequate haemoglobin content of the blood. Older people are often short of vitamins and plasma proteins. The addition of vitamins and a higher proportion of proteins in the diet is sometimes necessary.

Summary

The final result achieved by an injured patient depends very largely on the adequacy of the initial treatment. In severe injuries the initial treatment is directed towards saving the patient's life particularly by attention to the airway and the replacement of any blood loss. The next important factor in the treatment is accurate repair of damaged tissues (including any fractures), the prevention of infection and the prevention of loss of function. In this connection it should be stated that the aim of treatment is to return the patient to the level of function which he or she enjoyed before the injury. It must never be forgotten that restoration of function is as important as the primary treatment.

BIBLIOGRAPHY

Brown A A, Nicholls R J 1977 British Journal of Surgery 64: 397
Yates D Q W 1979 British Journal of Hospital Medicine 22: 323

21
Fractures and joint injuries

CAUSES OF INJURIES

Broken bones and injured or dislocated joints are very common results of trauma. There are however other conditions in which bones can be fractured and joints injured or dislocated. Fractures and joint injuries can therefore be divided into three types:
(a) traumatic,
(b) pathological,
(c) stress.

Traumatic

This group is by far the most common. The injury may be 'closed', i.e. the injury to the bone or joint does not communicate with the exterior, or it may be compound, i.e. the broken bone or injured joint is accessible to outside pollution and is therefore more likely to become infected. Such cases are always treated with antibiotics as well as the special treatment for the injury. Fractures may be of several anatomical types according to the severity of the injury and the direction of the force. If the bone ends are jammed together it is known as an impacted fracture. If the bone ends are splintered it is a comminuted fracture. If the bone is that of a young child it may well be only partially fractured. This is known as a greenstick fracture because it is similar to the way in which a living twig will break when a bending force is applied to it. If the fractured bone ends damage tissues close to the bones such as larger arteries or nerves, then the fracture is known as a complicated one (Fig. 21.1).

Pathological

A bone which is diseased will often fracture following a very minor trauma which would not break a normal bone. Such a fracture is known as a pathological fracture and arises in diseases such as malignant deposits in bones and in Paget's disease. Similarly a joint affected by diseases such as syphilis may dislocate spontaneously. There is a special

Oblique

Comminuted

Transverse

Impacted

Complicated
(Muscle between
fragments in this example)

Greenstick

Fig. 21.1 Varieties of fractures.

type of pathological dislocation of the hip seen in new born babies known as congenital dislocation. This is due to abnormal joint development and is discussed in Chapter 47.

Stress fractures

These arise in normal bones which have an undue and repetitive stress placed upon them. They usually start as partial fractures and as the stresses are repeated the fractures become complete, although some attempt at healing commences when the initial minor fracture appears.

The most common example of this rare condition is a fracture of the neck of the second metatarsal in young recruits to the armed services who are required to do a great deal of marching and foot stamping in their first few weeks of training. A stress injury of a joint is best exemplified by the development of arthritic changes in the joint following undue wear and tear.

CHANGES RESULTING FROM FRACTURE

In the traumatic fractures it must always be remembered that broken bones bleed and the blood loss can often be quite severe, for instance a patient with bilateral femoral fractures may well bleed six pints of blood into the muscles and soft tissues of the thighs. This accounts for the anaemia and severe pain and swelling which such an injury causes.

Fractured bones heal by the natural healing processes of the body. The blood clot between the ends of the bone becomes organised. This results in the formation of tissue known as callus in which special cells concerned with bone repair are found in plentiful amounts. One type of cell—the osteoblast—produces bone tissue whilst another cell—the osteoclast—removes and remodels excess bone so that eventually the healed bone adopts the same shape as it had prior to the fracture.

As a general rule bones take about 6 weeks to unite but the larger bones which take the full weight of the body such as the femur and the tibia will take as long again or even longer to become strong enough to take the body weight. The smaller bones and the non weight-bearing bones such as the humerus or the metacarpals may be strong enough to fulfil their normal function before the bone is fully united. It is a strange and unexplained freak of nature that those bones which can least easily be immobilised (e.g. the clavicle or the ribs) practically never fail to join whether or not they are immobilised, whereas the bones which are most easily able to be fixed (e.g. the humerus and the tibia) are the ones which most frequently fail to unite (Fig. 21.2).

Site of non-union

Fig. 21.2 Un-united fracture of the humerus.

SYMPTOMS AND SIGNS OF FRACTURES

1. Pain aggravated by movement.
2. Tenderness over the fracture line.
3. Swelling.
4. Deformity.
5. Shortening of the limb.
6. Loss of function.
7. Abnormal mobility at the fracture site.
8. Occasional crepitus or grating of the bone ends as they move on each other.

Sometimes all these symptoms and signs are obvious but in other cases only one or two of them may be present, depending upon the site of the fracture, the displacement and the leverage upon the fracture.

PRINCIPLES OF TREATMENT OF FRACTURES AND JOINT INJURIES

The important principles of treatment can again be classified under three headings as follows:
    1. Reduction.
    2. Rest until healed.
    3. Restoration of function.

1. Reduction

Unless a fracture is complicated (i.e. has damaged neighbouring important structures which need urgent treatment), then there is usually no urgency to reduce the displacement and the limb can often be splinted for several days if necessary until the final·method of treatment is decided. On the other hand a dislocated joint must be reduced as a matter of urgency because the longer the joint remains dislocated the more likely is the articular surface to become permanently damaged.

The usual method of reduction is by manipulation either with or without anaesthesia but in certain cases it may be necessary to perform a surgical operation in order to reduce the fracture or the dislocation. This procedure technically converts the injury into a compound type. It is therefore usual to cover the postoperative period with a course of antibiotic treatment.

2. Rest until healed

When considering the second principle of treatment it is important to know the various methods of splintage which are used. These vary from the most simple support such as a sling or a collar and cuff to the most complicated type of internal fixation or external splintage. A small, but important, point to note is that a sling is used to support the weight of the arm in such injuries as a fracture of the clavicle or a dislocation of the acromioclavicular joint; whereas a collar and cuff is used to allow the weight of the arm to hang down and thus aid the realignment of the bone. The latter is used in injuries such as fractures of the surgical neck of the humerus.

The most common method of external splintage used is plaster of Paris though recently other substances have been introduced which have all the advantages of plaster of Paris as well as other advantages, such as being water-resistant, lighter and allowing X-rays to pass through more easily than plaster. It must be remembered that any rigid cast applied to a limb encircles the limb and should the tissues swell beneath the plaster then the cast can restrict the circulation, sometimes with tragic results.

The indications that a plaster is too tight are:
    (a) pain which is persistent and increasing,
    (b) numbness of the extremities as the blood supply to the sensory nerves is cut off,
    (c) whiteness, paleness or duskiness of the extremities because of circulatory interference. The nurse should draw the sister's atten-

tion to any patient in whom she notices these signs presenting.
(d) increasing swelling of hand or foot.

It is much better to remove and reapply a plaster ten times than to leave on too tight a plaster which may cause loss of the limb. It must also be remembered that a poorly applied plaster cast may cause local soreness from pressure and that the sharp edges of the cast may also break the skin. The nurse must be aware of these possibilities and check plaster casts for comfort on frequent occasions.

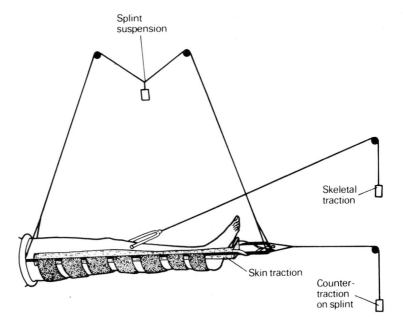

Fig. 21.3 The Thomas splint. The splint is suspended and *either* skin traction with counter-traction on the splint *or* skeletal traction is applied.

Special splints are also used in certain circumstances and perhaps the best known of these is the Thomas splint (Fig. 21.3). This splint was first devised by Hugh Owen Thomas (p. 647), in order to rest knee joints which were infected with tuberculosis. In more recent years it has become widely used throughout the world for the treatment of fractured femoral shafts. The ring of a Thomas splint is fairly rigid and can give rise to presure sores so it is common to apply counter traction from the bottom end of the splint over a pulley at the bottom of the bed in order to pull the ring away from the groin. A recent modification of the Thomas splint is the Povey splint which has a foam rubber ring round the upper part of the thigh which is much more comfortable than the Thomas splint. The whole splint is also much more manoeuverable for nursing purposes and the patient can easily be transported in the Povey splint. A further advantage is that the cumbersome frame needed to support a Thomas splint is unnecessary. In fractures of the femur, traction is commonly applied to the limb itself in order to keep the bone alignment in good position. Such traction can be applied through adhesive tape strapped to the sides of the lower limb (skin traction) or by means of a pin passed through the front of the upper end of the tibia (skeletal traction). Either type of traction may be fixed (i.e. fixed to the bottom end of a Thomas splint) or may be balanced (i.e. the traction is applied without fixation to the splint by means of a spring or a weight).

Any patient with fractures who is confined to bed for a long period (and this particularly applies to elderly people) is liable to pressure sores and careful nursing is essential in order to prevent these. Various types of mattress have been devised to reduce the risk of bed sores but by far the best method of preventing them is regular careful nursing care.

For a number of reasons the surgeon may decide to splint the fracture internally rather than use external splinting. Such a decision involves a surgical operation and the patient must be prepared for this in the same way as for any other major surgical operation. Particular care must be placed on preoperative shaving as an infected fracture or an infected joint as a result of unsterile surgery is a disaster for the patient. Internal fixation may be achieved by the use of bone screws, plate and screws, wire, rods within the cavity of the bone, or by a combination of one or more methods (Fig. 21.4). A useful method of fixation in dirty compound wounds is to insert threaded pins into the bone through the skin, and connect the free ends of the pins by an external bar. This fixes the fracture but allows the wound to be treated.

Fig. 21.4 Internal fixation. X-ray showing a fracture of the neck of the femur, fixed by a pin up the centre of the neck and a plate with screws holding it to the shaft.

Usually the safest method of treatment is conservative but operative reduction and fixation is often used in elderly people, so that they may be mobilised more quickly; in cases where the fracture or dislocation is completely unstable or for ease of nursing in multiple fractures.

Compound fractures, as opposed to closed fractures, require treatment within the first few hours but it is frequently wise to spend some time in treating the patient's general condition before turning one's attention to the local treatment of the compound fracture.

During the period of resuscitation the compound wound should be covered with a thick sterile dressing and left undisturbed until the patient is taken to theatre and anaesthetised. At operation all foreign material and non-viable tissue is excised from the wound which is then closed if possible.

If plaster is applied in such cases there is always some bleeding into the plaster and staining of the plaster from the exudate. Some surgeons like to cut a window in the plaster over the wound so that it can be re-dressed without disturbing the fracture, whereas other surgeons prefer to remove the plaster, dress the wound and re-apply plaster should this become necessary. Contaminated and compound wounds will heal quite adequately beneath the plaster. Sometimes it is not possible to close the wound and in cases where there is severe tissue damage it is sometimes wise to deliberately leave the compound wound open but clean and dressed with an appropriate antiseptic dressing. The limb is therefore encased in a plaster and final closure of the wound is then delayed for several days. It must not be forgotten that fractures of the base of the skull, fractures of the ribs, fractures of the jaw and sometimes fractures of the pelvis may be compound as they all may communicate with the exterior through the various body cavities. Complicated fractures which injure important organs close to the fracture site may also need fairly immediate treatment in order to repair or lessen the chance of permanent damage to the affected structure.

The treatment of pathological fractures follows the same principles as the treatment for traumatic fractures but in addition treatment may be instituted to deal with the underlying pathology. For instance it is quite common only to discover a secondary malignant deposit in the bone by the fact that a fracture has occurred. In this case, the fracture is often fixed internally and radiotherapy treatment given locally to kill off the cancer cells in the local deposit.

The rarely occurring stress fractures also call for the same principles of treatment as in traumatic fractures, though reduction is rarely required as it is unusual to find any displacement in stress fractures.

3. Restoration of function

The restoration of full functional activity following a fracture of a limb or dislocation of a joint is perhaps the most important principle of the three. It is no help to the patient to obtain a perfectly healed fracture in excellent position but be unable to use the limb because of stiffness. Restoration of function begins as soon as the primary treatment has been institued so the nurse must encourage the patient to use the muscles of the immobilised part as frequently and as actively as he can. The physiotherapist will see the patient perhaps once a day but the nurse may see the patient many times a day. A patient being nursed in a Thomas splint for a fractured femur who does not do his quadriceps exercises at least hourly and who does not exercise his calf muscles and his ankle, will find himself quite unable to walk when the splintage is finally removed, and his rehabilitation will be unduly prolonged. He may well develop a permanent limitation of movement of the joints of the limb if he has not conscientiously performed his rehabilitation exercises during the course of his treatment.

Restoration of function of course is not confined only to limbs. One of the most important aspects of treatment of fractures of the ribs is to keep the lungs fully expanded by deliberate breathing exercises. Head injuries may give rise to a certain amount of brain damage and this can affect the speech so that speech therapy becomes an important part of functional rehabilitation.

If a patient is confined to bed because of a fractured lower limb it is important not to let the muscles and joints of the other limbs become stiff, in order to achieve as early a restoration of function as possible. The patient must be continuously encouraged by the nursing staff to perform the exercises and treatment prescribed by the surgeon. There is nothing more rewarding than to see a seriously injured patient return to a full normal and active life.

IMPORTANT POINTS ABOUT PARTICULAR FRACTURES

FRACTURES OF THE SHOULDER GIRDLE AND UPPER LIMB

Shoulder girdle

Fractures of the clavicle are treated by 2 to 3 weeks rest in a broad arm sling or figure of 8 bandage, followed by mobilisation. There is rarely any difficulty in achieving union and full movement. Fractures of the scapula require rest in a sling until the pain and swelling subsides. No particular treatment other than this is necessary.

Fractures of the humerus

A fracture of the greater tuberosity of the humerus is commonly associated with a dislocation of the shoulder joint. The treatment for this is reduction of the dislocation as early as possible and this usually achieves a satisfactory position of the fracture of the greater tuberosity. Rest in a sling for 3-6 weeks followed by mobilisation of the arm is an acceptable form of treatment. Fractures of the surgical neck of the humerus are common in the elderly and are almost always impacted. Fractures of the mid shaft of the humerus are common and usually unite well. These usually require immobilisation by three splints together with a collar and cuff so that the weight of the arm keeps the humerus well aligned. An important point to check in all these fractures is that the radial nerve has not been damaged (Ch. 45). This is tested by asking the patient to dorsiflex the wrist.

Fractures around the elbow

These are common fractures in children. A supracondylar fracture of the humerus in children should be reduced by manipulation under general anaesthesia and supported in a collar and cuff with the elbow flexed beyond the right angle. One of the complications is compression of the brachial artery by swelling in front of the elbow and the nurse must check the radial pulse at hourly intervals as, if the pulse disappears, the flexion at the elbow must be lessened. As a general rule fractures around the elbow joint do not need to be immobilised in plaster but some complicated fractures do need open reduction and internal fixation.

FRACTURES OF THE FOREARM BONES

It is essential to obtain an accurate reduction in these cases as, if there is angulation or residual displacement after manipulation, the important function of rotation of the forearm will be limited. It is therefore quite common for fractures of the forearm bones to require open operation and internal fixation in order to get an absolutely accurate reduction.

Fractures of the distal forearm

The so-called Colles' fracture—an impacted fracture of the lower end of the radius with dorsal and radial angulation and displacement is one of the commonest fractures seen. It is particularly common in elderly people with frail bones and requires manipulative reduction followed by a plaster slab for 4 to 5 weeks.

Fractures of the wrist and hand

Because of the poor blood supply of this bone, fractures of the scaphoid may take many weeks to achieve full union and until union is achieved a scaphoid plaster cast is necessary. Fractures of the metacarpals usually do not present any difficulty and rarely require immobilisation but fractures of the fingers are most important and if badly treated will give rise to permanent deformities and limitation of movement.

FRACTURES OF THE SKULL

These are dealt with in the chapter on head injuries. The important feature of these injuries is whether there has been underlying brain damage or damage to the blood vessels which supply the brain. Occasionally one sees a depressed fracture when the skull has been struck with a hard round object which has the effect of depressing a circular portion of the skull below the general level of the skull, causing local injury to the underlying brain.

FRACTURES OF THE SPINAL COLUMN

Such injuries are becoming more and more common and, as with fractures of the skull, it is important to decide whether or not the fracture of the spinal column is associated with damage to the spinal cord.

Compression fractures of the vertebral bodies are the most common types of spinal fracture and are usually not associated with any spinal cord injury. They are treated by bed rest until the pain settles down. Extension exercises of the spine should be started as soon as the patient can comfortably perform them. Once the pain has diminished then the patient is allowed up and about.

Dislocations of the spine however frequently give rise to neurological complications and from the point of view of treatment and nursing it is important to decide whether such dislocations are stable or unstable. A stable dislocation without neurological damage is treated by reduction of the dislocation if possible followed by treatment in the same way as for a compression fracture. An unstable dislocation without spinal cord damage is uncommon but requires urgent reduction and operative fixation in order to prevent spinal cord injury during the various nursing procedures necessary whilst the patient is in hospital. Dislocations, whether stable or unstable, with neurological damage should be reduced although the amount of recovery to be expected is variable. As a general rule patients who are completely paralysed and have an unstable dislocation make no recovery of their spinal cord function distal to the level of the lesion (Fig. 21.5).

In these cases nursing care becomes most important as the patient will be confined to bed or a wheelchair for a long period and pressure sores develop very easily in skin without sensation. Two hourly turning is necessary and for this reason some surgeons will fix the dislocated spine by surgical means after reduction purely in order to facilitate the nursing care. Other important requirements are care of the bladder, breathing exercises and the prevention of fixed deformities in the paralysed part of the body. The most difficult cases to manage of course are those with the dislocation in the cervical spine where the legs, the intercostal muscles, and a variable proportion of the upper limb muscles are paralysed. However, it is surprising how well these people manage their ordinary lives if they receive skilled medical treatment and nursing in the first few weeks after injuries.

FRACTURES OF THE RIBS (See also Chapter 30)

The fractures of the ribs themselves are of little significance and no particular local treatment is performed for the fractures themselves. The major consideration is what damage has been done to underlying

Fig. 21.5 Dislocation of the cervical spine. Note the displacement of the bones and the severe angulation of the spinal cord.

structures. The fractured ends of the ribs may pierce the lungs giving rise to a haemothorax and pneumothorax. If the hole in the lung exerts a valvular effect so that air can escape from it but cannot be sucked back into the lungs then a particularly dangerous situation exists as a tension pneumothorax will develop. This requires urgent treatment otherwise the patient will die.

If a large segment of the chest becomes flail because of double fractures of several ribs then the mechanism of respiration is damaged and the flail piece of chest sinks in with inspiration and moves outwards on expiration. This is known as paradoxical respiration and is best treated by means of intermittent positive pressure respiration on a ventilator. Fractured ribs may also damage the spleen, the kidney, the stomach and the liver and laparotomy if often necessary in this case.

FRACTURES OF THE PELVIS

The pelvis surrounds internal organs which may be damaged by fractures of the pelvis. These organs include the urethra, the bladder and the bowel and urgent surgical treatment is necessary for these damaged organs.

Fractures of the pelvis which do not pass through the weight bearing area of the pelvis are treated merely by rest until the painful symptoms subside. Fractures of the pelvis involving the acetabulum or the sacroiliac joints require much longer periods of bed rest and sometimes need open reduction and fixation.

FRACTURES OF THE LOWER LIMBS

Fracture of the neck of the femur is one of the most common reasons for admission to hospital of elderly people. Because this is an injury of the aged it is almost always treated surgically in order to allow them to be up and about as soon as possible. Those fractures close to the femoral head are usually treated by removal of the femoral head and the insertion of a metallic prosthesis. This is because the head of the femur is likely to die as a result of damage to its blood supply and subsequent avascular necrosis. Fractures lower down the femoral neck are usually treated by means of a pin, which passes up the neck into the femoral head, attached to a plate which is screwed to the upper shaft of the femur (Fig. 21.4). It must be remembered that because patients with fractures of the femoral neck are usually old, they may well have other concurrent diseases. In addition the patient may be in a poor state of nutrition (often these old people live at home alone and eat poorly—in fact many of them are not found for some hours after the fall which has broken their femoral neck). They may be diabetic, in some degree of heart failure, myxoedematous or suffering from malignant disease. Many of them are anaemic and all these various problems must be considered preoperatively so that the patient's general condition is as good as possible before surgical treatment is undertaken.

Postoperatively, as much attention must be given to the patient's general condition as to the fractured femoral neck. It is usual to mobilise these patients as soon as possible after their operation taking partial weight on the injured limb, progressing to full weight-bearing as soon as they are comfortable.

Dislocation of the hip

Although dislocation of the hip is not common it is occurring with increasing frequency. The treatment is to reduce it as soon as possible and to make quite sure that the sciatic nerve has not been injured. A patient with a dislocated hip who cannot dorsiflex the foot on that side has very likely contused the sciatic nerve.

Fractures of the shaft of the femur

The safest way in which to treat these fractures is by immobilisation on a Thomas splint or other similar splint. The leg must rest snugly in the splint and must not lie on top of tightly stretched slings around the splint. Half the thickness of the limb must sit comfortable in suitable shaped slings under the splint whilst the other half should be visible above the splint. If skin traction is applied it is as well to shave the leg before application of the skin traction and to cover the skin with a Tinct. Benz. spray. This helps to prevent soreness of the skin and adds to the adhesiveness of the extension strapping. The care of a leg splint for the three months it takes until the fracture is solid requires regular attention and inspection by the nursing staff to check that the groin ring is not too tight, that the slings supporting the leg are at the right tension, and that the traction cords are kept taut.

Occasionally however a fractured shaft of femur is treated by surgical fixation either with a Kuntscher nail down the medullary cavity or by means of a heavy duty plate and screws.

Fractures of the patella

Crack fracture of the patella without separation of the fragments means that the extensor apparatus of the knee is still intact. The treatment required is aspiration of the knee joint to remove the blood and rest in a plaster of Paris cylinder for 6 weeks. However if the patellar fragments are widely separated then the extensor mechanism has been badly torn and requires surgical repair together with repair or excision of the patella. Once again plaster immobilisation is necessary for 6 weeks after this.

Fractures into the knee joint

These fractures should be treated by aspiration of the blood from the knee joint, manipulative reduction if possible or open reduction if indicated followed by immobilisation in a plaster cylinder for several weeks depending upon the age of the patient. Another useful method is by skeletal traction with a pin through the upper tibia.

Fractures of the tibia

These are best dealt with by means of plaster of Paris immobilisation but the plaster needs to extend from the upper thigh down to the toes in order to immobilise the tibia adequately. These fractures may take up to 4 or 5 months before solid union occurs. Fractures of the lower tibial shaft occasionally fail to unite for no very obvious reason. In this case bone grafting with internal fixation may become necessary. Some surgical centres treat fractures of the tibia initially by internal fixation although this increases the risk of infection.

Fractures around the ankle joint

The ankle joint is a hinge joint but there is also an element of gliding movement. The bony walls containing the talus are often fractured by forced rotation movement and, according to the force applied, one or more bones will fracture. These fractures are commonly known as Pott's fractures. They are usually treated by manipulative reduction and immobilisation in a plaster cast from the toes to just below the knee. The plaster is left in place for 8 to 12 weeks depending on the nature of the fracture. Occasionally they require open reduction and fixation with screws or wire.

Fractures of the heel bone

Fractures of the os calcis can be quite crippling injuries particularly if the fracture passes into the joint between the talus and the os calcis. This joint is responsible for accommodating the position of the foot to rough ground and a fracture which interferes with the movement of this joint will give rise to a permanent painful limp. Fractures of the os calcis are not therefore immobilised in plaster but the patient is kept from weight bearing until the fracture is united. During this period exercises to increase the mobility of the joint are performed regularly. Occasionally it is necessary to arthrodese the joint if it is badly damaged. Fractures of the mid foot and forefoot require immobilisation until united usually for 5 or 6 weeks but fractures of the toes can be treated without immobilisation.

22
Diseases of the skin

PRESSURE SORES

Pressure sores are an important complication which may develop from confining the patient to bed. In many cases they are preventable by skilled nursing, but in some cases no effort or skill can avoid their development, and the condition is frequently a terminal one.

Causes and predisposing factors

The cause is long-continued pressure. The pressure required need only be high enough to compress the blood vessels in conditions of hypotension resulting from shock or blood loss. Then otherwise tolerable pressure on the skin may cause a sore. Pressure causes discomfort, but in the debilitated and in paraplegics with a sensory loss, such discomfort may not be appreciated by the patient. The surface appearance of a pressure sore gives little indication of what may be its ultimate size.

General

    (a) Emaciation due to malnutrition or disease.
    (b) Senility.
    (c) Diabetes, anaemia, and other severe constitutional disturbances.
    (d) Immobility—e.g. paralysed patients.

Local

    (a) Pressure. The patient's body weight renders movement difficult if he is obese. In a thin subject the bony prominences are exposed to greater pressure (e.g. sacrum, greater trochanter, heels).
    (b) Loss of skin sensation. This is usually due to a lesion of the spinal cord or the peripheral nerves.
    (c) Incontinence is a potent cause of pressure sore formation, since the skin becomes moist and septic. Incontinence increases the risk of pressure sores five-fold.

Fig. 22.1 The pressure areas.

(d) Excessive sweating causes a moist skin—more liable to pressure sore formation.

(e) Friction such as too vigorous rubbing and the presence of foreign bodies—wrinkled sheets, breadcrumbs, etc.

(f) Impaired circulation (e.g. patients suffering from heart disease).

(g) Oedema.

The pressure areas

The pressure areas are those portions of the body on which the greatest weight is borne when the patient is recumbent, and it is at these sites that sores are liable to occur. They include the heels, buttocks, sacrum, scapular areas, elbows, the spinous processes of the vertebrae, the occiput, and the greater trochanters (Fig. 22.1).

The prevention of pressure sores

1. Pressure must be relieved by frequent change of posture, and the circulation revived by stimulation of the skin.

2. A carefully made bed, in which the sheets are pulled tight, smooth and freed from crumbs and wrinkles.

3. Sorbo or air rings and cushions are used if necessary, and the nurse should ensure that pressure is evenly distributed and that the patient is moved about in bed. Although frowned on by some authorities rubber rings are useful in the correct position.

4. The skin must be kept clean and dry.

All these objectives are ensured by:

(a) Attention to the skin. The skin should be washed with soap and water, rinsed and carefully dried. Massage which was carried out with apparent success is now very much frowned upon since research has shown that careful washing and drying alone is more effective. Silicone preparations are only of use as a barrier against incontinence.

(b) There are a number of sophisticated beds which are very effective but are extremely expensive. They include the Egerton net suspension bed in which the patient lies in a hammock, water beds and the Mediscus air bed.

The ripple bed was a considerable advance in the treatment and prevention of pressure sores. It has an alternating pressure-point pad used over the patient's ordinary mattress under the bottom sheet to provide regular, frequent automatic redistribution of the pressure areas. The pad consists of a vinyl plastic pad with alternating sets of air cells running transversely across the width of the regular mattress, with an air pump which automatically controls the cycle. Single pads are now available and a new twin pulsator will operate two pads.

(c) Immediately incontinence occurs, the patient must be washed from the waist to the knees and dried thoroughly. All soiled bedclothes are changed and zinc and castor oil ointment or silicones used to form a waterproof covering for the skin. An indwelling catheter is essential to prevent bedwetting in the persistently incontinent patient. 'Inco pads' may be used. These are made of several thicknesses of soft paper which can be easily changed and are disposable. They are useful only in as much as they protect bed linen. If left in position too long they can also aggravate the skin by causing friction.

(d) Seventy-eight per cent of all pressure sores occur in the ischial region and are consistently more common in chair-bound than in bed-fast patients with the same degree of helplessness. Bowker and Davidson have designed a cushion (Fig. 22.2) that is effective in relieving high pressure points by distributing body weight uniformly over a large area of the buttocks and thighs. It consists of a foam outer cushion fitted with a waterproof vinyl cover on a polyvinyl chloride bag containing five litres of the thixotropic gel.

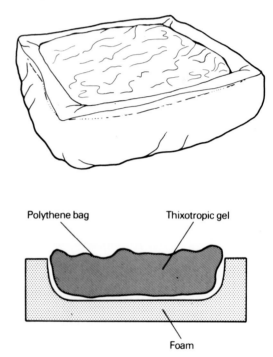

Fig. 22.2 Cushion containing thixotropic gell. (By courtesy of Bowker and Davidson.)

Established pressure sores

The first decision to be made is whether the sore is superficial or deep. Superficial sores which are painful, account for about 75 per cent of the total and will usually heal. A deep sore is painless, life-threatening and will not heal until the slough has been removed. Organisms colonise rather than invade the tissues so that antibiotics have no place in treatment.

When the lesion is still limited to an area of erythema of the skin, relief of pressure is most important. The patient's posture must be changed at least 2-hourly, and on occasions the patient may be allowed to sit out of bed with considerable benefit. The doctor in charge of the case should always be asked if this is possible in a case of threatened sores. Sitting out of bed may be substituting one form of immobility for another so frequent care is still necessary.

In some patients, particularly those in whom there has been complete transection of the spinal cord, the development of an ulcerated sore would appear to be inevitable, yet they almost never develop a pressure sore when they are cared for in special spinal injury units, perhaps because they appreciate the dangers of sitting-out.

If some part of the sore is healing by granulation, 1 per cent gentian violet or red lotion is of value. In the young subject who shows every sign of recovery from a long illness, and who has been unfortunate enough to develop a large pressure sore as a complication, a skin graft or rotated flap may be necessary to accelerate recovery. When ulceration has developed the same aseptic precautions should be followed as when dealing with a wound.

ULCERATION

An ulcer is a breach of an epithelial surface. Important in maintaining the discontinuity of the epithelium and preventing healing are pathogenic bacteria, defective oxygenation as a result of venous or arterial disease, oedema from circulatory defects or infection, a defective nerve supply, and continued trauma.

Types of ulcers

1. Traumatic
2. Inflammatory
   (a) Non-specific, e.g. carbuncle which has pointed.
   (b) Specific, e.g. tuberculosis, syphilis.
3. Trophic—due to impaired nutrition.
   (a) varicose ulcers (Ch. 24).
   (b) pressure or bed sores (p. 212).
   (c) ischaemic ulcers of feet or fingers.
   (d) ulcers due to anaesthesia (e.g. diabetic or other peripheral neuropathy, peripheral nerve injury).
4. Malignant
   (a) primary, e.g. squamous carcinoma, Rodent ulcer, malignant melanoma.
   (b) Secondary, e.g. direct invasion from carcinoma of breast, secondary deposits in skin.

The parts of an ulcer are:

The floor—the portion which can be seen.

The edge—side walls.

The base—the portion that can be felt.

COMPLICATIONS OF A SCAR

Wounds, ulcers, and burns which have involved the dermis leave a scar. Complications which may arise are:
1. Keloid formation. This is common after operations performed during pregnancy, following burns and after wounds in the Negro races and red heads.
2. Ulceration (from defective blood supply).
3. Contracture.
4. Neuroma (gives rise to pain).
5. Adherence to deep tissues.
6. Neoplastic changes.
7. Latent tetanus.

OTHER SURGICAL LESIONS OF THE SKIN AND SUBCUTANEOUS TISSUES

Injuries

Bee and wasp stings. The sting causes considerable pain. After removal of the sting by squeezing a compress of ammonia for a bee and vinegar for a wasp sting is applied. Bee and wasp stings cause 4 or 5 deaths a year in Great Britain due to anaphylaxis. A vaccine has been developed to nullify the effect of future stings in the estimated 60 000 people allergic to the stings.

Dog bites are treated with surgical toilet to the wound and the administration of tetanus toxoid and antibiotics. If the animal is suffering from hydrophobia (rabies), which is extremely rare in this country, the appropriate antitoxin must be obtained and administered as soon as possible to prevent the condition arising in the patient. The animal is isolated and kept alive to observe its behaviour before killing it, when its central nervous system is examined for rabies.

Foreign bodies. Needles, splinters of metal and wood, and fragments of glass frequently become embedded in the tissues. If the end of the foreign body is protruding it can usually be easily removed. Care must be taken to deal with injury to deeper tissues. If it is not protruding an X-ray is taken and the surgeon will advise if its removal is necessary. Most types of glass, because of their lead content, are opaque to X-rays and therefore cast a shadow on the film because the component materials have a high atomic weight.

If it has been decided to remove the foreign body, the part is kept splinted and at rest and a further X-ray is taken immediately before the operation to check that the foreign body has not moved.

Removal of a foreign body in certain sites may cause greater damage than if it is left alone. Many foreign bodies cause no trouble and become surrounded by and embedded in fibrous tissue.

The Burman metal detector is an electromagnetic detecting device which will locate quickly and accurately metallic foreign bodies. Location is based on the indications of a meter and of a small loudspeaker operating simultaneously. The instrument, which is set to give sound of uniform pitch, remains unchanged until the probe approaches close to the metallic foreign body when the sound and meter reading both rise sharply. When used following an incision the probe is covered with a specially designed rubber jacket which can be sterilised by autoclaving or can be boiled. Non-responsive retractors supplied with the instrument are used for retraction.

Localised infection of the skin

1. Boils. A boil is caused by infection of a hair follicle by the *Staphylococcus pyogenes*. The first symptom is a localised itching pimple which increases in size. The surrounding area becomes indurated and painful. As pus forms on the surface a yellow discharge occurs. Later there is sloughing, which is replaced by granulation tissue as healing commences. Should resolution occur without suppuration, the condition is known as a 'blind boil'.

2. Carbuncles. A carbuncle is a gangrenous process of the subcutaneous tissues. It is due to infection of multiple hair follicles. The commonest site is the back of the neck. Diabetics are particularly liable to develop carbuncles.

Treatment. The urine is tested for the presence of sugar. If the patient is a diabetic the dosage of insulin will usually have to be increased and the co-operation of the physician sought. The best method of treatment of a boil or carbuncle is by administration of the appropriate antibiotic; resolution is usual and the acute stage is greatly shortened. If pus forms drainage will be necessary.

3. Subcutaneous abscess is a common condition. It is a frequent termination of cellulitis. The classical signs of acute inflammation are present.

Treatment. When pus is present drainage is necessary.

Septic fingers

Infection of a tendon sheath is responsible for the crippling disability which may be seen in many cases as the end result of a septic finger.

Cause

Septic pinpricks and cuts from glass or other sharp objects are the usual causes.

Symptoms and signs

1. Pain in the finger, which is aggravated by movement.
2. The finger is swollen and throbbing.
3. Extension of the metacarpo-phalangeal joint is extremely painful.
4. Red lines on the arm (lymphangitis) and enlarged axillary lymphatic nodes (lymphadenitis).
5. General constitutional signs, flushed face, pyrexia, and loss of appetite, are present.

Fig. 22.3 Nail base removed for paronychia.

Treatment

1. Absolute rest. The arm should be kept supported in a sling.
2. Antibacterial therapy.
3. Incision and drainage followed by hypertonic sodium sulphate baths and active movement. Splinters or foreign bodies present will be removed at the same time. In addition, the general treatment of an acute infection is undertaken. Active movements of the fingers as soon as they are painless are very important.

Paronychia is the occurrence of infection around the nail bed. As soon as pus forms the bed is incised and the proximal half of the nail is removed to effect drainage (Fig. 22.3). The distal half is left covering the sensitive tissues. A new nail grows when the infection subsides and the portion of the old nail which has been left drops off. In a neglected case infection of the bone (the distal phalanx) develops.

Pulp space infection. The dense tissue of the finger tip is often infected by needle pricks. Unless early treatment is sought, necrosis of the underlying bone occurs. The pulp space may have to be drained surgically.

Diffuse infection of the spaces in the palm may occur as a result of a tendon sheath infection or a subcutaneous abscess which has not been drained adequately.

Tumours of the skin

Benign tumours, e.g. papillomas, haemangiomas, fibromas, are fairly common and may require excision.

Malignant tumours are:
1. Rodent ulcer.
2. Squamous-celled carcinoma.
3. Melanoma.
4. Secondary.

See Chapter 27.

BIBLIOGRAPHY

Bailey B N 1970 British Journal of Hospital Medicine 3: 223
Bowker P, Davidson L M 1979 British Medical Journal 2: 958
Gibbs J R 1977 Lancet 1: 174
Scales J T In: Bedsore biomechanics, Macmillan, Lond, p. 259

23
Oncology

DEFINITION

The science of new growth or tumour formation is known as oncology. A tumour, or new growth, is a mass of abnormal cells which grow unchecked by the normal body restraints. It consists of a mixture of cells undergoing division to form new cells and others which are differentiated and non-dividing. The ratio of dividing cells to the total number of cells in the tumour is called the growth fraction. When the rate of proliferation is higher than the rate of cell loss the tumour increases in size.

A new growth may be benign or malignant, and the difference is that unchecked a malignant growth will invariably kill the patient. Benign tumours are nonetheless important because, untreated, they may cause death by interfering with some vital function. A benign tumour of the meninges, for example, will cause cerebral compression and, unrelieved, the patient will die in a coma. A malignant growth is commonly known as a cancer.

THE CAUSE OF CANCER

The cause, or causes, of cancer are unknown, but there is, nonetheless, a vast amount of valuable information about the factors predisposing to its occurrence.

Predisposing factors

1. *Heredity.* Notable examples are the development of carcinoma of the colon in patients with familial polyposis and carcinoma of the oesophagus in the skin disease known as tylosis.

2. *Chronic irritation.* Chronic irritation has long been recognised as a predisposing factor. Constant irritation from coal-tar products or excessive exposure to sunlight may result in growths of the skin. Excessive cigarette smoking in bronchial carcinoma and ß-naphthylamine in

carcinoma of the bladder are well-recognised carcinogens.

Many pioneers of radiology lost their lives from skin cancer, the result of exposure to unprotected X-ray tubes.

3. *Chronic sepsis.* Tumours occurring in the tongue and buccal mucosa are less common nowadays than they were up to the middle of this century because of improvements in oral hygiene and the virtual disappearance of oral syphilitic ulceration.

Squamous carcinomas may occur at the site of chronic varicose ulceration of the legs. Bladder tumours may be associated with long-standing urinary stasis following prostatic hypertrophy or bladder stones.

4. *Viruses* may predispose to malignant new growth. In experimental animals a condition indistinguishable from carcinoma of the breast can be produced by a virus.

An increasing incidence of a particularly aggressive form of carcinoma of the uterine cervix is thought to be associated with widespread promiscuity amongst teenage girls. It has been suggested that a virus might be responsible.

5. *Immunity.* The rate of development of fatal malignancy amongst people suffering from AIDS (acquired immune deficiency syndrome) is currently of great interest. AIDS occurs especially in practising homosexuals, who may pass it to other people when they donate their blood for transfusion.

When the body's immunity is suppressed by disease or by the use of cytotoxic drugs (for the treatment of cancer or as part of a transplant programme) the risk of development of a (further) malignant tumour is greatly increased.

6. *Geographical variations.* There are fascinating geographical variations in the incidence of tumours. Japanese women have a much lower rate of breast cancer than American women, but when Japanese families emigrate to America and adopt a Western lifestyle the rate of breast cancer in their female offspring approaches that of American women.

There is a high incidence of cancer of the nasopharynx in Hong Kong and in men employed in the woodworking industry in Britain.

Cancer of the oesophagus is high amongst men in France who are heavy spirit drinkers, and stomach cancer predominates in Japan where raw fish is eaten.

THE DEVELOPMENT OF A MALIGNANT NEW GROWTH

Recent research on tumour viruses in animals has identified the presence of oncogenes. These are genes which become altered in structure or activity in cancer cells. Oncogenes have been found to be associated with malignant transformation of cells in tissue culture. In humans, oncogenes have been found at the site of abnormalities in chromosomes in tumour cells. Oncogenes affect the proteins in a cell and may play a vital role in the complex sequence of events that produce a malignant cell. As more is understood about these steps in the production of a malignant cell it may be possible to develop cytotoxic drugs which can prevent the malignant cell from developing and forming new malignant cells without at the same time damaging the normal cells of the body.

SCREENING FOR THE EARLY DETECTION OF CANCER

This may take the form of:

1. **Clinical examination.** Well women clinics should be promoted and women taught how to examine their breasts monthly.

2. **Exfoliative cytology.** Examples are:

(a) Cervical smear for detection of carcinoma cervix (p. 633).

(b) Screening of urine in rubber and dye workers who are liable to carcinoma of the bladder (p. 511).

3. **Needle biopsy** can be carried out in the outpatient department under local anaesthetic.

4. **Radiography.** A chest X-ray will detect a primary lung cancer or the presence of secondary deposits, but Mass Miniature Screening is not considered an economic screening procedure.

Mammography can be undertaken on a large scale although it is expensive. Speckled calcification may indicate the presence of a breast cancer. This procedure is not advised as a regular routine procedure in women of childbearing age as it gives a measurable dose of radiation to the ovaries.

BENIGN TUMOURS

Much confusion has arisen in following the terminology of tumour formation. The ending 'oma' simply means a new growth. A simple new growth is similar in substance to the tissue in which it arises and is named accordingly. Malignant new growths are named after the cells from which they arise.

Here are considered only the main types of simple new growths and the way in which they differ from malignant growths. Under the appropriate regions their clinical features are considered in detail.

Type of growth	Tissue of origin
Lipoma	Fat
Neuroma	Nerve tissue
Chondroma	Cartilage
Myoma	Muscle
Osteoma	Bone
Fibroma	Fibrous tissue
Angioma (naevus)	Blood vessels
Myeloma	Bone marrow
Odontoma	Teeth
Adenoma	Gland

A papilloma is a pedunculated tumour of the skin or of an epithelial lining. Some new growths are multiple. They have arisen separately and

not from metastasis. Common multiple simple new growths are:
Lipomas
Neurofibromas
Naevi.

Characteristics of benign tumours

1. The increase in size is slow. The tumour is limited by a capsule.
2. Spread into the neighbouring tissues does not occur. The tissue is pushed aside but not invaded.
3. They do not spread by the bloodstream or by the lymphatic system.
4. They may cause symptoms as a result of their size or by pressure on the neighbouring tissues.
5. There is no tendency to recur after excision.

The usual treatment is excision or in suitable cases treatment by cryosurgery (p. 226).

MALIGNANT NEW GROWTHS

The principal forms are:

1. **Those arising from the epithelial lined surfaces—carcinoma.**
   (a) *Squamous-celled carcinoma* (syn. epithelioma), which is a squamous-celled tumour growing from tissues covered by squamous cells, e.g. the tongue and skin.
   (b) *Adenocarcinoma* which is a glandular tissue tumour, e.g. breast, stomach, large intestine, salivary (Fig. 23.1).

2. **Connective tissue tumours (Fig. 23.2)—sarcoma.** These arise in bone (osteogenic sarcoma) or in fibrous tissues (fibrosarcoma). Other sarco-

Fig. 23.1   Carcinoma of the parotid gland (fungating).

Fig. 23.2   Sarcoma of the right buttock.

Fig. 23.3   Disseminated malignant melanoma.

mas include chondrosarcoma (arising from cartilage), liposarcoma (arising from fat), rhabdomyosarcoma (arising from striped muscle) and leiomyosarcoma (arising from smooth muscle).

3. **Pigment cells. Melanoma** (Fig. 23.3) arises in the pigmented layers of the skin and in the choroid of the eye. Simple pigmented moles may develop into malignant melanomas.

4. **Gliomas.** These arise in the central nervous system—the brain and spinal cord.

5. **Reticulo-endothelial tumours** involve the lymphatic system, e.g. Hodgkin's disease, non-Hodgkin's lymphoma.

In between simple and malignant growths there is a number of borderline growths, the best recognised being a rodent ulcer of the skin. They are locally malignant in that they destroy tissues, but rearely spread to remote sites or into the lymphatic system.

Papillomas of the urinary tract, which were always known to become malignant if untreated, are now believed to be the first manifestation of carcinoma of the bladder.

The spread of malignant new growths

Malignant new growths may spread:

1. **Locally.** The growth increases in size and invades the neighbouring tissues eroding blood vessels, the skin and bony tissues if adjacent.

2. **By metastasis** (i.e. by secondary growth formation).

(a) *By the lymphatic stream.* The local lymphatic glands enlarge as spread progresses.

(b) *By the blood stream.* The tumour may be widely disseminated to other tissues, and the deposit is also known as a metastasis or secondary new growth. This is a common method of spread of sarcomas, in particular, and this characteristic renders them rapidly fatal.

Secondary growths in bone are commonly the result of a primary growth in the breast, lung, prostate, kidney or thyroid. Many common carcinomas already have occult blood-borne metastases at the time of first diagnosis but symptoms may not manifest themselves for months or even for many years.

3. **Transcoelomic.** Tumour cells may spread within the peritoneal or pleural cavities leading to the production of ascites or a pleural effusion.

4. **By contact.** Where two surfaces of mucosa are in contact, e.g. in the vagina, a so-called 'kiss ulcer' may appear.

5. **Surgical implantation.** This is not a frequent occurrence, but is seen occasionally in the scar of an operation wound through which a new growth has been excised.

Characteristics of malignant new growths

1. Untreated, the patient usually dies from the disease.
2. Increase in size is progressive. They have no limiting capsule.
3. Spread occurs to the other tissues as described above and gives rise to secondary growths.

4. Ulceration and infection are common, and many of the symptoms and signs are due to infection of the growth. Infection is particularly liable to result in secondary haemorrhage.

Symptoms and signs of malignant new growths

The symptoms and signs described in this book, as we follow the course of new growths in each organ, are those of moderately advanced tumours. The early symptoms and signs are:

1. *A lump*—this should invariably be a cause for seeking medical advice.
2. *Bleeding*—from any part of the body. A few drops of blood lost even on only one occasion are important.
3. *Slight alteration in normal habits or functions*—to mention only a few: (a) increasing constipation; (b) difficulty with swallowing, walking, talking, or eating.
4. *Changes in metabolism.* Since some tumours such as those of the pancreas, the pituitary or the adrenal add to the function of these organs, a change in metabolism may be the first indication of tumour formation. Weight loss and lassitude may occur.

New growths in the early stages will be diagnosed only by careful clinical examination and painstaking investigation. When symptoms are marked the growth is usually well advanced.

Biopsy. In cases of doubt, a small portion of the growth is removed and examined under the microscope. This procedure is often of great value in diagnosis, but is not without danger because more rapid spread of the growth may result. The recovery of malignant cells from the interior of organs or in secretion or excretion is sometimes of great value in diagnosis.

Aspiration biopsy of lymph nodes or superficial tumours—sucking up a few cells into a syringe through a fine needle and making a smear on a glass slide to be stained and examined under the microscope—may aid diagnosis.

Exfoliative cytology is the process by which cells recovered from natural secretions like gastric juice or urine are centrifuged, sectioned in a paraffin block and examined under a microscope. Scrapings from organs like the cervix of the uterus may be treated similarly, and the opinion of an experienced pathologist is invaluable in the detection of cancer at a very early stage.

Biopsy and exfoliative cytology material will be examined by the pathologist. When a growth is malignant, certain terms are used. Anaplastic means that cell division has been rapid. Another term used in this connection is undifferentiated which means that cells are very poorly formed and bear little or no resemblance to the cells from which they arose. They are more malignant than a growth in which the cells are well differentiated and more like the cells of origin. It can be compared to drawing a square with a pencil on paper. The normal accurate square is drawn with a ruler—normal cells—it takes time. Drawn more hurriedly without a ruler but joined together it will still resemble a square—well differentiated but not an accurate square. Drawn still more rapidly it may have only two sides and be unjoined—poorly differentiated and anaplastic—rapid and bad.

TREATMENT OF NEW GROWTHS

Unfortunately neoplasia is all too often a generalised disease with many subclinical foci and it is these undetectable micrometastases which later become manifest. For many years surgery and radiotherapy were the main forms of therapy for most solid tumours with chemotherapy used as a last resort in disseminated cancer. Over the last two decades considerable advances have been made in the treatment of reticuloses, e.g. Hodgkin's disease and Burkitt's lymphoma.

Considerable efforts have been made to improve the survival of patients with carcinomas and sarcomas by the use of combination chemotherapy—several cytotoxic drugs used together. Multicentre trials are in progress to evaluate the success of chemotherapy. The chance of cure from chemotherapy is at its highest when the tumour mass is small, for at this stage the proportion of cells in division is highest. This is immediately after the apparently successful excision of a tumour or when there is only minimal residual tumour.

Immunotherapy, which builds up lost resistance, may be of value in the treatment of some tumours.

Joint consultations, where the surgeon, radiotherapist and chemotherapist, together with the radiologist and pathologist, discuss the investigation and treatment of individual patients with cancer, produce improved results.

The treatment of childhood cancer by a combination of surgery, radiotherapy and chemotherapy has already resulted in the cure of several thousands of children in Britain. With a long life span there is a proportionately greater chance of long-term damage to normal tissues and organs to emerge. The mutagenic effects of radiotherapy and chemotherapy on the gonads are an obvious hazard to any offspring. Some children are rendered sterile by chemotherapy or by radiotherapy directed, of necessity, to the gonads. Children treated successfully with radiotherapy or chemotherapy run a small but measurable risk of developing a second malignancy some years later.

Radical treatment

1. **Surgical excision** consists of removal of the growth and the whole of the area between it and the lymphatic glands, together with the glands themselves. The results are best when the glands are not invaded. Occasionally, a 'second look' operation is undertaken after a previously inoperable or recurrent tumour has been shrunk by chemotherapy or radiotherapy so that any residual tumour can be removed if possible. This 'second look' surgery is advocated for the treatment of advanced ovarian and testicular tumours and for some children's tumours, e.g. Wilms' tumour.

2. **Radiotherapy.** Radiation acts by destroying dividing cells. It is particularly useful for the radical treatment of primary tumours for which surgery is mutilating, e.g. cancer of the larynx or tongue. The modern treatment of early breast cancer consists of local excision of the mass followed by a radical course of external radiotherapy to the remainder of the breast plus the lymphatic drainage areas—the axilla, the supraclavicular fossa and the internal mammary chain. Bladder cancer is also frequently treated by a radical course of radiotherapy.

3. **Cryotherapy** is the destruction of living tissue by cold. The fundamental premise of cryodestructive surgery is that the living cells are first injured and later die from the results of freezing. A machine circulates liquid nitrogen through a partially insulated probe. A cryolesion is produced around a central freezing point.

The majority of skin tumours, benign and malignant, are best treated in this way. Postoperatively a slight haemorrhagic ooze may accompany the thawing process but ceases within a few hours. This may be followed by blister formation and subsequently by an eschar. This separates after several weeks and epithelialises.

4. **Laser beam treatment** is used for benign papillomata and early non-invasive squamous carcinoma of the larynx. It produces an excellent functional result. Dysplasia or early pre-invasive carcinoma of the cervix can be treated similarly in young women and does not affect subsequent childbearing.

5. **Adjuvant chemotherapy** implies the use of systemic agents in the destruction of disseminated microfoci of malignancy at a time when there is no clinical or investigative evidence of residual disease. In England and Wales 150 000 people die of malignant disease each year and it is estimated that 70 to 80 per cent die of metastatic disease. In the U.S.A. 700 000 new cases of malignant disease are registered each year and 50 per cent are estimated to have metastatic disease at the time of diagnosis or a high risk of recurrence following the presently available surgical or radiotherapeutic primary treatment (De Vita et al 1975).

The size of the total body burden of tumour has long been recognised as a factor influencing the response to chemotherapy. When the burden is reduced by surgical excision of the primary growth or shrunk by radiotherapy, chemotherapy is theoretically likely to be most effective in the destruction of micrometastases. The selection of patients will be determined only after the results of clinical trials now in operation. But already it is clear that for many children's tumours the results have been substantially improved with adjuvent chemotherapy. The possibility of long-term control of breast cancer and osteogenic sarcoma by adjuvant chemotherapy is still being investigated.

Palliative treatment

1. **Radiotherapy** is frequently of value in causing tumour regression and, in the advanced case, may delay deterioration. Radiotherapy is also a good method of relieving pain from secondary deposits in bone.

2. **Surgery.** Palliative operations are frequently undertaken to relieve symptoms such as obstruction.

The duty of a doctor or nurse is to relieve suffering, and, although not able to cure the patient of his disease, the treatment of his symptoms is all-important to him.

3. **Hormone therapy.** Oophorectomy or radiation ablation of the ovaries may produce a remission of recurrent breast cancer in young women.

Locally recurrent or metastatic breast cancer is frequently treated with hormones, the most commonly prescribed being the anti-oestrogen Tamoxifen in a dosage of 20–40 mg per day by mouth. This may produce good regression of a primary breast tumour in an elderly patient and also regression of local recurrence or lung metastases in women of any age but especially postmenopausal ones. Tamoxifen can also be used for recurrences in the very rare male breast cancer. Oral prednisolone is sometimes added to Tamoxifen. Stilboestrol or ethinyl oestradiol are far less commonly used now because they can cause cardiovascular symptoms.

A measurement of oestrogen receptors is sometimes made on a sample of the primary breast tumour. A high oestrogen receptor level may indicate a likely good response to hormone therapy.

Painful bony metastases in oophorectomised young women may respond to Deca Durabolin 50 mg intramuscularly every three weeks. Older postmenopausal women can be treated with Masteril (drostanolone proprionate) 100 mg intramuscularly three times a week. A newer hormone preparation for both soft tissue and bony metastases is Orimeten (aminoglutethimide) 250 mg orally q.i.d. This produces a 'medical adrenalectomy' and additional maintenance therapy of hydrocortisone 20 mg b.d. orally must be given.

Progesterones in the form of oral megestrol acetate or medroxyprogesterone acetate as either tablets or intramuscular injections are sometimes used in the treatment of painful metastases.

Metastatic prostatic carcinoma may be treated by oral stilboestrol 5 mg t.d.s. or Honvan tablets 100–300 mg daily. A newer preparation is Cyprostat (cyproterone acetate) 300 mg daily. Bilateral orchidectomy is also sometimes advocated.

4. **Cytotoxic agents** (cell poisons) destroy rapidly dividing cells, so they damage normal bone marrow cells as well as tumour cells. In addition they can damage the cells of the mucosa of the bowel, producing the side-effects of vomiting and diarrhoea. The superficial cells of the skin, including hair follicles, can also be damaged, resulting in alopecia. A very wide variety of cytotoxic drugs is now available. These may be administered as single agents or, more commonly, as combinations of three or more drugs. Combination chemotherapy should only be undertaken in specialised centres where experienced staff are able to deal with the severe complications which may arise in the neutropaenic patient.

5. **Antiviral agents** (Ch. 6). Interferon has been used but no conclusive results are yet available.

RADIOTHERAPY

As the name implies, treatment by radiation includes radium, 'X-irradiation', and radioactive isotopes.
The aim of radiotherapy is either:
1. Radical, to cure the disease.
2. Palliative, to relieve a symptom such as the pain of a bony metastasis, dysphagia in carcinoma of the oesophagus or bleeding from a carcinoma of the uterus.

Sealed radioactive isotopes

Radium and caesium emit several rays—alpha and beta particles, and gamma rays. Only gamma rays are used in the treatment of cancer. Radium is now being replaced by caesium which produces gamma rays of a lower penetrating energy than radium, making it easier to protect staff working with the patients from the harmful effects of radiation on normal tissues.

Fig. 23.4　Effect of radium.
A. Squamous-celled carcinoma of the nose before treatment.　　B. Same patient after treatment.

The forms of radiotherapy—classified by Paine (1980)

1. External beam irradiation

(a) Conventional X-ray therapy delivered from a superficial or deep X-ray set similar to diagnostic X-ray equipment. The energy output is relatively low (40-140 RV).
(b) Megavoltage radiation supplied by:
(i) X-ray sources from a linear accelerator with an output of 4-25 MeV.

(ii) Gamma ray sources, either cobalt (^{60}Co) or caesium (^{137}Cs). The energy output is 1.2 MeV.

2. Brachytherapy

The delivery of the radiation is relatively slow—the source being placed within or near the growth. It may be:

(a) Intracavitary. This is the usual treatment of malignant uterine tumours. Originally carried out with radium the treatment is now delivered with ^{137}Cs and can be afterloaded into a tube placed in the patient previously or by the Cathetron technique. In this technique the whole irradiation is carried out under general anaesthesia in a few minutes. The source holders are carefully placed by the operator and when all attendants have moved to an adjoining room from where the patient can be safely monitored then ^{60}Co sources are afterloaded mechanically.

(b) Interstitial therapy. Radium needles have been largely superseded by ^{192}Ir wires or ^{137}Cs needles (Paine 1972).

Radioactive isotopes

The radioactive isotope is a form of an element which behaves chemically in the same way as its normal form, but because of a different combination of particles within its nucleus, it is unstable and changes into a different element, releasing energy in the form of X-rays, gamma-rays, alpha and beta particles. The energy released enables them to be used in amounts small enough not to interfere with normal physiology and this is also the reason for their use in radiotherapy.

They are used in three ways.

1. Research.

2. Diagnosis. Radio-isotope imaging of bone with ^{99m}Tc-labelled phosphates is the most frequently performed scan in departments of nuclear medicine for pre-treatment assessment, staging and follow-up. One quarter of clinically early cases of carcinoma of the breast have a positive bone scan. Unnecessary surgery is avoided and early palliative treatment is commenced.

Radioactive iodine, which is concentrated in thyroid tissue, outlines the thyroid gland and will show if any gland tissue lies retrosternally. Scans using special isotopes are now common to outline the kidney, the lungs, the bones, the liver and the pancreas.

3. Treatment.

(a) Carcinoma of the thyroid—this sometimes takes up radioactive iodine and the radioactivity concentrated in the thyroid kills the carcinoma cells. Metastases from this tumour sometimes take up radioactive iodine. Radioactive iodine is also used to treat thyrotoxicosis.

(b) Polycythaemia rubra vera—radioactive phosphorus (^{32}P) is injected intravenously and destroys the excess red blood cells.

(c) Caesium or cobalt is used as a beam in place of deep X-rays.

All the substances actually injected into the body have a short life and the patient is not 'radioactive' for long. Also they are very local in their effects and other people can be in contact with them in safety.

Faeces and urine may need to be stored in protected containers until any radioactivity in them has diminished to a minimal quantity. This usually takes only a few days: then the excreta can be emptied into the drains in the usual way.

The mode of action of radiations

The gamma rays or X-rays destroy cells which are about to divide. Cancer cells divide frequently, hence the more rapidly growing the tumour the more radiosensitive it is likely to be. Some damage to the skin and tissues is inevitable with radical radiotherapy, and this is known as a 'radiation reaction'.

The care of the patient undergoing caesium/iridium treatment

Methods of afterloading with the caesium or iridium into hollow tubes inserted into the patient's body under anæsthetic have been developed. In the case of cancer of the cervix a hollow tube is inserted into the uterus and vagina. When the patient returns to the special side ward a computer-controlled machine called a Selectron pushes the ^{137}Cs pellets into the hollow tubes and removes them when the treatment has been completed. The patient is nursed flat in bed for the twenty hours or so that the treatment takes. When the nurse enters the room every two hours to check that the insertion has not slipped out of place, the machine removes the radioactive pellets into a shielded storage container so that the nurse is not exposed to radiation. As soon as the nurse leaves the room the isotope is returned to the patient and treatment continues. Patients are sedated and given adequate analgesia whilst the insertion is in place.

Hollow tubes can be inserted into the vulva or anus under anaesthetic for the treatment of squamous carcinomas arising in these areas. ^{192}Ir wires are then threaded into these tubes when the patient returns to the ward. Tumours arising in the tongue or floor of mouth can be treated by the insertion of iridium wires. These are left in place for about six days.

Radiotherapy reactions

Radiotherapy may give rise to general and local reactions.

General reaction

This may consist of nausea and general malaise. From its effect on the blood system anaemia and leucopenia may develop.

Local reaction (radiation reaction)

On the intact skin radium produces a painful erythema which, if severe, may lead to an indurated area of cellulitis. The stages are:

1. Erythema.
2. Dry desquamation.
3. Moist desquamation.

On the skin, zinc (in strapping) and mercurial lotions are avoided. The skin is kept dry and only baby powder applied. If desquamation occurs non-adherent sterile dressings (e.g. Melolin) or paraffin gauze are used. Gentian violet or proflavine cream may be soothing. Circulation of air round the irradiated site should be encouraged and the use of an electric fan for ten to twenty minutes a day is helpful. An infected ulcer may improve if oral metronidazole 200–400 mg t.d.s. is used. Tight clothing should be avoided and cotton should be worn next to the skin rather than synthetic garments.

In the mouth and throat sloughing and infection are common. A careful watch should be kept for secondary haemorrhage and blood cross-matched if it is suspected. Antibiotics may be necessary to control sepsis. Regular mouth washes with glycerine and thymol or Difflam are essential. Mucaine may alleviate dysphagia. Oral thrush is common and is treated with Nystatin suspension or Fungilin lozenges.

A soft diet and sometimes liquidised food is required. Plenty of fluids should be taken. Cigarette smoking should be actively discouraged.

The bladder. Regular bacterial examination of the urine is undertaken if frequency and dysuria persist. Antibiotics are prescribed as appropriate. Mist pot cit 10 ml t.d.s. or an anti-spasmodic such as Urispas or Cetiprin may help.

The rectum. Irritation and diarrhoea may develop. Proctitis may be relieved by Predsol suppositories or colifoam.

Complications of radiotherapy

Great care is taken to minimise the risk of dangerous complications of radiation therapy.

1. When the upper abdomen is irradiated the kidneys must be shielded either part way through or throughout the whole course of radiotherapy to ensure that nephritis, leading to hypertension and kidney failure, does not occur.
2. Radiation pneumonitis can occur following a course of radiotherapy to the chest wall or breast, leading to dyspnoea and a chronic cough.
3. Excessive radiation to the cervical spinal cord during the treatment of tumours in the neck can lead to myelitis and paralysis.
4. Radiation of limbs can lead to flexion deformity of joints.
5. Radiation is particularly dangerous to the bones and joints of growing children and can lead to curvature of the spine or premature fusion of joints if great care is not taken in prescribing the correct dose of radiation.
6. Damage to the rectum and sigmoid colon may occur after radiation

of the uterine cervix, leading either to stricture of the bowel or to perforation.
7. Radiation of the eye may lead to cataract formation or to corneal dessication.

Follow-up

The follow-up of patients suffering from cancer is important to the patient because recurrences are frequently treatable. It is also important to the hospital, so that the end results of treatment may be studied and correlated.

Protection of the nursing staff

All nurses working in a radiotherapy unit must be aware of the potential dangers of radiation. A radiation symbol (yellow on a black background) must be displayed prominently over the bed of every patient undergoing treatment with a radioactive implant or insertion. Heavy lead screens must be placed either side of the bed to protect the nurse as she attends to the needs of the patient. Speed is essential when carrying out these duties. No visitors are allowed at the bedside when a radioactive insertion is in place. Pregnant women visitors are not allowed to visit a ward in which radioactivity is present. It is advisable that a pregnant nurse should be re-assigned to another ward where no such radioactive insertions are undertaken. All nurses working in radiotherapy units must wear a radiation monitoring badge, which must be analysed fortnightly.

HANDLING OF CYTOTOXIC DRUGS

The administration of cytotoxic drugs has become an important part of the management of many patients with cancer. In some units specially trained nurses actually inject these drugs intravenously into the patients. In other units nurses assist the doctors in drawing up the correct amounts of the drugs into syringes and in setting up intravenous drips into which the drugs are inserted. Many of the cytotoxic drugs are very corrosive and cause vesiculation if spilt on to the skin. Considerable damage would be caused if droplets of these drugs fell into the eyes as the syringes were being filled. Nurses helping to draw up and administer cytotoxic drugs should wear surgical gloves, gown and goggles. Should spillage on the skin occur in spite of these precautions the area should be bathed copiously with cold water immediately.

Scrupulous care must be taken in recording the exact amount of each cytotoxic drug that is administered to the patient and the time it was given. Written records must be kept of any adverse side effects suffered by the patient during and after the administration of the cytotoxic drugs, such as pyrexia and rigors, mouth ulceration, vomiting and diarrhoea. Patients must be kept well hydrated and a chart of urine output maintained.

SYMPTOM CONTROL IN TERMINAL CANCER

Pain is usually the most predominant symptom in terminal cancer and it is essential that adequate analgesia should be given to keep the patient as free from pain as possible. This usually means that opiate drugs must be prescribed. Either morphine or diamorphine may be given orally, there being no difference in their effectiveness. Although for some patients a dosage of diamorphine of 10 mg four hourly may produce good pain relief, others may need dosages of the order of 60-100 mg or higher every four hours. Tablets of morphine or diamorphine mixture are given according to the patient's preference. There is no place for giving a complicated mixture of opiates, alcohol, honey and sedative, 'Mist Euphoria' or 'Brompton Cocktail' because this simply makes the patient drowsy without conferring any additional analgesic benefit. Most dying patients prefer to remain sufficiently alert to enjoy the company of their visitors.

The long-acting morphine preparation M.S.T.-I may be a useful alternative to four hourly diamorphine. It is given twelve hourly in a dosage ranging from 10 mg b.d. to 100 mg b.d. or far higher if required.

If the patient is nauseated or cannot swallow oral preparations, a useful alternative is proladone (Oxycodone) suppositories, one every eight hours.

Frequently it is beneficial to add anti-inflammatory drugs to the opiate regime when bone pain is a predominant feature. A wide range of proprietary preparations is available. The use of steroids, e.g. prednisolone 5 mg t.d.s. may also boost the analgesic effect and enhance the patient's general condition and boost his appetitie.

Almost all analgesics are severely constipating and very careful attention to the bowels is necessary. Regular laxatives must be given and suppositories and enemas used when indicated.

Patients with extremely severe persistent pain that cannot be controlled by oral or rectal opiates may benefit from the continuous administration of subcutaneous diamorphine via a syringe driver. Doses in excess of 1000 mg of diamorphine in 24 hours are likely to be required in patients who remain on the syringe driver for several weeks.

Several anti-emetic drugs are available but the persistent nausea and vomiting associated with some advanced malignancies may still be difficult to control. Stemetil (prochlorperazine), Maxolon (metoclopramide), Largactil (chlorpromazine) and Motilium (domperidone) can be given by mouth or by suppository. Suppositories can be inserted into a colostomy or even into the vagina if the rectal route is not available. Haloperidol is also an effective anti-emetic drug, as is Valoid (cyclizine). However, all the anti-emetic drugs have the disadvantage of causing drowsiness to varying degrees and may also cause extra-pyramidal symptoms of rigidity and twitching followed by nightmares and even by psychotic symptoms. As a last resort it may be necessary to give regular intramuscular injections of an anti-emetic.

Imodium (loperamide) is a useful drug in the control of intestinal colic and diarrhoea.

NURSING CARE OF PATIENTS WITH MALIGNANT DISEASE

In this chapter the nature, the diagnosis and technical aspects of treatment have been considered and in many of the pages which follow the management of malignancy in various regional sites is described. There is always a danger that the anxieties and fears of the patient are overlooked in our desire to effect a cure.

Many patients are investigated for symptoms which may be due to a malignant growth and while some are aware of the possibility others are quite oblivious. At this stage the nurse has every reason to be cheerful to the anxious patient. In many instances the patient suspects the worst, fears the consequences and loses all hope, when there is a possibility of cure. At this stage and at all stages in the management of the patient the nurse must be a good listener and however hurried she may be the patient must be given every opportunity to speak his thoughts. It is at this time that the staff can give the patient what is most needed, a sense of companionship and trust.

Once the diagnosis has been established a decision has to be made on the best method of treatment and the patient may be confronted by an increasing number of consultants as the decision is often a multidisciplinary one. All methods of treatment are almost always unpleasant either alone or in combination. Surgery is rarely of a minor nature and often radical and mutilating. Radiotherapy and chemotherapy to be effective have to be given in doses bordering on the toxic. A knowledge of the type of operation, the effects of irradiation at various sites as well as the toxic manifestations of chemotherapy with cytotoxic drugs is an essential background for the nurse. She can prepare the patient for the onset of unpleasant symptoms which may arise from treatment and if they occur he will feel reassured that they are transitory and not as he may otherwise presume due to extension of the disease.

The decision of how and to what extent a patient is informed is a medical one and the nurse must be aware of the decision of the doctor in charge of the patient. She should answer questions from the patient unhesitatingly within the general policy of the unit. Relatives should normally be taken into the picture but on occasions the patient wants to know the whole truth and insists that his relatives should not be distressed. On many occasions the patient almost certainly knows the diagnosis but obviously prefers no serious discussion.

The patient and his relatives need information and if possible reassurance on many aspects of his condition. The possibility of returning to a normal life or occupation is the first consideration and this varies with the site and extent of the lesion. All are anxious that pain be controlled and in the majority of patients this reassurance can be given (Ch. 5).

The maintenance of health is the first priority in a patient afflicted with malignant disease. The maintenance of nutrition, the correction of anaemia and the control of infection are essential. Nor should it be forgotten that the patient may develop nonmalignant disease which if not diagnosed and treated correctly may be lethal.

Quite as important with these patients as the length of life is the quality of life and good nursing care can do much to improve it. A check on body weight is a good general guide.

BIBLIOGRAPHY

Bush H 1978 British Journal of Hospital Medicine 20: 260
De Vita V T 1977. In: Salmon S E, Jones S E (ed) Adjuvant therapy of cancer, Elsever North Holland, Amsterdam, p. 640
Paine C H 1972 Clinical Radiology 23: 263
Paine C H 1980 British Journal of Hospital Medicine 23: 544

24

Diseases of arteries and veins

ARTERIES

Arteries (apart from the pulmonary artery) carry oxygenated blood to the tissues and therefore any impairment to the normal flow will lead to anoxia of the tissues. The blood flow within a vessel is governed by several factors including the diameter of the vessel, the cardiac output and the viscosity of the blood. The increased viscosity which may develop in some forms of blood disease such as leukaemia may lead to thrombosis. The flow in small vessels is much less than in larger ones and a critical closing pressure exists below which flow ceases, a point of importance in the development of thrombosis following vascular spasm and generalised hypotension.

Muscular activity plays an important part in the regulation of blood flow. When a muscle such as the calf muscle is exercised its demands for oxygen and glucose are increased. The waste products of metabolism act locally by producing vasodilation but if insufficient arterial blood is reaching the leg muscles these products accumulate in the tissues and lead to troublesome cramp-like pain felt within the calf. The pain, which is referred to as intermittent claudication, disappears with rest only to return with resumption of activity. As the degree of arterial obstruction increases, the claudication distance (i.e. the distance the patient can walk before getting pain) will diminish. Eventually the patient may complain of pain at rest which is sufficiently severe to keep him awake at night.

OCCLUSIVE ARTERIAL DISEASE

Arterial occlusion may occur suddenly, following an embolus or thrombosis, or gradually as in atherosclerosis (Fig. 24.1) and thromboangiitis obliterans. These conditions principally involve the lower limbs.

Embolism

This is due to the transmission of an organised thrombus from one part of

Old age   Youth

Fig. 24.1 Legs of old age showing absorption of the muscle mass due to the diminishing blood supply. Legs of youth showing good muscles.

the circulation to another where it becomes lodged, generally at the point of division of an artery. The embolus usually originates either within the left atrium, as in mitral stenosis, within the left ventricle as following myocardial infarction, or within an atheromatous aorta.

Impaction takes place at the site of division of peripheral vessels, the majority occurring within the common femoral artery at the origin of the profunda femoris.

While cerebral embolism is common and often fatal, embolism within the upper limb is less common and rarely produces any problem. Obstruction of the circulation produces sudden ischaemia of the affected part which, if not relieved, may proceed to gangrene.

Clinical features

Pain of sudden onset.
Pallor of the limb giving way eventually to a blotchy blue discoloration.
Paralysis of the affected limb.
Loss of cutaneous sensation.
Feeling of coldness.
Loss of pulsation within the artery distal to the point of occlusion.

Treatment

Early diagnosis and treatment are both important in saving limb and life. Whilst a small peripheral embolus may be treated conservatively with intravenous heparin to prevent propagation of the clot distal to the site of occlusion, an embolus which occludes a major artery such as the femoral is a surgical emergency. The operative management of arterial emboli has been revolutionised by the introduction of the Fogarty balloon catheter. The catheter may be introduced into the artery through a small arteriotomy and the thrombus retrieved in a 'chimney sweep' fashion from its site of impaction.

Anticoagulant therapy with intravenous heparin is commenced as soon as possible and continued postoperatively but because of the risk of bleeding it has to be carefully controlled (Ch. 18). The nurse should observe the colour and temperature of the toes as well as palpate the pulses in the arteries distal to the operation site to ensure that the blood supply is satisfactory and remains so. Absent pulsation or pallor and coldness of the toes should be reported without delay.

Atherosclerosis

The aetiology of this condition is unknown but it is characterised by the deposition of fatty material within the wall of the artery and predominantly within the subintimal layers. This deposition, together with the subsequent thrombus formation, leads to a narrowing of the lumen. The disease appears to be widespread throughout the circulatory system but tends to be concentrated at sites of bifurcation such as the aortoiliac region.

Clinical features

It is only when the blood flow is reduced to critical levels that the disease produces symptoms and these are gradual in onset. When it involves the main vessels to the leg the commonest symptom is that of intermittent claudication. In this condition, a cramp-like pain appears with exercise. It is generally felt within the calf but it may also be experienced within the thigh and gluteal region. The walking distance required to produce the pain gradually becomes shorter and within time proves to be incapacitating. Rest pain may become a distressing factor. It indicates marked ischaemia and, as it is often worse at night causing loss of sleep, leads to a rapid deterioration of morale. When it falls below a critical level death of tissue (gangrene) ensues.

Conservative treatment

The patient must learn to live with and within the symptoms.
Reducing weight will lead to some relief.
Stop smoking. Smoking is an important causative factor in the development of atherosclerosis. It also causes increased viscosity of the blood.
Avoid injury to the area of ischaemia. Nail trimming (Fig. 24.2) should be done with great care, the nails being kept long to avoid injury. As most sufferers have poor eyesight and tremulous hands they are advised not to attempt to cut their toenails.
Correct any anaemia.
Careful control of diabetes.

Fig. 24.2 Toe nails must not be cut short. Note the thin wasted limbs so characteristic of arterial insufficiency.

Surgical treatment

This should be considered only if the symptoms are severe and do not respond to conservative measures. Such symptoms are severe intermittent claudication interfering significantly with livelihood or lifestyle, rest pain or pre-grangrenous changes. The feasibility of such surgery will depend on the age and general health of the patient as well as arteriographic evaluation of the affected vessel. The latter involves the injection of radio-opaque material under local or general anaethesia into the arterial tree proximal to the site of obstruction. In the case of the lower limb the femoral artery may be punctured directly within the groin or the aorta may be punctured through the back, the needle passing to the left of the vertebral bodies. Bleeding from the artery or occlusion of the artery at the puncture site can occur. The patient must be left at rest for 4 hours after such an X-ray. Any pain or swelling at the puncture site must be reported. The colour and peripheral pulses of the legs should be checked regularly, as well as the patient's pulse rate and blood pressure.

Several types of operative procedure are available. The one used depends largely on the site and extent of disease.

1. Thromboendarterectomy. The inner diseased lining of the artery together with its contained thrombus is cored out either through a long incision or through several small incisions using a special ring stripper. The arterial incisions are then closed either by direct suturing or by incorporating a vein patch graft (Fig. 24.3).

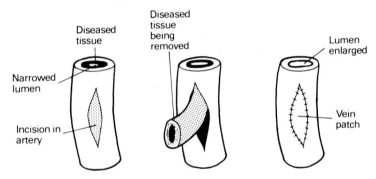

Fig. 24.3 Thromboendarterectomy through an incision made over the blocked segment. The inner core consisting of the diseased tissue is removed and the incision repaired by means of a vein patch graft.

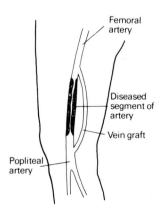

Fig. 24.4 A saphenous vein bypass graft.

2. Bypass grafts. The diseased segment may be left in situ and the region bypassed using the patient's own saphenous vein anastomosed, for example, to the femoral artery above and to the popliteal below (Fig. 24.4). Bypass grafts of synthetic material can be used in some circumstances.

Occasionally the only appropriate bypass procedure is to take blood via a graft from one site to another. For example, the common femoral artery on one side may be linked to the femoral artery on the other side or the axillary artery may be linked to the femoral artery on the same side. Synthetic graft material is usually used. Such a procedure may be sufficient to salvage a limb, preventing gangrene.

3. Angioplasty. This means plastic surgery on blood vessels. It usually involves widening the lumen or origin of an artery with a vein patch, with or without a local thrombo-endarterectomy. Profundaplasty (a plastic procedure on the origin of the profunda femoris artery) greatly improves the blood flow to the leg in selected patients.

4. Transluminal angioplasty. Short strictures in some arteries are suitable for stretching (or dilatation) with a special catheter. This is passed into the lumen of the vessel, usually via the femoral artery, under general anaesthetic. The catheter is advanced to the site of the stricture, where a small balloon at the end of the catheter is forcibly inflated, dilating the stricture. The procedure is performed under radiological control.

5. Lumbar sympathectomy. Interruption of the sympathetic chain reduces sympathetic tone in the arteries allowing vasodilatation to occur. This effect is not permanent and, in diseased arteries, may not be very great. However, it may result in relief of rest pain and recovery or arrest of pre-gangrenous changes in the skin. The sympathectomy can be done surgically or by injection, through the back, of sclerosant material around the nerve chain. The latter is known as chemical sympathectomy. It is a simple procedure (in the hands of an expert) done under local anaesthetic with minimal disturbance to the patient. Sympathectomy is used in patients who are generally unfit for major arterial surgery, those in whom direct arterial surgery is impossible, or those in whom the latter has failed to relieve symptoms.

Preoperative preparation

Preoperative preparation for major arterial surgery involves a careful assessment of the patient's general condition to ensure that he is fit for the procedure. Diabetes, if present, must be well controlled. Any infection, e.g. in chest or limbs, must be eliminated. Four to six pints of blood should be cross-matched. Some surgeons, when synthetic grafts are being used, treat the patient with prophylactic antibiotics, starting just before or during operation. The arterial X-rays must be available so that a check can be made of the disease to be treated. A urinary catheter should be passed on patients undergoing major abdominal arterial surgery.

Postoperative care

Postoperative care involves observation of the pulse and blood pressure (and central venous pressure if this is being measured) to ensure a stable circulation. No drains are placed in the abdomen but there may be a closed suction drain in limb wounds. Any excessive bleeding must be reported. The lower limbs are observed for colour, sensation and presence of pulses. Any change must be reported. In general the patient is kept at rest for one or two days and then gradually mobilised, unless there are instructions to the contrary. Thrombosis of grafts or arteries sometimes occurs, requiring re-exploration. Infection in the region of a graft can be disastrous, giving rise to secondary haemorrhage. Great care is taken with all the routine methods to avoid this. Paralytic ileus is a common complication of aortic operations.

ANEURYSMS

An aneurysm is a localised dilatation of an artery resulting from weakness

Diseases of arteries and veins / 241

of its wall, atherosclerosis being the commonest cause.

Degeneration of the whole of the arterial wall may give rise to a spindle-shaped enlargement of fusiform type whereas localised weakness of part of the wall may produce a saccular form. The weakness within the arterial wall may also be of a congenital nature such as the so-called berry aneurysm of the intracranial vessels (Ch. 44). Inflammatory changes in the arterial wall such as are found in syphilis may also lead to aneurysmal formation.

A traumatic aneurysm is really a false aneurysm with the development of an aneurysmal sac in a haematoma surrounding a damaged artery.

Clinical features

Presence of an expansile swelling which may be painful or painless. Palpable thrill and audible bruit.

Left untreated an aneurysm may rupture into the surrounding tissues or may thrombose with impairment of the peripheral arterial circulation.

Emboli may arise from the thrombus and block distal vessels.

Rupture of an abdominal aortic aneurysm is preceded by severe back pain. Profuse haemorrhage into the retroperitoneal tissues leads to severe shock and a tender abdominal mass is usually palpable. It may rupture into the peritoneal cavity.

Treatment

Aneurysms causing symptoms should be treated surgically. The considerable risk of rupture of an abdominal aortic aneurysm is the reason that most people treat such aneurysms with a diameter of 5 centimetres or more surgically. Age is a relative contraindication to this policy.

Complete excision of the aneurysm and its replacement by an arterial Dacron graft is the ideal procedure (Fig. 24.5). In the case of an aortic aneurysm the aneurysmal sac is usually sutured around the graft to stop other tissues sticking to the latter. The distal limbs of the graft are joined to the common or internal iliac or the femoral vessels, depending on the extent of the disease.

The general condition of a patient suffering from an aortic aneurysm is

Fig. 24.5 An abdominal aortic aneurysm containing a thrombus and its replacement by a Dacron arterial graft.

carefully assessed to assess their fitness for major surgery. The patient is prepared in the usual manner for an abdominal operation. A nasogastric tube has been found by some to be unnecessary, it's omission reducing postoperative pulmonary complications from 16 to 7.5 per cent. Six pints of blood should be cross-matched.

A ruptured abdominal aortic aneurysm is a very different and serious problem. Some patients die before reaching an operating table and amongst those who do undergo surgery there is a mortality of 45 per cent compared to 8.5 per cent when the aneurysm is unruptured. What the patient requires above all else is that the bleeding is controlled by placing a clamp across the aorta above the aneurysm.

A pressurised suit advocated by Lewis may be life-saving. On arrival at the hospital the patient is taken straight to the theatre. As rapidly as possible a nasogastric tube is passed (essential as the contents of his stomach are unknown), and the skin of the abdomen is prepared. An intravenous line (preferably two) is set up. Twelve units of blood are ordered.

If the patient's condition permits resuscitation is commenced but the systolic blood pressure is not raised above 100 mm Hg in case further bleeding occurs. The anaesthetist only induces the anaesthetic when the surgeon is ready to open the abdomen. As quickly as possible the surgeon opens the abdomen and puts a clamp across the aorta. Effective resuscitation is now possible and when the hypotension has been corrected by blood transfusion the patient is heparinised and the operation proceeds.

Postoperatively the patient is treated in an intensive care unit, where the blood pressure, central venous pressure, urine output, blood gases, serum electrolytes and all the other parameters which guide treatment are monitored. Paralytic ileus is a common complication.

The pulses in both lower limbs should be palpated half-hourly for the first 24 hours and any deficiency reported. The colour and sensation of the limbs should also be observed, any change being reported. As soon as the patient's general condition is stable and paralytic ileus, if present, is resolving mobilisation can commence.

THROMBOANGIITIS OBLITERANS

Although this condition is regarded by some to be simply an early form of atherosclerosis it is described here as a separate entity.

The disease tends to affect young men and is characterised by an inflammatory reaction which involves the arterial wall together with the adjoining vein and nerve. Remissions and relapses are often encountered with gangrenous changes appearing later in one or more toes and remaining localised for some time.

Treatment

Smoking should be stopped completely but although vasodilator drugs are often prescribed their efficacy is doubtful. The results of lumbar sympathectomy are variable but if pain is severe it is worthy of trial. Limited amputation of the toes is successful in this condition and major amputation should be withheld for as long as possible.

RAYNAUD'S DISEASE

This is an uncommon condition which affects the hands, women being affected much more commonly than men. There appears to be an exaggerated vasospastic response to cold, especially in the digital vessels, the attacks being characterised by blanching of the digits followed by blueness and pain and later by redness. Patches of gangrene may appear on the fingertips. The disease may be primary (or idiopathic) or secondary, being associated with a variety of underlying conditions including occlusive arterial disease, thoracic outlet syndromes, and collagen diseases such as scleroderma and rheumatoid arthritis.

Treatment

This is primarily directed towards protection from the cold by avoiding exposure, wearing warm clothing, and the use of electrically heated gloves, and the administration of vasodilator drugs may help. Cervical sympathectomy may lead to relief of symptoms. Local amputation of parts of digits is necessary if gangrene supervenes.

GANGRENE

This means death of tissue and may be massive in type as in the death of a whole limb (Fig. 24.6) or it may be localised in form as for example involving the fingertip.

Fig. 24.6 Gangrene of the foot.

Causes

Loss of blood supply as in atherosclerosis or emboli.
Physical or chemical violence as in burns.
Infection such as gas gangrene.

Types

Gangrene in general, apart from gas gangrene, may be of two types.
   1. *Moist gangrene.* The tissues are moist and infection spreads rapidly. Toxic products are absorbed in the tissues near to the gangrenous area. If the gangrene is moist the area must be treated as a septic wound and amputation is undertaken as soon as possible.
   2. *Dry gangrene.* This form is usually vascular in origin and the spread is slow. So long as the part is kept dry the gangrenous portion may separate at a line of demarcation, the tissues proximal to this being healthy and viable.

Treatment of the gangrenous limb

   (a) Keep the limb cool so that its metabolism is reduced.
   (b) Keep the affected part dry. This is best accomplished by complete exposure and the toes involved may be kept separated by dental rolls.
   (c) The limb should be protected from the weight of the bedclothes by a bed-cage and the heel supported on a foam pad.
   (d) Adequate relief of pain.
   (e) Lumbar sympathectomy may result in vasodilatation of the collateral blood vessels and an improvement in the cutaneous blood flow.
   (f) When gangrene threatens the patient's life amputation should be considered.

Gangrene of digits is a definite indication for direct arterial surgery because if this is possible, a major amputation may be avoided. If unsuccessful then some form of amputation is inevitable. Obviously this is a serious undertaking in an elderly feeble patient and the nursing care of such cases is of paramount importance. A constant anxiety is the healing of the amputation flaps in tissues which are obviously depleted of blood supply. A compromise has to be made. The higher the level of the amputation, such as midthigh, the better the chances of healing but against this must be placed the fact that amputation above the knee joint means that rehabilitation of the patient is going to be much more difficult. All amputations require careful skin preparation in the theatre and all should have intramuscular penicillin commencing on the day of surgery and continuing for five days after operation. These measures are essential to prevent gas gangrene in the amputation stump.

Postoperative management following amputation

Avoid injury to the stump.
The stump must be dressed and wrapped in crepe bandage (Fig. 24.7).

Fig. 24.7 Bandaging an amputation stump.

No pillow is placed behind the stump as a flexion deformity of the hip may develop.

Remove drain tube if present in 24 to 48 hours.

Exercise the stump from the second day.

Early mobilisation on crutches and fitting of the artificial limb.

Removal of skin sutures on the 10th day.

Investigate the home circumstances to effect physical changes necessary for a smooth return and maximum independance (e.g. bars in toilet, ramp to get into house in wheelchair, height of bed correct, etc.).

Complications following amputation

(a) Reactionary haemorrhage within the first 12 hours. This is uncommon. It is manifest by excessive bleeding into the dressing or via a drain and may be accompanied by the general signs of blood loss. It must be reported immediately. Surgery may be required to stop the bleeding.

(b) Secondary haemorrhage at 7–10 days. This is usually associated with infection or ischaemia of the tissues adjacent to the wound. The management is that of the infection or ischaemia.

(c) Ischaemia of the stump. The blood supply to the muscle or skin at the distal end of the stump may be inadequate, causing failure to heal of part or all of the wound. The affected tissues become necrotic. The skin changes through a dusky blue to black. Surgical excision of the dead tissue or re-amputation higher up may be necessary. If it is only a small area of skin that is necrotic this may separate spontaneously and the wound heal by granulation.

(d) Infection. This is more common in diabetic patients than in others. The stump becomes painful, swollen, red and hot. It may be necessary to open the wound and excise dead tissue to provide adequate drainage. The bone end may become involved in the infection. Sometimes the end result is an irregular tethered scar with a persistent sinus. This makes fitting of an artificial limb difficult. Surgical revision is necessary.

(e) Phantom pains. The patient may still complain of pain in the foot or hand which has been amputated.

(f) Amputation stump neuroma. This is a painful condition in which one of the nerve ends, remaining as a result of the amputation, becomes swollen or tethered in the scar. Avoidance of local pressure or excision of the area is the treatment.

Prognosis

Seventy per cent of all amputations performed are on patients over 70 years of age and half of all unilateral amputees who survive 3 years will lose the other leg.

VEINS

Anatomy in the leg

The internal (or long) saphenous vein runs in front of the medial malleolus, ascends the leg within the subcutaneous tissue just behind the medial border of the tibia, passes behind the posterolateral aspect of the knee and then continues along the medial aspect of the thigh to perforate the deep fascia at the saphenous opening to join the femoral vein. The main vein has many tributaries, the principal one being the posterior arch vein.

The short saphenous vein runs up the back of the calf from behind the lateral malleolus to perforate the deep fascia behind the knee and join the popliteal vein. These superficial veins communicate with the deep intramuscular veins via communicating channels which perforate the deep fascia. The natural flow of blood is from the superficial veins via the perforating channels into the deep veins, the valves present within the veins directing the flow and preventing any tendency to back-flow.

VARICOSE VEINS

A varicose vein is one which is elongated, tortuous and dilated. Destruction of the valves, either in the perforating veins or at the junction of superficial with deep veins, allows for back-flow into the superficial veins and as a result elevation of the pressure (especially during exercise) within the superficial veins. This eventually leads to the varicosities (Fig. 24.8).

The cause of the initial valve damage is often unknown. However, increased intra-abdominal pressure or pressure on the pelvic veins may be important (e.g. pregnancy, pelvic tumours, constipation). Previous destruction of valves in the deep veins due to deep venous thrombosis results in increased pressure in these veins. This in turn results in

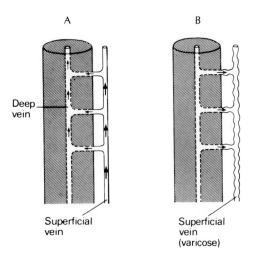

Fig. 24.8 A. Normal flow of venous blood through competent communicating veins from the superficial system to the deep system. B. Reversal of flow following incompetence of the communicating veins with the development of varicosities within the superficial system.

increased pressure, valvular damage and reversal of flow in the perforating veins, leading on to superficial varicose veins. Such patients may have the post-thrombotic syndrome (see below).

Clinical features

Small varicose veins give rise to no symptoms. The principal symptom in the more prominent veins is a dull aching pain towards the end of the day. Women often complain of the unsightly appearance (Fig. 24.9). Enlargement of the vein at the saphenous opening may produce a soft swelling often 2 cm in diameter which has a well-marked cough impulse and empties on lying down. This is known as a saphena varix. Slight ankle swelling towards the end of the day is not uncommon.

Investigation

The site of valvular damage is determined clinically by the doctor using one or more tourniquets applied at different parts of the leg. These are applied with the patient supine and the leg elevated. The patient stands and the control of backflow in the veins is noted. Ascending venography may be necessary to determine the state of the deep veins or the site of incompetent perforating veins.

Treatment

1. Elastic support stockings may be used to provide relief in patients unfit or unwilling to undergo surgery or in those in whom surgery is inappropriate. The stockings should exert a graduated compression from the ankle up the leg, the pressure being highest at the ankle and lowest at

Fig. 24.9 Varicose veins.

Fig. 24.10 Varicose ulcer.

the top of the leg. The stockings may be below knee, above knee or in the form of tights, depending on need. The patient must be measured and fitted with the correct size, as well as having two of any stocking to enable him to wash and change it.

2. Injection sclerotherapy. This is suitable for the milder varicosities, varicosities below the knee and for incompetent perforating veins. The aim is to induce a phlebitis within the vein. The agent used is sodium tetradecyl sulphate. It is injected at one or more sites in the vein, which is emptied by elevation of the leg. Pressure pads over the sites of injection, crepe bandages and elastoplast are then applied from the foot to the thigh; a full-length elastic stocking is worn for support. This is all left untouched for 6 weeks. The patient is encouraged to walk 2 or more miles per day.

3. Surgery. This approach is the most successful for large varicosities and those extending above the knee. It consists of tying the internal or the short saphenous vein at its junction with the deep veins and stripping the appropriate vein from the ankle to this point. Incompetent perforating veins are also tied.

Preoperative preparation includes the routine general measures, plus shaving of the appropriate leg and accurate marking of the veins to be treated surgically (this is done by the surgeon).

Postoperatively the leg is supported by a crepe or elastic bandage. The foot of the bed is elevated for 24 hours. Early mobility is encouraged. The patient should walk, or rest with the legs elevated. Stitches are removed between the 7th and 10th postoperative day.

The popular use of the saphenous vein as a bypass vascular graft may influence the surgeon in his decision to resort to surgery.

Complications

1. Phlebitis. This is often associated with thrombosis (thrombophlebitis). It presents as a tender lump at the site of varicosities. Initial treatment is bed rest with elevation of the foot of the bed and analgesics as necessary. Local application of lead and opium or glycerine and ichthyol dressings may give symptomatic relief. Once the acute pain has gone mobility with an elastic stocking is encouraged.

2. Haemorrhage. This is due to local trauma to a varicosity around the ankle. Treatment is immediate elevation of the leg with the patient supine. Local pressure is applied and maintained before mobility is resumed.

3. Liposclerosis. This occurs in the lower third of the leg as a result of incompetent perforating veins. Haemosiderin escapes into the subcutaneous tissues causing pigmentation and subsequent fibrosis. The skin becomes thickened, hard, brown and inflexible. It may become scaley, inflamed and itchy (varicose eczema). The treatment is that of the underlying abnormal veins, especially the incompetent perforators, together with a good elastic stocking. Stanozolol may reduce the fibrosis and pigmentation.

4. Ulceration. This usually occurs secondary to liposclerosis (Fig. 24.10). The commonest site for such varicose (or gravitational) ulceration is the lower third of the leg medially. A variety of treatments is available but each consists of a combination of one or more of the following—maintaining a clean granulating base with, for example, saline or hydrogen peroxide soaks; bed rest with elevation of foot; maintenance of local pressure and support by pad or silastic foam on ulcer and crepe or elastic bandage or elastic stocking on leg; application of icthopaste, viscopaste or similar bandage; treatment of incompetent perforating veins; treatment of liposclerosis; local application of zinc, as zinc sulphate, or oral administration of zinc; skin grafting.

5. Post-thrombotic syndrome. This results from damage to the deep veins as a result of previous deep venous thrombosis but may only be diagnosed when the patient presents with varicose veins. It is characterised by a heavy or bursting feeling in the leg, particularly towards the end of the day, and swelling of the ankle. Varicose veins, liposclerosis or ulceration may be present. Treatment is symptomatic, consisting of elevation of the foot of the bed at night and the wearing of graduated compression stockings.

BIBLIOGRAPHY

Lewis D G, McKenzie A, McNeil I F 1973 Annals of the Royal College of Surgeons of England 52: 53–58

25

The lymphatic system and the spleen

Lymph is a tissue fluid which collects within the prelymphatic extracellular spaces from where it is conveyed to the larger lymphatic channels and by these eventually to the blood stream. It passes to the lymph nodes which are structurally adapted to filter and sample the lymph passing through them. This enables the system to isolate infection and when necessary triggers off host defence mechanisms. This response is mediated through lymphoid follicles contained within each node.

The principal sites of lymph nodes are indicated in Figure 25.1. Individual areas of the body drain to regional or primary groups of nodes. Efferent vessels from these lead to secondary groups of lymph nodes and may communicate with channels leading to the larger main ducts which join the venous system at the root of the neck.

Enlarged lymph nodes maybe demonstrated by the shadow they cast on straight X-rays (e.g. in the mediastinum) or by the displacement they cause of other structures (e.g. displacing the ureter laterally).

Both the lymphatic channels and the nodes may be displayed radiographically following the injection of contrast media into a small subcutaneous lymphatic, a technique known as lymphangiography. Lymphatic structures can also be examined by ultrasound scanning, radioisotope scanning, CT scanning and open excision biopsy of the node. These techniques are now applied to the clinical investigation of oedema and malignant disease.

THE LYMPHATIC GLANDS

INFLAMMATORY CONDITIONS

Acute lymphadenitis. This is commonly due to an acute septic focus, such as a boil, tonsillitis, or a septic wound.

The primary cause must be treated. Locally, a counter-irritant relieves pain, and in many cases the infection subsides without very much trouble. Occasionally suppuration occurs and incision and drainage may be necessary.

Chronic lymphadenitis. *Tuberculous.* This is now a comparatively rare

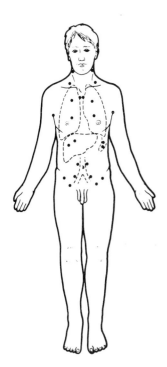

Fig. 25.1 The principal sites of the lymphatic glands.

condition. The commonest site is in the neck. Resolution usually occurs with rest and antituberculous chemotherapy. If the glandular mass enlarges, excision of the glands is performed. A cold abscess may be aspirated or drained and the gland removed by curettage. In the abdomen, tuberculous glands usually heal by calcification, and may give rise to symptoms on account of mechanical interference with the functions of the intestine.

Other causes of chronic lymphadenitis include sarcoidosis, infectious mononucleosis and syphillis.

MALIGNANT TUMOURS OF LYMPH NODES

These may be primary or secondary.

1. Secondary malignancy is by far the commonest, the lymph node being the first 'port of call' of most malignancies once it moves outside its primary site.

2. Primary malignancy i.e. lymphoma (Fig. 25.2). This is less common, Hodgkin's disease being the commonest variety. Once a definite diagnosis has been made by open lymph node biopsy the patient is thoroughly investigated to determine the extent of the disease before treatment is planned. Lymphoma may be found wherever there is lymphoid tissue e.g. the liver, the spleen, the gastrointestinal tract as well as the lymph node areas. The extent of involvement determines to a large extent the choice of therapy and has a direct relationship to the prognosis. It is determined by clinical examination of all the lymphatic drainage areas, a chest radiograph, ultrasound scanning, lymphangiography, CT scanning, and in some cases an exploratory 'staging' laparotomy.

Fig. 25.2 Lymphoma. The glands of the neck are visibly enlarged.

Many patients with Hodgkin's disease and other malignant lymphomas can look forward to a normal span of life following radiotherapy or chemotherapy.

LYMPHATIC VESSELS

Several clinical syndromes associated with oedema of unknown aetiology affecting infants, children and young adults are related to congenital developmental abnormalities of the lymphatic vessels demonstrated by lymphangiography. These conditions are usually difficult to treat and only the most severe cases should be subjected to surgery. This consists of excision of the oedematous subcutaneous tissue with the construction of skin graft procedures.

Lymphoedema from lymphatic obstruction also occurs as a result of:
(a) invasion of the lymphatics by cancer cells,
(b) surgical removal of the lymph nodes,
(c) parasitic infestation of the lymph channels, e.g. filariasis.

THE SPLEEN

The spleen is closely allied to the lymphatic system and it is frequently enlarged in lymphatic disorders, e.g. Hodgkin's disease and infective mononucleosis. It may also be enlarged in conditions unrelated to the lymphatic system such as portal hypertension, thrombocytopenic purpura, chronic myeloid leukaemia, and myelofibrosis.

INDICATIONS FOR SPLENECTOMY

1. Rupture is the commonest indication. The spleen is damaged in a crush injury of the left hypochondrium. The patient complains of left sided abdominal pain and exhibits all the signs of internal bleeding. Left shoulder tip pain may also occur due to irritation of the diaphragm by blood.

Immediate laparotomy and splenectomy is life-saving. The injury may result in a subcapsular haematoma which can rupture any time up to 3 weeks after the injury.

2. Hereditary spherocytosis is a condition in which the red blood cells are fragile and are broken down by the spleen leading to anaemia and jaundice.

3. Thrombocytopenic purpura is a bleeding disorder caused by a reduction of circulating platelets. The site of platelet consumption (the spleen) is removed.

4. In certain rare cases of **leukaemia** and **myelofibrosis** in which the spleen is breaking down red cells faster than they are being made, thus causing anaemia.

5. As part of a **staging laparotomy** for lymphomas.

6. In certain cases of **portal hypertension.**

Preparation for splenectomy

In an emergency situation in which the patient is shocked an intravenous infusion is set up, with uncross-matched 'O' negative blood if necessary, a blood sample is sent for urgent cross-matching, a nasogastric tube is passed and the patient taken straight to the operating theatre.

In an elective case the preparation is similar to that for any major abdominal operation. Anaemia is corrected, blood is cross-matched and the blood platelet count performed. If the operation is for thrombocytopenic purpura and the platelet count is low, fresh platelets should be available for transfusion once the splenic vessels have been ligated.

The spleen is situated in the left hypochondrium, and access is difficult if the stomach is distended. For this reason a nasogastric tube is passed before the patient leaves the ward and left in position during the operation and for 24 hours afterwards.

Postoperative care

The pulse and blood pressure must be recorded until stable. A drain is usually placed in the splenic bed. Reactionary haemorrhage may occur giving rise to signs of shock and excessive blood loss via the drain. This should be reported immediately. Surgical intervention may be required. The drain can be removed in 24 to 48 hours.

Collapse or pneumonia of the lower lobe of the left lung is an occasional complication and may be prevented by deep-breathing exercises. Acute dilatation of the stomach is prevented by leaving the nasogastric tube in position and aspirating the stomach until it is emptying normally.

Thrombosis, particularly venous, may occur due to the rise in platelets which follows splenectomy. The measures previously described to prevent it should be energetically pursued.

In the long term, patients who have had a splenectomy are more liable to develop acute infections, particularly with the pneumococcus, than are normal people. Children appear to be especially at risk. Some doctors treat such children prophylactically with penicillin over a long period or advocate immunisation with a pneumococcal vaccine.

26

Organ transplantation

When an organ ceases to function owing to disease it can occasionally be replaced by artificial materials or by an organ taken from another individual.

Artificial materials introduced into the human body encounter a hostile environment and no material has yet been devised which combines ideal mechanical properties with perfect compatibility with human tissues. Having said this, many prostheses enjoy a considerable measure of success, good examples being the hip joint prostheses in joint replacement surgery and Dacron arterial grafts in vascular surgery.

The replacement of a diseased organ by one removed from another individual has, in recent years, become a reality although the potential rejection by the body of the transplanted organ remains a major obstacle.

TYPES OF TRANSPLANT

1. Autograft. (Fig. 26.1). Tissue taken from one area of the body and placed in another. A good example of this is skin grafts.

2. Allograft. Tissue taken from one individual in a species and placed in another of the same species. Examples are renal and hepatic transplants.

3. Xenograft. Tissue from one species transplanted into a member of another species.

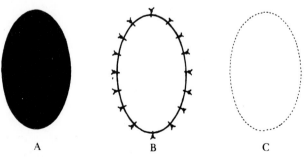

A   B   C

Fig. 26.1 Autograft. Skin defect (A) is closed by autograft of skin (B) and remains healed when the graft has 'taken' (C).

TISSUE REJECTION

The process is essentially an immunological one. When skin of guinea pig A is grafted on to guinea pig B the grafted tissue is initially accepted but at about the 10th day thrombosis occurs within the blood vessels which have grown into the grafted tissue, and the skin dies (Fig. 26.2). This phenomenon is known as tissue rejection. If a second piece of skin is grafted on to guinea pig B rejection is more rapid, occurring in 3-5 days.

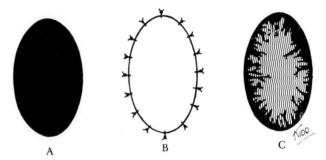

Fig.26.2 Homograft reaction. Skin defect (A) is closed by homograft of skin (B) and gradually withers away (C) owing to the homograft reaction.

The process of rejection is accompanied by the features of an inflammatory response with infiltration of the area with leucocytes and exudation of fluid into the intercellular space. Within the cell membranes of the grafted organs are a number of factors called transplantation antigens. These antigens are recognised as foreign by the recipient lymphocytes. A generation of lymphocytes is produced which are specifically committed to the destruction of the grafts. The lymphocytes enter the blood stream and infiltrate the graft. This reaction on the part of the lymphocyte represents the cellular component of the immune response. In addition there is a humoral component in which the lymphocytes produce and release into the circulation antibodies which act upon the foreign antigens on the cell membranes of the graft.

Modification of rejection process

In order that any allograft procedure may succeed, the process of rejection must be modified. At present this may be accomplished in two ways, both of which are used particularly in renal transplantation.

A. Donor matching. This is done to determine histocompatibility of donor and recipient. Transplantation antigens are inherited characteristics. If donor and recipient are of the same genetic make-up, as in identical twins, no rejection will occur and the graft may survive indefinitely. Attempts have, therefore, been made to determine compatibility between the antigens of the donor and recipient—an assessment called tissue matching.

The first and most important part of the matching process is to ensure blood group (ABO) compatibility between the donor and the recipient. Following this other antigens like HLA (Human Leukocyte Antigen) are matched for each individual. A good tissue match of HLA, A B, and DR (D-related) loci is compatible with long survival of the grafted tissue. Therefore the most compatible donor on the basis of tissue typing is chosen.

B. Immuno suppression. It is also possible to modify the production of antibodies by suppressing their manufacture.

In clinical practice the objective of immunosuppression is to obtain complete acceptance of the grafted organ without depressing the immune defences. Such an ideal has not yet been achieved. However, immunosuppression can be achieved by:

1. Donor specific immunosuppression—this form of immunologic tolerance is not yet available in clinical transplantation, but very interesting results are seen in animal experiments.

2. Non-specific immunosuppression—can be achieved by:

(a) Organ grafting following high doses of total body X-irradiation. This led to a high complication rate and in most cases failed to prevent rejection. This method was used in earlier days of organ transplantation.

(b) Antilymphocyte preparations. Products like antilymphocyte serum, antilymphocyte globulin and antilymphoblast blobulin, when injected into a recipient, reduce the number of circulating lymphocytes and thus modify the process of rejection by impairing the immune response. These preparations are also used in the treatment of episodes of rejection in clinical transplantation on renal and cardiac allograft recipients.

(c) Pharmacological immunosuppression. Drugs are used to suppress the immune response e.g. azathioprine, steroids and cyclosporin A. Azathioprine acts by interfering with the metabolism of lymphocytes where as steroids (prednisone and hydrocortisone) diminish the inflammatory response. Comparitively recently cyclosporin A (an antibiotic fungal product) has been used. It is a very potent but toxic drug, which seems to act on T-cell differentiation at an early phase, possibly interfering with the signal for T-cells to proliferate. (T-cells are those lymphocytes whose maturation depends on the thymus.)

Clinical applications

Renal transplantation has now been clinically acceptable for nearly twenty five years. More than 35 000 cases of renal transplantation have been carried out in various centres of the world.

In the United Kingdom, of the total number of renal transplants carried out, approximately 90 per cent of the kidneys are obtained from cadavers whereas 10 per cent are from live related donors.

The sources of cadavaric kidneys are mainly from patients dying in hospitals after road traffic accidents or subarachnoid haemorrhage, who are usually on ventilators.

In the United Kingdom, the combined Colleges of Surgeons and Physicians in 1976 have laid down very clear-cut and strict criteria for the certification of brain death (= acceptable as clinical death). This, after a lot of debate, is now accepted by the clinicians and is practised in the day-to-day management of patients on life-support machines.

Certification of brain death is done by two senior doctors (one of whom must be of consultant rank) who have been involved in the treatment of the patient. Having obtained the consent from relatives for the removal of organs and the consent from the Coroner, in Coroner's cases, and before the ventilator is switched off, the transplant team is contacted. They then remove the organs in a proper surgical operating theatre.

Fig. 26.3   A transplanted kidney in position.

The donor kidney is transplanted into the right iliac fossa (Fig. 26.3) of the recipient, the renal vessels being anastomosed to the iliac vessels, whilst the ureter is implanted into the dome of the bladder.

Although both liver and heart transplants have been carried out at many centres the results do not compare favourably with those of renal transplantation. The concensus of opinion, therefore, is that until the rejection problem has been finally conquered both liver and heart transplantation should be confined to a few international centres.

The results of liver transplantation are showing improvement as a result of better surgical technique. Rejection episodes are easily controlled with immunosuppressive drugs and hypothermic preservation will keep the donor liver in good condition for ten hours.

In recent years, with the advent of better tissue matching, newer immunosuppression and repeated pre-transplant blood transfusion to the recipient, the success rate of organ transplantation has improved considerably. At present the one year graft survival in cadaveric kidney transplant has improved from 50 per cent to 80 per cent and in live related donor transplant from 85 per cent to 95 per cent.

Although the method of immunosuppression is still far from ideal a donor specific immunosuppression with minimum side effects is probably the best hope for future improvement.

27

The face, the mouth and the tongue

A patient suffering from a surgical lesion of the face or lip usually seeks medical advice in the early stages of the disability. The mildest lesion of the face is usually of some concern even to the most self-effacing individual, and facial disease or deformity can depress the morale of a patient out of all proportion to the size or severity of the lesion. Unsightly scars or naevi will effect profound changes in the attitude and outlook of the patient. They may affect his whole life, and the importance of the work of the plastic surgeon lies in reducing his disabilities.

WOUNDS

Wounds of the face, because of the abundant blood supply to the part, heal rapidly. Thorough cleansing and the removal of grit is important, as failure to do this results in an ugly discoloured scar. The fine stitches inserted should be removed on the third or fourth day to avoid permanent stitch marks. Sepsis is rare, dressings are unnecessary and the wound may be left exposed.

A depressed fracture of the malar bone is not uncommon, and early elevation is undertaken so that the cheek prominence is restored.

INFLAMMATORY CONDITIONS AND CYSTS

Cellulitis and carbuncle. The lips may be affected. Infection of the upper lip, once regarded as a most dangerous condition, is now easily resolved by the use of antibiotics.

Chancre of the lip. A primary syphilitic lesion (chancre) may appear on the lip. The glands in the neck are enlarged.

Chronic inflammatory conditions. Chronic inflammatory conditions are not common. The rhagades of congenital syphilis may be seen as healed scars in the adult.

Cysts of the face. Sebaceous cysts (Fig. 27.1) are common, particularly on the nose and around the ears. They are due to blockage of the duct of

Fig. 27.1 Sebaceous cyst below the left clavicle.

a sebaceous gland. The pent-up secretion of sebum is responsible for the swelling, and the lining of the cyst is the stretched sebaceous gland. The treatment is excision.

Dermoid cysts may form at the line of fusion of the skull and face and may be found at the root of the nose or over the external angular process of the orbit (Fig. 27.2).

Fig. 27.2 External angular dermoid cyst. The overlying skin is freely movable.

NEW GROWTHS OF THE FACE AND LIPS

Simple tumours

Simple tumours, particularly naevi, may be disfiguring. They are usually treated by surgical excision. Destruction by cryosurgery or with carbon dioxide snow may be used.

Basal cell carcinoma (Syn. Rodent ulcer)

A rodent ulcer (Fig. 27.3) usually occurs on the upper part of the face, and is frequently situated dangerously near to the eyes. It is locally malignant and, untreated, will erode the bones of the face and skull until a septic meningitis kills the patient. Its progress is very slow at first.

Radium to the surface, excision or cryodestruction are effective. In late cases the eyeball may have to be removed.

Fig. 27.3 Rodent ulcer.

Squamous-cell carcinoma

Cancer is commoner on the lower than on the upper lip, and used to be frequently associated with a long-standing habit of smoking a hot clay pipe.

Clinical features. The growth appears as a hard nodule which later becomes either papilliferous and warty in appearance, or it assumes the characteristics of a typical malignant ulcer. The base is fixed and the edge is hard and everted. The lymphatic glands underneath the chin and the lower jaw enlarge as spread occurs. Untreated, the tumour erodes the lower jaw.

Treatment. Surgical excision, radiotherapy or cryosurgery may be used. The glands are treated by subsequent block dissection.

CLEFT LIP AND CLEFT PALATE

Cleft lip and cleft palate are congenital deformities due to the failure of fusion of the various tissues forming the lips and the palate. Cortisone

Fig. 27.4   Example of cleft lip and palate (a) at birth, (b) aged 4 months, (c) aged 16 months.

intoxication, virus infections such as rubella, oxygen and vitamin deficiency, as well as radiation damage during foetal life, are now known to be causal factors. Cleft lip almost invariably affects the upper lip, and may involve one or both sides. It may occur alone or in association with a cleft palate. In most cases there is some deformity of the face and nose. A cleft palate may involve the hard and the soft palate or only a portion of the soft palate. The disability of these lesions may be summarised as follows:

1. The obvious cosmetic deformity.
2. Feeding is difficult with a cleft palate but a cleft lip causes no interference.
3. Nasal catarrh and respiratory infections are common because the mouth and the nose communicate. There is a high incidence of hearing problems.
4. The speech is seriously impaired.

Fig. 27.5   Example of dental obturator for temporary closure of palatal defect.

Treatment

A cleft lip is repaired as soon as possible usually at about 3 months. This is done surgically. There are various techniques employed for obtaining a good cosmetic result. Figure 27.4 shows an example of cleft lip and palate.

The orthodontist by making a plate (Fig. 27.5), similar to a dental prosthesis, for the newborn baby with the cleft palate can aid the baby to suck. Furthermore modification of the plate can mould the cleft into correct alignment before surgical closure is undertaken. This has given vastly superior cosmetic results; in particular, deformity of the nose is very much reduced.

The cleft palate is repaired surgically about the age of 1 year. The palate must be repaired if good speech is to be attained.

Preoperative care of a case of cleft lip

The infant must be trained to take food from a special spoon (Fig. 27.6) or dropper although a normal spoon is often quite satisfactory. His reaction to this form of feeding must be satisfactory before operation is contemplated. Sucking with a soft teat is preferable if a dental plate can be fitted. He should be gaining weight. The blood haemoglobin should be not less than 12 g/dl. Preoperatively, systemic antibiotics will usually be prescribed to counteract any infection which may develop.

Swabs of the nose and throat should be taken before operation and the child should be in hospital for at least a week.

Postoperative care of cleft lip

1. Antibiotics will be continued postoperatively. The wound is left exposed. The mouth and nose are frequently cleansed so as to avoid infection. The sutures are removed on the fifth day after operation or earlier as the surgeon directs.

A Logan's bow may be applied for 14 days to keep the lip in the normal pouting position and to take tension off the suture line.

2. The arms are splinted lightly to prevent the infant 'picking' the dressing.

3. Feeding must be as careful as before operation.

4. Rest is essential. Crying must be reduced to a minimum, since it tends to stretch the suture line. Sedatives, such as chloral hydrate, may be necessary.

Preoperative care of cleft palate

This is similar to that outlined above for a cleft lip.

Postoperative care of cleft palate

1. The arms are splinted to prevent the child injuring the suture line in the mouth. The patient is propped upright in bed.

Fig. 27.6 Spoon adapted for feeding infant with cleft lip or cleft palate.

2. Feeding is carefully carried out. Since the mouth is now smaller than previously, and also very tender, there may be considerable difficulty in feeding. The diet should consist of milk, jelly, blancmange, fruit juice, and soup. Rusks, vegetables, and toast are avoided lest the suture line in the mouth should be injured.

3. The mouth is cleansed with several spoonfuls of sterile water before and after every feed.

4. The stitches do not require removal, since catgut is usually employed and will dissolve spontaneously. Wire sutures, if inserted, will be removed by the surgeon.

Continual supervision and further operations to correct associated deformity are necessary until adult life.

A long convalescence is necessary, and the child must be under the care of a speech therapist.

THE MOUTH AND THE TONGUE

The most serious disease inside the mouth is a carcinoma originating in the buccal mucosa or in the mucous membrane of the tongue. The condition is frequently associated with chronic irritation, and is rarely seen inside a clean mouth.

Glossitis

The commonest cause of inflammation of the tongue is antibiotics causing vitamin B_2 deficiency. Tobacco or undiluted spirits are important causes while cytotoxic drugs are an occasional cause.

Chronic glossitis in which the tongue is firm, fissured and later white and cracked on the surface (leukoplakia) is a pre-cancerous condition. Excisional biopsy and cryosurgical excision of the affected area is undertaken.

Cysts in the mouth

1. Simple mucous retention cysts are not uncommon.
2. A ranula is a cystic swelling of the floor of the mouth.
3. A dermoid cyst may protrude into the floor of the mouth.
Excision is the usual treatment.

Ulceration of the tongue

Ulceration of the tongue may be:

A dental ulcer. A dental ulcer is always situated on the side of the tongue in the neighbourhood of a jagged tooth.

Syphilitic ulceration is painless, and the ulcer has a typical punched out appearance.

Malignant ulceration is discussed below.

Aphthous ulcers. Aphthous ulcers are characterised by the development of single or multiple erosive lesions in the oral mucosa surrounded by an area of oedema and hyperaemia. They vary in size from 2 to 10 mm and may be episodic. In women, characteristically they occur premenstrually. The cause is unknown, but oestrogen therapy is effective in healing most patients with premenstrual aphthous ulcer as well as in some in whom the ulcer is not related to the menstrual cycle. Stilboestrol 3 mg daily is a suitable dosage.

NEW GROWTHS OF THE TONGUE

Simple new growths

1. Papilloma.
2. Angioma.

The patient feels the nodule. In the case of angiomas slight haemorrhage is usually present. These growths are excised with a diathermy knife.

Malignant new growths

The incidence of carcinoma of the tongue has been greatly reduced by routine dental care and the effective treatment of syphilis.

Symptoms and signs

Pain may be present in the tongue or referred to the ear.

Haemorrhage. Small haemorrhages are common once ulceration has occurred. A massive fatal secondary haemorrhage is a not unusual termination.

Ulceration. Ulceration has usually occurred by the time the patient seeks advice. It takes the form of a sloughing ulcer with a firm, indurated base and a large everted edge (Fig. 27.7). As the disease advances the patient may be unable to protrude the tongue from his mouth. Salivation is excessive as a result of irritation, and the exudation of pus which results from secondary infection of the growth. Secondary deposits may occur in the lymphatic glands in the neck.

Course of the disease

Untreated, death occurs from:
1. Broncho-pneumonia, which results from the inhalation of the infection in the growth.
2. Secondary haemorrhage.
3. Starvation and exhaustion as a result of pain, and extension of the growth into the tissues of the neck and mouth.

Treatment

Dental treatment is undertaken before any surgical treatment can be attempted. The teeth and gums are invariably septic.

Fig. 27.7   Squamous-cell carcinoma of the tongue.

Radiotherapy. Interstitial radium can be applied to the primary growth, but radiotherapy has given disappointing results in the treatment of the glandular field.

If the glands are invaded they are treated by what is known as a 'block dissection' of the neck. This is usually undertaken after the primary growth has been treated by radium.

Surgical excision. Alternatively the primary lesion can be excised together with the neck glands in continuity. If the glands are not invaded a careful watch is kept on their condition. For this operation the skin is prepared from about 15 cm below the clavicle up to the hair line.

Nursing care. The patient with radium in the mouth requires very special care. *The threads of the needles* must be securely fixed on the face with strapping and regularly inspected and counted to ensure that a radium needle has not been swallowed. All excreta are inspected before disposal. Frequent bland mouthwashes must be given, and a fluid diet, as rich as possible in protein and other nutrients, must be provided. Meat soups, eggs, milk, jellies and fruit juice to which glucose has been added can all be taken. Peanut butter is very useful to keep the mouth moist.

The mouth is septic and irrigation with hydrogen peroxide or eusol diminishes foetor.

The patient should be nursed upright in bed and provided with:
1. A bowl into which saliva can drain.
2. Gauze swabs or disposable tissues to wipe his lips. The bowl for salivation and the swabs should be checked in case they contain a radium needle.
3. A pencil and paper to communicate his wishes.

Pain is usually severe, and morphia may be necessary for its relief. Earache, although not due to an organic cause in the ear, may be treated by the instillation of phenol drops (5 per cent) into the ear and a cotton-wool plug. They act as a counter-irritant at the site to which pain is referred.

The radium reaction is frequently severe, and secondary haemorrhage is most liable to occur 2 or 3 days after the radium has been removed. Its risk is minimised by frequent cleansing of the mouth and encouraging the patient to wash out the mouth as often as possible. Chemotherapy may be prescribed to control infection. Should bleeding occur, the nurse must pull the patient's tongue well forward with the tongue forceps. This frequently controls the haemorrhage temporarily. If this is not successful, the common carotid artery pressure point at the root of the neck must be compressed at once and medical aid summoned without delay.

THE SALIVARY GLANDS

The normal healthy mouth, apart from cleansing of the teeth, does not require mouthwashes. The mouth of the patient who is toxic, dehydrated or forbidden to take fluid becomes dry and more septic than usual. He has little stimulus to excite salivation. The result is that infection creeps up the ducts down which saliva normally flows profusely, and an inflammatory condition develops in the gland. It is for this reason that moistening of the mouth, and mouthwashes, are so important in preventing infection in the conditions just mentioned. Even better than moistening the mouth is to stimulate the flow of saliva, and this can be achieved by giving the patient chewing gum or barley sugar.

Acute sialadenitis (acute inflammation of a salivary gland)

This is due to the conditions which we have mentioned above, and is common only in the parotid glands.

The face is tender and swollen over the affected parotid gland. The patient complains of difficulty in opening his mouth.

The prevention and treatment have already been indicated, namely, mouthwashes, chewing gum and drinking plenty of fluids, if they are allowed. Should suppuration develop, incision will be necessary.

Acute non-suppurative parotitis (mumps)

This is a virus infection and an entirely separate condition. Both parotid glands are usually swollen. Orchitis and very rarely pancreatitis may occur as complications.

Chronic sialadenitis and salivary calculi

The secretion from the parotid gland is thin and serous; that from the submandibular gland is thick and mucoid. As a result of obstruction or stricture of the duct, a low-grade chronic inflammation may arise in a gland. In some cases a calculus forms and blocks the duct. Because of the thicker secretion, 95 per cent of calculi are formed in the submandibular gland.

Symptoms and signs

The patient complains of a swelling in the submandibular region which increases in size at meal times and diminishes in the periods between meals. The enlarged gland can be palpated. A radiograph is taken to prove the presence of a calculus.

Treatment

Treatment may consist of:
1. Removal of the calculus.
2. Dilatation of Wharton's duct with lacrimal probes.
3. Excision of the gland.

A calculus in Wharton's duct is removed from inside the mouth. No special local preoperative preparation is necessary. Postoperatively, these patients may be sent from the theatre with a small swab in the mouth, which is attached outside to a pair of Spencer Wells forceps. The patient is usually coughing by the time he leaves the theatre, and the swab can be removed shortly afterwards. It is unusual for severe haemorrhage to develop. Stitches in the mouth are usually of catgut and do not require removal.

Dilatation of Wharton's duct is usually undertaken for strictures; dabbing the surface with local anaesthetic may suffice, or no anaesthetic may be necessary. The preparation for an excision of the gland is similar to that for excision of the lymphatic glands of the neck.

Fig. 27.8 Mixed parotid tumour.

Parotid tumours

1. Mixed parotid tumour (Fig. 27.8)—75 per cent are benign. The superficial lobe of the parotid gland is excised.

2. Carcinoma—the facial nerve is invaded. It is treated by total removal of the parotid.

3. Some rarer tumours, such as adenolymphoma, may occur.

THE TEETH AND THE JAWS

In the first or deciduous dentition there are 20 teeth which erupt at intervals from about 6 months to 2 years of age. The permanent teeth, which number 32, follow the deciduous teeth and commence to erupt at the age of 6 years. They continue their eruption until the age of 12, when only the third molar (wisdom) teeth are unerupted. Their eruption occurs in the late teens. The roots take three years to develop completely after the teeth have commenced to erupt. Failure to erupt may result in impaction (Fig. 27.9)

Fig. 27.9 Impacted third molar (wisdom tooth).

Each tooth forms a firm joint with the jaw, being held in its socket in the alveolar bone by a fibrous ligament, the periodontal ligament, which is attached to the tooth root and to the bone.

ABSCESSES ARISING FROM THE TEETH

An abscess arising from a tooth may be the cause of infection at remote sites in the body. Infection arising from teeth may be of two types:

1. *Open sepsis.* Open sepsis occurs almost invariably from infection of

the gum margins and from decayed teeth and roots. It is commonly caused initially by the deposits of calculus (tartar) which irritate and inflame the gum margins. It is known as open sepsis because the infected material drains into the mouth. The pus forms in the pocket between the gum margin and the root of the tooth and drains into the mouth producing halitosis (bad breath). Infection may spread to the sinuses, tonsils and stomach. Open oral sepsis predisposes to chest infections after general anaesthesia.

2. *Closed sepsis*. Closed sepsis is considerably more important than the open type. Infection almost invariably commences as dental caries (decay) and if this is untreated it spreads and infects the pulp of the tooth, from which it is but a short step to the jaw and the venous blood stream, through which it is passed around the body. Such bacterial spread (bacteraemia) is dangerous in patients suffering from congenital or rheumatic heart disease because it can lead to bacterial endocarditis.

Dental abscess

1. *Acute.* An acute dental abscess (alveolar abscess) arises from an infected tooth. The onset is heralded by acute pain, increasing in severity. Swelling is not marked at this stage.

About the third day there is characteristically a sudden remission of the pain as the inflamed, congested tooth pulp dies. Soon the infected material escapes through the root end and produces inflammation of the periodontal ligament. This makes the tooth tender to touch and to bite on, and pain returns in the jaw. With the pus tracking through the periosteum into the soft tissues, a generalised swelling occurs. The patient feels unwell, looks ill and the temperature, which should not be taken in the mouth, is elevated.

Fig. 27.10 Apical abscess.

Treatment consists of extraction of the offending tooth. This will usually provide sufficient drainage, but in the presence of extensive facial swelling with pus, external drainage may be necessary in addition. Antibiotics will be used in severe cases. Nursing treatment, apart from vigorous hot mouth-washes, is on the general lines of an acute toxic condition.

2. *Chronic.* A chronic abscess may follow an acute abscess which has pointed in the mouth, leaving a sinus which has failed to heal. More commonly they are chronic from the beginning, caused by low grade infection from the dead pulp of a tooth over a prolonged period (Fig. 27.10).

Odontomes

Odontomes are cysts or tumours arising from the cells from which teeth are formed. Excision and removal of the epithelial elements is undertaken, together with malformed dental hard tissued—i.e. masses composed of enamel, dentine and cementum in differing proportions.

Dental caries

Dental caries is a very common disease in civilised peoples and its treatment is a matter for the dental surgeon. It is the progressive destruction of the enamel and dentine of a tooth by acids produced by oral bacteria. The bacteria (which are part of the normal flora of the mouth) convert carbohydrates such as sugar and starch to acid— e.g. lactic acid, which can slowly dissolve the hard tooth tissues. The dental plaque, a film lying on uncleaned teeth, is the site where bacteria act to produce the acid. It follows that in simple terms, caries can be controlled by (a) reduction of the amount of sugar in the diet, and particularly by cutting down the duration of time it is present in the mouth; (b) removal of the dental plaque by brushing between the teeth conscientiously; (c) making tooth structure more resistant to acid attack by applying fluoride gels to the teeth or, better still, incorporating fluoride in the developing tooth through the intake of fluoridated drinking water. The addition of minute quantities of fluorine (as sodium fluoride) to water supplies where this element is naturally lacking significantly reduces the incidence of dental caries.

A nurse should never advise a patient to have his teeth extracted, however bad they may appear—only to seek dental advice. Conservative treatment may well be possible.

Haemorrhage following the extraction of teeth

As we would expect, this may be primary, reactionary or secondary. Reactionary, or intermediate haemorrhage, occurring a few hours after extraction is by far the most common and is probably caused by excessive vigorous rinsing of the mouth or by licking the clot and dislodging it.

Treatment

The head is raised on pillows and the mouth cleaned and examined with a good light. A pressure pack is placed over the bleeding socket. A gauze swab soaked in hot water and wrung out is placed over the socket and the patient is instructed to bite on it. 'Surgicel' gauze may be packed into the socket before applying the pressure pack. If this fails, the gum will probably have to be sutured, usually after giving a local anaesthetic. Make sure the patient does not suffer from a constitutional bleeding disorder—e.g. purpura, haemophilia or is on anticoagulants. Morphia 15 mg may be useful to reduce apprehension and agitation.

FRACTURES OF THE JAW

Almost all fractures of the jaw are caused by violence—e.g. the car accident victim or the boxer. Pathological fractures occasionally occur as a complication of osteomyelitis or as a complication of a large dental cyst or neoplasm.

The immediate treatment is to ensure a free airway. The muscular control of the tongue, because of its dependence on an intact lower jaw, may be lost in a fracture and if the patient is laid flat on his back there is a considerable risk of the tongue falling back, causing asphyxia. This may be prevented by placing a suture through the tongue, by tongue forceps, or by nursing the patient lying on the face until either the mandible has been immobilised in a forward position or the patient's control of the tongue has returned.

All patients suffering from a fracture of the jaw are transported in the prone position.

Treatment of fractures of the mandible

The aims of treatment are reduction of the fracture, its immobilisation and the prevention of infection. It may be immobilised by:
1. Gunning splints (in the edentulous patient).
2. Eyelet wiring.
3. Cast metal splints.

The teeth are fixed together either by wires or metal cap/splints to ensure correct relationship upper to lower. If they occlude correctly then the bone, of necessity, must be in correct alignment. Maintaining the teeth in occlusion may be necessary for 5 to 6 weeks. The mouth is syringed with sodium bicarbonate 1.60 using a 20 ml plastic syringe, and as soon as possible, the patient is encouraged to clean his teeth with a small toothbrush and paste. Corsodyl mouth wash (containing 0.2 per cent chlorhexidine gluconate) 10 ml twice daily, is a useful antiseptic and cleansing agent which reduces dental plaque and helps good oral hygiene. Food, which has to be in liquid form, may be given by a catheter and plastic funnel, or by flexible straw. Meals should be small and given frequently.

Actinomycosis

This is an example of chronic infection due to a fungus which may occur in the jaw. Classically, an extensive brawny swelling develops and in the later stages multiple sinuses which discharge sulphur granules are present. An alternative form simulates an acute dental abscess, but healing is delayed. Infection usually arises following a dental extraction or any lesion involving a breach of the oral mucous membrane. The organisms are present in normal mouths, but can occasionally enter the tissues and produce a persistent infection.

Treatment consists of the administration of penicillin or tetracycline for 6 weeks. Surgery is confined to providing free drainage from the abscess.

TUMOURS OF THE JAW

Simple tumours

Simple tumours are usually osteomata. They are not very common. Simple tumours of the mouth such as fibromas are often seen, particularly if an irritant factor such as an ill-fitting denture is present.

Malignant tumours

These may be:

1. Sarcoma. A sarcoma may develop in the upper or lower jaw but is much less frequent than a carcinoma.

2. Carcinoma. A carcinomatous growth may arise in the lining of the maxillary antrum which extends in all directions—upwards towards the eye, inwards to block the nostril, downwards eroding the hard palate and forwards into the muscles and skin of the face. Carcinoma may arise in the oral epithelium, for example in the floor of the mouth or cheek, and spread to involve the jaw bones. When well established it presents as a large ulcerated lesion which is painful and bleeds easily.

Treatment

Radiotherapy and surgery are usually combined in the treatment, the affected half of the jaw being removed in the case of carcinoma arising from the maxillary antrum. The dental surgeon may make an appliance to repair the loss of tissue. However, there are now sophisticated surgical techniques available which effect very good repair of the defects created.

THE NECK

Wounds

Wounds in this area bleed freely, and deep wounds may open massive blood vessels, like the carotid artery or internal jugular vein. A further danger of a wound in this area is damage to the larynx or trachea with resulting respiratory obstruction. Tracheostomy may be necessary.

Swellings in the neck

Swellings in the neck are common. They are:

1. Lymphatic glandular swellings.
2. Goitre (Ch. 28).
3. Sebaceous cyst.
4. Thyroglossal cyst, which arises in the midline above the prominence of the thyroid cartilage. It arises on a vestigial tract running from the tongue to the thyroid. Excision is the usual treatment.
5. A branchial cyst, which arises high in the neck near the angle of the lower jaw. It is a developmental abnormality. Excision is usually performed and it may be quite an extensive operation.
6. Cystic hygroma is a condition of dilatation of the lymphatic vessels. It occurs in children and frequently becomes mildly infected. Infection sometimes results in recession. Excision is the usual treatment.
7. Ludwig's angina, which is a dangerous condition of cellulitis of the floor of the mouth. Rapid swelling appears even before pyrexia. Tracheostomy instruments should always be ready in case of respiratory obstruction. The patient should be kept very still as heart failure may cause sudden death.

28

The endocrine glands

Apart from the thyroid gland the majority of the endocrine glands are small in size and deeply situated in the body. Their vital role in all disease processes as well as in sustaining the patient during and after operations is well recognised although an enormous amount of research has still to be done to unravel their complex functions.

Excessive or diminished function of a gland usually gives rise to well recognised clinical manifestitations.

Investigations

Investigations are undertaken where appropriate in an attempt to:

1. Outline the gland anatomically and functionally by X-rays, including angiography and CT scanning and by radioisotope scanning

2. Measure the level of a hormone in the blood directly or by radio immuno-assay or bio-assay techniques.

3. Assess the target organ response where one hormone stimulates the secretion of another. The administration of adrenocorticotrophic hormone (ACTH) stimulates the normal adrenal cortex to secrete cortisone. Failure of secretion is indicative of adrenal insufficiency.

4. Detect the level of substances in the blood or urine which may be in excess or diminished as a result of hormonal dysfunction. The electrolytes, glucose, calcium and the 17 ketosteroids are examples.

Endocrinology is a rapidly expanding science and, as a result of many sophisticated tests, some of which are mentioned in outline above, disease can be diagnosed much earlier, in many cases when the patient has very few symptoms and no physical signs. This is particularly fortunate since the physical appearance of some of these patients is a cause of great distress to the patient and his relatives. In the more florid stages of some endocrine diseases the signs are not easy to conceal. We should treat these patients as human beings, which they are, and with the special sympathy which they deserve. Many of the conditions are controlable or curable and, as far as possible, this hope should be conveyed to the patient in our conversation and attitude. Patients with thyrotoxicosis may be irritable, moody and demanding while the patient with acromegaly is usually embarrassed.

THE PITUITARY

The pituitary gland, weighs about 0.6g and lies in the sella tursica (pituitary fossa) in the sphenoid bone. The roof of the fossa, formed on dense dura mater, is pierced by a stalk which connects the gland to the hypothalamus. The optic chiasma lies above the roof and upward extension of a growth of the gland may press on the nerve fibres causing defects in the visual field. There are two active lobes, an anterior and a posterior.

The secretions of the two lobes and their function are shown in Figure 28.1. The page cross references in the table after each hormone are to the pages in this book where their action is relevant to the topic under discussion in that place. Perhaps in a small measure this stresses the importance of a knowledge of their action in general surgical management where the gland itself is not the site of disease or dysfunction.

Hormone	Physiological action
From the Anterior Lobe	
1. Growth hormone (GH) (Somatotrophin)	Skeletal and connective tissue growth-antagonises the action of insulin.
2. Thyrotrophic hormone (TSH) (p.279)	Regulates secretion of thyroxine.
3. Adrenocorticotrophic hormone (ACTH) (p.293)	Controls adrenocortical activity and secretion of cortisol.
4. Gonadotrophic hormone	Essential in development of the sexual organs in both sexes.
(i) Follicle stimulating hormone (FSH) (p.618)	Stimulates ripening of the ovarian follicle in the female and spermatogenesis in the male
(ii) Luteinising hormone (LH) (p.618)	Maintains the corpus luteum which secretes progesterone. In the male stimulates testosterone.
5. Prolactin (p.297)	Stimulates milk production.
From the Posterior Lobe	
1. Pitressin (antidiuretic hormone)	Antidiuretic (the action on smooth muscle contraction is pharmological rather than physiological).
2. Oxytocin (p.297)	Contracts uterine muscle. Propulsive action on milk ducts in the breasts.

Fig. 28.1 The pituitary hormones and their action.

SURGERY OF THE PITUITARY GLAND

Pituitary dysfunction arises from oversecretion or undersecretion of one or more hormones. This may arise from tumour formation, vascular diseases, trauma, or be a sequal of an infective process. It also follows surgical removal or destruction of the gland by irradiation. The lesions in which surgical intervention may be advised are:

1. Chromophobe adenoma which, by pressure on the cells which secrete thyrotrophic and gonadotrophic hormones, produce widespread effects. The patient is over weight, sluggish and the metabolic rate is depressed. Amenorrhoea is usual. The tumours are radioresistant and surgery is undertaken.

2. Acidophil adenoma results in gigantism in the young or acromegaly (Fig. 28.2) in the adult, from excess of growth hormone. Radiotherapy to destroy the gland is the usual treatment. Alternatively surgical removal is undertaken.

Fig. 28.2 Acromegaly—note the coarse features.

Hypophysectomy (Removal of the pituitary)

Preparation

The patient is admitted a few days before operation and the urinary excretion of 17-ketosteroids estimated. The uptake of radioactive iodine is estimated for subsequent assessment of thyroid function.

Cortisone or prednisone is administered preoperatively as ordered by the doctor.

Pleural or ascitic collections are aspirated.

The usual preparation for craniotomy (Ch. 44) is undertaken for a transfrontal approach. An alternative approach either for excision or for the implant of yttrium-90 is transphenoidal. In some circumstances the pituitary gland can be destroyed by the transphenoidal injection of alcohol.

Postoperative care

The pituitary controls all the other ductless glands so that removal causes widespread effects and the postoperative care reflects some of the methods of dealing with this upset. Consciousness is quickly regained. Steroids are administered in the dose and by the route ordered by the doctor. If the blood pressure drops an intravenous dose of 100 mg of hydrocortisone may be required.

The wound heals uneventfully. 300 mg of DOCA may be implanted beneath the sheath of the rectus muscle in the abdominal wall before discharge from hospital.

Special dangers
1. Lassitude.
2. Anorexia.
3. Low blood pressure.
4. Danger of infection.
5. Electrolyte imbalance—salt depletion, retention of potassium and a rise in blood urea.

Salt capsules, 4 g daily, may be given if the blood pressure is low. If the blood pressure is raised salt is forbidden.

Occasional complications
1. Fits. The risk may be diminished by administering antiepileptic drugs.
2. Diabetes insipidus. 40 mg of post-pituitary snuff, once to three times daily, may be advised.
3. Hypothyroidism. Thyroxine may be given but it is to be avoided if possible on account of the danger of stimulating the neoplasm.

After hypophysectomy or adrenalectomy vomiting is a most important symptom and is usually due to lack of cortisone.

DISEASES OF THE THYROID GLAND

A goitre is an enlargement of the thyroid gland. The thyroid gland is an endocrine gland situated at the root of the neck in front of and at the sides of the trachea and oesophagus (Fig. 28.3). The diseases to which it is subject are unusual in that they do not conform to the pattern of those to which we are accustomed elsewhere.

The thyroid secretes three hormones:
Thyroxine
Tri-iodothyronine
Calcitonin.

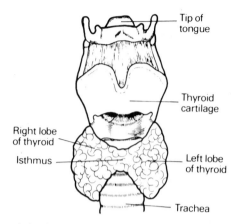

Fig. 28.3 The thyroid gland consists of two lobes joined in front of the trachea by an isthmus.

The first two hormones, of which thyroxine accounts for 90 per cent, are essential for normal growth in infancy and for the maintenance of a balanced metabolism in adult life. If iodine is deficient in the diet, or if the demands of the body for thyroxine are temporarily in excess of the gland's capacity to produce it, the gland substance may enlarge in a attempt to compensate. Later, the enlargement may subside evenly and smoothly, but frequently it is so large or retrogression so patchy that the patient is left with an irregular nodular goitre. The absence of the gland, or the failure to produce sufficient thyroxine, results in cretinism in infants (Fig. 28.4) and myxoedema in adults (Fig. 28.5). The whole tempo of the activities of the body is depressed in these conditions. On the other hand, an excessive amount of secretion results in the condition known as thyrotoxicosis, with the result that the whole pace of the patient's activities is accelerated.

Fig. 28.4 An untreated cretin in adult life.

Fig. 28.5 Myxoedema showing thin hair and dry skin.

A thyrotropic hormone (thyroid stimulating hormone) in the pituitary regulates the production of thyroxine which is manufactured in the secretory cells of the vesicles of the thyroid. Iodine is taken up from the blood and when the hormone is released into the blood stream it combines with the plasma proteins. This is known as the protein-bound iodine (PBI). An increase is a manifestation of excessive thyroid secretion and a diminution occurs in myxoedema but it is now more usual to estimate the level of thyroxine in the serum, the normal level being 3.0-7.5µg per 100 ml.

Secondarily, as a result of enlargement, symptoms due to pressure on the neighbouring organs may occur.

Calcitonin—a serum calcium-lowering hormone which inhibits bone destruction—is now known to be secreted in the thyroid, in addition to thyroxine.

Fig. 28.6   Simple nontoxic goitre.

Investigation of thyroid disease

(a) Thoracic inlet X-ray. This may demonstrate tracheal compression and displacement as well as a retrosternal goitre.

(b) Serum thyroxine (T_4) estimation.

(c) Serum tri-iodothyronine (T_3) estimation. Some cases of thyrotoxicosis are due to a raised (T_3) in the presence of a normal T_4.

(d) Thyroid stimulating hormone (TSH) estimation. This is raised in cases of hypothyroidism.

(e) Thyroid antibody measurement. Thyroid antibodies are present in the serum in significant concentration in cases of autoimmune thyroiditis as well as in some cases of thyrotoxicosis.

(f) Radioactive iodine uptake and scan.

Radioactive iodine is used in the diagnosis and treatment of thyroid gland diseases. This material disintegrates with the emission of energy in the form of gamma ray, which can be detected by Geiger counters. In diagnosis, a small (tracer) dose is given orally or intravenously and the amount in the thyroid and in the urine measured. A high thyroid uptake with low urinary excretion is indicative of hyperthyroidism, whilst a low thyroid uptake and high urinary excretion suggests hypothyroidism. The scan will demonstrate whether a goitre is diffusely enlarged or multi-nodular and whether all or only parts of the gland are over or under-active.

(g) Radioactive technetium scan. This is similar to a radioactive iodine scan but does not provide quantitative functional information. The anatomy of the gland can be demonstrated. Whether or not all or part of it is functional or non-functional can be seen.

(h) Ultrasound scan. This will demonstrate the size of thyroid enlargement as well as its consistency (i.e. solid or cystic).

SIMPLE ENLARGEMENTS OF THE THYROID

Simple or non-toxic enlargement of the thyroid is fairly common (Fig. 28.6). The gland usually enlarges in the neck, but occasionally the enlargement occurs behind the upper portion of the sternum (retrosternal goitre).

Causes

During periods of special stress, such as puberty, the calls for thyroxine are greater, and a diffuse enlargement of the gland may occur. It is physiological in origin, and the colloid goitre of puberty requires no special surgical intervention.

Since iodinised salt has been used, endemic goitres with a definite geographical distribution have almost disappeared.

The simple enlargement may subside if not excessive, or subsidence may occur in one portion of the gland and not in another. This process results in the production of nodules in the gland. They may be single or multiple (multinodular goitre).

Symptoms and signs

The most obvious and frequently the only complaint is the goitre itself. A goitre always moves on swallowing because it is attached to the larynx. Surgical interference is indicated if the patient complains of:
1. Pressure symptoms which may be:
    (a) Dysphagia (difficulty in swallowing).
    (b) Dyspnoea (difficulty in breathing—the trachea, which is normally C shaped and thinner posteriorly because there is no cartilage, is so compressed on both sides that it may be 'scabbard' in shape).

(c) Hoarseness due to pressure on the recurrent laryngeal nerves.
2. Cosmetic disfigurement.
3. Symptoms suggestive of toxic or malignant change.
4. The goitre is retrosternal.

Investigations

1. Serum thyroxine to confirm that thyroid function is normal.
2. X-rays of chest and thoracic inlet to determine the degree (if any) of the deformity of the trachea resulting from pressure.
3. Radioactive isotope scan may be necessary to determine the anatomy and position of the goitre (e.g. whether one nodule or multinodular, whether retrosternal or not).

Treatment

Surgical operation consists of partial thyroidectomy. The after-care is similar to that of toxic goitre, but antithyroid drugs are unnecessary.

Complications of a simple goitre

1. The onset of toxic symptoms.
2. The occurrence of haemorrhage into an adenoma with the sudden onset of severe dyspnoea. This may require emergency thyroidectomy.
3. Malignancy.

THYROTOXICOSIS

Toxic goitre is a condition in which the secretion of thyroxine is excessive in quantity. The disease is more common in women.

The disease may commence in a gland which was previously normal, or it may develop in a thyroid already subject to simple enlargement. The former is described as primary thyrotoxicosis or Graves' disease and the latter as secondary thyrotoxicosis. The main distinction is that the patient is usually older in the secondary type and the heart muscle is less fit to withstand being driven so much faster. The other clinical distinction is that the eye signs, particularly exophthalmos, are nearly always present in Graves' disease.

Symptoms and signs

The onset of toxic symptoms may follow a severe mental shock or anxiety. The thyroid gland may be very large, or there may be almost no enlargement at all. There is often a systolic bruit to be heard with a stethoscope over the gland. This is due to the increased vascularity. The severity of the symptoms bears no relationship to the size of the goitre. The symptoms are those of an accelerated metabolism. The body is being driven faster than normal.

Fig. 28.7 Thyrotoxicosis.

General symptoms and signs

1. The skin is moist and hyperaemic. Sweating may be profuse, and cold weather is preferred to a warm sunny day.

2. The eyes are protruding (exophthalmos), staring, and have a frightened look. This is common in Graves' disease (Fig. 28.7) but unusual in secondary thyrotoxicosis in the older patient.

3. Loss of weight is marked but the appetite is good.

4. A fine tremor of the fingers is present.

5. Mentally, the patient is hyperexcitable, nervous, and difficult to get on with. Frequently the patient with a toxic goitre will insist on leaving hospital in the midst of treatment.

6. Diarrhoea and vomiting may be present, and are due to overactivity of the intestinal tract.

7. Menstrual disturbances may occur, particularly amenorrhoea.

Cardiovascular symptoms

The heart rate is always increased and palpitations are a common complaint. The systolic blood pressure is raised and the diastolic pressure lowered, with the result that the pulse pressure is increased and the pulse is full and bounding.

Later, irregularity of the heart beat may occur usually in the form of atrial fibrillation. Unrelieved, the patient dies of cardiac failure, which is usually associated with acute mania.

Investigations

1. Serum thyroxine—this is raised.

2. Radioactive-iodine uptake studies and scan may be necessary to reveal thyroid over-activity in atypical cases.

3. X-rays of thoracic inlet to detect any pressure deformity of the trachea.

4. Indirect laryngoscopy—to inspect movement of vocal cords and detect any paralysis (due to pressure on recurrent laryngeal nerve).

Treatment

There are three forms of treatment available.

1. *Anti-thyroid drugs.* They interfere with the production of thyroxine by the gland. Carbimazole is the commonly used drug, starting with a dose of 10 to 20 mg t.d.s. When the patient's weight is rising and signs of toxicity are gone the dose is reduced to a maintenance level. Agranulocytosis is a rare complication of these drugs but must always be considered as a possibility. The white blood count should be checked regularly. The disadvantage of all anti-thyroid drugs is that they often lead to an increase in the size of the gland.

This treatment is used in: (a) patients with mild disease, (b) those with minimal goitre, (c) children and young adults, (d) sometimes in pregnancy, (e) in patients being prepared for surgery. If used as definitive treatment the drugs should be continued for up to one year and then stopped. One third of the patients will remain well while, of the rest, some will become toxic almost immediately and others will develop recurrent thyrotoxicosis in the future.

2. *Radioactive iodine therapy.* Radioactive iodine is given as a drink. It is taken up by the thyroid gland, which is destroyed by the effect of the local irradiation.

It is indicated for:

(a) Patients with a minimal or small goitre.

(b) Recurrent thyrotoxicosis (after surgery) where a second operation carries a much higher risk of damage to the recurrent laryngeal nerves.

(c) In patients with concurrent medical disease which precludes safe operative intervention.

It is contra-indicated in:

(a) Patients under 40 years of age for fear of causing carcinomatous change in the thyroid. Many people now consider this risk to be minimal and treat patients of a younger age.

(b) Pregnancy.

With the passage of time an increasing number of patients following this therapy develop hypothyroidism, requiring hormone replacement therapy.

3. *Sub-total thyroidectomy.* The majority of the gland is removed, leaving about 5 g on each side.

It is indicated for:

(a) Severe cases not easily controlled by drugs.

(b) Patients with moderate or large goitre.

(c) Recurrent thyrotoxicosis following drug treatment.

(d) Patients unsuitable for radioactive iodine therapy.

(e) Patients unwilling to take or intolerant of drugs.

(f) Sometimes in pregnancy.

A small number of patients following surgery develop recurrent thyrotoxicosis. A larger number, with the passage of time, develop hypothyroidism.

THE GENERAL AND NURSING CARE OF A PATIENT FOR THYROIDECTOMY FOR THYROTOXICOSIS

All patients require a period of medical treatment before operation can be undertaken.

The operation is performed when the patient is in a euthyroid state, that is a condition of normal thyroid function. The patient is now feeling better, less excitable (the heart rate is about 80 per minute) and gaining weight. This is confirmed by the serum thyroxine reading returning to normal.

Preoperative preparation

Drugs which are used in the preoperative stage are:

(a) Carbimazole is given for several weeks before admission but its administration is stopped 10 days before the operation. Some surgeons continue antithyroid drugs up to the day of the operation.

(b) Propanolol (120–160 mg daily in divided doses) may be used as the only preoperative preparation for thyroidectomy or in combination with carbimazole. It is a beta-blocking drug which inhibits the peripheral action of thyroxine. As it acts on the heart and target organs the serum thyroxine is not lowered. Therefore it must be continued on the day of operation and for the subsequent 5 days because there may be a high level of thyroxine in the circulation.

(c) Lugol's iodine (0.3 to 0.9 ml t.d.s.) in milk may be given for the 10 days before operation as it is thought to reduce the vascularity of the gland. Some surgeons omit it.

(d) Diazepam 5 mg b.d. quietens the patient and ensures sound sleep.

(e) Digitalis may be given if atrial fibrillation is present. This is given in the form of digoxin (0.25 mg) sufficiently frequently to control the fibrillation.

The above preparation can be done as an outpatient. The patient should be admitted 2 or 3 days preoperatively for rest and to confirm the euthyroid state.

Observations:

(a) The sleeping pulse rate is the most important guide of progress.

(b) The *heart rate* must be counted if the patient is fibrillating (Fig. 28.8).

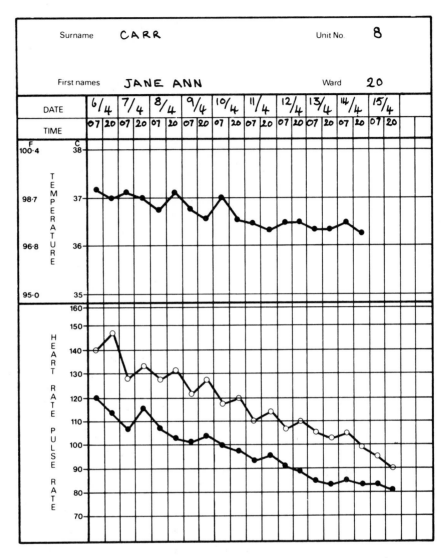

Fig. 28.8 The pulse and heart rate must be recorded in artrial fibrillation (o—o = heart rate, ●—● = pulse rate).

Immediate preoperative care

(a) Check haemoglobin.

(b) Cross-match 2 units of blood.

(c) X-ray chest and thoracic inlet.

(d) Indirect laryngoscopy (by ENT surgeon) to check movement of vocal cords.

(e) The skin of the neck, the upper half of the chest, the axillae and the upper arms are shaved and washed with 2 per cent hexachlorophane soap.

(f) The hair should be fixed away from the ears and neck with a suitable cap.

The operation

Up to nine-tenths of the gland is removed at operation which is usually performed under general anaesthesia. The wound is closed and drained, either with a tube brought out through a separate stab incision or with a corrugated or similar drain through the lateral ends of the wound.

Fig. 28.9 Position for thyroid operation. Note shoulder support.

The postoperative care

Position in bed

If a general anaesthetic has been administered, the patient is laid in the lateral position until recovery takes place and is then propped up as soon as possible supported by a back rest. This relieves venous congestion. In all movements the head is supported and extension of the neck is avoided.

Treatment immediately on return from the theatre

(a) The respirations are frequently shallow and slow. A careful watch is necessary, and oxygen administered if required.

Difficulty with breathing may be caused by haemorrhage. An excess of blood in the drainage bottle, on the dressings, or swelling of the neck should be reported at once. Respiratory obstruction may develop some hours postoperatively due to oedema in the subglottic area of the larynx, i.e. just below the vocal cords and intubation may be necessary to avoid brain damage from hypoxia. Respiratory difficulty may also arise if there has been damage to the recurrent laryngeal nerves. Any respiratory difficulty must be reported immediately.

(b) The patient should swallow a little fluid as soon as possible, as it serves to clean the mouth. She should speak only in a whisper so as to decrease the pain in the neck.

(c) The bedclothing should not be too heavy. Frequent cold sponging is important if the patient is sweating. A room which is too warm must be cooled by a fan.

During the night

(a) *Haemorrhage*. A careful watch must be kept for excessive bleeding. It is important to remember that the site to look for haemorrhage is at the back of the dressing or on the pillow, if an open drain has been used.

(b) *Drugs* to encourage sleep are prescribed and given before the patient is too lively.

Care of the drain and sutures

The drain in usually removed at 24 hours after the operation unless there is excessive drainage. The stitches should be removed on the third or fourth day. If clips or staples have been used, alternate ones should be removed on the second day and the remainder on the third day. Thereafter plastic, spray is all that is necessary. If serum collects in the wound aspiration may be necessary.

Complications and their treatment

Haemorrhage. Some bleeding is usual, but excessive haemorrhage must be notified at once. Severe haemorrhage will cause bulging of the wound and severe dyspnoea due to formation of a haematoma. Reopening of the wound may be necessary.

Thyroid crisis. In the immediate postoperative period the patient may become acutely toxic with a rapid pulse, raised temperature, profuse sweats and confusion. This is due to the sudden release of a large amount of hormone into the blood as a result of surgical manipulation. With good preoperative preparation this is a rare occurrence. Any suggestion that such a problem may be arising must be reported immediately. The treatment is with propranolol, sedation and tepid sponging.

Tetany. Removal or trauma to the parathyroid glands may result in tetany. The patient complains of a tingling and numbness of the face, lips and hands, and twitching of the muscles. Most cases subside spontaneously, but calcium gluconate usually gives rapid relief. The blood calcium is estimated. More remotely a high dosage of vitamin D and oral calcium supplements are used.

Apart from tetany, it is advisable to estimate the blood calcium three months after thyroidectomy. It has been shown that latent parathyroid deficiency may give rise to such distressing conditions as bilateral cataracts.

Respiratory complications. Soreness of the throat and neck are almost invariable complaints, and are soothed by giving the patient blackcurrant pastilles to suck. Chest infections are unusual.

Hoarseness is usually due to the trauma of the operation, and clears up rapidly. Occasionally it is caused by damage to the recurrent laryngeal nerve. This will be diagnosed by indirect laryngoscopy when one or both vocal cords are seen not to be moving. In cases where both nerves have been damaged, the paralysed vocal cords lie almost in apposition so that the space between them is negligible. The result is that the patient has acute respiratory distress and tracheostomy must be performed without delay. The vocal cords should be inspected in all patients postoperatively before discharge from hospital.

Hypothyroidism may occur as a remote complication in about 10 per cent of patients. They should thus be followed up regularly. It is common in the early postoperative period (often up to 6 months) for the serum thyroxine to be low but this frequently returns to normal as the gland remnant functions more satisfactorily.

Recurrent thyrotoxicosis.

Instructions to the patient on leaving hospital

Two or 3 months are necessary to gain the full benefit from the operation. Weight increases and, 3 months later, most patients are fit to lead a normal life. The patient can be reassured that a necklace will adequately conceal the scar and that the latter will fade over 12 months. Some lanolin rubbed into the scar will make it more supple. Many patients now feel the cold and must wear warmer clothing.

At a follow-up 1 and 3 months later the serum calcium and thyroxine are estimated. Laryngoscopic examination is undertaken if there has been any problem with the vocal cords. An assessment is made to detect early hypothyroidism or recurrent thyrotoxicosis.

NEW GROWTHS OF THE THYROID

Benign new growths

An adenoma is the commonest new growth. It presents as a solitary lump in the thyroid gland. A radioisotope scan is done to confirm that it is a solitary lump and not one nodule in a multinodular goitre. Some may undergo cystic change. The treatment is excision, removing the majority of the lobe of the thyroid in which the lump is situated. About 10 per cent of such lumps turn out histologically to be malignant.

Malignant new growths

There are three main histological types of malignant new growth which occur in the thyroid gland.

(a) Papillary—
predominantly younger age group (20–30 years)
female more than male
slow growing
spreads to cervical lymph nodes

(b) Follicular—
predominantly younger age group (20–30 years)
female more than male
slow growing
spreads via blood stream to bones
may take up radioactive iodine

(c) Anaplastic—
predominantly older age group (50–60 years)
often rapidly progressive
local pressure symptoms common

spreads by local invasion, to local lymph nodes
and via blood stream
may invade recurrent laryngeal nerve causing vocal
cord paralysis

The treatment of papillary and follicular tumours is by total thyroidectomy, preserving the parathyroid glands and recurrent laryngeal nerves.
Involved cervical glands are removed. If the follicular tumour takes up
radioactive iodine this is used to treat any bone metastases. The patients
are given thyroxine, not only as replacement therapy but also to suppress
pituitary secretion of TSH, thus avoiding stimulation of any remaining
thyroid tissue.

The treatment of anaplastic tumours is more difficult and much less
satisfactory. The gland is often irremovable because of local invasion of
surrounding tissues. Treatment consists of a combination of partial or
total thyroidectomy, radiotherapy, thyroxine and local palliative procedures. The prognosis is poor.

INFLAMMATIONS

A rare but interesting type of chronic inflammation of the thyroid gland is
Hashimoto's thyroiditis which is thought to be an auto-immune disease.
In this condition the body reacts to some of its constituent proteins which
escape from the thryoid gland. It may resemble carcinoma. It is diagnosed on a high thyroid antibody titre in the blood and histological
biopsy.

An acute thyroiditis, thought to be of viral origin, occasionally occurs.
It is self-limiting and called de Quervain's thyroiditis.

A diffuse iron hardness of the gland sometimes occurs and is known as
Riedel's thyroiditis. Its main importance lies in its tendency to resemble
carcinoma.

THE PARATHYROID GLANDS

The parathyroids are two pairs of tiny glands situated behind the
posterior border of the thyroid gland (Fig. 28.10). The upper parathyroids
are fairly constant in position but the lower two are much more variable
in position and may even be situated in the mediastinum. The secretion,
parathormone, acts by:
1. Mobilising calcium and phosphate from bone;
2. Increasing calcium absorption from the gut;
3. Increasing the reabsorption of calcium from the renal tubules.

HYPERPARATHYROIDISM

Excessive secretion of parathormone may be due to an adenoma or
hyperplasia and may present as:

1. *Bone disease* varying from decalcification to cystic formation (osteitis fibrosa cystica). This may present as bone pain.
2. *Urinary stone* formation. All patients with urinary stones are investigated for overactivity of the parathyroids. About 5 per cent of such patients will be found to have hyperparathyroidism.

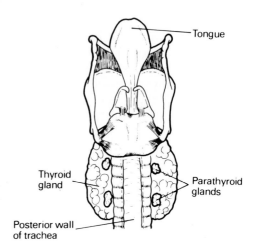

Fig. 28.10 The four parathyroid glands are situated on the posterior border of the thyroid. Also illustrates that the posterior wall of the trachea is weak because it has no cartilage.

3. *Dyspeptic symptoms.*
4. *Mental agitation.*
5. *Incidental hypercalcaemia.* This may be noted on a routine blood test for some other condition.

Investigations

These include:
1. Estimation of the
  (a) fasting serum calcium level (normal 2.25-2.62 mmol/l).
  (b) serum phosphate level. Calcium and phosphate levels are inter-related.
  (c) serum proteins. Calcium is bound to albumin in the blood.
  (d) serum alkaline phosphatase.
  (e) calcium and phosphate excretion in the urine over 24 hours.
  (f) detailed calcium balance studies in a metabolic unit.
  (g) serum parathormone level.
2. Radiography of the skeleton and urinary tract.
3. Localisation of adenoma by
  (a) selective angiography via thyroid arteries.
  (b) radioisotope scanning techniques.
  (c) selective venous sampling techniques to measure parathormone level in venous blood draining from each side of the neck.

Treatment

An adenoma is removed. In hyperplasia three whole parathyroid glands and one half of the remaining one are removed. The operative approach is the same as for a thyroidectomy. A parathyroid is a minute gland and even a tumour is tiny in size and soft in consistency. Not only is a parathyroid not palpable clinically, it is rarely palpable at operation. To add to the surgeon's difficulties the lower glands are variable in position and may be situated in the mediastinum so that exploration of the chest may be necessary to find the tumour. Even in the most experienced hands there is sometimes failure to find the tumour. The possibility should be discussed with the patient before he consents to the operation.

The nursing care is similar to that of a patient undergoing thyroidectomy, in the care of the wound and general management.

Special observations

The sudden withdrawal of excess parathormone from the blood in the immediate postoperative period may result in hypocalcaemia and tetany. The serum calcium level is monitored at frequent intervals, 4 hours after operation and twice daily thereafter, but the nurse should be specially alert to note any symptoms suggestive of tetany and test clinically for the classical signs discussed below. Intravenous calcium gluconate may be prescribed. When the condition is stabilised the patient is given a high calcium diet or calcium supplements as ordered by the surgeon after further studies of the patient's calcium metabolism.

HYPOPARATHYROIDISM

Lack of sufficient parathormone causes a fall in the serum calcium with great irritability of the nerves. This is manifested by spasm and twitching of the muscles and is known as tetany. It may be caused by conditions other than lack of parathormone, such as excessive vomiting or hyperventilation (usually of hysterical origin) which cause a lowering of ionised serum calcium.

The common surgical cause is removal or damage to the parathyroid glands. The clinical features are:

1. Paraesthesia. The commonest site is around the side of the neck, the mouth, the fingers and toes.

2. Muscle twitching which may affect all muscles but particularly those of the forearm and hand as well as those of the leg and foot (carpopedal spasm). Two signs may be elicited by the nurse:

(a) *Chvostek's sign*—tapping over the skin just above the angle of the jaw will stimulate the branches of the facial nerve to produce twitching of the eyelids and the angle of the mouth.

(b) A sphygmomanometer cuff applied to the arm and inflated above the systolic pressure for not more than 2 minutes will cause carpal spasm.

In most severe cases the respiratory muscles are involved with stridor and fear of suffocation. Generalised twitching may be mistaken for epilepsy but there is no loss of consciousness. *Investigations* of parathyroid function are undertaken. *Treatment* is as outlined for tetany complicating thyroidectomy as well as treatment of the cause.

THE ADRENAL GLAND

The adrenal glands are two flat, canary yellow, structures lying above the upper pole of each kidney (Fig. 28.11). Each gland consists of a cortical and a medullary portion which, although anatomically joined, are physiologically separate. Blood containing the secreted hormones drains into the adrenal veins—the right draining directly into the inferior vena cava, the left into the left renal vein which, in turn, joins the inferior vena cava.

Disease of the adrenal glands may cause over or under activity of the cortex or of the medulla. Under activity from disease or surgical excision for therapeutic reasons will require replacement therapy.

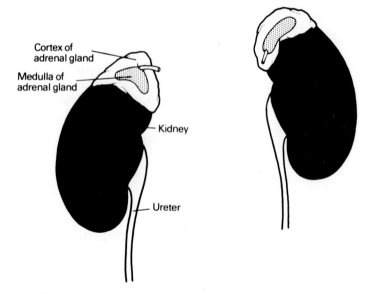

Cortex of
adrenal gland

Medulla of
adrenal gland

Kidney

Ureter

Fig. 28.11 The adrenal glands.

THE CORTICAL HORMONES

These are very numerous, at least 50 have been discovered. The principal groups are:

1. The mineralocorticoids which regulate water and electrolyte balance, the most important being aldosterone which conserves sodium in the body.

2. The glucocorticoids which convert body protein to carbohydrate. In addition hydrocortisone (which is converted in the body from cortisone) enables the body to respond to stress, inhibits the action of insulin and is important in maintaining blood pressure. In excess it inhibits the inflammatory reaction and also the rejection reaction in tissue transplantation.

3. The sex hormones. Androgens and oestrogens are secreted. ACTH stimulates the adrenal cortex to secrete glucocorticoids and the sex hormones. Excess of hydrocortisone in the blood inhibits the secretion of ACTH. The secretion of the mineralocorticoids is independent of the pituitary.

THE MEDULLARY HORMONES

These are:
  1. Noradrenalin
  2. Adrenalin
  Both hormones stimulate the sympathetic nervous system including the blood vessels causing vasoconstriction. Noradrenalin which is shorter acting than adrenalin accounts for 20 per cent of the secretion but in phaeochromocytoma the proportion is reversed.

HYPOCORTICISM

Acute adrenal failure is most commonly a sequence of bilateral adrenalectomy where the patient has failed to take the prescribed amount of cortisone or has been vomiting. Sudden and unexpected postoperative collapse due to an adrenal haemorrhage is a rare occurrence.

The clinical picture is one of muscular weakness, severe shock, hypotension and vomiting. The immediate administration of hydrocortisone intraveneously is essential.

Chronic adrenal insufficiency (Addison's disease) is caused by tuberculous infection of the adrenal or atrophy of the tissues of the gland. Muscular weakness, a persistent low blood pressure and skin pigmentation occur. Replacement therapy and antituberculous drugs are indicated if necessary.

HYPERCORTISM

Hypercortism is due to a tumour or hyperplasia of the cortex. The clinical features are similar to those resulting from the administration of excessive doses of cortisone or excessive secretion of ACTH and is known as Cushing's syndrome (Fig. 28.12). The moon shaped face, obesity from water and salt retention, hypertension, muscular wasting and hirsutes are all characteristics. The treatment is removal of the tumour if present or, in cases of hyperplasia, subtotal adrenalectomy.

Rare tumours occur in the adrenal cortex which secrete aldosterone or sex hormones. They give rise to specific syndromes and require treatment by surgical removal.

Fig. 28.12 Cushing's syndrome in the adult, showing buffalo hump (side view), acne, hirsutes, plethoric appearance.

MEDULLARY OVER-ACTIVITY

This is almost always due to a tumour—a **phaeochromocytoma**. The symptoms and signs are those of excessive secretion of adrenalin and noradrenalin. They arise from hypertension and are headache, palpitation, dyspnoea and weakness. The treatment is excision but special care is necessary to neutralise the effects of increased adrenalin secretion before and during the operation as well as to counter hypotension postoperatively. The nursing care and postoperative checks are similar to that described below for adrenalectomy with the following additional precautions, the details of which will be prescribed by the surgeon. Preoperatively phentolamine is administered by mouth for some days to suppress the secretion and immediately preoperatively it is given intravenously. During the operation it is given when the gland is handled by the surgeon as this results in flooding the circulation with adrenalines. Following excision, dangerous hypotension may occur and noradrenalin should always be available to counteract the fall in blood pressure. These patients should be handled with the greatest gentleness, particularly when being positioned on the operating table since any pressure on the loin or abdomen is liable to cause a further increase in adrenalin secretion.

ADRENALECTOMY

Bilateral removal of the adrenals may be indicated in disseminated carcinoma of the breast or prostate when it is beyond other methods of control. Other indications for bilateral removal of the adrenals are selected cases of Cushing's syndrome.

Preoperative management

Patients selected for adrenalectomy for disseminated carcinoma of the breast are always at an advanced stage of the disease. The extent of the malignancy must be mapped out carefully. A low haemoglobin must be corrected by transfusions. Hydrocortisone is given by intramuscular injection of 100 mg one hour before operation. Both adrenal glands are usually excised at one operation but if it is decided to remove one at a time the opposite one is removed 10 days later. Because of danger of delay in healing and trauma on the table to a healing wound, the stitches from the first wound are not removed until the second operation has been completed. Pethidine, 50 to 100 mg, is preferable to morphia because of the danger of liver damage from secondary deposits.

The striking benefit of adrenalectomy is immediate relief of pain in most cases of secondary deposits in bone. After 18 months to 2 years most patients relapse.

Postoperative care

Following operation hydrocortisone is given in 100 mg doses, intramuscularly 6-hourly, for one day. Close observation of the blood pressure is essential, and if the patient becomes hypotensive the dosage and/or frequency of hydrocortisone must be increased. This is reduced to two doses of 100 mg on the next day after operation and continued orally as cortisone acetate in 25 mg doses 6-hourly for 2 days. On the fourth day cortisone is reduced to 75 mg and from the sixth day most patients are maintained on a dose of 50 mg a day. It is explained to the patient that the adrenal glands, which produce a substance called cortisone, essential to life, have been removed. Cortisone must be taken in tablet form for the rest of the patient's life. The patient should take a normal diet with plenty of salt. A few patients require in addition fludrocortisone (a mineralocorticoid) 0.1 mg daily. If she is not feeling well or gets tired, she should return at once. If she vomits, cortisone can be given by injection. If she goes abroad, she must make sure that she can get a maintenance dose of cortisone or she will die. It is essential that patients should carry 'steroid cards' to indicate that they are on maintenance cortisone therapy.

When adrenalectomy is performed for carcinoma of the breast the ovaries are also removed so that no oestrin-producing tissue remains in the body. The patient who has had only one adrenal removed requires replacement therapy—the other adrenal may be functionless from secondary deposits.

THE SURGICAL SIGNIFICANCE OF CORTICOSTEROIDS

Patients who have been on corticosteroids for any length of time usually have a medically induced adrenal insufficiency due to the suppressive action of the administered steroids on the pituitary gland.

The dose of cortisone should be increased before, during and immediately after operation to cover the increased demands made by anaesthesia and surgical intervention. Failure to observe this principle may lead to death of the patient from acute adrenal insufficiency.

Corticosteroids may be used as:

1. Replacement therapy, e.g. Addison's disease, hypopituitarism, and after bilateral adrenalectomy.
2. Therapeutically. Apart from adrenal insufficiency, cortisone is widely used in the group of diseases known as the collagenoses: notably rheumatoid arthritis, scleroderma, polyarteritis nodosa, and lupus erythematosus. In addition it may be used in such diseases as iritis, thrombocytopenic purpura, and status asthmaticus.

Corticosteroids given in a dose beyond what is normally required for the maintenance of life cause the body to: (1) retain sodium salts, (2) excrete potassium salts. If more than 50 mg is used potassium chloride (3 g daily) should be given to make good the increased excretion of potassium salts. In addition a low salt diet is necessary. The patient who has undergone bilateral adrenalectomy, on the other hand, should take a normal salt diet because her replacement dosage of cortisone is equal to the normal secretion of the hormone.

Many patients receiving corticosteroid therapy may come for urgent surgical intervention and the dosage of steroids has to be increased before and after operation.

There are many complications of cortisone which may be of surgical importance. The commonest are:

1. Reactivation of a latent pulmonary tuberculous focus.
2. Bleeding from a peptic ulcer.
3. Development of silent fulminating infections, for example, appendicitis.
4. Rapid development of cardiac failure.
5. Oedema including 'moon'-shaped face usually due to overdosage.

Other complications include thrombosis, osteoporosis, psychosis, and skin reactions such as acne and mild hirsutism.

BIBLIOGRAPHY

Wade J S H 1978 British Journal of Hospital Medicine 20: 456.

29

Diseases of the breast

ANATOMY AND PHYSIOLOGY

The protuberant portion of the breast lies on the anterior chest wall but breast tissue extends towards the midline, to the lateral chest wall and towards the axilla (the axillary tail). The alveoli which produce milk ultimately empty by lactiferous ducts whose orifices are situated in the apex of the nipple. The areola which surrounds the nipple contains sweat glands, sebaceous glands and accessory mammary glands. The lymphatic drainage of the breast is mainly to glands situated in the axilla but it is also along the internal mammary artery, which runs down behind the costal cartilages in the anterior mediastinum to the internal mammary nodes, and to the supraclavicular nodes.

The breast has a rich blood supply and this increases in pregnancy. After delivery the anterior pituitary releases the hormone prolactin which stimulates the alveoli of the breast to produce milk. The sucking stimulus of the child initiates the release from the posterior pituitary of oxytocin which causes contraction of the alveoli and results in the flow of milk along the ducts.

The breast differs from other exocrine glands in experiencing full physiological activity only periodically during reproductive life, i.e. when lactation is established.

SYMPTOMS OF BREAST DISEASE

Breast disease usually presents itself in three ways:

1. A palpable lump is frequently the only complaint. The general physical upset is slight but the mental anguish may be overwhelming.

When a patient confides to a nurse that she has discovered a lump in her breast the only advice she can be given is to consult her doctor without delay. The nurse can add the small consolation that four out of five lumps felt by patients are simple and non-malignant.

2. Discomfort within the breast. This may be cyclical, occurring with menstruation, or continuous.

3. A discharge from the nipple. This may be bloodstained as in the case of a duct papilloma or carcinoma, milky following lactation, or a clear brown or greenish fluid in the case of fibroadenosis. A discharge from the nipple should be tested for the presence of haemoglobin.

BENIGN CONDITIONS OF THE BREAST

CONGENITAL ABNORMALITIES

These are uncommon apart from retraction of the nipple. One occasionally encounters an accessory nipple situated in the same longitudinal plane as the normal nipple and even more rarely an accessory breast.

INFECTION OF THE BREAST—ACUTE MASTITIS

This is not uncommon during lactation, when cracks or fissures are likely to develop in the nipple and areolar regions. Acute lactational mastitis also develops in an area of milk engorgement due to a blocked lactiferous duct. A breast engorged with milk is an excellent medium for the proliferation of organisms, usually *Staphloccocus pyogenes*.

Symptoms and signs

The affected portion of the breast is painful, tender, warm and indurated. The patient feels ill and the general signs of inflammation may be present. As pus develops, throbbing pain occurs and the patient is pale and tired from lack of rest and toxic absorption.

Treatment and nursing care

Prevention

Breast abscess is best prevented by careful preparation of the nipple in the last 2 months of pregnancy and the institution of scrupulous hygiene during lactation. The nipples should be massaged with a good toilet soap and water. Rolling the nipples between fingers may get them accustomed to the friction of sucking. Any suitable ointment may be applied twice weekly but is not really necessary.

Treatment of established infection

1. In the early stages the administration of flucloxacillin may control the inflammatory reaction. The infant should be weaned from the affected breast, which should be elevated and supported. A sedative is usually prescribed to promote sleep. The infant, of course, is fed at the other breast. The practice of manual expression of milk from the breast if excessive milk production occurs whilst breast feeding avoids galactocele formation.

2. Drainage is necessary as soon as pus forms. An incision is made, under general anaesthetic, to release the pus and a drain is usually inserted. Pus is sent for culture. At this stage weaning is inevitable from both breasts.

Lactation is best suppressed by a tight binder. The nurse must show that she understands that the engorged breast will be initially uncomfortable and that an occasional sedative may be required. Without the stimulation of suckling the high prolactin concentrations in the blood fall to normal and lactation ceases within a week. Fluid restriction is unnecessary, causes further discomfort and has little effect on milk secretion. Oestrogens so long used for suppression have been abandoned because of the risk of thrombo-embolism. In the occasional patient in whom stronger measures are necessary bromcriptine may be prescribed. To overcome the occasional nausea which it may cause it is advisable that it be taken with meals.

Antibioma

Occasionally an acute mastitis treated with antibiotics forms an encysted abscess, the pus is buried beneath a thick firm wall and a month later the patient is worried because she has a large lump in her breast. Simple incision and drainage are all that is necessary.

Drugs and breast feeding. Whether a drug prescribed for the mother will conflict with breast feeding is not a question that can be answered reliably and what information there is is often conflicting. In general prescribing is avoided and, if not, advice from the nearest drug information centre may be sought.

FIBROADENOSIS

The breasts enlarge and develop their adult characteristics at puberty, due to hormonal influences generated in the pituitary, the ovary, and possibly in the thyroid gland. During each menstrual cycle, some slight enlargement of the breasts occurs, to be followed by retrogression until the next cycle. Normally this periodic enlargement and retrogression occurs evenly throughout the whole of both breasts. Occasionally, however, due either to the excessive enlargement of one segment or the failure of another to subside evenly, irregularity may occur in the breast substance, with the result that the patient complains of a lump, which is usually painful in the days immediately before menstruation. These lumps, or masses, are known as fibroadenosis. They may be:

1. Generalised. The whole of one or both breasts may be hard and irregular. There may be a discharge of clear or greenish coloured fluid from the nipple.

2. Segmental. May be limited to one segment or a quadrant of one or both breasts.

Fibroadenosis has three histological features. There is increase in the glandular tissue (adenosis), interstitial fibrosis increases (fibrosis) and cysts may form. One or other of these features may be predominant in an area of fibroadenosis.

Treatment

If the lump is thought to be a cyst, aspiration is undertaken in outpatients. Fluid aspirated is sent for cytological examination. If the lump disappears on aspiration the patient is reassured and re-examined in a few weeks. If the lump aspirated does not completely disappear or reappears it must be excised.

If the mass is localised and not cystic it is usually excised and examined under the microscope so that the diagnosis can be confirmed with certainty. Nothing reassures the patient more. The cavity in the breast is almost obliterated with stitches, but a small drain may be brought out through a separate stab incision. The main wound in the skin is closed. The drain is removed in 24 to 48 hours. To prevent separation of the wound and consequent broadening of the skin scar the sides of the incision must be supported by gauze and strapping or elastoplast drawn up from the sides so that the wound is not flattened (Fig. 29.1). The stitches are removed in 7 days. Many benign breast lumps can be removed under general anaesthetic as day cases without the need for drainage.

Fig. 29.1 Diagrammatic cross-section of wound (incision) showing correct method of applying strapping over gauze to pull edges together as indicated by arrows.

SIMPLE TUMOURS OF THE BREAST

These are always best excised so that the diagnosis can be confirmed by pathological examination and the patient's anxieties arrested. They are:
  1. Fibroadenoma.
  2. Duct papilloma. This is a benign tumour which arises in one of the terminal lactiferous ducts. It causes a blood-stained discharge from the nipple. As these tumours are liable to develop into duct carcinoma, excision is advisable.

TRAUMA

Injuries to the breast may result in:
  1. A haematoma which may organise to form a swelling. Exploration may be necessary to settle the diagnosis and drain the haematoma.

2. Fat necrosis. A hard, craggy mass which is frequently adherent to the skin appears. The diagnosis may be suspected clinically but excision is mandatory so that a scirrhous carcinoma is excluded.

CARCINOMA OF THE BREAST

Every woman who discovers a lump in her breast has a not unnatural dread that it is a carcinoma. Unfortunately, this dread too often results in concealment of her condition until it is too late, yet the breast remains one of the most favourable sites for the treatment of a new growth. The earlier treatment is instituted, the greater the chances of cure.

One in seventeen of all women acquire the disease and many eventually die from it irrespective of the form of treatment. There is an overall mortality of 8 per cent per year with a higher rate in the first three years. One half are dead in five years and three-quarters succumb eventually even as long as 20 years from diagnosis.

Carcinoma of the breast should be regarded as a systemic disease until it is proved otherwise. No big improvement in survival can be expected until a method is found to combat micrometastases at the time of diagnosis of the lesion in the breast. Hence the potential importance of scanning clinics.

It used to be believed that cancer of the breast in old women was a fairly benign condition and for that reason labelled as an atrophic scirrhous growth. Mullen has shown that most women in the age group 71-100 are likely to die of their cancer and that this justifies a more aggressive approach to treatment.

Evidence to date suggests that the use of oral contraceptives is unrelated to the risk of breast cancer. Nonetheless it should be remembered that it must be many years before the possible relationship between oral contraceptives and breast cancer is finally settled. Oral contraceptives do increase the incidence of non-malignant lumps in the breast.

Screening for carcinoma of the breast

The effectiveness of screening has still to be evaluated. Clinical examination will discover a palpable lump but the mass may be too small to be felt with the hand. Mammography will show an area of calcification if present but repeated mammograms expose the patient to radiation hazards. Screening requires back up services for biopsy.

Varieties of carcinoma of the breast

1. Scirrhous carcinoma. This is the commonest form. It is hard in consistency.

2. Encephaloid carcinoma is a softer growth and spreads more rapidly than the scirrhous type.

3. Duct carcinoma. The rarest growth is characterised by bleeding from the nipple and is occasionally associated with an eczematous-like condition of the nipple and areola (Paget's disease). It is a favourable growth to treat.

4. Acute carcinomatosis of lactation is fortunately rare. The patient develops a growth while lactating, and the great vascularity of the breast at this time causes rapid spread.

The spread of carcinoma of the breast

1. *Locally* spread occurs by invasion of the skin overlying the growth and invasion of the pectoral muscles of the chest wall.

2. *Lymphatic spread* occurs to the axillary lymphatic glands and later to the supraclavicular group. Spread to the lymphatic glands in the chest may occur early in growths of the inner segments of the breast.

3. *Spread by the blood stream* may result in invasion of the bones (particularly the vertebrae) the liver and the lungs.

Clinical staging of carcinoma of the breast

Stage 1. A small growth with no localised spread.

Stage 2. Evidence of local extension such as a skin attachment and enlarged mobile lymph glands.

Stage 3. Fixed lymph glands and pectoral fascia or skin involvement.

Stage 4. Disseminated spread.

Although clinically a growth may be stage 1, undetected secondary deposits may already be well established and the disease already well advanced.

The TNM international classification gives a more accurate clinical assessment. The size of the tumour (T) is measured and graded 1 to 4. The presence or absence of palpable lymph nodes (N) and presence or absence of metastases (M) is noted as 0 or 1.

Symptoms and signs

1. A painless, hard, irregular mass in the breast is the usual complaint. It has been noticed while washing, or as a result of a trivial knock. It is easily felt with the flat of the hand. There is usually some elevation of the breast. With a lump in the breast, as in vaginal bleeding, the greatest service a nurse can do is to refer the patient immediately to her doctor.

2. Attachment to the skin and the deeper structures, namely, the pectoral muscles and the ribs, occurs as the growth extends.

3. Recent retraction of the nipple may be present. This sign is diagnostic.

4. A coarsening of the skin, known as *peau d'orange,* may be present, due to blockage of the subcutaneous lymphatic vessels (Fig. 29.2).

5. Ulceration of the skin and fungation occur in late and untreated cases (Fig. 29.3).

6. The lymphatic glands in the axilla may be enlarged and hard. The supraclavicular glands may be similarly enlarged.

7. There may be tumour deposits in the skin overlying the breast and on the adjacent chest wall.

Fig. 29.2 Carcinoma of breast showing elevation and retraction of the nipple *(top)* and peau d'orange *(below)*.

Fig. 29.3 Advanced fungating carcinoma of the breast.

8. There may be evidence of distant spread, e.g. enlarged liver or ascites.

Investigations

Clinical examination enables the correct diagnosis to be made in well over 80 per cent of patients. The following investigations may be used to diagnose the nature of a breast lump and, if it is carcinoma, to assess the extent of spread of the disease.

1. Mammography. This is a soft tissue X-ray of the breast. The presence and nature of a lump can be determined by its appearance.

2. Aspiration cytology. A small bead of fluid and cellular debris can be aspirated from a lump with a needle and syringe. A smear is made on to a slide which is placed in a special fixative and then stained. Histological examination of the cells indicates the nature of the lump.

3. Needle biopsy (using a Tru-cut or Menghini needle) or high speed drill biopsy provides tissue for histological examination. This can be done as an outpatient.

4. Excision biopsy of a lump under general anaesthetic can be done as a day-case. This is not appropriate if the lump is thought to be malignant.

5. Frozen section biopsy. The lump is excised and examined immediately by a frozen section technique. If malignancy is confirmed, definitive surgery is carried out under the same anaesthetic.

6. X-rays of the chest and axial skeleton (skull, spine, pelvis). These may show spread of disease to lung or bone.

7. Isotope bone scan. This is a more sensitive method of detecting bone metastases than straight X-rays. It may still not detect very small metastases (micro-metastases).

8. Estimation of urinary hydroxyproline excretion. This is raised if bone metastases are present.

9. Serum calcium estimation. This may be raised when considerable bone destruction is occurring.

10. Liver function tests. These may indicate liver involvement.

11. Ultrasound scan. This is used to detect liver metastases.

MANAGEMENT

Management of early disease

The management of the patient will depend on the local extent of the primary disease and the presence or absence of metastases.

If the disease is apparently localised to the breast the following avenues of treatment are available. There is no great difference in the long-term results between the first four methods of treatment.

(a) Radical mastectomy i.e. removal of the breast, the overlying skin, the pectoral muscles and the axillary lymphatic glands. This procedure is not as popular as it was in the past because of the disfigurement produced.

(b) Patey mastectomy (Fig. 29.4) is the same as a radical mastectomy

Fig. 29.4 External rotation of the shoulder joint is the only movement which it is important to recover in the first week following mastectomy. If this is full, abduction will also be full. This patient has had a Patey mastectomy performed.

with the exception that the pectoralis major muscle is preserved. It provides adequate tumour clearance without the obvious deformity that results from removal of the muscles.

(c) **Simple mastectomy,** removing just the breast, and axillary node biopsy. This is followed by radiotherapy if the axillary nodes are found to be involved.

(d) **Wide excision of the lump** followed by radiotherapy.

(e) **Radiotherapy** may be used alone for those cases with locally inoperable primary disease.

(f) **Immunotherapy,** using B.C.G. vaccine as a non-specific stimulus of the immune defence mechanisms may be prescribed.

(g) **Adjuvant chemotherapy.** Some people advocate the use of cytotoxic drugs at the time of surgery in an attempt to prevent or treat undetectable micro-metastases.

Care of the mastectomy patient

Preoperative preparation

1. Local. Both axillae are shaved, the affected one because it comes into the incision, and the opposite one because the bandages pass around it. The area of both breasts, the arms to the wrists, and the abdomen to below the umbilicus, are washed with 2 per cent hexachlorophane soap.

2. The thigh. The ipsilateral thigh should be shaved and washed so that it is ready as a donor area should a skin graft be required.

3. Blood. Blood should be grouped and serum saved. Two units of blood should be cross-matched for a radical mastectomy.

4. Marking. The lump to be excised should be clearly marked on the skin.

5. Consent. The patient must understand the nature of the operation to be performed. Care and sensitivity is necessary in explaining this. It is helpful for the doctor and nurse to speak to the patient together, perhaps with a close relative present.

The operation

The prepared area is generously towelled off.

The care of the arm during the operation. The arm is held by a nurse until the patient is towelled for operation. It is held abducted, one of the nurse's hands holding the patient's wrist and the other hand resting on the table to protect the patient's radial nerve on the lower third of the humerus. The nurse must be careful not to over-abduct the arm for fear of causing damage to the large nerve-trunks. It is then fixed on a suitably padded side arm of the operating table (Fig. 29.5).

A transverse elliptical incision is usually used. The skin is stitched and the dead space drained, commonly with a tube to suction apparatus. If the skin will not come together, a skin graft is used to close the defect.

If suction drainage is used, only a light dressing is necessary. If an open drain is used then dressing gauze is applied and the chest bandaged.

Fig. 29.5   Position for operations on the breast.

Postoperative care

When recovery from the anaesthetic has taken place, the patient is propped up and a pillow is placed at the bottom of the bed, so that she can push against it with her feet. She is mobilised the next day.

Haemorrhage and care of the drainage tube. In the first 24 hours oozing of blood and serum always occurs. The amount collecting in the drainage apparatus should be carefully observed. If a bandage is used it must be firmly secured. Any excessive haemorrhage should, be reported at once. The tube is removed after 48 to 72 hours as long as drainage is not excessive. Some surgeons insert two drainage tubes.

Pain is relieved by morphia (15 mg) or similar analgesic on the night following the operation and as required.

Care of the wound. The edges of the wound should be inspected for undue tension during dressing, and stitches are released if necessary.

Ballooning of the flaps may occur due to collection of serum. This is evacuated by aspiration or by the gentle insertion of sinus forceps. The flaps themselves must be observed for sloughing, and, should it occur, eusol compresses are applied.

The sutures are removed as follows: alternate sutures are removed on the tenth day and the remainder on the 12th day. Many surgeons remove them earlier than this.

If a bare area has been grafted great care must be taken to 'float off' with sterile saline the innermost dressing, which is usually a small piece of tulle gras.

Care of the arm. It is important to commence arm movements on the second day after operation, but it is unwise to insist on much abduction for 4 or 5 days. The wound is disturbed and serum oozing increases. The patient must be encouraged to externally rotate the shoulder joint gently, and by the tenth day should have no trouble in touching the back of her head with her hand. If she has full external rotation at once she will have no difficulty in achieving full abduction. This is important, since her greatest disability will be in fastening her clothes at the back and doing her hair.

The nurse must remember that in the early days the patient will require some assistance with drinks and food because of the disability of the arm. Her locker or bed-table should be placed on the side opposite to that on which the operation was performed.

Complications

1. Respiratory complications. Respiration may be impaired by the trauma of the operation and the restriction of chest movements caused by the firm bandaging. Deep-breathing exercises, although difficult in this situation, must be encouraged.

2. Sloughing of the flaps. Should extensive sloughing occur, skin grafting must be undertaken later, when the area has granulated cleanly. Sloughs must be removed and sepsis reduced to a minimum as soon as possible. Eusol compresses are valuable before and just after the sloughs have separated.

3. Oedema of the arm may occur immediately if ligation of the axillary vein has had to be performed. More remotely, it may be due to lymphatic obstruction following removal of the axillary contents, constriction of the axillary vein from fribrosis or to recurrence of the growth. It is a most distressing symptom. Elevation of the arm at night may control moderate swelling.

4. Thrombosis of the axillary vein may occur occasionally.

Cosmetic deformity

This is easily concealed by a suitable prosthesis attached in the patient's clothing. There is a large variety of prostheses available in different sizes. The patient should be measured and fitted by an expert.

The management of advanced carcinoma of the breast

Advanced carcinoma of the breast is defined as extensive local disease (judged by size and fixity of tumour, fixity of axillary lymph nodes) or spread of disease beyond the breast and axillary lymph nodes. There is no cure for such disease. The objective of treatment is to maintain the best possible quality of life with as little disturbance to the patient as possible. There are a number of treatments available. There is little evidence that the use of any one of these early in the course of the disease as opposed to later makes any difference to the eventual outcome. If there is a good response to one form of treatment there is more likely to be a good response to any subsequent treatment and (vice versa). In general, treatment is reserved for the control of symptoms and is either local or systemic.

1. *Local surgery.* A 'toilet' mastectomy, if technically possible, will alleviate ulceration, discharge and bleeding from locally advanced disease.

Laminectomy and spinal cord decompression may relieve symptoms secondary to vertebral metastases.

Internal fixation of pathological fractures through metastases in long bones may be necessary.

2. *Local radiotherapy.* This can be used to treat the symptoms of local disease (e.g. ulceration) or bone metastases.

3. *Endocrine (hormone) therapy.* This may be by ablative (removing glands) or additive (prescribing drugs) methods.

(a) Ablative methods. Bilateral oophorectomy (removal of ovaries) is the first line of treatment for recurrent or advanced disease in pre-menopausal women or those not more than 2 years past the menopause. This involves a relatively minor lower abdominal operation under general anaesthetic. The same effect can be achieved by irradiation of the ovaries (but this may reduce the total dose of irradiation remaining available for treatment of disease elsewhere). Bone pain may be dramatically relieved. If a good response is obtained then adrenalectomy (p. 294) or hypophysectomy should be performed if symptoms recur. The pituitary can be destroyed more simply by implantation of radioactive substances or alcohol injection. Pituitary ablation is also used in post-menopausal women with bone pain unresponsive to other treatment.

(b) Additive methods. The drugs used are either androgenic, oestrogenic or progestogenic in their action. The latter have been used but are without any great benefit. Androgenic drugs are used in pre-menopausal women when other treatments have failed. However their virilising effect puts a severe limitation on their value. Oestrogenic drugs are used in post-menopausal women, often as a first line of treatment for recurrent or advanced disease. Tamoxifen, which has anti-oestrogenic properties, is superior to oestrogens in its effect and is currently regarded as the best drug available.

The presence or absence of oestrogen receptors in the primary tumour can be measured. Their presence is to some extent a measure of the hormone dependence of the tumour and an indication that the tumour is more likely to respond to endocrine manipulation than one in which receptors are absent.

4. *Chemotherapy.* Cytotoxic drugs are valuable, in selected cases, for control of locally advanced or recurrent disease unresponsive to other treatment. Several agents are usually used in combination on a cyclical basis. The gastrointestinal upsets, loss of hair, leucopenia and other side-effects are disadvantages which have to be weighed against the possible benefits of such treatment.

5. *Other palliative treatment.* Drainage of a pleural effusion or ascites is sometimes necessary for symptomatic relief.

Hypercalcaemia, resulting from metastatic bone destruction, can cause severe generalised symptoms. It requires special treatment prescribed by the medical staff.

Mastectomy and the patient

The surgeon is well aware of the psychological insult that may arise from mastectomy. Some surgeons seek to avert this by subcutaneous implant of a silicone prosthesis at the time of mastectomy or, more commonly, at a later date. This can provide a very good artificial breast. A latissimus dorsi skin flap can be used to provide adequate skin cover when inserting such a prosthesis. The fear that adequate primary treatment or subsequent local treatment may be hindered by the insertion of an implant is the reason that many surgeons have no enthusiasm for its use. This fear has yet to be allayed, Some surveys show that healthy women, should they develop carcinoma of the breast, are more concerned about the adequacy of the clearance of disease than resultant deformity. Self-confidence is more likely to be restored by faith in their treatment and the provision of an adequate prosthesis than the pursuit of cosmetic surgery.

DISEASES OF THE MALE BREAST

Since the male breast is a vestigial organ, disease is uncommon.

Fibroadenosis is the most common simple lesion and is frequently due to pressure from braces. It may require excision.

Gynaecomastia (excessive development of the male breast) may occur in the newborn infant or at puberty. It can be unilateral or bilateral. It is sometimes very painful. It occurs as a complication of drug therapy (numerous drugs including many antibiotics and tranquillisers can cause it); as a complication of oestrogen therapy for carcinoma of the prostate; in association with liver disease and excess alcoholic intake, probably due to excess oestrogen in the blood; and in association with rare oestrogen-secreting tumours of the adrenal gland or testicle. It often resolves spontaneously. If symptoms persist the treatment is subcutaneous mastectomy, preserving the nipple.

Carcinoma of the male breast occurs occasionally, accounting for 1 per cent of all breast cancer. The symptoms and signs are the same as in women, but because there is almost no breast tissue for the growth to invade, fixation to and invasion of the underlying muscle and ribs occur very early.

BIBLIOGRAPHY

Baum M 1976 British Medical Journal 1439
Mueller C B et al 1978 Surgery 83: 123
Rolland and Schellens L J 1973 Obstetrics and Gynecology 80: 945
Williams E M, Baum M, Hughes L E 1976 Clinical Onocology 327

30
Lungs, chest wall and pleura

PNEUMOTHORAX

There are two types of pneumothorax—(a) spontaneous and (b) traumatic. Either kind can develop into a 'tension' pneumothorax.

Spontaneous pneumothorax

This is the more common variety and is seen more frequently in males than females, often between the ages of 20 and 40 years. Air escapes into the pleural cavity as a result of rupture of a small emphysematous bulla on the surface of the lung, usually at the apex. The bulla ruptures quite spontaneously and there is not usually any associated history of straining or sudden exertion. The patient complains of pain in the chest and dyspnoea, the severity depending on the size of the pneumothorax. The lung is separated from the chest wall by the air in the pleural cavity and the underlying lung is progressively reduced in size. If adhesions are present, or if the air leak stops, the underlying lung may only partially collapse.

Treatment

A small pneumothorax probably requires no active treatment and the patient is advised to remain quiet and to restrict his activities. The air is gradually absorbed over the following 7 to 10 days and the underlying lung re-expands. If the lung should fail to re-expand, or if the pneumothorax occupies more than 20 per cent of the thoracic cavity, an intercostal drainage tube is inserted through the second intercostal space anteriorly, and connected to an underwater-seal drainage bottle (Fig. 30.1). With each expiration, air bubbles will be seen to escape down the tube and through the water. Air cannot re-enter the tube and pleural cavity because of the water seal. So long as the air leak in the lung persists, bubbles of air will escape. However, if the lung can be made to expand fully, and this may require applying suction to the drainage system, the lung will begin to stick to the pleural lining of the chest wall and the hole will be gradually sealed off. When this happens, the escape of air ceases and the intercostal tube is normally removed 24 hours later. Many patients will develop a second pneumothorax weeks, months or even years after the first. These patients are very likely to go on and develop further recurrent pneumothoraces on the same side and, therefore, more active treatment than simple intubation is normally recommended after the second pneumothorax. There is some debate as to which is the best method of treating recurrent pneumothorax. The instillation of various irritant solutions into the pleural cavity has been recommended, e.g. tetracycline solution and iodised talc powder. The aim of these is to promote adhesions between the lung and the chest wall, thus preventing further collapse of the lung. A more certain way of achieving the same effect is to submit the patient to parietal pleurectomy. Through a standard thoracotomy, the parietal pleura is stripped off the chest wall leaving the raw surface of ribs and muscles exposed. The lung sticks to this surface extensively and recurrent pneumothorax is most uncommon after this procedure. However, it is a major operation. It does, though, have the advantage that any emphysematous bullae on the surface of the lung can be ligated or plicated and thus further reduce the risk of future pneumothoraces. Occasionally, thoracotomy, pleurectomy and ligation of bulla is essential for a persistent air leak that is not responding to conservative treatment.

Partially collapsed lung

Pneumothorax

Underwater seal drainage bottle

Fig. 30.1 Pneumothorax. Intercostal tube in situ.

Traumatic pneumothorax

This is most commonly associated with fractured ribs when the surface of the lung is punctured by the sharp edge of a broken rib. It can, however, result from an external blow with no apparent rib injury. Traumatic pneumothorax is frequently associated with bleeding into the pleural cavity resulting in a haemopneumothorax. Tension pneumothorax is more likely to develop after trauma because the air leak is usually larger and may, indeed, be from a tear in the trachea or major bronchus.

Treatment

Treatment is similar to that for spontaneous pneumothorax except that active intervention is usually more frequently necessary. An intercostal tube is inserted and suction applied to draw the lung out against the chest wall in the hope that it will stick and the air leak become sealed. A large air leak suggests fracture of the trachea or bronchus. This can be confirmed at bronchoscopy and thoracotomy. Repair of the tear is indicated. Similarly, a large tear in the lung substance will produce a large air leak and thoracotomy may be required to suture the lung. If a haemothorax is also present, two tubes will usually be necessary—one at the apex to evacuate air and the other at the base of the pleural cavity to evacuate blood.

Tension pneumothorax

Normally when air escapes into the pleural cavity, a balance of pressures is achieved with the lung either partially or fully collapsed. Some times, however, when the air leak is large, air continues to escape into the pleural cavity, even after the lung is fully deflated. With each inspiration more air is sucked into the cavity and gradually the heart and mediastinum are pushed to the opposite side. As the mediastinum moves over to the good side, the underlying good lung becomes compressed so that eventually the lung on the pneumothorax side is completely collapsed and the good lung is seriously compressed. The patient is intensely cyanotic and the circulation is grossly embarrassed. Death ensues unless urgent measures are taken.

Treatment

The tension can be easily and quickly relieved by insertion of an open needle through the chest wall into the pneumothorax. Air whistles out, the heart begins to return to the midline and the compression of the good lung is reduced. An intercostal tube should be inserted as soon as possible and connected to an underwater sealed drainage bottle. Subsequent treatment is as described above.

Tension pneumothorax presents a serious, life-threatening emergency which responds to simple urgent measures.

CHEST INJURIES

A patient with a major chest injury can present a frightening situation to an inexperienced nurse or doctor. However, many of the injuries though serious can be simply and effectively treated. A cool head and a know-ledge of the structures within the chest which are liable to injury and the types of injury which can occur to each, can be of considerable help to those who have to deal with this type of patient.

Structures which may be injured

1. Chest wall, ribs, sternum, costal cartilages and soft tissues.
2. Lungs, bronchi, trachea
3. Oesophagus
4. Diaphragm
5. Heart and great vessels
6. Abdominal viscera
7. Other injuries (head, limbs, spine etc.)

Types of injuries

(a) Bruising and lacerations are dealt with as in any other part of the body. A penetrating injury through the soft tissues into the pleural cavity can result in a sucking wound, so that on each inspiration air is drawn into the pleural cavity through the chest wall. The air is not able to escape because on expiration the soft tissues fall together again. A pneumothor-ax develops which can progress to a tension pneumothorax. The hole can be sealed in an emergency situation by application of a finger, or preferably a wad of jellynet gauze. An intercostal tube can then be inserted and the wound in the chest wall later repaired.

(b) Fractured ribs. Simple fractures of the ribs can be very painful. Treatment consists in relieving the pain until they heal. However, in the elderly patient or chronic bronchitic, serious complications can develop following simple fractured ribs. These patients are reluctant to cough because of the associated pain and do not, therefore, clear their bronchi-al secretions adequately. Patchy collapse develops in the lungs which can progress to pneumonia. It is essential in this type of patient that pain is adequately relieved so that vigorous chest therapy can be applied. Regular analgesia is given, particularly before physiotherapy. Fractured ribs may be complicated by pneumothorax or haemothorax and these are dealt with on their merits.

If several ribs are fractured in two places, a flail segment can develop. An area of chest wall loses its rigidity and fixation to the remainder of the chest wall and begins to move paradoxically with respiration (Fig. 30.2). Normally, on inspiration the chest wall expands but the loose flail segment moves inwards, sucked in by the negative pressure within the thorax. On expiration, the flail segment moves out again as the remain-der of the chest wall moves in. The portion of lung underlying the flail segment cannot expand with inspiration. This is not important if the flail segment is small, but a large flail segment will result in collapse of a wide area of underlying lung. This lung is not properly ventilated and the patient becomes cyanosed with a falling arterial blood P_{O_2}. If this reaches critical levels, active intervention is essential: This will normally consist in passing an endotracheal tube and putting the patient on positive pressure ventilation. The lungs are then expanded by positive pressure and the flail segment moves synchronously in and out with the remainder of the chest wall. This is continued for between 10 and 20 days, by which time the fractures have begun to heal, the chest wall moves as one piece again and the patient can be weaned off the ventilator. If thoracotomy is necessary to deal with internal injuries, the fractured ribs can be wired together so that the period of ventilation required is considerably shortened.

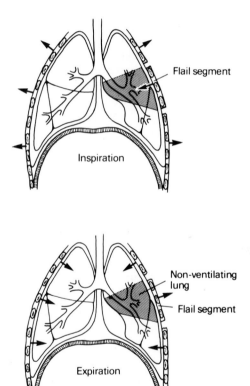

Fig. 30.2 Flail segment. Paradoxical movement on respiration.

Fractures of the costal cartilages and a stove-in sternum can behave like a flail segment and the treatment is similar.

(c) Pneumothorax. This has already been dealt with earlier in this chapter.

(d) Haemothorax. Bleeding can occur into the pleural cavity following injury from three common sources. An intercostal artery can be ruptured in association with a fractured rib, a tear of the lung may be associated with bleeding therefrom and injuries to the aorta may also occur.

Aspiration of the blood from the pleural space is usually indicated. If the bleeding continues an intercostal tube should be inserted and the bleeding monitored. Thoracotomy is indicated for persistent or profuse bleeding.

INFECTIONS OF THE CHEST

Lung abscess

A lung abscess is formed by the development within the lung tissue of a cavity filled with pus. Abscesses may be single, or multiple, large or small, and involve one or two lungs. The condition is much less common nowadays since the advent of antibiotics, with improved anaesthesia and dental care. It may be due to specific infections of the lung such as staphylococcal pneumonia and tuberculosis, or to occlusion of the bronchus supplying the affected portion of lung, e.g. by carcinoma or foreign body. Aspiration of vomit following anaesthesia or intoxication with alcohol is another common cause of lung abscess. An abscess can also develop in the lung following pulmonary embolus, or lung trauma.

Patients complain of cough, fever and malaise and may have pleuritic pain. Weight loss is common and patients may be very ill. If the abscess communicates with the bronchial tree, purulent sputum will be expectorated. Chest X-ray shows one or more cavities in the lung field, often with a fluid level and tomograms can be helpful in distinguishing between a breaking-down carcinoma and a simple lung abscess. Treatment consists of bronchoscopy to exclude bronchial occlusion by carcinoma or foreign body and, if possible, to obtain secretions for culture. Antibiotics are given on the basis of culture sensitivities and these should be continued so long as the condition appears to respond. Lung resection is indicated if the lesion fails to respond to medical treatment, if a neoplasm is suspected, if haemoptysis is troublesome or if a broncho-pleural fistula develops. Occasionally patients are too ill for major chest surgery and the abscess is then simply drained externally.

Bronchiectasis

Bronchiectasis, like lung abscess, is much less frequently seen since the advent of antibiotics. The condition is caused by a combination of bronchial obstruction and pulmonary infection. A common cause is enlargement of hilar lymph glands during an infection in childhood. The infection which occurs distal to the obstruction damages the walls of the smaller bronchi which lose their elasticity and become dilated. The mucosa of the bronchial wall is damaged and secretions collect in the dilated bronchi. These secretions are prone to infection, giving rise to the symptoms and complications of bronchiectasis.

Patients complain of a chronic cough productive of purulent sputum. The amount and degree of infection of the sputum varies. Haemoptysis is common, as are acute exacerbations of infection in the surrounding lung tissue. Infection of the pleural space can lead to empyema and embolism of infected material can reach the brain causing cerebral abscess. Clubbing of the fingers is often seen in patients with bronchiectasis. Chest X-ray may appear normal, or show increased vascular markings with a honeycomb-like appearance in the affected areas. Bronchoscopy should be carried out to exclude bronchial obstruction and a broncho-gram is essential to define the extent of the disease.

Medical treatment consists of postural drainage with short courses of antibiotics for bouts of acute infection. Surgery is indicated if the bronchiectasis is localised to one area of the lung. Removal of this part of lung results in complete cure. Surgery is not indicated, however, when the disease is extensive in both lungs.

Empyema

An empyema is a collection of pus within the pleural cavity. It may be secondary to an infective condition in the lung, e.g. simple abscess, bronchiectasis, pneumonia or tuberculosis. It may also be seen after thoracotomy, or following perforation of the oesophagus. Chest wall injuries may also give rise to empyema and a secondary empyema may develop in relation to a sub-phrenic abscess.

Patients may complain of cough and chest pain and are usually toxic with a fever. Chest X-ray reveals a pleural effusion and aspiration of this confirms the presence of pus. Because the abscess is usually walled off by a thick layer of fibrous tissue, systemic antibiotics are not usually effective, though they may be indicated to control toxicity.

Treatment consists initially in aspiration of the pus and injection of appropriate antibiotics into the pleural space. Many will resolve in this way, but it the pus becomes too thick for aspiration, surgical drainage by rib resection and insertion of a large drain is essential. Excision of the empyema and decortication of the underlying lung may be necessary for chronic empyema. Occasionally, when the underlying lung is grossly diseased, pleuropneumonectomy is indicated.

Tuberculosis

Most patients with pulmonary tuberculosis respond to medical treat-ment and do not require surgery. However, there are still a few indica-tions for lung resection and these include the following:

1. When the sputum is still positive for tubercle bacilli 3 to 6 months after starting treatment, especially if the organism is resistant to one of the major drugs.
2. When the affected lobe or lung is destroyed by the disease.
3. Persistent haemoptysis, or troublesome bronchiectasis.
4. A persistent cavity, in spite of treatment.
5. When a neoplasm is suspected in addition to the tuberculosis.
6. When a patient proves very unreliable in taking drugs, or attend-ing follow-up.

Surgery will usually consist of lobectomy but occasionally a totally destroyed bronchiectatic lung will be removed by pneumonectomy.

TUMOURS OF THE BRONCHI AND LUNGS

Bronchial adenoma

Bronchial adenomata are rare tumours which may occur in either sex, commonly between the ages of 20 and 40 years. They are of low grade malignancy and grow slowly but may metastasise. They usually occur in the central air passages and cause their effects either by bleeding and causing haemoptysis, or by occluding one major bronchus with collapse of a lobe. Most bronchial adenomata are usually visible at bronchoscopy and treatment is surgical. The tumour is removed together with the portion of lung supplied by the affected bronchus. The reported survival rates vary between 50 and 95 per cent at 5 years.

Hamartoma

A hamartoma is a benign tumour consisting of several different elements normally found in lung tissue, e.g. cartilage, fibrous tissue, epithelium. This type of tumour does not give rise to symptoms and is usually found by chance on a routine chest X-ray. However, it may be difficult to differentiate a hamartoma from a carcinoma and thoracotomy and surgical removal is usually indicated.

Carcinoma

At least 30 000 people die every year in England and Wales from carcinoma of the lung. The disease affects men more commonly than women but the ratio between the two is narrowing. The cause of lung cancer is not known, but there is a strong relationship to the number of cigarettes smoked. There may also be an increased incidence among people who work in arsenic and cobalt mines, or in the chromate and nickel industry.

Pathology

The three main pathological types are squamous carcinoma (50 per cent), undifferentiated carcinoma (30 per cent) and adeno-carcinoma (20 per cent). There is another type of lung cancer which is only infrequently seen and this is the alveolar cell carcinoma.

Squamous growths grow more slowly than the other varieties and metastasise later. Tumour tissue in the centre of the growth may break down and the appearances on chest X-ray then resemble a lung abscess. Undifferentiated growths, particularly the oat cell variety, metastasise early and carry a poor prognosis. Adenocarcinomata tend to occur in the periphery of the lung and their growth rate is intermediate between the other types.

Spread of lung cancer occurs either directly to the surrounding structures, e.g. mediastinum or chest wall, or along lymphatic channels to central lymph nodes or directly via the blood stream to distant organs. The most common sites of metastases are brain, bone and liver, though secondary deposits may occur anywhere.

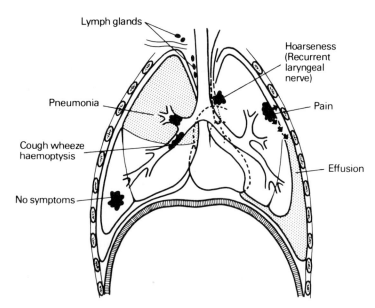

Lymph glands

Hoarseness (Recurrent laryngeal nerve)

Pneumonia

Pain

Cough wheeze haemoptysis

Effusion

No symptoms

Fig. 30.3 Symptoms and signs of lung carcinoma in relation to location of tumour.

Symptoms

One of the difficulties in the successful treatment of lung cancer is that there is an initial latent period during which a tumour may grow for a long time before producing any symptoms. When symptoms do occur the condition is already frequently inoperable. Symptoms will depend on the location of the tumour (Fig. 30.3). Involvement of the bronchus may cause cough, haemoptysis, wheezing and dyspnoea. Occlusion of a bronchus may produce pneumonia with fever and toxicity. Weight loss is common and involvement of the chest wall causes pain. Dysphagia results from obstruction of the oesophagus either by the tumour itself or by glands which may also compress the superior vena cava, resulting in superior mediastinal obstruction with swelling and cyanosis of the head and neck and dilatation of the veins over the upper chest wall. Hoarseness may develop from involvement of the recurrent laryngeal nerve supplying the vocal cord, and involvement of the pericardium may produce cardiac symptoms. Tumours of the lung can secrete hormones into the circulation producing an endocrine disorder or peripheral neuropathies. Headaches and vomiting may result from cerebral secondaries, pathological fractures from involvement of bone and abdominal pain and swelling from liver metastases.

Investigation

Examination of the sputum for malignant cells will give a high incidence of reliable results if a good specimen of bronchial secretions is presented to an expert pathologist. Chest X-ray, including a lateral film, will frequently allow a confident diagnosis, but tomograms of the suspicious area will give clearer definition and will help to differentiate a simple pneumonia or abscess from a neoplasm. Bronchoscopy should be carried out in all suspected cases and if the lesion is within range of the instrument, a biopsy should be taken. If a pleural effusion is present, this should be aspirated and a specimen sent for cytological examination. A blood stained effusion invariably implies malignant involvement of the pleura. If cytology of the fluid is negative and neoplasm is still suspected, thoracoscopy can be a useful method of obtaining a biopsy from the surface of the lung or pleura. Mediastinoscopy may also be indicated in order to obtain a mediastinal gland for examination if it is suspected that these are involved by growth.

Surgery

At least 75 per cent of patients with carcinoma of the lung are already inoperable by the time they first present to the doctor either because they have distant metastases, or the tumour has spread locally to involve the chest wall or mediastinum. Sometimes the lesion is still resectable, but the patient's respiratory function is so poor that lung resection is contraindicated. About 20 per cent of patients, however, will be considered suitable for operation when all investigations have been completed.

Preoperative preparation is most important. Since most patients have been smokers and many of them have bronchitis, it is essential to start chest physiotherapy before operation. They must also stop smoking and if the sputum grows pathological organisms on culture, this is treated with appropriate antibiotics. The operation is explained to the patient and his relatives and every effort made to gain the patient's confidence for the difficult postoperative period. Operation is performed through a thoracotomy on the side of the lesion. The tumour is assessed for position, size and evidence of spread. Approximately one fifth of patients who are operated on will prove to be inoperable at operation. If the

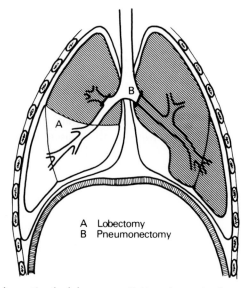

A   Lobectomy
B   Pneumonectomy

Fig. 30.4   A. Line of resection for lobectomy.   B. Line of resection for pneumonectomy.

tumour is removable, a decision is made as to whether it can be completely removed together with any involved glands by lobectomy or pneumonectomy. The pulmonary arteries and veins are ligated and divided individually and the bronchus is then dealt with. This is divided close to the trachea for a pneumonectomy, and near the origin of the lobar bronchus for a lobectomy (Fig. 30.4). The open end is closed with either interrupted nonabsorbable sutures, or with a stapling clamp. If possible, the bronchial stump is covered with a flap of parietal pleura to reduce the risk of postoperative bronchopleural fistula.

Fig. 30.5   Arrangement of tubes following lobectomy.

Following lobectomy, two tubes are left in the chest (Fig. 30.5) one at the apex to evacuate air and to allow the remaining lobe to expand to fill the space and one at the base of the thorax to evacuate any blood drainage. The basal drain can usually be removed within 48 hours, but the apical drain is left until all air leak has ceased, and this may take several days. Following pneumonectomy, a single tube is left in the pleural space to evacuate blood drainage and to equalise pressures on both sides of the chest. This tube can usually be removed within twenty four to forty eight hours.

In the immediate postoperative period it is most important to observe the behaviour of the chest tubes. Excessive blood drainage should immediately be reported and the decision to remove an apical tube will often depend on the observations of a nurse regarding air leakage. Tubes should be removed quickly and cleanly to prevent entry of air or infection into the thoracic cavity.

After operation, the patient's colour, respiratory rate, blood pressure and pulse rate and rhythm are carefully monitored and any abnormalities reported. A thoracotomy wound is painful and regular analgesia is essential. Because of the pain, patients often have difficulty in coughing and clearing their secretions, and although chest physiotherapy will regularly be given by a trained physiotherapist, it will always be necessary for the nurse taking care of the patient to encourage and help him to clear his secretions between the visits of the physiotherapist. This is particularly important at night. Retained secretion can lead to serious complications with collapse and infection in the residual lobe or lung. Occasionally bronchoscopy is necessary to clear the secretions when chest physiotherapy cannot cope, and tracheostomy may even be required if bronchoscopy is insufficient to keep the airways clear.

Without operation, 99 per cent of patients with lung cancer are dead within 2 years. Even with surgery, the 5 years survival is limited. Prognosis depends on several factors but mainly the histological type of the carcinoma, the size of the lesion and the degree of involvement of the lymph glands. Approximately 40 per cent of patients undergoing resection for squamous cell carcinoma, 15 per cent of patients with adenocarcinoma and 10 per cent of patients with oat cell tumours will live 5 years or more.

Radiotherapy

Radiotherapy seldom cures a patient with carcinoma of the lung. It can also cause unpleasant side effects and patients are usually quickly aware of their diagnosis when referred for this treatment. It should, therefore, on the whole, be reserved for specific indications and not offered to every patient with carcinoma of the lung who is unsuitable for surgery. Radiotherapy can be very effective in controlling certain symptoms such as pain, dyspnoea, haemoptysis, dysphagia and superior mediastinal obstruction so that, if these symptoms are significant, it is often worthwhile referring them for radiotherapy. There are also some patients with an operable lesion who, for some other reason, are not suitable for surgery and these may also be treated. Generally speaking, however, long term survival is not improved by radiotherapy and patients should be carefully selected.

Chemotherapy

The use of drugs in the treatment of lung cancer is continually progressing and for the future this perhaps holds the best hope of improvements in prognosis. However, at the present time, survival is not significantly affected by chemotherapy and the use of drugs, like radiotherapy, should be for selected patients only.

31
Surgery of the heart

...The blood is passed through the lungs and the heart by the pulsation of the ventricles, is forcibly ejected to all parts of the body, therein steals into the veins and porosities of the flesh, flows back everywhere through those very veins from the circumference to the centre, from small veins into larger ones and hence comes at last into the vena cava, and to the auricles of the heart...

Harvey 1628

STRUCTURE

The heart consists of a connective tissue framework of four fibrous rings (Fig. 31.1). The atria, ventricles, valves and roots of the pulmonary artery and aorta are attached to this framework. It is enveloped in a serofibrinous sac called the pericardium.

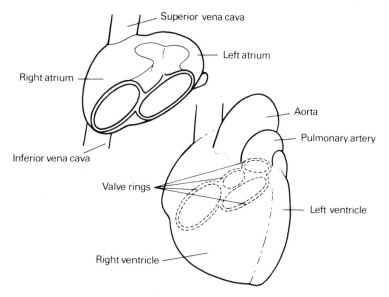

Fig. 31.1 The relationships of the cardiac chambers to the arterial roots and fibrous skeleton of the heart.

The ventricles are the pumps which provide most of the energy for the circulation of the blood. The right ventricle is like a bellows useful for propelling a large volume against a low resistance. The left ventricle is spherical and thus efficient at pumping against a high resistance.

Each atrium lies behind and to the right of its corresponding ventricle. The atria transfer blood from the veins (pulmonary and systemic) into the ventricular pumps. They may be likened to booster pumps.

Cardiac valve movements are passive. The atrioventricular valves (mitral and tricuspid) are funnel shaped. The chordae tendineae extend like guy ropes from the valve cusps into the papillary muscles. The semilunar valves (aortic and pulmonary) consist of three symmetrical cups attached to the roots of the great vessels.

The pericardium with its fluid lubricates the heart, holds it in a fixed anatomical position and separates it from the other mediastinal structures.

The heart's blood supply is provided by two coronary arteries which arise from the sinuses of Valsalva of the aortic root. The left main coronary artery (Fig. 31.2A) divides 2 cm from its ostium into two main divisions, the anterior descending and the circumflex. The anterior descending branch runs down the anterior interventricular groove, round the apex and ascends for a short distance in the posterior interventricular groove. The circumflex branch courses around the base of the left ventricle. The right coronary artery (Fig. 31.2B) passes beneath the left atrial appendage to the atrioventricular groove to reach the posterior interventricular groove. The venous drainage of the myocardium consists of a superficial and deep system. The very extensive superficial system of veins converge to form the coronary sinus which terminates in the right atrium. The deep system of veins communicates directly with the atria and ventricles through the thebesian veins.

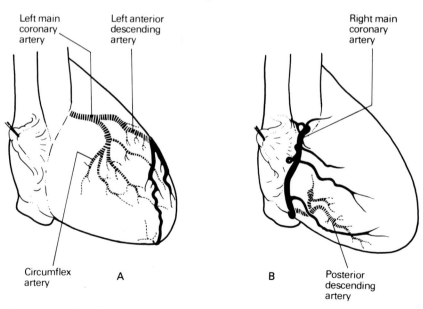

Left main coronary artery

Left anterior descending artery

Right main coronary artery

Circumflex artery

A

B

Posterior descending artery

Fig. 31.2 A and B The superficial coronary arteries.

FUNCTION

The delivery of blood to all organs of the body is accomplished by the pumping action of the heart.

Systemic circulation

The systemic circulation consists of three functional divisions—the arterial pressure reservoir, the capillaries and the venous volume reservoir.

The left ventricle ejects blood into the aorta and other elastic arteries. When the ventricles relax the flow of blood from the ventricles ceases but the elastic wall tension in the arteries continues to drive the blood through the capillaries (Fig. 31.3).

The velocity (speed) of blood flow through the capillaries is less than elsewhere in the circulation because of the very great cross section area of the capillary bed. Thus the blood comes into close contact with the extravascular tissues. These features of capillary flow provide ideal conditions for the rapid transfer of substances by diffusion.

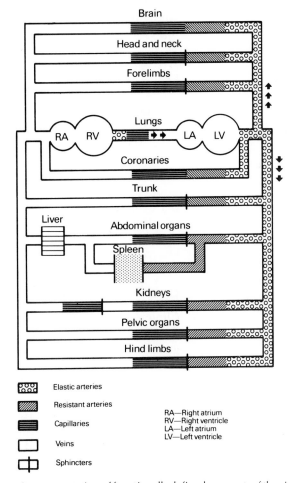

Fig. 31.3 Schematic representation of functionally defined segments of the circulation.

The systemic veins provide a mechanism whereby the volume can be varied over wide limits with only slight changes in pressure. The venous return is a most important regulator of cardiac output. If the pumping action (contractility) of the heart is unimpaired an increased venous return will increase cardiac output; conversely a decreased venous return will decrease cardiac output.

The systemic circulation may be described as a high pressure, high resistance system which supplies the variable requirements of many different tissues, thus it requires many controls. 'Central' control is mediated through the sympathetic nervous system and governed largely by the vasomotor centre of the medulla oblongata. In addition blood flow through various tissues may be adjusted locally in response to their metabolism and oxygen requirements.

Pulmonary circulation

The right ventricle pumps mixed venous blood through the pulmonary arteries and arterioles into the pulmonary capillary bed where gas exchange takes place. The pulmonary circulation in contrast to systemic circulation may be seen as a low pressure, low resistance circuit supplying a single function to one organ.

PREOPERATIVE ASSESSMENT AND CARE OF THE PATIENT

Cardiac disease is a source of great anxiety to the patient and the family. It is essential that the surgeon should explain the nature of the disease, the proposed surgical procedure and the likely outcome of treatment to both patient and family.

All members of the caring team should likewise ensure that they understand the nature of the patient's disease and the operation to be performed. They can then make it easy for the patient and family to ask questions which will be answered in simple nontechnical language. This gives the patient confidence in those who are caring for him and a knowledge that his welfare is their primary objective.

Cardiovascular system

Clinical assesment (history and examination) is of prime importance in the diagnosis of cardiac disorders, but is supplemented by special investigations.

Echocardiography

Echocardiography uses ultrasound to examine the structure of the heart. The position of the pericardium, heart and cardiac chambers and valves is recorded and the size and movements of these structures are studied. The recent development—two dimensional echocardiography—provides a motion picture of the heart similar to an angiocardiogram.

Stress test

Blood pressure and electrocardiogram are continuously monitored as the patient performs varying levels of work on a treadmill or bicycle. Changes in heart rate, blood pressure and the electrocardiogram provide an assessment of the heart's response to work.

Cardiac catheterisation

Cardiac catheterisation provides the surgeon with precise anatomical information. The catheter is a flexible tube about 100 cm long. It is connected to a continuous infusion drip containing heparin to prevent intravascular clotting. It It is usually passed under local anaesthesia.

Right heart catheterisation

The catheter is passed through the antecubital vein to enter in succession the right atrium, right ventricle and pulmonary artery.

Left heart catheterisation

The left heart chambers may be entered in an antegrade fashion by passing a catheter into the right atrium, and then penetrating the atrial septum, the catheter enters the left atrium and may be advanced into the left ventricle.

A catheter may be introduced into the brachial or femoral artery and passed retrogradely up the aorta and into the left ventricle.

The pressures in all the chambers of the heart may be measured (Fig. 31.4).

Changes in pressures show the presence of disease, e.g. a high left ventricular pressure with a simultaneous low aortic pressure shows a pressure drop (gradient) across the aortic valve, thus revealing the presence and severity of aortic stenosis (Fig. 31.13).

Blood samples can be withdrawn from the different chambers. Measurements of the oxygen saturation and tension may show the presence of abnormal communications (shunt) between the systemic and pulmonary circulations.

	Systole	Diastole	Mean
Right Atrium (RA)	–	–	0 to 8
Right Ventricle (RV)	15 to 30	0 to 8	–
Pulmonary Artery (PA)	15 to 30	3 to 12	9 to 16
Left Atrium (LA)			1 to 10
Left Ventricle (LV)	100 to 140	3 to 12	–
Aorta ((AO)	100 to 140	10 to 80	70 to 105

Fig. 31.4 Normal resting pressures (mmHg)

Selective angiocardiography

Radio-opaque dye is injected through a catheter into a selected cardiac chamber. This will show the shape and size of the chamber and helps to detect any abnormality of cardiac contraction. The presence of a thrombus or a tumour within the chamber will be revealed. Regurgitation of the dye from one chamber to another confirms the presence of a valve leak or abnormal communication and is helpful in assessing the severity of the leak.

Selective coronary arteriography

Specially shaped catheters are inserted into the brachial or femoral artery and passed up the aorta, and then directly into the orifice of the coronary arteries. Dye injected through these catheters outlines the coronary arteries and this is essential for the precise localisation of coronary artery disease.

Specialised catheters

Specialised catheters have been devised for specific functions:
  1. Endomyocardial biopsy—for the diagnosis of acute rejection following cardiac transplantation.
  2. Dilation of coronary arterial stenosis.

Pulmonary function

Pulmonary function requires careful evaluation: chest X-ray, spirometry and blood gas analysis are essential investigations.

Patients who smoke must be encouraged to abstain for as long as possible preoperatively. The physiotherapist will provide education in deep breathing manoeuvres and the use of incentive spirometric devices.

Renal function

Serum urea and creatinine are measured and if they indicate any impairment of renal function a creatinine clearance is performed.

Gastro-intestinal tract

A history of dyspepsia should be carefully evaluated and if necessary barium studies and fibreoptic gastroscopy should be performed.

General care

Particular attention is given to the elimination of infection which may be the cause of postoperative bacterial endocarditis. Careful dental inspection and radiographic studies will reveal any septic foci and these are eradicated. Cultures of throat, nose, skin, hair and urine are obtained and any infection found is treated appropriately.

The patient will be admitted a few days prior to surgery. Very ill patients will require a longer period of intensive medical and nursing care.

CARDIOPULMONARY BYPASS

Cardiopulmonary bypass is a technique which allows the pumping function of the heart and the gas exchange function of the lungs to be temporarily replaced by a pump oxygenator (heart-lung machine). The heart is exposed through a median sternotomy incision, in which the sternum is split down the middle and spread widely by a mechanical retractor.

Heparin is given to prevent the blood clotting as it passes through the pump oxygenator. Tubes are inserted into the superior and inferior vena cava and the patient's venous blood is drained into the pump oxygenator. The oxygenated blood is pumped back into the patient usually

Fig. 31.5 (a) Normal circulation. (b) Circulation on cardiopulmonary bypass.

PA = pulmonary artery. PV = pulmonary vein. AO = aorta. RV = right ventricle. LV = left ventricle. I.V.C. = inferior vena cava. S.U.C. = superior vena cava.

through a tube placed in the ascending aorta, but occasionally into the femoral artery (Fig. 31.5). Thus the patient's heart and lungs are bypassed and the surgeon is able to operate inside the cavities of the heart. When the surgeon has closed the cardiac chambers the heart and lungs resume their normal function, and the tubes are removed from the vena cava and aorta. Any excess heparin is neutralised by the appropriate dose of protamine sulphate.

Operations which do not require cardiopulmonary bypass are marked with an asterisk in the subsequent text.

MYOCARDIAL PROTECTION

Most heart operations require a dry, quiet heart; it is, therefore, necessary to interrupt the coronary blood flow and arrest the heart. The heart, unlike other organs, must resume full funtional activity before the patient is disconnected from the the pump oxygenator. Protection of the myocardium during the operation is critical to the survival of the patient. The principles of modern myocardial protection can be summarised under two headings.

1. Energy conservation—rapid diastolic arrest produced by chemical cardioplegia.

This achieved by infusing a solution containing 20 mmol of potassium per litre into the coronary circulation.

2. Hypothermia—lowering cardiac temperature slows all metabolic processes. Hypothermia is achieved by:

(a) Cooling the cardioplegic infusate to 6°C.

(b) Cooling the surface of the heart by spraying it with Hartman's solution at 4°C.

(c) Moderate reduction of general body temperature to 20–27°C. This prevents rewarming of the heart by the surrounding tissues.

CONGENITAL HEART DISEASE

Congenital abnormalities of the heart result from an arrested or defective embryonic development. The eight most frequently encountered anomalies which account for 85 per cent of all congenital cardiac lesions will be described.

It may be useful for the student to group congenital heart defects as follows:

1. Abnormal communication between the pulmonary and systemic circuits which permits the passage of blood from the systemic to the pulmonary circulation, i.e. left to right shunt. This leads to overloading of the pulmonary circulation. Examples of this are patent ductus arteriosus, atrial septal defect and ventricular septal defect.

2. Abnormal communication between the pulmonary and systemic circuits which allows passage of blood from systemic veins to systemic arteries without first traversing the lungs. This leads to arterial hypoxaem-

ia and cyanosis. Examples are the tetralogy of Fallot and transposition of the great vessels.

3. Lesions not associated with shunts. Examples are coarctation of the aorta, pulmonary stenosis and aortic stenosis.

Patent ductus arteriosus

The ductus arteriosus connects the pulmonary and systemic circulations in foetal life, so that blood is short-circuited away from the lungs where it is not required. At birth spontaneous closure usually takes place, but occasionally the ductus remains open and the blood flows from the systemic to the pulmonary circulation. Congestive cardiac failure and bacterial endocarditis are the commonest complications. The operation* to close the patent ductus is performed through a left thoracotomy. The ductus may be ligated, but some surgeons prefer to divide it and suture the ends to avoid the possibility of recanalisation.

The operative mortality is 2 per cent.

Atrial septal defect

The secundum-type atrial septal defect is one of the most common congenital cardiac malformations. Females are affected almost twice as frequently as males.

The communication between the two atria results in a flow of blood from left to right atrium.

Children

The increase in pulmonary blood flow is well tolerated. Many are asymptomatic. Fatigue and exertional dyspnoea are the most common symptoms.

Closure of the defect is advised in those who have a significant left to right shunt.

Adults

Adults may present with dyspnoea, atrial arrhythmias, pulmonary hypertension or cardiac failure.

Age is not a contraindication to surgery but pulmonary hypertension associated with a small left to right shunt is a clear contraindication to surgery.

Surgical treatment

The defect is usually closed by direct suture, but a patch of pericardium or Dacron is required to close very large defects.

The operative mortality is 1 per cent.

Ventricular septal defect

Defects may occur anywhere in the ventricular septum, may be single or multiple, and may vary in size from the very small to the almost complete absence of the ventricular septum.

It is important to understand that the defect may occur as an isolated lesion (approximately 55 per cent) or associated with other malformations. This latter complex group will not be discussed.

Pathophysiology

The communication between the two ventricles results in a flow of blood from the left chamber to the right. The size of the shunt is related to the size of the defect.

The increased pulmonary blood flow leads to dyspnoea, recurrent pulmonary infections, pulmonary hypertension and cardiac failure.

Natural history

Defects show a tendency to close spontaneously. In about 40 per cent of those born with a ventricular septal defect it will have closed by three years of age.

Bacterial endocarditis is rare.

A large left to right shunt predisposes the patient to develop increased pulmonary vascular resistance and pulmonary hypertension, which tends to worsen as the patient gets older.

Surgical treatment

This is not advised in infancy unless very severe symptoms make it essential. Children with normal pulmonary artery pressures do not require surgery as the risk of endocarditis is small. Elective surgery is advised in children with large shunts. The defect is repaired with a patch. The operative mortality is 1 per cent.

Coarctation of the aorta (Fig. 31.6)

This is a narrowing of the aorta just distal to the origin of the left subclavian artery, which causes a high blood pressure in the cerebral circulation and the arms. The blood to the lower two-thirds of the body reaches it by way of a series of anastomotic channels, which run back into the aorta via the intercostal vessels.

Fig. 31.6 Coarctation of aorta. AO = aorta.

Surgical treatment *

The coarctation is exposed through a left thoracotomy incision. The narrowed segment is excised and the cut ends of the aorta are sutured together. A tube graft of Dacron is inserted if the ends will not come together.

The operative mortality is 6 per cent.

Pulmonary stenosis

There is a dome-like fusion of the cusps of the pulmonary valve with a central perforation often only 2–4 mm in diameter. The pressure in the right ventricle is increased and the pressure in the pulmonary artery is reduced. This leads to right ventricular hypertrophy, and eventually to right ventricular failure.

Surgical treatment

Open valvotomy—the commissures are incised to produce a complete opening of the valve.

The operative mortality is 1 per cent

Valvular aortic stenosis

Pathology

The thickened valve is usually bicuspid with a single fused commissure.

Pathophysiology—see Figure 31.13.

Surgical treatment

This is indicated when symptoms are confirmed by haemodynamic evidence of critical stenosis. The aorta is opened and the fused commis-

Fig. 31.7 (a) Tetralogy of Fallot. RA = right atrium RV = right ventricle PA = pulmonary artery LA = left atrium LV = left ventricle AO = aorta. (b) Blalock Taussig shunt. The left subclavian artery is anastomosed to the pulmonary artery. AO = aorta PA = pulmonary artery.

sure is incised. Follow-up studies suggest that most patients will require valve replacement in later life.

The operative mortality is 2 per cent.

Tetralogy of Fallot

The original description of the tetralogy included pulmonary stenosis, ventricular septal defect, dextroposition of the aorta, and right ventricular hypertrophy. The important features are illustrated in (Fig. 31.7a).

The obstruction caused by the pulmonary stenosis reduces the blood flow to the lungs, and thus the blood is shunted from the right ventricle through the ventricular septal defect to the left ventricle and into the aorta. The ingress of 'venous' blood to the aorta causes hypoxaemia and cyanosis.

Surgical treatment

Complete correction of the defect may not be possible in infants; temporary improvement may be produced by increasing the blood flow to the lungs. This is achieved by performing a Blalock Taussig shunt* (Fig. 31.7b).

Complete correction is achieved by relieving the obstruction to the pulmonary blood flow and closing the septal defect with a patch.

The operative mortality is 5 per cent.

Transposition of the great vessels

The great arteries arise from the anatomically inappropriate ventricles; the aorta from the right ventricle and the pulmonary artery from the left

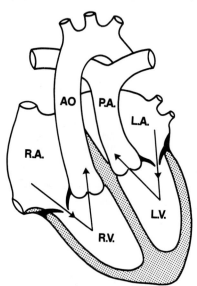

Fig. 31.8 Transposition of the great arteries, RA = right atrium RV = right ventricle AO = aorta LA = left atrium LV = left ventricle PA = pulmonary artery.

ventricle (Fig. 31.8). Thus venous blood enters the right ventricle and is then pumped into the aorta and systemic arteries causing hypoxaemia and cyanosis.

Surgical treatment

(a) *Palliation—balloon septostomy Rashkind procedure.* A special catheter is passed across the atrial septal defect. The balloon is inflated and pulled back into the right atrium. This enlarges the defect and improves mixing of arterial and venous blood.

(b) *Atrial correction—Mustards' technique.* The right atrium is opened and the atrial septum excised. A large patch of pericardium or Dacron is inserted so that oxygenated blood from the pulmonary veins is directed to the right ventricle and then pumped to the aorta; and the systemic venous blood directed into the left ventricle and pumped into the pulmonary artery.

The operative mortality is 9 per cent.

(c) *Anatomic correction.* In certain forms of transposition it is possible to perform an anatomic correction at the arterial level.

ACQUIRED HEART DISEASE

Mitral stenosis

Aetiology and pathology

Rheumatic valvulitis causes:
(a) Scarring, thickening and deformity of the valve cusps.
(b) Thickening and fusion of chorda tendinea.
(c) Calcification of cusps and chorda.

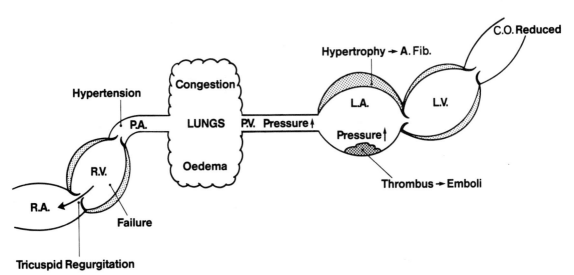

Fig. 31.9 Mitral stenosis—pathophysiology. LA = left atrium PV = pulmonary vein PA = pulmonary artery RV = right ventricle RA = right atrium A. Fib. = atrial fibrillation LV = left ventricle AO = aorta CO = cardiac output.

Pathophysiology

The left atrial pressure rises as the valve orifice becomes smaller, leading to a series of functional and structural changes illustrated in Figure 31.9.

Surgical treatment

A valvotomy is performed when the valve cusps are pliable and there is no significant regurgitation.

Closed valvotomy*. Exposure of the heart is by left thoracotomy. A finger is inserted into the left atrium through a small incision in the auricular appendage and a Tubbs' dilator is inserted into the left ventricle through a small incision in the left ventricular apex. The finger in the left atrium guides the tip of the dilator into the valve orifice and the fused cusps are separated by opening the dilator (Fig. 31.10).

Fig. 31.10 Closed mitral valvotomy. The surgeon's index finger is in the left auricle—the Tubbs' dilator through the apex of the left ventricle.

Open valvotomy. The left atrium is opened and the valve commissures are incised with a scalpel. Most surgeons prefer the open procedure as a more effective valvotomy can be performed, regurgitation can be recognised and corrected, and any thrombus present can be removed.

The operative mortality is 2 per cent.

Mitral regurgitation

Aetiology and pathology

Rheumatic valvulitis causes fibrosis, retraction and rigidity of the cusps, and fusion and shortening of the chorda tendinea and papillary muscles. Myocardial ischaemia may result in papillary muscle dysfunction. Bacterial endocarditis and chordal rupture are other causes.

Pathophysiology

Regurgitation of part of the left ventricle's blood volume into the left atrium raises left atrial pressure and reduces cardiac output (Fig. 31.11).

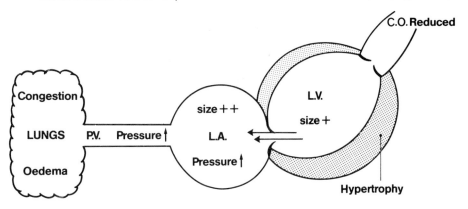

Fig. 31.11 Mitral regurgitation—pathophysiology. LA = left atrium LV = left ventricle PV = pulmonary vein AO = aorta CO = cardiac output.

Surgical treatment

(a) *Annuloplasty.* In a small select group of patients it is possible to remodel and narrow the mitral annulus. A Carpentier ring (Fig. 31.12) may be used.

The operative mortality is 4 per cent.

(b) *Valve replacement.* When the principal lesion is mitral regurgitation or if the mitral stenosis is not suitable for valvotomy, then the valve is excised and a new valve is inserted.

Fig. 31.12 Carpentier rings and valve sizers.

Aortic stenosis

Aetiology and pathology

  (a) Rheumatic valvulitis.
  (b) Congenital bicuspid valve.
  (c) Idiopathic calcification.
  The valve cusps are thickened and rigid and may eventually calcify. The valve orifice is narrowed.

Pathophysiology (Fig. 31.13)

Fig. 31.13 Aortic stenosis—pathophysiology. LA = left ventricle AO = aorta.

Surgical treatment

When angina pectoris, blackouts, or left ventricular failure occur, treatment should not be delayed.
  Valve replacement—the aorta is opened and the diseased valve excised and replaced by an artificial valve.
  The operative mortality is 5 per cent.

Aortic regurgitation

Aetiology and pathology

  (a) Rheumatic valvulitis causes fibrosis and retraction of the cusps.

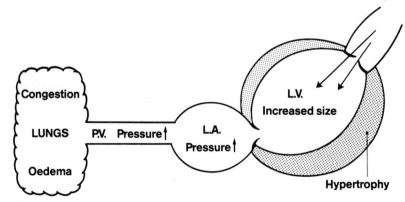

Fig. 31.14 Aortic regurgitation—pathophysiology. LA = left atrium PV = pulmonary vein.

(b) Bacterial endocarditis results in destruction or perforation of the cusps.

(c) Other causes include: dissecting aneurysm of the aorta and Marfan's syndrome.

Pathophysiology

The regurgitation of a large volume of blood from the aorta into the left ventricle leads to left ventricular dilatation and hypertrophy (Fig. 31.14).

Surgical treatment

Patients with aortic regurgitation remain asymptomatic for many years. Valve replacement (see Aortic stenosis) is indicated by the onset of symptoms.

Multi-valvular disease

Involvement of more than one valve is not uncommon, particularly in patients with rheumatic heart disease. Thus it may be necessary to replace both mitral and aortic valves.

The operative mortality is 10 per cent.

Tricuspid valve stenosis is sometimes associated with mitral and aortic valve disease and these patients require triple valve replacement.

The operative mortality is 20 per cent.

The increased risk of surgery is acceptable because otherwise these patients have a dismal prognosis.

Artificial cardiac valves

Two types are available:
1. Mechanical valves have an excellent record of durability but all are associated with the risk of thromboembolism. The three types caged ball, tilting disc and bileaflet, are illustrated in Figure 31.15.

| (a) | (b) | (c) |

Fig. 31.15 Mechanical valves. (a) Caged ball valve—Starr Edwards (b) Tilting disc—Bjork Shiley (c) Bileaflet—St. Jude.

2. Biological valves (tissue) were introduced in an effort to overcome the problem of thromboembolism. The long-term durability of these valves remains in question:
   (a) Homograft—a human aortic valve removed as soon as possible after death, sterilised and stored in a preservative solution.
   (b) Heterograft—an animal valve (porcine) which is sterilised, mounted on a frame and stored in glutaraldehyde (Fig. 31.16).

Fig. 31.16   Heterograft—animal valve—mounted on frame.

Endocarditis

This occurs in about 1 per cent of patients.

Early endocarditis. This is due to organisms introduced at the time of surgery or in the early postoperative period. Wound, respiratory and urinary tract infections, reoperation and contamination of intravascular catheters increase this risk. Prevention is the responsibility of all members of the caring team. The prognosis in early endocarditis is poor.

Late endocarditis. This results from transient bacteraemia which may be caused by genitourinary surgery, dental extractions and upper respiratory tract infections. It is essential that patients with artificial valves should have antibiotic prophylaxis if they are to undergo procedures known to predispose to endocarditis.

Thromboembolism

Thrombosis and subsequent thromboembolism is related to the artificial valve and sometimes to abnormalities of the cardiac chambers, e.g. atrial fibrillation.

Mechanical valves require long-term oral anticoagulants.

Biological valves require anticoagulation for twelve weeks. Patients with a predisposition to thromboembolism (large left atrium, atrial fibrillation, and those with preoperative thrombosis) require long-term anticoagulant therapy.

When non-cardiac surgery is indicated in patients with artificial valves who are receiving anticoagultants, the drugs can be stopped for three days with minimal risk to the patient. Heparin can be substituted for the oral anticoagulant in the immediate postoperative period.

Biological valves should be used in women in the child-bearing age who require valve replacement as there is a risk of fetal malformation due to the teratogenic effects of warfarin.

Angina pectoris

Stable angina is a condition in which chest pain 'with a sense of strangling and anxiety' is produced by exercise or emotion, and relieved rapidly by rest.

Unstable angina—severe prolonged episodes of angina which occur at rest or with minimal exercise.

Aetiology and pathology

Atherosclerotic coronary stenosis is the commonest cause of angina pectoris. The stenosis restricts blood flow to the affected coronary artery resulting in myocardial ischaemia and hypoxia.

Surgical treatment

This is indicated when unacceptable limiting angina is not relieved by medical therapy.

Selective coronary arteriography provides an assesment of the site and severity of stenoses. Luminal obstructions of 70 per cent or greater indicate the need for bypass operation.

Aorto-coronary saphenous vein bypass—a length of saphenous vein is removed from the leg. The vein is reversed and anastomosed proximal to the aorta and distal to the coronary artery beyond the stenosis.

The operative mortality is 1–2 per cent.

Internal mammary coronary artery anastomosis—the internal mammary artery (usually the left) is dissected from the posterior aspect of the sternum and its distal end is anastomosed to the coronary artery (usually the left anterior descending). The operative mortality if 1–2 per cent.

Relief of angina

Sixty per cent of patients report complete relief of symptoms and a further 25–30 per cent experience a substantial reduction in the frequency and severity of their symptoms.

Effect on survival

Surgical treatment improves survival in patients with left main coronary artery disease. Randomised trials have shown that life is also prolonged in patients with three vessel (left anterior descending, right coronary artery and circumflex) disease. Survival is also improved in patients with two vessel disease, in whom the stenosis of the left anterior descending artery is proximal to the first diagonal branch.

Fig. 31.17 Percutaneous transluminal coronary angioplasty.
  (a) Catheter approaching lesion
  (b) Balloon straddling lesion
  (c) Balloon inflated
  (d) Stenosis abolished.

Percutaneous transluminal coronary angioplasty

A small group of patients, whose symptoms make them candidates for coronary bypass surgery, can be treated by this technique. A special catheter incorporating a balloon (Fig. 31.17a) is introduced under local anaesthetic. It is passed into the diseased coronary artery so that the balloon straddles the stenosis (Fig. 31.17b). The atherosclerotic lesion is disrupted by inflating the balloon (Fig. 31.17c) and the stenosis is abolished (Fig. 31.17d). The mortality is 0.5–1 per cent.

Thoracic aneurysms

Fusiform or saccular aneurysms may involve the ascending, transverse arch or descending thoracic aorta; the latter two being the more common.

Aetiology and pathology

Arteriosclerosis, cystic medionecrosis or syphilis lead to weakening of the aortic wall.

Surgical treatment

Aortography is essential for the precise definition of the site and size of the aneurysm. The aneurysm is excised and a Dacron tube graft is inserted. The surgical approach is dictated by the site of the aneurysm. The operative mortality is 20 per cent.

Fig. 31.18 Aortic dissection. (a) Proximal or ascending (b) Distal or descending.

Aortic dissection

A tear in the intima of the aorta allows blood to enter the aortic wall. The arterial pressure forces the blood inwards separating the layers of the aorta for variable distances.

Aetiology and classification

A dissection is an acute spontaneous event and an exact cause is usually not discovered. It is associated with hypertension and left ventricular hypertrophy.

In about 60 per cent of patients the intimal tear is located in the ascending aorta just distal to the aortic valve (Fig. 31.18a); in a further 30 per cent the tear is located just beyond the left subclavian artery (Fig. 31.18b).

Treatment

Relief of pain and reduction of systolic blood pressure are the basis of emergency treatment. Once the patient has been stablised definitive diagnosis by aortography is essential.

Surgical treatment

The aorta is opened, the tear excised and the region of the false lumen is obliterated. Aortic continuity is restored by direct suture or by inserting a Dacron graft.

Chronic constrictive pericarditis

The thickened pericardium and its inflammatory exudate encase the heart and impede the relaxation of the ventricles.

Aetiology and pathology

Almost any form of acute pericarditis may result in chronic pericarditis. Despite the most careful investigation the aetiological agent is not identified in over 50 per cent of patients.

The patient presents with signs of right heart failure, i.e. raised venous pressure, ascites, hepatomegaly and oedema. Cardiac output is reduced.

Surgical treatment

Pericardiectomy is the only definitive treatment. The thickened pericardium and exudate which prevent ventricular relaxation must be completely excised.

CARDIAC PACEMAKERS

Types of pacemakers

The type of pacemaker is best indicated using the three-letter identification code (Fig. 31.19) suggested by the Inter-Society Commission for Heart Disease Resource. To assist the student the older terminology is translated into the three code system in Figure 31.20.

1st letter— chamber paced	2nd letter— chamber sensed	3rd letter— mode of response
V, A, or D	V, A, D, or O	I, T, D, or O
V = ventricle	A = atrium	D = Double (both atrium & ventricle)

O = No sensing function or not applicable
I = Inhibited (output blocked by sensed signal)
T = Triggered (output discharged by sensed signal)

Fig. 31.19 Three letter identification code.

Three-letter code	Description	Old terminology
V O O	Ventricular pacing No sensing	Fixed rate
V V T	Ventricular pacing & sensing Triggered mode	R. synchronas demand
V V I	Ventricular pacing & sensing Inhibited mode	Demand R. Inhibited

Fig. 31.20 Pacemaker identification—new and old codes.

Temporary pacing

Indications:
1. Complete heart block.
2. Myocardial infarction.
3. Arrhythmias.
4. Cardiac surgery.

Transvenous (endocardial)

An electrode is inserted through a vein and passed into the right atrium or right ventricle.

Trans-thoracic (myocardial)

Leads may be inserted in cardiac surgical patients before the wound is closed. One lead is attached to the base of the atrial appendage, and two to the ventricular myocardium. These leads are usually effective for only a few days.

Fig. 31.21 External pacemaker.

An external pacemaker (Fig. 31.21) may be used in VOO/AOO or VVI/AAI modes.

The patient must be protected from electromagnetic interference as temporary systems are much more vulnerable than permanent implants.

Permanent pacing

Indications:

Bradycardia—
1. Acquired atrioventricular block
2. Congenital atrioventricular block
3. Sinus node dysfunction (sick sinus syndrome)
4. Atrial fibrillation with ventricular bradycardia.

Tachycardia—certain forms of tachycardia will respond to pacing techniques. The techniques may be summarised as follows—

(a) Over-drive suppression—the faster the pacing the less heart tissue is excitable and capable of generating premature beats.

(b) Under-drive termination—fixed rate stimulation at less than the arrhythmia rate which by chance produces an appropriately timed stimulus to interrupt the rhythm.

(c) Programme—by trial and error the precise termination point is found and then through a memory process the termination stimulus is delivered at the effective point.

Method of insertion

Permanent pacing may be achieved by transvenous (epicardial) or transthoracic (myocardial) electrode placement. The transthoracic approach requires a thoracotomy for lead attachment, and, therefore, the transvenous route is preferred because it is associated with a lower morbidity and mortality.

The pacemaker pocket

The pacemaker (Fig. 31.22) is usually placed in the upper part of the chest wall, below the junction of the inner and middle third of the clavicle. The procedure is performed under a local anaesthetic.

Fig. 31.22 Implantable pacemaker.

Transvenous electrode

The cephalic vein is the preferred site of insertion. The electrode is inserted under fluroscopic and electrocardiographic control.

The introducer technique

The introducer technique is now used with greater frequency. A needle is inserted into the subclavian vein and a guide-wire is passed through the needle and positioned in the superior vena cava under fluroscopic control. The needle is withdrawn and a sheath and dilator is passed over the guide-wire. The guide-wire is removed and the electrode is passed through the sheath.

Complications

Epicardial. Early postoperative complications are usually those associated with a thoracotomy.

Transvenous (endocardial). Infection, phlebitis or haematoma may occur at the site of the venous cut-down. The electrode may perforate the myocardium causing tamponade, or allow stimulation of extra-cardiac structures such as the diaphragm. Thrombosis associated with the electrode may give rise to pulmonary emboli.

A wide variety of *arrhythmias* may complicate the insertion of any type of pacemaker.

Failure may present as a cessation of pacing, aberrant stimulation, or change in timing characteristics. Failure may be due to:

(a) Failure of the battery
(b) Fracture of an electrode
(c) Displacement of an electrode
(d) Increase in pacing threshold.

Pacemaker clinic

Regular checks for the patient and the electronic device are essential. This is best achieved by a special Pacemaker Clinic which is fully equipped to assess pacemaker function. In such a setting the goals of maximum pacemaker longevity, minimum surgical procedures and maximum patient safety can be achieved. Early pacemakers can be suppressed by non-cardiac energy resources, e.g. hair dryers and electronic drills. The modern pacemaker is protected by shields and filters and the sensitivity to electromagnetic interference has been markedly reduced.

POSTOPERATIVE CARE FOLLOWING CARDIOPULMONARY BYPASS

The patient will return to a specialised cardiac surgical intensive care unit. Electrocardiogram, blood pressure, central venous pressure and skin temperature are constantly monitored and electronically displayed.

Pericardial and mediastinal drainage tubes are connected to a calibrated collecting system and blood loss is recorded every fifteen minutes. Excess blood loss may be due to technical surgical factors or clotting difficulties. Treatment is directed to eliminating or correcting the cause.

Serial measurements of haematocrit, serum electrolytes and arterial blood gases are performed. Cardiac isoenzymes, serum urea and creatinine are measured daily.

Renal function

A urinary catheter is attached to a calibrated collecting system and urine output is recorded hourly. Nephrotoxic drugs should be discontinued when renal function is impaired and many other drugs will require appropriate revision of dosage. Peritoneal dialysis is required if the patient is aneuric; hypercalcaemia and acidosis may indicate urgent dialysis. Haemodialysis is employed if peritoneal dialysis is ineffective. Renal failure after open-heart surgery is associated with a high mortality.

Cardiovascular system

Cardiac output is normal when it supplies the metabolic needs of the body. A Swan-ganz catheter is inserted if arterial pressure, skin temperature and urine flow indicate reduced cardiac output, and cardiac output is estimated using the thermo-dilution technique. Early recognition and treatment of low cardiac output is essential as it is the most frequent cause of postoperative death. Low cardiac output may be due to:

1. Hypovolaemia
2. Cardiac tamponade (compression of the heart by blood in the pericardial cavity).
3. Reduced myocardial contractility resulting from:
   (a) Inadequate intraoperative myocardial protection
   (b) Acute myocardial infarction
   (c) Preoperative left ventricular dysfunction
   (d) Hypoxaemia
   (e) Acid-base imbalance.

Treatment is directed to eliminating or correcting the cause. Inotropic drugs such as dopamine, isoproterenol and dobutamine are the first line of defence when cardiac output is reduced because of depressed myocardial contractility. These drugs are delivered with the assistance of a continuous battery powered infusion pump. Intra-aortic balloon counterpulsation is instituted if the inotropic drugs fail to improve cardiac output.

Arrhythmias

Cardiac arrhythmias may complicate the patient's recovery. The most frequently encountered arrhythmias and an outline of the approach to their treatment is provided in Figure 31.23.

Arrhythmias	Treatment
Premature ventricular contraction	(a) Potassium supplement if serum potassium is reduced (b) Xylocaine (c) Pacing
Atrial fibrillation	(a) Digoxin (b) Cardioversion
Atrial flutter	(a) Cardioversion (b) Digoxin
Atrioventricular block	Pacing

Fig. 31.23 Commonest postoperative arrhythmias.

The respiratory system

A chest X-ray is taken and arterial blood gases estimated when the patient is admitted to the Unit. The endotracheal tube is removed when the patient is alert and has an adequate cough reflex. Patients require adequate analgesia to control pain and permit effective coughing and deep breathing. The nurse and physiotherapist help and encourage the patient with deep breathing and coughing. Sputum is checked daily and frequent cultures are made to permit the early recognition of any infection.

Intermittent Positive Pressure Ventilation (IPPV). Some patients require prolonged intermittent positive pressure ventilation to achieve satisfactory gas exchange. The gases must be warmed and humidified. Frequent percussion of the chest wall and aspiration of the endotracheal tube after forceful use of the Ambu bag are essential to clear tracheobronchial secretions. The patient is turned at regular intervals.

Central nervous system

Damage to the nervous system is the most feared complication after cardiac surgery. Age, and the presence of preoperative neurological dysfunction, indicate an increased risk. Importance of perfusion technique and the use of arterial blood filters have significantly reduced their incidence.

THE SCOPE OF CARDIAC SURGERY

Surgical correction of most of the serious congenital and acquired heart lesions is now possible. The patient is usually returned to a useful and active life.

BIBLIOGRAPHY

Braimbridge M V 1981 Post-operative cardiac intensive care. Blackwell Scientific Publications, Oxford

Neutze J M, Moller C T, Harris E A, Horsburgh M P, Wilson M D 1982 Intensive care of the heart and lungs—A text for nurses and other staff. Blackwell Scientific Publications, Oxford

Underhill S L, Woods S L, Sivarajan E S, Halpenny C J 1982 Cardiac Nursing. Lippincott, Philadelphia

32

Diseases of the oesophagus

ANATOMY

The oesophagus is a hollow, muscular tube which extends from the cricopharyngeus muscle in the neck, at the level of the sixth cervical vertebra, through the posterior mediastinum and oesophageal hiatus in the diaphragm to the stomach. (There is, therefore, a short length of cervical oesophagus and a short length of intra-abdominal oesophagus.) Most of the organ, however, lies within the thoracic cavity, running down behind the trachea, heart and pericardium. The aortic arch crosses it to the left in the mid-thoracic region. Behind the oesophagus lie the thoracic vertebra in the upper part and the descending aorta in its lower part (Fig. 32.1).

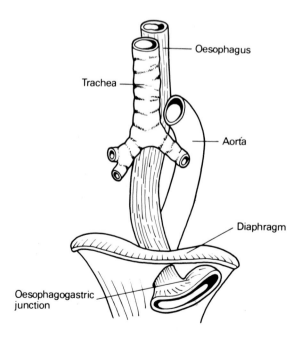

Fig. 32.1 Anatomy of the oesophagus.

The oesophagus receives its arterial blood supply from branches of the inferior thyroid artery in the neck, from branches of the aorta in the thorax and from branches of the left gastric artery below the diaphragm. Venous drainage mirrors the arterial supply to a large extent. There are, however, numerous communications between the venous plexuses throughout the oesophagus and these are important in the development of oesophageal varices (Ch. 36). The veins draining the thoracic part of the oesophagus to the azygos veins communicate freely with those draining the intra-abdominal oesophagus to the portal system. Lymphatic drainage is to the glands in the neck, the central glands in the mediastinum and the coeliac glands below the diaphragm. Again, there are extensive communications between the lymphatic channels.

PHYSIOLOGY

The oesophagus is not an inert tube, but is a physiological organ and disturbances in the nervous mechanism controlling it can result in distressing symptoms. Parasympathetic control is through the vagus nerves and sympathetic from the thoracic sympathetic chain. The oesophagus has a physiological sphincter at both upper and lower ends which is under nervous control. Their relaxation is controlled during the act of swallowing and after the bolus of food has passed they regain their tone, preventing reflux and regurgitation of the swallowed food. As the muscles of the pharynx contract on swallowing, the upper sphincter relaxes to allow the food through and then contracts again. A peristaltic wave passes down the oesophagus, taking the bolus with it. Immediately prior to the arrival of the peristaltic wave at the lower oesophageal sphincter, the sphincter relaxes and opens the way for the food to enter the stomach. It then closes again, preventing reflux of gastric contents into the oesophagus. Disturbances of this finely coordinated mechanism, as occurs in, for example, achalasia and hiatus hernia, can result in serious difficulties of swallowing (dysphagia).

Investigation

   1. Radiology. Screening of the oesophagus on swallowing barium suspension can give much information on the movements of the oesophagus and will also demonstrate the presence of tumours, strictures and foreign bodies. If a perforation is suspected, a water soluble contrast medium (e.g. Gastrografin) is normally used since this is absorbed from the tissues into which the medium might escape.

   2. Oesophagoscopy. This can be done under either general or local anaesthesia depending on the preference of the patient and the endoscopist. It can also be done with the larger rigid metal oesophagoscope or the flexible fibre-optic instrument. The rigid oesophagoscope allows for better suction, removal of food debris and larger biopsy. The flexible instrument (Fig. 35.1) is less bulky to pass and probably give better views of the intra-abdominal oesophagus and the junction with the stomach. In addition, it can be passed on in to the stomach and duodenum for examination of these areas if this is indicated.

3. Manometry. If a soft, fine bore catheter is passed into the oesophagus and connected to a pressure transducer, the pressure within the lumen of the oesophagus at different levels can be measured and a pressure trace produced on paper. There is a normal 'pressure profile' for the oesophagus which demonstrates the presence and position of the upper and lower sphincters and which records the contraction and relaxation in these sphincters and in the remainder of the oesophagus as the peristaltic wave passes down in response to swallowing. Certain abnormalities in this pressure profile have been recognised in different disease states and these characteristic abnormalities are sometimes diagnostic in difficult cases when radiology and oesophagoscopy are negative.

HIATUS HERNIA

A hiatus hernia is a hernia of the stomach through the oesophageal opening (hiatus) in the diaphragm.

There are two main types of hiatus hernia:
1. Sliding (Fig. 32.2),
2. Rolling (or para-oesophageal Fig. 32.4).
A combination of the two can occur.

Many people have a hiatus hernia and are either unaware of it or have few or no symptoms.

1. SLIDING HIATUS HERNIA (Fig. 32.2)

This is by far the commonest type comprising 85 to 90 per cent of all hiatus

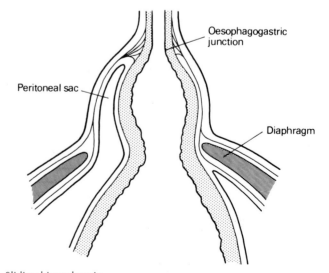

Fig. 32.2 Sliding hiatus hernia.

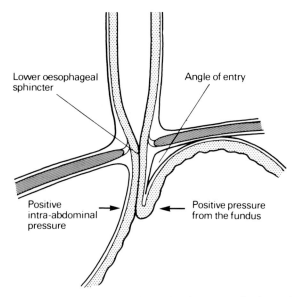

Fig. 32.3 Normal control of gastro-oesophageal reflux. Control is lost in hiatus hernia.

herniae. The essential problem in sliding hiatus hernia is that the mechanism preventing reflux of gastric contents into the oesophagus breaks down. The normal control is illustrated in Figure 32.3. Food can be regurgitated into the mouth and the oesophageal mucosa is bathed in acid secretions. The symptoms of sliding hiatus hernia result either from this gastro-oesophageal reflux, or from impaction of the hernia in the oesophageal hiatus. Inflammation of the oesophageal mucosa gives rise to the pain of heartburn or oesophageal spasm. Healing of the inflammation can result in scarring of the oesophagus which may eventually produce a stricture. Dysphagia may be due to either oesophageal spasm, stricture formation or impaction of the hernia.

Investigation

1. Barium swallow and meal will, in most cases, demonstrate the presence of the hernia and of any gastro-oesophageal reflux, although small hernias can be difficult to demonstrate. The location and severity of any associated stricture will also be shown.

2. Oesophagoscopy is necessary to determine the degree of inflammation of the oesophageal mucosa (oesophagitis) and to assess any stricture present.

3. Manometry can be helpful in patients with persistent symptoms and negative barium studies and oesophagoscopy.

Treatment

Many patients will require no treatment because they have few or no symptoms. If symptoms are present, medical treatment should normally be tried in the first place. Medical treatment consists of three basic components:

1. Weight reduction. Many patients will find that their symptoms are completely relieved simply by losing weight. This takes the pressure off the abdomen and allows the herniated stomach to fall back into place.

2. Posture. Since the symptoms of reflux are frequently made worse by lying down or bending over, patients should be advised to avoid sleeping flat and stooping. The head of the bed should be raised on blocks or at least the patient should be supported with several pillows.

3. Drugs. Numerous drugs have been used to alleviate the symptoms of reflux and these fall into three broad categories:

(a) antacids which neutralise the gastric acid,

(b) drugs which form a bland neutral layer on top of the gastric contents so that when reflux occurs it is this bland, non-irritating fluid which is refluxed and

(c) drugs which reduce the acid-secretion of the stomach. None of these drugs will do anything to relieve symptoms of regurgitation or impaction of the hernia, but they do help to relieve acid heartburn and may reduce the degree of oesophagitis. They do, of course, have to be continued indefinitely.

4. Other measures which are of value are to stop smoking, to avoid wearing tight garments, to eat smaller meals and to avoid eating and drinking before going to bed.

Surgery

Surgery is indicated in the following circumstances:

1. Patients in whom the above medical treatment has failed to relieve distressing symptoms.
2. Patients who either cannot or will not accept medical treatment indefinitely and who have significant symptoms.
3. Patients who have developed complications of hiatus hernia, e.g. stricture.

The hiatus can be approached either from below the diaphragm through an abdominal incision, or from above the diaphragm by thoracotomy. The advantages of the thoracic approach are better exposure of the region of the hiatus and, more importantly, it is possible by this approach to mobilise the oesophagus, to free it from its adhesions and thus to carry out a repair which is devoid of tension. As oesophagitis develops, the oesophagus usually becomes thicker and shorter and mobilisation, therefore, becomes increasingly important to obtain a tension-free repair. A number of operations have been described for the repair of hiatus hernia and all the successful ones have the aim of reducing the hernia, restoring the intra-abdominal segment of the oesophagus and the lower oesophageal sphincter to their normal positions below the diaphragm, and to recreate the angle of entry of the oesophagus into the stomach. When these have been achieved, the margins of the hiatus are narrowed down around the oesophagus.

Postoperative care

Following thoracotomy, the patient will have an intercostal drain which should be connected to an underwater seal drainage bottle and left unclamped on open drainage. This is usually removed after 24 to 48 hours. A nasogastric tube is usually unnecessary and the patient is allowed small amounts of fluid the day after operation, progressing over the next few days to free fluids, semi-solids and a normal diet. Chest physiotherapy is important to prevent respiratory infections and early mobilisation is encouraged. Pain should be relieved by analgesics, initially by intra-muscular injections and later by oral administration. The patient is normally discharged from hospital between 10 and 14 days after operation.

Management of peptic stricture

Peptic stricture is a late complication of reflux oesophagitis. Persistent inflammation leads to the formation of scar tissue in the oesophageal mucosa and wall. The patient usually gives a history of hiatus hernia for several years with the onset of slowly progressive dysphagia. The condition has to be distinguished from carcinoma of the oesophagus and this is done on the basis of the clinical history, barium examination and oesophagoscopy. There are three ways of dealing with the problem:

1. Repeated oesophagoscopy and dilatation. This is usually reserved for elderly and infirm patients who are not considered suitable for major surgery.

2. Repair of the hiatus hernia with one or two dilatations. This method of treatment is only suitable if the stricture is still relatively soft and easily dilated. In this situation, repairing the hernia and stopping the acid reflux can prevent the stricture progressing and one or two dilatations are sufficient to open up the way through.

3. Resection of the stricture and replacement of the removed oesophagus with a segment of colon. Alternatively, the whole oesophagus can be removed and the stomach brought up through the chest to the neck and anastomosed to the cervical oesophagus. Both these operations give good relief of dysphagia.

ROLLING (PARA-OESOPHAGEAL) HIATUS HERNIA (Fig. 32.4)

Although this type of hiatus hernia occurs through the same opening in the diaphragm as the sliding variety, the symptoms and complications of the two conditions are completely different. The intra-abdominal segment of the oesophagus retains its proper position below the diaphragm and gastro-oesophageal reflux does not occur. The hernial sac is present in front of the oesophagus and through this the fundus of the stomach enters the chest. As the hernia enlarges, the greater curvature of the stomach also rolls up into the chest and may take with it the greater omentum and the transverse colon.

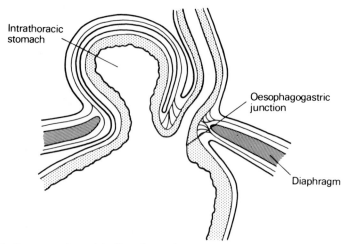

Fig. 32.4 Para-oesophageal (rolling) hiatus hernia.

Symptoms

Because gastro-oesophageal reflux does not occur, the symptoms are not those of reflux oesophagitis. In fact, there may be few symptoms associated with this type of hernia though if they do occur they may consist of vague indigestion and discomfort in the epigastrium after meals. Patients may also complain of retrosternal or chest pain, and nausea and vomiting. The complications of this type of hernia are serious and can be life threatening. Bleeding is common and may take the form either of chronic blood loss, leading to an iron deficiency anaemia, or haematemesis of sufficient severity to require blood transfusion. The contents of the hernia are liable to the same complications as, for instance, an inguinal hernia. The stomach may become twisted (volvulus) and this can lead to strangulation. Other abdominal viscera pulled up into the chest may become incarcerated and obstructed.

Treatment

There is no useful medical treatment for rolling hiatus hernia. Since gastro-oesophageal reflux does not occur, the medical measures advocated for sliding hiatus hernia are ineffective. Elderly or infirm patients with few symptoms are usually left alone without treatment. However, because of the risk of serious complications, the patient with a rolling type of hernia is normally recommended to have a surgical repair. The preparation of these patients for operation and their post-operative care is similar to that for a sliding hernia. The actual operative technique differs only a little.

ACHALASIA

The word achalasia means 'failure to relax' and the disease is so called because the main problem is a failure of the lower oesophageal sphincter to relax on swallowing. This normally relaxes to meet a peristaltic wave carrying a bolus of food down the oesophagus. In achalasia, the sphincter remains in tone so that when the bolus of food reaches it, it remains closed and forms a functional obstruction to the passage of food. The condition can occur at any age and its cause is not known for certain. Examination of the oesophagus shows degeneration of the nerve cells and plexuses in the wall of the oesophagus which coordinate the movements of the oesophagus. The muscular wall of the oesophagus usually becomes hypertrophied and thickened in an attempt to overcome the obstruction at the lower end, but the wall gradually becomes weaker and weaker and the oesophagus dilates until it is no more than an inert, thin-walled tube containing a great deal of fluid and food residue (Fig. 32.5).

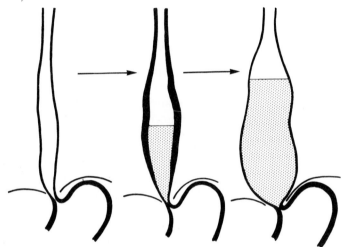

Fig. 32.5   Achalasia. Progression of changes in oesophagus.

Symptoms

The principal symptom is dysphagia which usually comes on slowly but the patient may complain of a sudden onset of symptoms after an emotional shock. The food tends to stick behind the lower sternum and the patient has trouble with both fluids and solids. The patient may experience retrosternal pain after eating caused by incoordinated spasms of the oesophagus. As the oesophagus dilates and fills with fluid and food, the patient may complain of regurgitation particularly on lying flat or bending over. Sometimes the oesophageal contents are aspirated into the trachea causing respiratory symptoms. Weight loss is common and may be severe.

Investigation

The X-ray appearances on barium examination are typical with a dilated oesophagus narrowing down to a taper point at its lower end. Even air has difficulty in passing into the stomach and the gastric bubble is frequently absent.

Oesophagoscopy is not usually necessary to establish the diagnosis, but is usually done to exclude other diseases such as carcinoma and to clean out the oesophagus before operation.

The muscular disorder in the oesophagus in achalasia can be clearly demonstrated by oesophageal manometry and this is a useful method of confirming the diagnosis.

Treatment

There are no drugs of value in the treatment of achalasia and patients are usually managed either by intra-luminal dilatation of the lower oesophageal sphincter, or by operation. Dilatation is frequently followed by recurrence of the achalasia and is accompanied by a certain risk of perforation. Surgery is, therefore, generally preferred.

Operation

Prior to operation, the patient should be kept on a liquid diet for 48 hours and the oesophagus emptied by a large bore nasogastric tube the night before and morning of surgery. Surgery is carried out through a left thoracotomy and the operation of choice is a Heller's myotomy. This consists of a vertical incision dividing the circular muscle at the lower end of the oesophagus rather like a Ramstedt's operation for pyloric stenosis (Fig. 32.6). The muscle is divided down to the mucosa which is allowed to pout through. The encircling fibres are thereby divided and the efficiency of the lower oesophageal sphincter is destroyed. This interference with the lower oesophageal sphincter will usually result in postoperative reflux of gastric secretions into the oesophagus unless an anti-reflux operation is carried out at the same time. Therefore a repair of the hiatus hernia is usually combined with the Heller's myotomy.

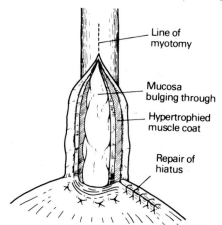

Line of myotomy

Mucosa bulging through

Hypertrophied muscle coat

Repair of hiatus

Fig. 32.6 Heller's myotomy for achalasia with repair of hiatus hernia.

Postoperative care

An intercostal tube will be in place and this should be connected to an underwater seal drainage bottle. The tube can usually be removed 24 to 48 hours after operation. Oral fluids can often be commenced the day after operation with progression to semi-solids and a solid diet over the following 5 to 7 days. Dysphagia is usually markedly improved but may never be quite normal again due to the generalised muscular incoordination and weakness of the remainder of the oesophagus.

CARCINOMA OF THE OESOPHAGUS

Carcinoma of the oesophagus is a condition more common in men than women, which presents more frequently in later life. Its cause is unknown. The incidence and sex distribution of the disease varies considerably in different parts of the world, and dietary factors have been implicated. Certain disorders, such as achalasia, the Plummer-Vinson syndrome and caustic burns of the oesophagus, are associated with a higher incidence of the disease.

Pathology

Most of the tumours are squamous cell carcinomas, but some of those arising near the oesophago-gastric junction are adeno-carcinomas. Tumours can occur in any part of the oesophagus but are most common in the lower third. Tumours spread by direct invasion of surrounding structures. to the lymph glands in the neck, the mediastinum and along the course of the left gastric artery to the coeliac axis. Widespread dissemination of the disease can occur through the blood stream, particularly to the liver.

Symptoms

A carcinoma is usually present in the oesophagus for some time before it produces symptoms and it is this early latent period which hinders successful treatment. The main symptom is dysphagia which is experienced at first with certain types of solid food, but is steadily progressive until the patient has difficulty even with liquids. The poor dietary intake is associated with weight loss and bleeding may also occur.

Investigation

A barium swallow will demonstrate the presence of an obstructive carcinoma. The lesion can then be visualised at oesophagoscopy and a biopsy taken. A liver scan is sometimes helpful in determining whether spread has occurred to the liver. Oesophageal manometry has no place in the diagnosis of malignant tumours of the oesophagus.

Treatment

Surgical resection offers the only real prospect for cure in the present state of knowledge. In addition, removal of the tumour is often the best form of palliative treatment and the patients are able to eat and swallow their own saliva until they die. If the tumour is not removable or if widespread metastases are present and the patient is not expected to live for more than a few weeks, palliation is obtained by the insertion of an indwelling tube through the growth (Fig. 32.7).

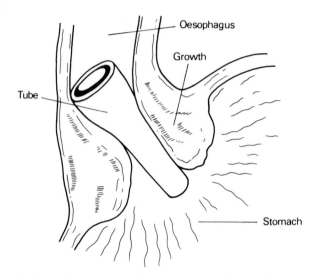

Fig. 32.7   Indwelling tube for inoperable carcinoma of the oesophago-gastric junction.

Preoperative preparation

Many patients with carcinoma of the oesophagus are in a poor nutritional state with disturbances of fluid and electrolyte balance. These should be corrected with a nourishing fluid diet, or, if necessary, with intravenous fluids. Anaemia, if present, should be corrected and vigorous chest physiotherapy commenced, since many patients have poor respiratory function and may even have developed areas of aspiration pneumonitis due to tipping over of fluid from the obstructed oesophagus into the bronchial tree.

Operation

The amount of oesophagus and stomach removed will depend on the location of the tumour. For tumours in the lower third of the oesophagus, the whole of the oesophagus below the tumour plus approximately 5 cm above the upper limit of the tumour together with the upper third of the stomach, the spleen and the associated lymph glands will be removed (Fig. 32.8). A similar amount of oesophagus, but less stomach is removed for tumours of the middle third. Almost the entire oesophagus is removed for tumours of the upper third of the oesophagus within the chest. Continuity is restored by anastomosing the cut end of the oesophagus to the remaining portion of the stomach which is brought up through the hiatus into the chest. For tumours of the upper third of the

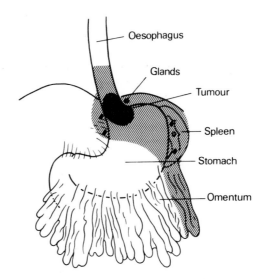

Fig. 32.8 Oesophagogastrectomy for carcinoma. Extent of resection.

oesophagus, this anastomosis will usually be in the neck to the cervical oesophagus.

The incision used will vary with the preference of the surgeon. For tumours at the lower end of the oesophagus, most surgeons will use a left thoraco-abdominal incision extending from the chest across the costal margin on to the left upper abdomen (Fig. 32.9). When the ribs are spread and the costal margin and diaphragm divided, an excellent exposure is obtained of the whole region. For tumours higher in the oesophagus, resection can be carried out through an extension of this incision on the left side together with a separate cervical incision if necessary. However many surgeons prefer the Ivor Lewis procedure in which an incision is first made in the abdomen to mobilise the stomach and when this has been closed the patient is turned on the left side and an incision is made in the right chest for resection of the tumour and construction of the anastomosis. Since the vagus nerves are necessarily divided during the resection, a drainage procedure is frequently carried out on the pylorus to prevent gastric stasis. A formal pyloroplasty may be done or a more simple pyloromyotomy with division of the encircling muscle layer.

Umbilicus

Costal margin

Fig. 32.9 Thoraco-abdominal incision for oesophagogastrectomy.

Postoperative care

An intercostal drain will be present and this should be connected to an underwater seal drainage bottle. A nasogastric tube will be left in the stomach and this is aspirated at hourly intervals. The nasogastric tube should be treated with great care; it will have been carefully placed in position at operation and if it becomes dislodged will need to be passed again blindly with the risk of pushing it through the newly constructed anastomosis. The tube should therefore be securely taped to the patient's nose and great care exercised in handling it. The amount of aspirate usually diminishes over the first 3 to 4 days after which the tube can be removed. The incision is a painful one and regular analgesia is required postoperatively. Chest physiotherapy is of considerable import-ance, particularly since many of the patients are elderly and have poor respiratory function.

The patient is allowed nothing by mouth for several days after opera-tion. The normal period is 4 days, after which the patient is allowed small amounts of clear fluid and if this is tolerated he will progress to free fluids, a sloppy diet and solid food over the next 5 or 6 days. During the period of nothing by mouth, fluid and electrolyte balance is maintained by an intravenous drip.

Sutures are removed after 10 days and the patient is usually able to return home 2 weeks after operation by which time he should be able to manage a reasonable diet. However, because of the reduction in the size of the stomach, many patients find that they cannot eat normal quantities of food and they should be encouraged instead to eat smaller amounts more frequently. The mechanisms which normally prevent reflux of gastric contents into the oesophagus have been removed at operation, and patients are likely, therefore, to complain of regurgitation or vomit-ing on lying flat. These symptoms can usually be controlled if the patient sleeps propped up on several pillows.

Results of surgery

Patients with adeno-carcinoma do less well than those with squamous cell carcinoma, and patients with squamous growths in the upper and mid-oesophagus do less well than patients with squamous growths at the lower end. In the majority of patients, surgery is purely palliative and allows them to eat and swallow their own saliva. Only 10 to 15 per cent of patients live for 5 years or more after resection. These results are poor and are not likely to improve until either earlier diagnosis can be made, or alternative forms of treatment are discovered. Irradiation is sometimes combined with surgery but generally speaking irradiation is ineffective in the treatment of oesophageal carcinoma. However, tumours of the upper oesophagus, particulary the cervical oesophagus, do very poorly with surgery and many people consider that irradiation should be the first line of treatment for tumours situated in this region. Chemotherapy has little place at the moment in management of carcinoma of the oesophagus, but drugs and different combinations of drugs are being developed all the time and it is likely that improvements in this form of treatment will be made in the next few years.

Palliative intubation

Several different kinds of tubes have been manufactured for the pallia-tive treatment of carcinoma of the oesophagus in patients considered unsuitable for resection. Some of these can be inserted from above through an oesophagoscope, but others require a laparotomy and opening of the stomach to pull the tube through and fix it in position.

The most commonly used tubes which are inserted through a laparoto-my are the Mousseau-Barbin tube and the Celestin tube. The stomach is opened through a short incision and the tube is fed down from above by the anaesthetist and pulled through the growth by the surgeon, so that its upper wide mouth lies above the tumour. The lower end is cut short by the surgeon and fixed to the side wall of the stomach. The stomach is then closed and the wound repaired.

Patients are normally able to take fluids 48 hours after such a procedure and progress quite quickly to a sloppy type of diet. More solid food can be taken provided the patient chews it well and washes it down frequently with a fizzy drink. The tube can become blocked by food or by the growth growing up and around the orifice. Displacement can also occur as well as ulceration of the lining of the oesophagus or stomach by the edge of the tube. Generally speaking, however, these types of tubes provide a reasonable palliation for the short length of time the patient survives.

FOREIGN BODIES

Foreign bodies can become lodged in the oesophagus at any age, but are more common in children and in elderly people with either no teeth or poorly fitting dentures. The object may lodge in the oesophagus, either because of its bulk or because of a pathological narrowing of the oesophagus itself. In the normal oesophagus there are three narrowed areas: at the cricopharyngeus, the arch of the aorta and the diaphragm. Pathological narrowing is usually due to a peptic stricture but may be due to a carcinoma.

The patient will often complain of pain in the chest and an inability to swallow either solids or fluid. Perforation of the oesophagus may occur with all the serious complications associated with this. Plain P.A. and lateral X-rays should be done together with a gastrografin swallow to localise the foreign body and identify any leak from the oesophagus.

Management

If a foreign body has lodged in the region of the cricopharyngeus there may be associated respiratory obstruction. A child should be tipped head down and given a sharp blow between the shoulder blades. In the adult, a similar blow may dislodge the foreign body but failing this the patient should be grasped from behind with the arms encircling the lower chest and the hands gripped together in the epigastrium. A sudden bearhug in this situation is often effective in dislodging the foreign body. There is no urgency usually about removing foreign bodies further down the oesophagus. This is done at oesophagoscopy under general anaesthesia.

Perforation of the oesophagus by a foreign body is a serious complication. After removal of the foreign body, the patient is turned on the side and through a thoracotomy the hole in the oesophagus is repaired. Mediastinitis and infection of the pleural space develop very rapidly after perforation of the oesophagus and treatment is urgent. Without treatment, the patient invariably dies and if treatment is delayed recovery is, at the best, prolonged and complicated.

PERFORATION OF THE OESOPHAGUS

Aetiology

1. Instrumental. Perforation of the oesophagus is not uncommon after oesophagoscopy, particularly if this is done inexpertly or with undue force. A tear may occur in the cervical oesophagus in trying to pass the instrument through the cricopharyngeus muscle. Lower down the oesophagus, perforation is usually due to either inexpert dilatation of a stricture or carcinoma, or to an unduly generous biopsy.

2. Foreign body. A sharp foreign body can perforate the oesophagus at any level but is more likely to do so at the three narrowed regions of the oesophagus, as described under 'Foreign bodies'.

3. Spontaneous. Perforation of the oesophagus can occur spontaneously during violent vomiting, particularly after a heavy meal or excessive alcohol intake. A tear develops usually in the lower third of the oesophagus on the left hand side, but may occur in the mid oesophagus on the right side.

Consequences of perforation

(a) Cervical perforation. Air escapes into the tissues of the neck giving rise to surgical emphysema. If the condition is untreated, an abscess will subsequently develop in the neck.

(b) Intra-thoracic perforation. Air escapes into the mediastinum and pleural space. The air can track up the mediastinum into the neck and again produce surgical emphysema. Air in the pleural space results in a pneumothorax. The communication between the oesophagus and the mediastinum and pleural space allows infection to develop and mediastinitis and empyema ensue (Fig. 32.10). If the patient has vomited on a full stomach, part of the vomit will find its way into the pleural cavity. The infection following this is particularly severe and rapidly developing. Untreated, the patient will die and the chances of the patient surviving are poor if the diagnosis is delayed for more than a few hours.

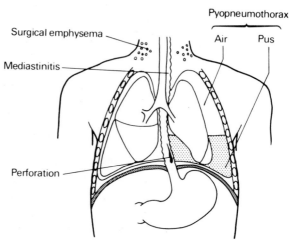

Fig. 32.10 Complications of perforated or ruptured oesophagus.

Management

(a) **Cervical perforation.** If recognised early, this type of perforation can usually be managed quite simply with antibiotics and nil by mouth for several days. Infection of the cervical spaces does not occur and the tear usually heals. If this condition is not recognised and an abscess develops, this will have to be drained.

(b) **Intra-thoracic perforation.** It is important that the condition is recognised quickly. Chest X-ray will show a pneumothorax and perhaps also a fluid level in the pleural cavity. A gastrografin swallow will demonstrate the site of the perforation.

An intercostal tube is inserted to relieve the pneumothorax and oesophagoscopy performed to carry out toilet of the oesophagus, to remove any foreign body and to verify the position of the perforation. Thoracotomy is performed immediately to drain the mediastinitis and empyema and to repair, if possible, the tear in the oesophagus. If surgery has been delayed by more than a few hours, the tissues of the oesophagus around the tear become very soft and will not hold sutures, in which case the best that can be done is to place a large drainage tube to the site of the perforation.

Postoperative recovery can be quick if surgery is carried out soon after the perforation, otherwise recovery is prolonged and it is several weeks before the perforation closes and the empyema settles down. Until the fistula is closed the patient is allowed nothing by mouth and is fed either intravenously or by gastrostomy or jejunostomy. If the perforation is associated with a stricture or tumour of the oesophagus, it is unlikely to close unless the obstruction is removed and this is usually done at the first operation if the patient's general condition permits.

OESOPHAGEAL ATRESIA

This is a congenital abnormality. The oesophagus ends blindly in the upper chest. Usually the lower end communicates normally with the stomach and has a proximal fistula into the trachea (Fig. 32.11). The baby is often born to a mother who has had hydramnios. The child is unable to swallow normally, continually dribbles mucus from its mouth and may have cyanotic attacks. If atresia is suspected no feed should be given, to prevent inhalation into the lungs. A soft radio-opaque catheter should be passed into the pharynx and if it will pass no further than 4 inches it is likely that the baby has an atresia. An X-ray, with the catheter in position, confirms the diagnosis. Until operation can be performed the baby should be nursed on its abdomen in the head-down position, but some believe that in order to prevent gastric juice entering the trachea the baby should be propped up and the mucus extractor should be taken on the journey to the hospital. The nasopharynx is aspirated and no feed of any kind given. An intravenous infusion is set up and blood cross-matched. At early operation, usually through a right thoracotomy, the fistula is closed. It may be possible to join the two ends of the oesophagus. If they are too far apart primary anastomosis may not be possible.

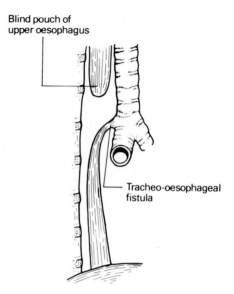

Blind pouch of
upper oesophagus

Tracheo-oesophageal
fistula

Fig. 32.11 Oesophageal atresia.

The upper pouch is brought out into the neck to allow saliva to dribble away and the baby is nourished through a gastrostomy tube. Later, when the baby is stronger (perhaps several months old) an isolated length of colon with its blood supply intact is passed up through the anterior mediastinum and is anastomosed to the oesophageal pouch above and to the stomach below.

33

Pathophysiology of the gastrointestinal tract

The surgical anatomy of the gastrointestinal tract is outlined in Figure 33.1. The liver and biliary apparatus on the one hand and the pancreas on the other develop as diverticula of the gastrointestinal tract to which they remain connected by the common bile duct and the pancreatic duct. Their external (exocrine) secretions are discharged into the second part of the duodenum, usually through a common opening guarded by the muscular sphincter of Oddi into the biliary papilla.

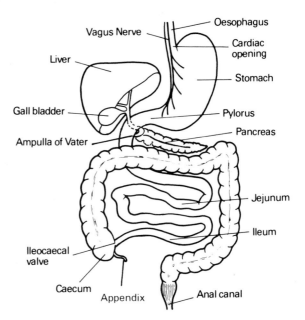

Fig. 33.1 Normal anatomy of the gastrointestinal tract.

The remainder of the gastrointestinal tract runs in continuity (apart from the appendix) from the cardiac sphincter of the stomach to the anal canal. The stomach with its thick muscular walls and deep mucosal lining is in continuity with the oesophagus. The cardiac sphincter prevents the reflux into the oesophagus of acid and pepsin which are secreted in the cells of the fundus and body of the stomach. The pyloric antrum which is not acid-secreting leads to the pyloric canal which is guarded by the pyloric sphincter—the distal opening being the pylorus. The rich blood supply comes from the coeliac axis and the venous drainage is ultimately to the portal vein. The nerve supply is from the vagus nerves and the sympathetic plexus.

The small intestine consists of the C-shaped duodenum, the jejunum and lower small intestine, known as the ileum. The last part of the ileum is the narrowest portion of the bowel and enters the caecum through the ileo caecal valve. The total length of the small intestine is about 3.6 to 3.9 m (10 to 11 feet); the older estimates of 23 feet which were made on postmortem specimens are now thought to be erroneous. The jejunum accounts for about 60 per cent of the total length, the ileum about 40 per cent. The duodenum receives chyme, acid and pepsin from the stomach, through the pylorus, and bile and pancreatic juice through the biliary papilla. Digestion and absorption take place predominantly in the jejunum. The products absorbed ultimately enter the portal circulation.

The large intestine from the caecum to the rectum is about 121 cms (4.5 feet) in length, the rectum 11.25 cm (5 inches) and the anal canal 4.75 cm (1.5 inches).

The functioning of the gastrointestinal tract is under nervous and hormonal control. The complex churning movements of the stomach mix the food and prepare the mixture for the duodenal action of enzymes. They are secreted in an alkaline medium which neutralises the acid chyme from the stomach. Peristalsis is the characteristic movement of the small intestine and reflex mass peristalsis occurs once or twice daily in the large intestine.

The hormonal control of secretions is shown in Figure 33.2.

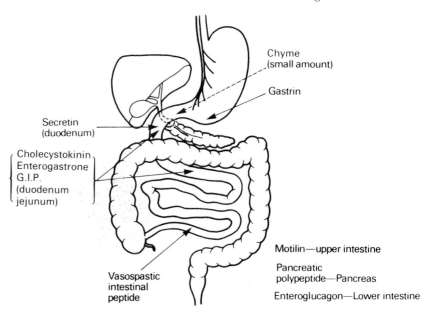

Fig. 33.2 Sites of origin of gastrointestinal hormones (G.I.P. now stands for glucose dependent insulin releasing peptide).

Acid pepsin

Acid pepsin secretion is stimulated by:

1. Vagal action. The cephalic phase of secretion in which the thought and taste of food initiate the stimulus.

2. Gastrin—a hormone secreted into the blood from the pyloric antrum which continues the second phase of the secretion of acid and enzymes; it is released by the presence of food in the stomach and intestine, some foods being more potent stimulants than others.

The stomach takes minutes to fill with food but hours (3 to 6) to empty. The trickle of chyme which occurs through the pylorus stimulates the release of hormones in the duodenum. As the pyloric sphincter relaxes a little bile enters the stomach and can be detected in gastric juice of all patients in which the pyloric canal is not obstructed.

The duodenal hormones

Those released are:

1. Secretin which stimulates the flow of pancreatic juice containing the powerful enzymes which digest protein, fat and carbohydrates. It also diminishes the secretion of gastric juice.

2. Cholecystokinin, which is secreted in response to the presence of fatty food in the duodenum. It relaxes the sphincter of Oddi and contracts the gall-bladder, which discharges its bile (concentrated 50 times) into the common bile duct and thence into the duodenum.

3. Enterogastrone, which diminishes gastric secretion and gastric emptying.

The small intestine secretes intestinal juice (succus entericus) but it is weak in enzymes and comparatively unimportant in digestion.

Digestion of food into aminoacids, glucose and fatty acid is virtually completed in the jejunum and absorption which begins in the duodenum is almost entirely completed in the jejunum. The ileal contents are almost entirely a fluid faecal residue but the terminal ileum is the area for the absorption of vitamin B_{12} and of bile salts.

The colon removes water and salts from the residue to produce semi-solid faeces but it should be noted that the majority of the body's water is *absorbed from the small intestine.*

Vasospastic intestinal peptide (V.I.P.)

This occurs in the nerve plexus of the small and large intestine. It is believed to control blood flow, secretion, and motility in the intestine. Oversecretion of the hormone may produce the clinical syndrome W.D.H.A. (Watery Diarrhorea, Hypokalaemia and Achlorhydria). Such excessive production may result from a tumour of the islet-cells of the pancreas.

Gastric inhibiting peptide (G.I.P.)

This is secreted in the mucosa of the small intestine and was originally thought to inhibit gastric acid secretion. Subsequent work has shown that its physiological action is to stimulate the release of insulin when glucose is taken by mouth. However it retains the initials G.I.P. which now stand for glucose-dependent insulin-releasing peptide.

Three other peptides have been identified in the gastrointestinal tract, pancreatic polypeptide, motilin secreted in the upper small intestine and enteroglucagon secreted in the lower intestine. The action of these hormones is undecided.

PATHOPHYSIOLOGICAL CHANGES

Normal function is altered by the effects of disease or surgical intervention.

DISEASE

Mucosal damage

Lesions which result in extensive involvement of the mucous membrane result in loss of function. A carcinoma of the stomach destroys its power to secrete acid and enzymes while gastroenteritis not only prevents digestion and absorption but results in dehydration and loss of electrolytes. Extensive proctocolitis causes haemorrhage from ulceration, absorption of toxins occurs in the large areas of denuded mucosa and fluid loss may be considerable.

Perforation

This results in leakage of the contents. Outside the confines of the gastrointestinal tract all the contents are irritant and if not highly infected soon become so. The possible results are:

(a) **General peritoneal contamination** resulting in general peritonitis (Fig. 33.3). This is the usual result in peptic ulcer perforation and unless 'sealing' (described below) comes into play the same result is inevitable from perforation of the lower reaches of the gastrointestinal tract. Widespread paralysis of the bowel results and bacterial infection causes death if the condition is unrelieved.

(b) **Sealing by omentum or adjacent bowel** may occur. This gives rise to an abscess which localises the disease and may result in resolution, or it may require drainage.

(c) **Fistula formation.** A gastric ulcer may perforate into the transverse colon giving rise to a gastro-colic fistula (Fig. 33.4B). Food passes undigested into the colon but more important is that colonic contents pass into the stomach and then circulate in the duodenum and small intestine causing severe infection which is life threatening. Another very dangerous fistula is where the diseased colon forms a fistula with the bladder (Fig. 33.4C). Infected flatus causes a urinary infection and the symptom of pneumaturia (gas in the urine). The other fistula which may

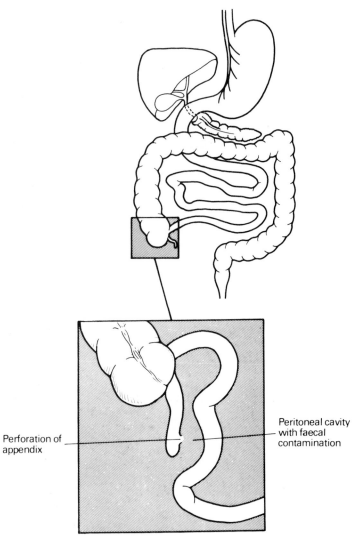

Perforation of appendix

Peritoneal cavity with faecal contamination

Fig. 33.3 Perforation of the appendix causes faecal peritonitis.

develop is one between the fundus of the gall bladder and the duodenum (Fig. 33.4A). This causes no trouble in itself since bile is still delivered where it is required, namely into the duodenum, but a gallstone, if present, is passed into the gut—if it is large then it lodges in the lumen of the terminal ileum (the narrowest portion of the bowel). An acute intestinal obstruction results.

Obstruction

Figure 33.5 illustrates the effects of obstruction. Common to all obstructive lesions are:
  (a) dilatation of the segment above, accumulation of secretions, reverse flow and stagnation with resultant infection.
  (b) collapse and loss of function beyond the site of obstruction.

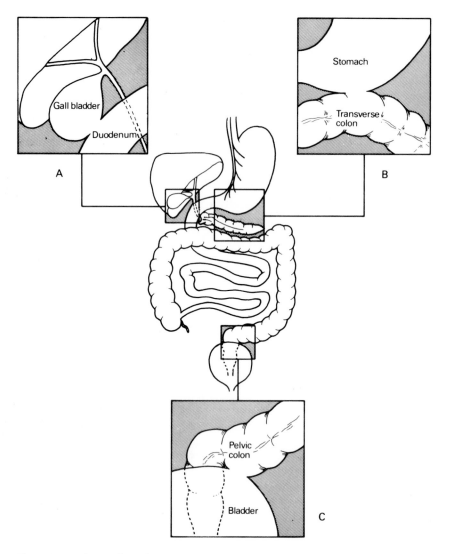

Fig. 33.4 Fistulas involving the gastrointestinal tract: A. Gall bladder to duodenum. B. Stomach to colon. C. Colon to the bladder.

The common sites of obstructions are:

(a) **The pyloric end of the stomach.** The stomach is dilated, filled with fluid and food (consumed perhaps days before). Bile is absent in the secretion. The patient is unable to eat, vomits copiously and, therefore, loses weight, becomes dehydrated and goes into electrolyte imbalance. Since no chyme passes to the duodenum there is weight loss from lack of nutrition.

(b) **The small intestine.** The great volume of material in the jejunum— chyme from the stomach, bile, pancreatic and intestinal juices well up. The bowel dilates, the contents regurgitate into the stomach and are vomited. It is important to note that because the contents are vomited abdominal distension is *minimal*. Gross dehydration and electrolyte imbalance result.

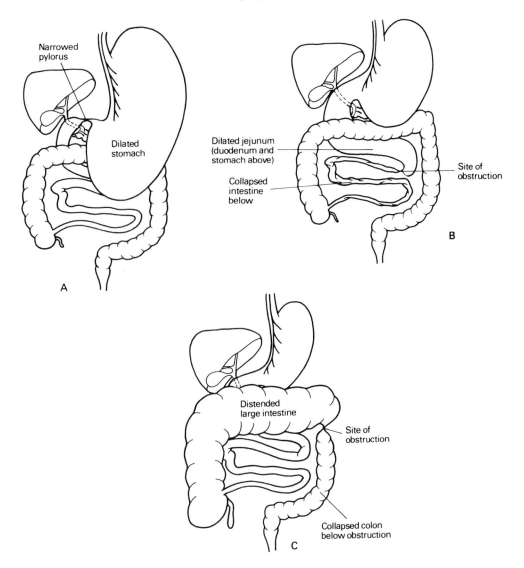

Fig. 33.5 Obstruction in the gastrointestinal tract: A. Pyloric stenosis. B. Small bowel obstruction. C. Large bowel obstruction.

(c) The large intestine. The large intestine contains much less fluid than the small intestine but a large quantity of gas which, denied exit, causes enormous abdominal distension. The dominant symptom is the inability to pass this flatus as well as faeces. Regurgitation of the large bowel contents into the ileum occurs only minimally and at a very late stage. Therefore, vomiting, so marked in small bowel obstruction, is rare in obstruction of the large intestine.

(d) The biliary tract. Figures 36.4 and 36.5 show the sites of obstruction.

(i) The cystic duct. A stone impacted in the cystic duct prevents the gall bladder emptying into or filling from the common bile duct. The gall bladder, as in all obstructions, distends and the retained contents become infected. Jaundice does not develop because bile from the liver

can still flow along the common bile duct into the duodenum and digestion is unaffected.

(ii) The common bile duct may be blocked by a stone or neoplasm. The whole duct system into the liver is dilated. Jaundice develops and if unrelieved deepens each day. Because bile is absent from the intestine the faeces are pale. Bile pigments are excreted in the urine. Retained bile salts cause pruritus of the skin. Infection (cholangitis) is heralded by the onset of rigors. Unrelieved the bile escretion by the liver ceases but mucus secretion continues (white bile).

(e) Pancreatic obstruction alone will cause steatorrhea.

SURGICAL INTERVENTION

All surgical intervention in the gastrointestinal tract, with the exception of appendicectomy, may cause physiological changes. Some are relatively mild and well within the powers of the body to compensate, others are more profound. The principal operations are:

Vagotomy

Total or truncal vagotomy diminishes:
   (a) Gastric secretion—the beneficial effect.
   (b) The motility of the stomach so that it distends and cannot empty adequately. A pyloroplasty or gastrojejunostomy is necessary to ensure it drains.

The effect on the intestine is variable. A significant proportion of patients have a more frequent bowel action but a small number suffer from attacks of uncontrollable diarrhoea.

The purpose of the more selective vagotomies (Ch. 35 and Fig. 35.4) is to cause the inhibition of gastric secretion without the undesirable side effects.

Gastrectomy

The various forms of gastrectomy are shown in Figure 35.5. The most physiological is a Billroth I in which the stomach is rejoined to the duodenum. Even in this case more rapid emptying of the stomach may occur in the absence of a pyloric sphincter.

The effects of a Polya gastrectomy are:
   (a) The absence of a reservoir—'dumping into the jejunum' en mass.
   (b) Food may empty into the efferent loop before bile or pancreatic juice mix with it with the result that digestion is inadequate.
   (c) Bile may rush into the stomach instead of into the efferent loop, the stomach is irritated and bile may be vomited separately from food.
   (d) The efferent loop may be obstructed.
   (e) Loss of intrinsic factor from the stomach and rapid passage of intestinal content may prevent absorption of vitamin B_{12} with resulting macrocytic anaemia. Poor absorption of iron may cause microcytic anaemia.

The results will be undernourishment, loss of weight, anaemia, vitamin deficiency, and the danger of reactivation of a healed tuberculous lesion in the lung.

Enterectomy

Resection of moderate lengths of the small intestine produces very little physiological change but loss in excess of 75 per cent may cause rapid transit of intestinal content, diarrhoea and malabsorption. Extensive resection of the ileum may result in megaloblastic anaemia from failure to absorb vitamin B_{12}. Bile salts are absorbed in the terminal ileum and if not absorbed may irritate the colon with resultant diarrhoea.

Colonic resection

Total colectomy results in a semi-fluid continuous motion through an ileostomy but digestion and absorption are unaffected. Right hemicolectomy (Fig. 39.5) may cause more frequent bowel action partly because the faeces are less solid and partly from the reduced ability to reabsorb bile salts as the terminal ileum is resected as part of the operation.

Cholecystectomy

This causes no significant changes—bile still flows into the duodenum.

Pancreatectomy

Total pancreatectomy produces diabetes and insulin replacement is required. The absence of pancreatic secretion causes steatorrhoea as well as diminished digestion and absorption.

Shortcircuiting (by-pass) procedures

Most by-pass operations produce significant changes. A gastrojejunostomy may occasionally give rise to syndromes similar to those which occur following gastrectomy. If the upper jejunum is by-passed malabsorption may develop and by-passing the terminal ileum may cause vitamin B_{12} deficiency. One risk of all by-pass procedures is that a 'blind' loop may be left in which stasis occurs. Infection of the contents occurs, fouls the intestine and gives rise to malabsorption. Surgical correction is necessary.

34

The acute abdomen

Nowhere is surgical progress more obvious than in the management of the acute abdomen. Before the turn of the century surgical intervention was rare (although Lawson Tait performed the first successful appendicectomy in 1880). For the first half of this century it was well recognised that the progress of the primary condition had to be halted without delay before the secondary manifestations of shock, dehydration and toxaemia overwhelmed the patient making spontaneous recovery unlikely. Operation was undertaken with the least possible delay, anaesthesia by modern standards was poor and antibacterial substances were unknown. Dehydration and electrolyte imbalance was not corrected and the value of nasogastric suction was not recognised.

The progress of the primary condition has still to be halted by operation without unnecessary delay but it is now recognised that the dangerous secondary manifestations can be largely avoided by preoperative corrective treatment. If they are, the chances of a successful outcome are greatly increased. Because of the fear that operation may be delayed even a few hours all analgesics were forbidden until the operating surgeon saw the patient. Nowadays an analgesic, the dosage of which is measured against the severity of the patient's pain, is given by the first doctor to see the patient. It enables the patient to give a coherent history, local tenderness may be even easier to detect and a mass, if present, is more easily palpable than in an abdomen with extreme rigidity.

All acute abdominal catastrophes can be resolved into three groups:

1. Peritonitis.
2. Intestinal obstruction.
3. Intra-abdominal haemorrhage. (This forms a small group of which the symptoms and signs are those of peritonitis in addition to those of internal haemorrhage.)

    These conditions almost invariably require emergency operation for their relief. The problem, however, is not as simple as that because many other conditions cause acute abdominal pain. The differentiation of those which require operation from those which do not is of vital importance.

The most important of these lesions which do not require operation are:

1. The colics
    (a) Intestinal—gastroenteritis ⎤
    (b) Ureteric (p. 493)   ⎬ Rarely require urgent operation.
    (c) Biliary (p. 425)   ⎦

2. Extra-abdominal causes of abdominal pain
    (a) Pleurisy and pneumonia ⎤
    (b) Coronary thrombosis
    (c) Spinal lesions
    (d) Uraemia
    (e) Certain blood diseases ⎬ Operation harmful and unnecessary.
    (f) Arteriosclerosis
    (g) Diabetic hyperglycaemia
    (h) Herpes zoster
    (i) Porphyria ⎦

ACUTE PERITONITIS

The peritoneum is a continuous, thin, shiny, avascular membrane which lines the abdominal cavity. The portion behind the muscles of the anterior abdominal wall and in front of those on the posterior abdominal wall is known as the parietal peritoneum and is richly endowed with nerve endings. Irritation of this portion of the peritoneum gives rise to pain at the site at which it is stimulated.

The visceral peritoneum is the portion which is reflected to envelop most of the abdominal organs. It forms the outer or serous coat of organs like the stomach and the intestines. It has few nerve endings and is almost insensitive.

The peritoneal cavity (Fig. 34.1), which is the space between the parietal and visceral layers, contain a fine film of sterile fluid. Infection or inflammation of this cavity is known as peritonitis. Peritonitis may affect part or all of the peritoneal cavity (producing local peritonitis or general peritonitis).

General causes

The general causes of peritonitis are:
    1. Blood-borne (rare).
    2. Penetrating wounds.
    3. Closed abdominal injury—causing rupture of an organ (e.g. spleen, liver, gut).
    4. Inflammation of an organ—local peritonitis (e.g. appendicitis, cholecystitis).
    5. Escape of gastrointestinal contents or contents of another organ— general peritonitis (e.g. perforated peptic ulcer, ruptured gall bladder, ruptured ovarian cyst).

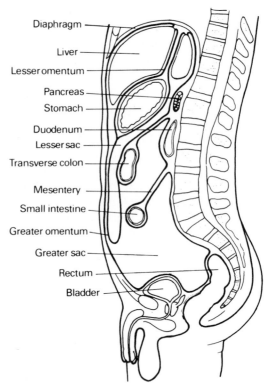

Fig. 34.1 The peritoneal cavity.

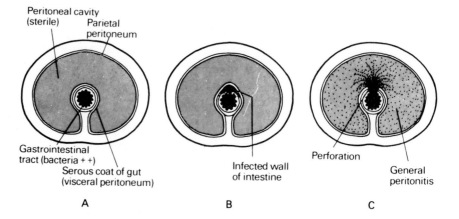

Fig. 34.2 The mechanism of peritonitis.
(A) Healthy peritoneal cavity.
(B) Infected wall of bowel, bacteria spreading in the wall.
(C) Perforation of gastrointestinal contents into peritoneal cavity.

The last is much the most frequent cause. If the gastrointestinal tract is healthy its irritant and infected contents make no contact with the peritoneal cavity, from which they are protected by the mucus, muscular and serous coats of the stomach or intestine. If a portion of these organs becomes diseased and their walls infected this infection may spread to the serous covering coat which becomes inflamed (Fig. 34.2B). The serous covering coat is part of the visceral peritoneum. If this is inflamed it irritates the adjoining parietal peritoneum and pain is felt at the spot where this is inflamed. This is known as a local peritonitis.

If the disease progresses and the organ ruptures the infected contents leak into the peritoneal cavity and a general peritonitis has developed (Fig. 34.2C). The peritoneum responds in the ordinary way to inflammation, including an enormous outpouring of fluid. The infection can be overcome provided the supply of toxic material from the gastrointestinal tract is sealed off.

If it is not, the result is:
1. Widespread absorption of toxins.
2. Paralysis of the intestines. Nature tries to limit the out-pouring of septic contents by rest.

Specific causes

The commonest causes (Fig. 34.3) of general peritonitis are:
1. Perforated acute appendicitis.
2. Perforated gastric or duodenal ulcer.
3. Perforated diverticulitis.
4. Acute pancreatitis.
5. Rupture of the intestine, the rectum, or the bladder secondary to inflammation, trauma, obstruction, neoplasm.
6. Ruptured ovarian cyst. Rupture of the uterus or Fallopian tubes.
7. Ruptured spleen or liver—closed abdominal trauma.
8. Abdominal wounds penetrating the peritoneal cavity.
9. Haematogenous (blood-borne) infection.

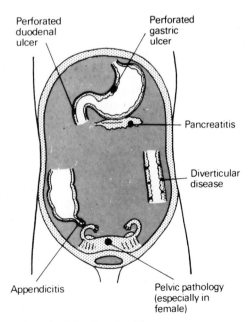

Fig. 34.3 Common sites of origin of peritonitis.

Investigations

The nature and extent of investigation will vary with the condition of the patient, whether the underlying cause of the condition can be readily diagnosed clinically and whether the investigations will add any information which will assist in management of the patient. Investigations considered necessary are ordered in the admission room, specimens are taken and if the patient is to be X-rayed this is done before admission to a ward bed so that unnecessary movement is avoided. Routine examination of the urine is mandatory. Other investigations which may be ordered are:

1. Radiography of the chest and abdomen. These X-rays must be taken not only with the patient supine but also with the patient erect (or sitting). If this position is too painful then a lateral shoot-through X-ray must be taken. This is so that any gas free in the peritoneal cavity will be seen just under the diaphragm or under the anterior abdominal wall. X-rays will be inspected for the presence of free gas in the peritoneal cavity, dilated loops of bowel, urinary calculi or gall-stones.

2. Laboratory examination of the urine for the presence of red blood cells and pus, which may be seen in the presence of ureteric stones or in a urinary infection, and to exclude diabetes.

3. Serum amylase, which is raised in acute pancreatitis.

4. Serum electrolytes, which are particularly liable to be disturbed in vomiting.

5. Electrocardiograph and an estimation of the serum transaminase to exclude coronary infarction as a cause of abdominal pain.

6. A white blood cell count.

7. Blood for haemoglobin and for grouping and cross matching.

8. Peritoneal aspiration may reveal the presence of bile, pus or blood. This may be done with a syringe and needle or a peritoneal cannula.

Treatment

The principles of treatment are:

1. To terminate, if possible, lesions which threaten to cause general peritonitis before this becomes established.

2. To treat shock. The fluid loss is mainly plasma, water and electrolytes. These are replaced intravenously.

3. To rest the gastrointestinal tract—food and purgatives are forbidden and aspiration of the stomach contents is undertaken.

4. To counteract infection. All patients apart from those with recently perforated peptic ulcer are candidates for bacteraemia. Treatment with gentamicin and intravenous metronidazole should be commenced before operation.

5. To cut off the source of irritant or infection e.g. suture of a perforation or removal of a perforated appendix.

6. To cleanse or drain the peritoneum of septic contents and pus. This involves not only sucking out pus at operation but also intraperitoneal lavage with saline so that all pus, faecal material and fibrin are removed. A long vertical incision may be necessary to do this.

Clinical features of peritonitis

In the pages which follow the clinical features and management of peritonitis are discussed. Acute appendicitis is taken as an example not only because it is fairly common but the course it may follow illustrates:

1. The importance of removing a potential cause of peritonitis.
2. The nature in which the disease may be localised.
3. That diffuse peritonitis results if it perforates and contaminates the peritoneal cavity. The faecal peritonitis which results is identical to that caused by any lesion in which the bowel perforates. The basic management, complications and high mortality are the same.

ACUTE APPENDICITIS

The cause

The cause is unknown. Infection commences in the appendix. It may be blood-borne or arise because the lumen of the appendix is blocked by, for example, a faecolith. This prevents the drainage of mucus and pus into the caecum. The organ may dilate and burst (perforate), with leakage of faecal material into the peritoneal cavity. In a smaller percentage of older patients the obstruction of the appendix may be due to a carcinoma of the caecum. Rarer causes are a carcinoid tumour or matted worms.

The course of the disease

Without treatment the disease may take several courses:

1. Resolution may occur.
2. A localised mass or abscess may form.
3. General peritonitis may develop.

If the attack subsides, recurrence is likely. Early in the attack no one can forecast with certainty how it will progress and, for this reason, the wisest course is to remove the appendix before peritonitis has had time to develop. In children and the very old resolution is less likely to occur, while progress of the disease is often more rapid.

Early symptoms and signs of acute appendicitis

Sudden colicky pain around the umbilicus is the first symptom (Fig. 34.4). The patient is frequently awakened with pain which comes on in attacks lasting a minute or two. It increases in severity, then passes off completely, only to recur. Vomiting may occur with considerable relief, but as the hours pass by the attacks of pain become more frequent and more severe. Later, the pain settles in the right iliac fossa, where it is no longer intermittent but constant in type. It is sharp and aggravated by movement. This is local peritonitic pain. The temperature may be normal or slightly raised (37.2°C; 99°F), and the pulse rate shows a slight increase. The tongue is usually furred but moist, and no flatus is passed per rectum from the commencement of the attack.

Should the appendix be pelvic in position, diarrhoea may be present, and if it is adjacent to the bladder frequency of micturition may occur.

On examination the abdomen is tender, with muscle guarding in the right iliac fossa, but elsewhere it is soft and painless. Digital examination of the rectum may reveal tenderness on the right side of the pelvis.

Fig. 34.4 The pain of acute appendicitis is first felt around the umbilicus and later settles over the appendix.

The clinical features of appendicitis with established peritonitis

The symptoms become more severe and the general condition of the patient deteriorates. The pain is constant and severe in the right iliac fossa, but it may ease suddenly when the appendix perforates, only to return over the whole abdomen. Rigidity and tenderness are widespread, and vomiting is frequent and profuse. Movement aggravates the pain.

As the patient becomes weaker from lack of sleep, toxaemia and fluid and electrolyte disturbances, the pain and rigidity give way to painless distension of the abdomen. Diarrhoea may be profuse.

The general appearance, so typical of late peritonitis, sets in. The face is shrivelled and flushed, but the eyes are glistening and bright. The mind is usually clear, but at this stage the patient is frequently too weak to give a coherent account of his illness. The result is that it may be impossible to decide with certainty the cause of his peritonitis. The temperature is always raised (38° to 39°C; 100° to 102°F) and the pulse is rapid, irregular, and of poor volume. This very serious clinical state should be avoided nowadays by the early treatment of conditions likely to lead to general peritonitis and the immediate treatment of the latter once it is recognised.

Appendix mass

An attack of appendicitis may terminate in the formation of a localised mass in which may form an abscess. The surrounding coils of small intestine and omentum are bound together around the caecum and appendix by a fibrinous exudate. This is nature's way of localising the disease. This inflammatory mass may gradually resolve spontaneously.

Alternatively, if the appendix perforates, instead of contaminating the whole of the peritoneal cavity, the infection is limited to the area around the appendix by the greater omentum and small intestine. This, in turn, may resolve or enlarge and leak into the general peritoneal cavity. In cases where a mass is present, and also in cases of over 48 hours' duration which appear to be subsiding, it is sometimes decided to observe the patient but to operate at once should their condition deteriorate. The method of observation usually used is known as the Ochsner-Sherren regime.

The Ochsner-Sherren regime

This method should be carried out only in the hospital, so that operation can be undertaken at once if it is considered necessary. It is a technique of observation of an acute attack and not a radical cure. The appendix will usually be removed after the attack has subsided:

1. Sedatives or analgesics are usually unnecessary at rest. The size of the swelling in the right iliac fossa should be observed and its limits marked on the skin of the abdominal wall so that increase or diminution in size can be detected.

2. The patient is nursed in whatever position he is most comfortable.

3. Vomiting or pain is reported at once.

4. Only sips of water are allowed by mouth for 48 hours. Fluid and electrolyte balance is maintained by intravenous infusion.

5. The mouth is rinsed out frequently and the teeth kept clean.

6. A fluid balance chart is kept.

7. The pulse is charted hourly and the temperature two hourly for the first 12 hours. After this time a four-hourly pulse and temperature reading is substituted, so as to diminish the disturbance which hourly readings would cause to the patient.

Treatment of acute appendicitis

The most satisfactory case to treat is one in which the appendix is removed early in the attack. The convalescence is almost invariably smooth, and restoration of the patient to health is rapid. An oblique incision in the right iliac fossa is used, splitting (not cutting) the muscles to gain access to the peritoneum. The stitches are removed between 5 and 7 days.

If general peritonitis is present, removal of the appendix and peritoneal toilet are performed. A drain may be inserted. If a large abscess is present drainage only may be undertaken leaving the appendix to be removed 3 to 6 months later.

Preparation of the patient with an acute abdomen for operation

This is similar to the preparation of a patient for any abdominal operation but as the time is limited the approach must be orderly so that nothing essential is omitted. Many of these patients are admitted in the small hours of the morning when the ward is relatively under-staffed.

When the patient is in bed and a final decision to operate has been made, the nature of his condition is explained and consent obtained and, if he desires it, a Minister of religion summoned. A patient may ask what will happen if he refuses operation and while this is something the medical staff must answer the nurse should bear in mind that in some conditions such as peptic perforation death is almost certain. In others, such as appendicitis which has not yet caused peritonitis, the mortality is 20 per cent if untreated so it is untruthful and foolish to say to the patient that unless he has an operation death is inevitable. The truthful answer is that at that stage no-one knows whether he is in the unfortunate 20 per cent or the 80 per cent who will recover.

ethics

An intravenous line is usually instituted and electrolyte imbalance if present is corrected. Further serum electrolyte estimations may be required. The blood haemoglobin is measured and blood cross-matched if necessary.

A nasogastric tube is passed, aspirated as often as ordered and left on free drainage into a bag. In acute intestinal obstruction the stomach may be refilled with fluid every few minutes. The nature and quantity of fluid aspirated is recorded.

The skin preparation. The supra pubic area and the abdominal wall is shaved, washed with 2 per cent hexachlorophane soap and water and dried. The whole area from the nipples to the knees is prepared. Sometimes a second abdominal incision may be necessary. On the other hand a very ill patient in severe pain is kept still and all skin preparation, including shaving, is left until he has been anaesthetised.

Antibiotics. In some diseases prophylactic antibiotics reduce the incidence of complications. Thus wound infection following acute appendicetomy is less common if metronidazole is administered, usually as a suppository (or intravenously), immediately before operation and eight-hourly thereafter for 24 hours. In patients with faecal peritonitis, antibiotics are part of the treatment, commencing just before or during operation and continuing for 2 to 5 days.

Premedication is given as ordered. In many cases the anaesthetist prefers to give it in the theatre.

The bladder is emptied and a further check is made that the urine has been examined and the results recorded.

Immediate preoperative ward preparation includes covering the patient's head with a disposable paper theatre cap and wrapping him in a theatre gown. The patient's identification label should be written out, checked, and attached to the wrist on admission. Dentures are removed and kept in a place of safety.

On the journey to the theatre. The patient is lifted carefully onto a trolley protected by warm blankets. On arrival at the theatre the ward blankets are changed for theatre blankets. A small bowl and the patient's case notes and radiographs are taken to the theatre.

After the operation the ward nurse returns to the theatre and accompanies the patient back to bed, keeping a careful watch for any change in colour and his breathing. She must see that the nature of the operation and any special instructions of the surgeon or anaesthetist are recorded and understood before she leaves.

Postoperative care

Once sufficient fluid is being taken orally the intravenous infusion is discontinued. Progress to a light diet is allowed as soon as it is tolerated. As soon as the patient recovers from the anaesthetic he should be allowed to assume whatever position he finds most comfortable. As soon as possible, and usually by the following day, he is mobilised.

Intravenous infusion. The type of fluid infused and the speed of infusion are as ordered by the medical staff. If the patient is suffering from established peritonitis intravenous fluid replacement is always necessary. Oral fluids are commenced as soon as the bowel sounds recover.

The patient with faecal peritonitis recovers more slowly. Intravenous nutrition is often needed. This should be considered in any event if oral nutrition cannot be recommenced within 2 or 3 days of operation.

Nasogastric tube. This should initially be left unspigotted on continuous drainage and aspirated hourly. The nature and quantity of fluid is recorded. Once the quantity of fluid diminishes and bowel sounds return, the tube is spigotted and aspirated less frequently (unless other instructions are given by the medical staff). The tube is usually removed fairly soon thereafter.

Antibiotics. If being used these are administered as prescribed.

Pain. Postoperative analgesics, usually morphia (10 mg) or pethidine (50 mg), are given regularly or as necessary to prevent or control pain.

The bowel. The passage of a flatus tube twice daily may prevent the usual 'distensive' pain of which many of these patients complain. About the third day a suppository is administered if the patient has not had a bowel action.

Drains. These are removed when ordered by the surgeon. They may need to be rotated and shortened a little each day to prevent one becoming adherent to a loop of intestine. Shortening is performed by cutting the external stitch, withdrawing the tube slightly, and transfixing the remainder with a sterile safety pin. Removal of a drain should be recorded.

Records
1. An hourly pulse for 12 hours.
2. A four-hourly temperature reading.
3. Blood-pressure chart.
4. A fluid balance chart.

Complications of emergency abdominal surgery

In most patients complications are few. Retention of urine (Ch. 43) or chest infection is treated as necessary. The patient with established peritonitis is more likely to develop complications.

Paralytic ileus. This is an important and not infrequent complication due to temporary loss of motor tone in the smooth muscle of the gut. Not only is this a normal response to surgery but it is also due to the inflammation or infection of the peritoneum. The intestines are paralysed and dilated. Their contents may regurgitate into the stomach, which may itself be dilated. Vomiting does not occur until the stomach is overdistended with fluid. No flatus is passed per rectum. Factors responsible for prolonged ileus are:

1. Excessive handling of gut.
2. Unrelieved intestinal distension.
3. Attempts to stimulate intestinal activity by means of drugs when paralysis is still present.
4. Overdosage of drugs producing hypotension, or hypotension secondary to disease process.
5. Infection (intraperitoneal).

It is worth noting that paralytic ileus may complicate major trauma, or surgery of the spine or retroperitoneal space.

Paralytic ileus is in large measure preventable. In cases where it is anticipated that it may develop, treatment is commenced from the end of the operation until the bowel has recovered.

Symptoms and signs. The abdomen is distended, but usually there is no pain. The distended abdomen makes breathing difficult and embarrasses the action of the heart. The pulse rate is always rapid, and in severe cases the patient is very toxic in appearance. Bowel sounds are absent.

Treatment. Given time and rest the intestines will recover their tone. A flatus tube may be passed per rectum four-hourly or left in the rectum continuously. The stomach contents are aspirated continuously or every half-hour through a nasogastric tube and the volume recorded. Some surgeons use instead a Miller-Abbott tube, which is similar to a nasogastric tube and has an inflatable balloon to facilitate its passage into the intestine for a considerable distance. The mouth is kept clean but nothing given orally. Some cases of paralytic ileus are due to loss of potassium. The serum electrolytes are estimated and any electrolyte deficiency corrected.

Analgesics are administered if necessary and intravenous infusion commenced so that the fluid balance is maintained. Intravenous nutrition may be needed.

The sign of recovery. The return of the bowel sounds and the passage of flatus per rectum, normally or by a flatus tube, are the signs that the bowel has recovered its tone. The function of the flatus tube is to overcome the resistance of the anal sphincter.

Residual abscesses (Fig. 34.5). The commonest site for a residual abscess is in the wound and the patient improves immediately if it is drained adequately. The next most likely site is the pelvis. The onset of a pelvic abscess is heralded by pyrexia and the passage of mucus per rectum. The inflammatory swelling can be felt on rectal examination. Drainage, which is performed through the anterior rectal wall in the male

Subphrenic abscess

Subhepatic abscess

Pelvic abscess

Fig. 34.5 Sites of some residual abscesses.

or the posterior vaginal wall in the female, leads to immediate improvement.

A subphrenic (beneath the diaphragm) abscess is more difficult to diagnose. There may be difficulty in breathing, high temperature—evidence of general toxicity. A straight X-ray of the diaphragm may reveal a cavity filled with fluid and gas. Ultrasound examination is probably the best way of detecting an intraperitoneal collection of pus. The abscess is drained by a small incision below the subcostal margin if placed anteriorly but one sited posteriorly may require a rib resection. The postoperative care is that of a pyothorax (Ch. 30).

Abscesses may also arise in the subhepatic space (just under the liver), in either paracolic gutter or around the site of the surgery (e.g. right iliac fossa following appendicectomy).

Faecal fistula. A gangrenous appendix frequently involves a portion of the caecal wall in the inflammatory process. After operation a small portion of the wall may slough, and faecal contents contaminate the wound and excoriate the skin. The vast majority heal spontaneously in 2 or 3 weeks, but the skin must be protected from the discharge by stomadhesive or similar preparation (Ch. 38). The persistence of the fistula with 'sulphur granules' in the effluent suggests that actinomycosis may have been the underlying cause. Nowadays this is rare.

A faecal fistula may similarly arise from the site of an emergency intestinal anastomosis or a colonic perforation.

Burst abdomen. This is an occasional complication of any abdominal operation. It is very rare following a gridiron incision (used for appendicectomy) but much commoner after longitudinal incisions. The first sign is a sero-sanguinous discharge from the wound, which separates allowing the intestines to prolapse on to the abdominal wall. It is predisposed to by:

(a) Severe coughing.
(b) Infection of the wound.
(c) Deficiency of vitamin C, resulting in failure of the wound to heal.
(d) Removal of stitches before the wound has healed.
(e) Anaemia and malnutrition.
(f) Cortisone therapy preoperatively.
(g) Abdominal distension for any reason.
(h) Malignant disease.

Treatment. The prolapsed intestines are wrapped in a sterile towel which has been soaked in warm saline, and the surgeon is informed at once. The patient is taken to the theatre, anaesthetised, and the wound is resutured. It is remarkable that the condition usually causes little or no circulatory failure, and the patient has an uneventful convalescence.

If a wound has not actually burst but there is a danger of this happening, a corset dressing is advisable.

Remote complications

Intestinal obstruction. This complication occurs as a result of adhesions. It can occur a few weeks or months, or several years, after operation. It is more common after extensive peritonitis but can occur after any laparotomy. Occasionally it occurs a few days after the operation. The treatment is further operation to relieve the obstruction.

Incisional hernia. An incisional hernia may occur after any operation. Wound infection, burst abdomen, and pulmonary complications predispose to its development.

Intraperitoneal lavage

The value of intraperitoneal lavage in the treatment of peritonitis is now well established. It may take one of two forms after the cause has been dealt with. The first would seem to be the method of choice.

Intraoperative. In advanced peritonitis 'radical surgical debridement' is undertaken. Thorough cleansing of the whole peritoneal cavity, including every corner of the abdomen and in between loops of bowel, is undertaken with large volumes of saline to remove pus, faeces, fibrin and food. A long vertical incision is necessary. Post-operatively intestinal obstruction is a risk and in severe cases a long intestinal tube is passed through a proximal jejunostomy to the caecum to act as an internal splint. An antibiotic may be added to the fluid but this is not considered essential by Hudspeth (1978). The results are extremely good and complications are few.

Antibiotic lavage. A triple mixture of gentamicin, cephalothin and lincomycin, of which 10, 50 and 30 mg are dissolved in a litre of 1.5 per cent Dianeal, a solution used for peritoneal dialysis. At the end of the operation at which it was sought to control the contaminating source, Portex drains (which must have a rounded cup) are inserted into the subhepatic pouch, the subsplenic area and the pelvis. Each is used in turn, the others being spigoted and through it 1 litre of solution is infused every hour, left for 30 minutes and then drained for 25 minutes. The process is continued for 72 hours. Stephen and Loewenthal claim:

(a) The maintainance of adequate antibiotic concentrations in the blood and peritoneal fluid.

(b) The dialysing fluid maintains normal serum electrolyte values.

(c) Body temperature is controlled so that the patient is rendered afebrile. The authors warn that this is a procedure only for severe peritonitis with intraperitoneal faecal leakage.

PERFORATED PEPTIC ULCER

An ulcer developing on a surface exposed to the action of acid-pepsin is known as a peptic ulcer, and includes gastric and duodenal ulcers. Perforation of a gastric ulcer is usually a more severe condition than perforation of duodenal ulcer. This is because the acid gastric juice is extremely irritant to the peritoneum and a much larger quantity of fluid leaks from a perforation in the stomach than from a similar perforation in the duodenum. Apart from this, the clinical features and treatment are the same. Fluid from the stomach or duodenum leaks through the perforation into the peritoneal cavity causing general peritonitis.

A chronic ulcer may perforate but an acute ulcer which is part of a widespread gastritis may also perforate. Aspirin and alcohol are recognised causes of acute ulceration. Steroid therapy is liable to reactivate a latent peptic ulcer. The most dangerous place for a patient to perforate is in hospital while being treated conservatively for peptic ulcer. This is because the pain is assumed to be simply an exacerbation of ulcer pain and the perforation may not be immediately recognised.

Symptoms and signs

The sudden onset of violent, constant, generalised abdominal pain is the outstanding symptom. The patient lies perfectly still where he has been smitten with pain. He feels as though he has received a powerful blow in the abdomen. Vomiting may occur. The face is pale and anxious and the skin feels cold and clammy. The temperature is invariably subnormal at first and the pulse rate is elevated. The whole abdomen is tender and extremely rigid or board-like. It does not move with respiration and there is no distension. If unrelieved the pain ceases after about 24 hours as the abdomen distends from general peritonitis. Not all patients give a history suggestive of previous indigestion.

Treatment

The tempo of deterioration is much faster in this condition than in a case of acute appendicitis. After 24 hours the patient suffering from acute appendicitis is still in a comparatively early stage because peritoneal contamination has not usually occurred. The mortality rate in patients suffering from untreated perforated peptic ulcer of 24 hours' duration is about 90 per cent.

Treatment is urgent surgery. The perforation is closed with stitches and peritoneal toilet performed. If the symptoms before perforation were such that definitive surgical treatment for the ulcer was indicated this may sometimes be carried out in the emergency situation.

Preoperative treatment

An intravenous line is set up and fluid replacement is commenced. A nasogastric tube is passed and the stomach emptied. Every millilitre of gastric contents recovered lessens the damage to the peritoneal cavity. The pain is relieved by an injection of morphia. As soon as possible the patient receives the usual preparation for an acute abdominal operation.

Postoperative treatment

The general treatment is similar to that for acute appendicitis.

The hygiene of the mouth is even more important in this condition, since fluids by mouth are usually forbidden for the first 24 hours after the operation.

Diet. For the first 24 hours only parenteral fluid is given. After this a fluid diet is prescribed on return of the bowel sounds and is gradually increased to include suitable proportions of carbohydrate, fat and protein.

The immediate postoperative complications are similar to those following acute appendicectomy (p. 385), and more remotely to those of a case of peptic ulcer treated surgically (Ch. 35).

Instructions to the patient on discharge

It should be explained that the operation was a life-saving measure and that there is a 70 per cent chance that he will have further trouble. He can improve his chances of cure by avoiding undue stress and tobacco.

POSTOPERATIVE PERITONITIS

Postoperative peritonitis is a very important condition. It is one of the major causes of fatality following abdominal operations. It is peculiarly difficult to diagnose and in not a few cases postmortem examination reveals that deaths which have been attributed to cardiac failure and respiratory infection are, in fact, cases of true peritonitis from leakage of an anastomosis or rupture of the intestine. The real difficulty is that the severe pain and dramatic suddenness with which most peritoneal symptoms commence are clouded by:

1. Postoperative analgesics and hypnotics.
2. Some pain in the abdominal wound ⎤ which are usual
3. Some degree of pyrexia ⎦ postoperatively.

The important observations are:
1. Any complaint of undue pain should be reported.
2. Tenderness after the second day should be minimal.
3. Abdominal distension should be either responding to the usual measures or, if it is becoming worse, peritonitis should be suspected.

At an advanced stage these patients pass into acute circulatory failure and die very rapidly.

ACUTE INTESTINAL OBSTRUCTION

There are few conditions in which the real gravity of the patient's condition is more belied by his apparent well-being than in acute intestinal obstruction. The obstruction may affect the large or the small intestine. Obstruction of the small intestine is always more severe than obstruction of the large intestine because of the great loss of fluid by vomiting in the former.

There are innumerable causes of intestinal obstruction, which are considered in Chapters 37 and 39, but to illustrate the two main types a typical case of obstruction in each of the two portions of the intestine is discussed here.

SMALL BOWEL OBSTRUCTION

Symptoms and signs

Colicky abdominal pain commencing around the umbilicus is the first symptom. The pain waxes and wanes, is temporarily relieved by vomiting, but recurs again and again, and never moves from the centre of the abdomen.

Vomiting is constant. At first food is returned, later bile-stained gastric juice, and, in the late stages, the foul infected contents of the intestine above the obstruction. This fluid smells of faeces and is described as 'faeculent' vomit.

The loss of fluid, rich in chlorides, is considerable.

The bowels. There is usually absolute constipation, i.e. no flatus is passed after the administration of an enema or a Dulcolax suppository.

On examination the temperature is normal but the pulse is rapid. Tenderness is unusual, unless gangrenous gut is present in the abdomen, but there is fullness of the central and lower abdomen. Only in very late cases is gross distension present.

Peristalsis (worm-like movements) of the bowel may be visible through a thin abdominal wall.

If an external strangulated hernia is the cause of the obstruction a tense, tender, painful irreducible swelling which has no impulse on coughing will be felt over one of the hernial sites. On the other hand, if the obstruction is due to some other cause, for example, a peritoneal band, the signs previously described will be present alone.

LARGE BOWEL OBSTRUCTION

The commonest cause is a growth narrowing the lumen of the bowel. The acute attack develops when a faecal mass blocks the already narrowed lumen.

Symptoms and signs

Obstruction in the large bowel is much better tolerated than obstruction in the small bowel. The main complaint is a feeling of abdominal distension and sometimes breathlessness, for the distension impairs the action of the heart and lungs.

Intestinal colic and vomiting appear only when a fair degree of distension has already occurred preventing the contents of the small intestine from flowing through the ileocaecal valve to the large intestine. A history of increasing constipation is almost invariable before the 'acute stoppage'.

The physical contents of the large intestine can be compared to a coal fire which consists of smoke and embers. If the chimney is blocked the real trouble arises in the room from the smoke. In the large intestine it is the gas which fills the bowel and all the striking symptoms are due to the retention of flatus and not to the presence of faeces.

The treatment of acute intestinal obstruction

The mortality rate of this condition is high, so that every care must be taken if it is to be reduced. Resuscitative measures must be instituted at once. Fluid depletion and electrolyte imbalance, which is usually severe in small bowel obstruction, has to be corrected.

A Dulcolax suppository or a disposable phosphate enema is given on admission. This serves the dual purpose of confirming the diagnosis and of clearing the bowel below the obstruction so that there is no unnecessary difficulty in the passage of the intestinal contents after the obstruction has been relieved.

A patient suffering from intestinal obstruction is given nothing by mouth before the operation.

If the obstruction is subacute, and there is no sign of gangrene an obstruction may be treated for a trial period by nasogastric suction and intravenous fluid replacement. Some patients with multiple adhesions may recover if the obstruction is due to a kinking of a loop of bowel.

Very occasionally a volvulus of the pelvic colon may be reduced by passing a rectal tube through a sigmoidoscope. An intussusception (Ch. 37) may also be reduced by retrograde pressure from a barium enema given under X-ray screening control.

Immediate preoperative preparation

This is similar to the preparation for any acute abdominal operation, but special stress is laid on fluid and electrolyte replacement.

A nasogastric tube to aspirate the stomach contents is left in the stomach for 24 hours or longer after the operation. This relieves vomiting while the patient is being prepared, and prevents vomiting during the induction of anaesthesia. The aspiration of vomited material into the lungs may be fatal. If the obstruction is so severe that fluid is welling up in the stomach very rapidly, the patient is placed on the operating table in the slightly head-down position and the theatre nurse must aspirate the stomach contents even while the anaesthetist is inducing anaesthesia.

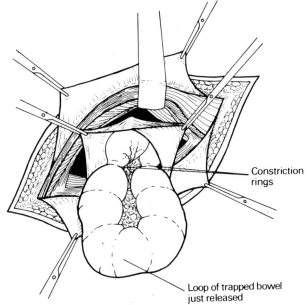

Fig. 34.6 Strangulated hernia. The intestine which has been released is viable. Note the released loop as well as the intestine above it is distended.

Fig. 34.7 Gangrenous small intestine. The obstruction has been relieved but as the gut is gangrenous it must be resected and continuity restored. The gut above is still distended.

The operation

This is always confined to the simplest and quickest procedure necessary to relieve the obstruction. Division of a band or reduction of a strangulation is all that is necessary if the bowel wall is not gangrenous (Fig. 34.6). If gangrene is present (Fig. 34.7), resection will be necessary.

In the large intestine the most frequent method of relief is to form an artificial, 'anus', proximal to the obstruction, usually a colostomy—on rare occasions a caescostomy. The care of these fistulae is described in Chapter 38.

Postoperative treatment

Parenteral fluid replacement is continued. Continuous aspiration of the stomach for 24 hours is frequently necessary, and the passage of a flatus tube per rectum is also important. These patients are sometimes very breathless from abdominal distension and are more comfortable when nursed sitting upright.

The general care of the patient and his wound is similar to that in any abdominal operation.

Postoperative complications. Particularly important in acute obstruction are:

1. Recurrence of the obstruction. The symptoms are similar to the original lesion.

2. Paralytic ileus is very common, since, although the mechanical obstruction has been relieved, the bowel wall may have developed paralysis as a result of the distension.

INTRA-ABDOMINAL HAEMORRHAGE

INTRAPERITONEAL HAEMORRHAGE

Intraperitoneal haemorrhage is not a very common cause of an acute abdomen. The only common lesion is an ectopic gestation. This is fully described in Chapter 50. Traumatic causes include laceration of the spleen and of the liver.

The principles of treatment are:
1. Replacement of blood.
2. Control of haemorrhage by suture or removal of the affected organ.

RETROPERITONEAL HAEMORRHAGE

The commonest causes of *retroperitoneal* haemorrhage are:
1. A ruptured aneurysm of the abdominal aorta (p. 241).
2. Acute haemorrhagic pancreatitis (p. 429).

ANTEROPERITONEAL HAEMORRHAGE

The only common cause of a haemorrhage in front of the peritoneal cavity is rupture of the inferior epigastric artery which may cause sudden swelling behind the lower rectus sheath and in front of the peritoneal cavity. It is sometimes associated with severe coughing or handle-bar injuries.

OTHER CONDITIONS OF PERITONEUM

CHRONIC PERITONITIS

General acute peritonitis has already been described. Chronic disease of the peritoneal cavity is described briefly to complete diseases of the peritoneal cavity.

It is usually tuberculous in origin. This is now very rare in the U.K. but is still a problem in underdeveloped areas of the world. It may take three clinical forms:

1. Diffuse tuberculosis of the surface of the intestines and parietal peritoneum with the exudation of free clear fluid.

2. Diffuse adhesive changes which may cause intestinal obstruction. A similar condition known as sclerosing peritonitis may be caused by the drug practolol.

3. Multiple cold abscesses and fistulae usually pointing at the umbilicus.

Operation is only indicated if intestinal obstruction develops. Otherwise the treatment is rest and anti-tuberculous chemotherapy.

CARCINOMA OF THE PERITONEUM

Carcinoma of the peritoneum is common, and is almost invariably secondary to growths elsewhere in the abdomen. The whole peritoneal surface may be studded with nodules of growth, and ascites is frequently abundant. No treatment of a curative nature is possible, but symptomatic relief may be given by tapping the abdomen and allowing the fluid to drain away. Radioactive gold and cytotoxic drugs are now being used in the relief of the ascites associated with this condition. A suspension of the colloidal form of the metal or drug is introduced through the aspirating needle. In 50 per cent of cases there is relief of the ascites. It does not cure the primary condition. Sometimes an artificial shunt, in the form of a valved tube running subcutaneously, is inserted between the peritoneal cavity and a major neck vein to allow continuous drainage of fluid.

ASCITES

A collection of free non-purulent fluid in the peritoneal cavity is known as ascites. The term 'free' means that the fluid can move around the peritoneal cavity instead of being contained in one part of it—when it is described as encysted.

Causes

1. Carcinoma peritonei.
2. A failing heart.
3. Certain forms of renal failure.
4. Cirrhosis of the liver and portal hypertension.
5. Some forms of tuberculous peritonitis.
6. Portal vein thrombosis.
7. Inferior vena caval obstruction.
8. Meigs' syndrome (ovarian fibroma with ascites).
9. Escape of chyle.

Treatment

The treatment is that of the cause where possible. Oral diuretics may improve the condition a great deal. Locally, tapping (paracentesis) may be performed. A small trocar and disposable cannula or peritoneal dialysis cannula are inserted into the peritoneal cavity after the injection of a local anaesthetic (1 per cent Lignocaine). The bladder must be emptied in preparation for the operation, and the skin of the abdominal wall is prepared in the usual way. The cannula is inserted in the mid-line below the umbilicus or in one or other iliac fossa, so as to avoid major blood vessels in the abdominal wall. Several pints of fluid may be withdrawn and a specimen is sent both for biochemical and cytological examination. A firm binder is applied after the operation to lessen further collection and assist with the drainage of fluid. An artificial peritoneo-venous shunt, as outlined above, may be of value in some patients.

Nursing procedure for paracentesis abdominis

A basic dressing trolley is prepared, additional items on the bottom shelf are:

Local anaesthetic and syringe	Drainage bag
Scalpel	Green Savlon
Trocar and cannula (or other apparatus)	Iodine
Extra tubing	Green towels
Adjustable clamp	Gown, mask, gloves
Receiver	Specimen jars
Binder or many-tailed bandage	

The nature of the procedure is explained to the patient, and his cooperation is obtained.

The doctor prepares himself. The trolley is taken to the bedside. Privacy is ensured. The patient is made comfortable in the semi-recumbent position.

The bladder is emptied. If the patient cannot pass urine this is reported to the doctor. Catheterisation may be necessary.

The binder (or many-tailed bandage) is placed in position. The bed-clothes are turned down.

The nurse opens the outer wrappings of the basic dressing pack, opens other packets as required, and assists the doctor to assemble the apparatus. The doctor performs the procedure, assisted by the nurse. The nurse observes the patient, giving help and reassurance.

The tubing is connected to the cannula and to the drainage bag. The clamp is adjusted to allow the rate of flow ordered by the doctor. The binder is fastened in position, and readjusted as necessary.

The nurse looks after the patient whilst the drainage continues. Special observations are made on the general condition of the patient, the rate and flow of the fluid, the amount and the nature of the fluid.

The apparatus is taken down on instruction from the doctor. The wound is sealed, e.g. with plastic spray. The trocar and cannula are rinsed in cold water, placed in the appropriate container and returned to CSSD.

PSEUDOMYXOMA PERITONEI

This is a most unpleasant condition which occurs following rupture of a pseudomucinous cyst of the ovary.

BIBLIOGRAPHY

Hudspeth A S 1975 Radical surgical debridement in the treatment of advanced peritonitis. Archives of Surgery 110: 12-33
Stephen M, Loewenthal J 1979 continuing peritoneal lavage in high risk peritonitis. Surgery 85: 603-606

35

The stomach and duodenum

The surgical anatomy and physiology of the stomach and duodenum have been considered in Chapter 33. Investigation to detect the presence of an organic lesion and to assess gastric secretory function is spread over several days. This adds to the patient's anxiety and the reason for each procedure should be explained.

INVESTIGATIONS OF GASTRO-DUODENAL DISEASE

The investigations performed are:

Radiographic examination

Radiographic examination is performed after a barium meal preferably of the double contrast variety.

An aperient should be given two evenings before the barium meal examination. No food or drink is taken from midnight before the examination so that the stomach is empty of food at the time of radiological examination (say 10.00 hours).

After the barium meal is given no further solids or fluids must be given to the patient until the radiologist is satisfied with the X-rays.

Tests of gastric secretory function

In all these tests a gastric tube is passed, preferably orally, into a fasting stomach (fasting for 12 hours). An X-ray is taken to ensure that the tube is in the body of the stomach.

All specimens collected in these tests must be clearly labelled.

The patient is now positioned in bed on his left side. A low grade suction pump is used to withdraw the stomach contents at regular intervals, air being pumped in through a bleeder tube if the tube appears to be blocked.

Resting juice is aspirated and put into the first container—three quarter-hour basal specimens are then collected under continuous suction.

1. Pentagastrin. A subcutaneous injection of pentagastrin is then given (6 µg per kg body weight). Six further specimens are then collected at quarter-hour intervals. Pentagastrin has virtually no side effects. It stimulates the mucosa of the body and fundus of the stomach directly to produce acid. It provides a measure of the maximal acid output.

2. Insulin. This procedure is similar to the pentagastrin test. Three quarter-hour basal specimens are collected, a blood sample being taken with the third. Intravenous injection of soluble insulin 0.25 units per kg body weight is given. Eight quarter-hour specimens are again collected and blood samples are taken half an hour and three-quarters of an hour after the insulin injection. The patient may become hypoglycaemic and sweat profusely after insulin injection. Oral or intravenous dextrose should be available but is rarely necessary. Insulin causes hypoglycaemia, which causes central stimulation of the vagus nerve and thus stimulation of gastric acid secretion. This test is a measure of the vagal component of gastric acid secretion.

3. Night secretion volume. After a suitable tranquilliser such as Valium, the total amount of gastric juice secreted over a period of the 12 hours of the night is aspirated hourly or by continuous suction and the acidity is estimated. A volume in excess of 400 ml is suggestive of a duodenal ulcer while a volume of a litre suggests a gastrin-secreting pancreatic tumour.

Gastric secretion tests are particularly indicated for:

(a) Preoperative assessment. They can be of some help in deciding which operation to use (though not many surgeons use them for this) and may be useful for later comparison with postoperative results.

(b) Recurrent dyspepsia after vagotomy and drainage.

(c) If the diagnosis of the Zollinger-Ellison syndrome is considered. In this condition the level of serum gastrin is greatly raised.

(d) Occassionally in X-ray negative dyspepsia.

Four terms are used to describe the nature of gastric juice:

Hyperchlorhydria—excess of hydrochloric acid (more than normal)
Hypochlorhydria—hydrochloric acid less than normal
Achlorhydria—no hydrochloric acid
Achylia—no pepsin.

Tests for occult blood in the faeces

Red meat and green vegetables must be excluded from the diet for 3 days previous to the collection of the specimen. It is not necessary to submit the patient's entire stool for testing. A disposable plastic container should be used, with a tin spoon attached to the under surface of the lid.

Oesophagogastroduodeonoscopy (Fig.35.1)

The modern fibreoptic endoscope enables the oesophagus, stomach and duodenum to be viewed, photographs to be taken and specimens to be taken for biopsy. In preparation for gastroscopy (as it is commonly called) no food or drink is allowed for six hours. It may be necessary to empty the stomach via a tube (e.g. because of bleeding, pyloric stenosis).

Fig. 35.1 Oesophagogastro-duodenoscopy

The examination is carried out as an outpatient under local anaesthetic. The throat is anaesthetised by administration of a local anaesthetic lozenge 20 minutes before examination or with local anaesthetic spray.

Anxiolytic agents (e.g. diazepam) may be administered intravenously to produce light sedation and amnesia. The patient lies in the left lateral position with the neck bent well forward, chin on chest, while the instrument is passed. No food or drink is allowed for half an hour after the examination because the pharynx is anaesthetised and fluid may run into the larynx.

Fibreoptic instruments are expensive and delicate. They require special handling and care. Only nurses specifically trained should be involved in this.

Cytological examination of gastric contents

The fasting stomach is aspirated (or washed out) via a nasogastric tube. The fluid is filtered or spun down and then examined by the pathologist, who looks at the nature of the cellular content to detect the presence of malignant cells.

NASOGASTRIC INTUBATION AND ITS USE

The passage of a nasogastric tube for investigation and in perioperative care is a common nursing procedure. It will therefore be discussed here.

A stomach tube is usually passed through the nose although some nurses and doctors who have undergone gastric surgery have felt that intubation was less intolerable by having it placed through the angle of the mouth. A further point to be borne in mind about passing the tube nasally is that staphylococci are often harboured in the nose and if a nasal tube is to be indwelling for some days it is advisable to take a nasal swab to make sure staphylococci are not present.

In the discussion which follows reference to the nasogastric route is equally applicable to a tube passed by mouth with two exceptions. A stomach full of retained solid foodstuff such as occurs in pyloric stenosis or one full of blood clots can be emptied only through a large bore tube and this can be passed only through the mouth.

Indications for intubation

1. Stomach wash out. Pyloric stenosis or poisoning.
2. Aspiration of excessive fluid accumulation. Pyloric stenosis, acute intestinal obstruction and acute dilation of the stomach.
3. To prevent gastric dilation in a stomach paralysed after surgery.
4. Removal/prevention of blood clots in haematemesis.
5. Gastric secretion tests.
6. Recovery of gastric juice for cytological examination.
7. Feeding where a patient who is unable to take food orally, has a functioning stomach and small intestine.

The advantages to be gained from intubation are considerable but it should not be overlooked that it is an unpleasant experience and a further discomfort following major surgery. The incidence of pulmonary complications is diminished where its use can be avoided. The gastric contents may become infected while the tube is present. Oesophageal strictures have occurred following nasogastric intubation.

Nursing procedure for passing an intragastric tube

Equipment required:
Tube—Ryle's, oesophageal (Lenin), stomach or other
Paper towel or roll
Cleansing material for nose—sinus forceps
　　　　　　　　　　　　　　　　—cotton wool swabs
　　　　　　　　　　　　　　　　—sodium bicarbonate solution
　　Lubricant—KY jelly
　　Spatula and torchlight
　　Litmus paper
　　Vomit bowl, mouthwash
　　Medical wipes
　　Strapping
　　20 ml Syringe
　　Receiver
　　Spigot
　　Local anaesthetic spray

Other specific apparatus according to reason for procedure.

The procedure is explained to a conscious patient, and his cooperation obtained. Privacy is ensured. Dentures are removed, if necessary.

When possible, the patient sits straight up, supported by pillows, with his head tilted well forward. An unconscious patient lies in the semi-prone position. A paper towel is placed under the chin. If he can do so, the patient is asked to blow his nose, otherwise the nurse carefully cleanses the nostrils.

The nose and throat may be sprayed with local anaesthetic (under medical supervision). The tip of the tube is lubricated. When the nasal route is used, it is gently inserted along the floor of the nose into the pharynx. When the oral route is being used, the tongue is depressed and the tube is passed over the side of the mouth and tongue into the pharynx, care being taken not to touch the uvula. When the tube is in the pharynx, the patient is asked to swallow, and the tube is gently pushed each time he does so. Sips of water may be given to assist in swallowing. In between swallows he is encouraged to take a deep breath. The nurse observes the patient for any coughing, apnoea, cyanosis or vomiting. If the tube is entering the larynx or trachea, it is removed, and the nurse passes it again when the patient has recovered from the coughing etc.

To ensure that the tube is in the stomach, the mouth is opened, the tongue depressed and the torch used to see the position of the tube in the pharynx. Using the syringe, some of the contents of the stomach are aspirated and tested with litmus paper. An acid reaction would most probably indicate that the tube is in the stomach.

A spigot is inserted into the end of the tube, and the tube is attached to the face with a piece of strapping.

When a patient has an indwelling nasogastric tube, it is necessary to attend to the cleanliness and condition of the nares and the mouth at regular intervals.

Gastric aspiration

A nasogastric tube is passed as described above.

1. Intermittent aspiration. A tray is prepared containing:

Receiver	Medical wipes/tissues
20 ml syringe	Disposal bag.
Measure jug	

It is kept on the patient's locker, covered by a paper/green towel.

The patient is advised of what is to happen. The nurse holds a tissue around the end of the tube, she removes the spigot and places it in the receiver. She ensures that there is no air in the syringe, attaches the tip to the tube and applies gentle suction. She holds the end of the tube and detaches the syringe. The aspirate is measured while still in the syringe, and then emptied into the jug. The aspiration is repeated until no fluid is aspirated. The spigot is reinserted. The total amount of aspirate is charted. The nurse leaves the tray clean, placing used tissues in the disposal bag. She reports to the nurse in charge.

2. Continuous drainage. The tube is connected to a drainage bag. The amount of drainage is measured and charted as instructed, e.g. hourly or when the bag is emptied or changed. Intermittent aspiration is also necessary to check that the tube is not blocked.

Removal of nasogastric tube

The patient is advised of what is to happen. The adhesive tape holding the tube is gently detached. The nurse tells the patient to take a deep breath, rapidly and smoothly withdraws the tube, and places it in a disposable bag. The patient's face is cleaned and his oral hygiene attended to. Used equipment is discarded.

Gastric washouts

Equipment required. This includes that for passing an intra-gastric tube with the following addition:

Tubing 24 inches in length
Connector (from tubing to stomach tube)
Funnel
Small jug—1 litre
Large jug containing 4 litres fluid (e.g. tap water) at 100° F (37.8°C)
Bucket
2 Large polythene sheets.

The procedure is carried out very much as detailed for passing an intragastric tube (p. 402).

When the patient is unconscious, the position of the patient may be semiprone, prone or recumbent, with the head lower than the trunk. Usually, in such patients, the doctor intubates the patient and carries out the stomach lavage.

The polythene sheets are spread to protect the patient, bedding and floor. The bucket is placed on the floor. The stomach tube is passed into the stomach.

The small jug is filled with fluid. The funnel, tubing and connector are assembled. Some fluid is run through to expel air, and then stopped. The connection is attached to the stomach tube. The funnel is raised above the level of the head (or stomach if the head is low); 300 ml (half pint) of fluid is run into the stomach. Before the funnel is empty it is inverted over the bucket, and the fluid siphoned back. A specimen of the first washing is sometimes saved for analysis of gastric contents, particularly drugs.

The process is repeated until the fluid returns clear, or the 4 litres of prepared fluid have been used.

Afterwards, the tube is compressed and withdrawn quickly. The patient's face is wiped, he is given a mouthwash and left comfortable in bed. An unconscious patient is kept under observation, and any alteration in the level of unconsciousness noted and reported.

Used equipment is discarded. The siphoned contents are measured and recorded, and saved for inspection.

The nurse washes and dries her hands and makes a report to the nurse in charge.

PEPTIC ULCER

A peptic ulcer is an ulcer which occurs on a surface exposed to the action of acid pepsin.

The common sites (Fig. 35.2) *are:*
1. The first part of the duodenum—duodenal ulcer.
2. The lesser curvature of the stomach—gastric ulcer.

Less common sites (Fig. 35.2) *are:*
1. The jejunum after anastomosis of the stomach to the jejunum—stomal ulcer.
2. Lower oesophagus, usually associated with hiatus hernia causing a reflux oesophagitis and going on to an oesophageal ulcer.
3. An ulcer in the ileum adjoining a Meckel's diverticulum which contains ectopic fragments of gastric mucosa.

All peptic ulcers are similar in pathology, basic clinical features and complications with the exception that a gastric ulcer may become, or may be mistaken for, a malignant (carcinomatous) ulcer of the stomach.

The cause of a peptic ulcer is unknown, but certain conditions are said to predispose to its formation in susceptible patients or to aggravate an existing ulcer:
1. There is a higher incidence of duodenal ulcer amongst patients of blood group O than in the population in general.
2. Excess of acid and pepsin secretion—in duodenal ulcer.
3. Loss of the protective action of gastric mucus—in gastric ulcer.
4. Drugs, smoking and alcohol.
5. Irregular meals with stomach empty for long periods—duodenal ulcer.
6. Endocrine factors—a pancreatic gastrin secreting tumour which stimulates excessive acid secretion in the stomach is the best known.

Clinical features of an uncomplicated peptic ulcer

(a) Burning epigastric pain appearing half an hour to 2 hours after

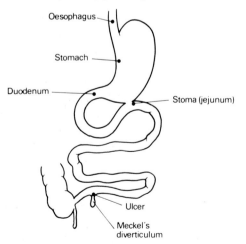

Oesophagus

Stomach

Duodenum

Stoma (jejunum)

Ulcer

Meckel's diverticulum

Fig. 35.2 Sites of peptic ulceration (a gastrojejunostomy is illustrated in this diagram).

food. Food may relieve the pain of a duodenal ulcer but aggravates that of a gastric ulcer.

(b) The appetite of a patient with a duodenal ulcer may remain good whilst the patient with a gastric ulcer is afraid to eat.

(c) Although nausea and heartburn are common features vomiting is unusual except in complicated cases.

(d) Remission and exacerbation are characteristic especially in duodenal ulcer.

(e) Pain at night—duodenal ulcer.

Investigations

Barium meal
Gastric secretion tests
Endoscopy—with biopsy if necessary

The complications of a peptic ulcer

The principal ones are:
(a) Perforation—pp. 370, 389.
(b) Haemorrhage
(c) Pyloric stenosis and hour-glass contracture —see below
(d) Carcinomatous change in a simple gastric ulcer—rare.
(e) Penetration of adjacent organs. A chronic ulcer may invade locally the pancreas, the liver, or the intestine (usually transverse colon). If the pancreas is penetrated the pain is more constant and more severe than usual, and referred to the back. If the colon is penetrated a gastrocolic fistula may occur (Ch. 33).

Penetrating ulcers usually require surgical treatment.

Treatment

The principles of treatment of a peptic ulcer are the same whether medical or surgical measures are employed. Basically they aim at the dilution, neutralisation or diminution of acid pepsin.

1. Dilution by frequent meals, milk drip or short circuit operation, for example, gastrojejunostomy.
2. Neutralisation:
    (a) Alkalis.
    (b) Buffers, such as milk.
3. Diminution:
    (a) Drugs inhibiting vagal action, including sedatives which diminish anxiety. Rest in bed has similar effect.
    (b) Drugs inhibiting acid secretion locally, e.g. cimetidine.
    (c) Vagotomy.
    (d) Gastrectomy.
    (e) Avoidance of smoking.
4. Increasing mucosal resistance—agents such as carbenoxolone sodium stimulate protective mucorrhoea in gastric ulcer.

The prostaglandins secreted in the stomach modulate the response of the acid secreting cells to stimulants such as gastrin and histamine. This protective function is blocked by drugs such as cortisone or phenylbutazone. The administration of synthetic prostaglandins is complementary to the action of drugs like cimetidine.

Indications for surgical treatment are:

(a) The occurrence of complications—perforation, haemorrhage, stenosis, malignant change.

(b) The failure to respond to careful medical treatment. This is a relative indication and requires fine judgment. The frequency, severity and duration of symptoms are the criteria considered. If a gastric ulcer fails to heal in 4 to 6 weeks medical treatment is deemed to have failed. The treatment of an uncomplicated ulcer requires a multidisciplinary approach including close co-operation between the physician and surgeon.

Surgical measures are either a vagotomy or a partial gastrectomy (see below).

HAEMATEMESIS AND MELAENA

HAEMORRHAGE FROM PEPTIC ULCER

This occurs due to erosion of a blood vessel in the base of an ulcer, releasing blood into the lumen of the stomach or duodenum. It may occur from a previously diagnosed peptic ulcer or be the first indication of the presence of an ulcer. Corticosteroids may have activated a latent ulcer. Some drugs taken by mouth are liable to cause erosions of the gastric mucosa (e.g. aspirin, non-steroidal anti-inflammatory drugs). Such acute erosions may bleed.

When blood accumulates in the stomach the colour changes rapidly from red to black due to the action of gastric acid. It may be vomited (**haematemesis**) as black coffee-ground material or, if the haemorrhage is so severe that no mixing with gastric acid occurs, fresh red blood may be vomited. Alternatively the blood may pass from the stomach or duodenum into the intestine, passing rapidly to the rectum from which it is excreted as a tarry stool (**melaena**).

All patients with such bleeding require admission to hospital however mild the symptoms and signs, because no one can forecast the outcome. It may be a trivial incident or it may be the beginning of a haemorrhage that will never cease until it is controlled by surgical measures.

Management of patient

Such patients should be managed by physician and surgeon together. The aims of management are to correct, if necessary, the consequences of the bleeding and to stop or prevent further bleeding. It can be considered under the following headings.

1. Assessment of severity of blood loss and continued bleeding.
   (a) History. The length of the history and the amount of haematemesis and melaena will provide an indication of the amount of

blood lost. If the patient has collapsed at any time the blood loss is severe.

(b) Examination. The signs of shock—pallor, sweating, rapid pulse, low blood pressure—indicate severe blood loss.

(c) Haemoglobin estimation—on admission and repeated daily—aids in assessment.

(d) Pulse and blood pressure records—kept half-hourly (or more frequently in severe cases). A rising pulse rate and falling blood pressure indicate continuing haemorrhage, or, following a period of stability, re-bleeding.

(e) Central venous pressure monitoring. This is done in more severe cases.

(f) Record of blood loss. Any haematemesis and melaena, including quantity, is recorded on a chart.

(g) A wide-bore nasogastric tube is passed and the stomach emptied continuously to assess bleeding and prevent accumulation of clot. Not all medical staff agree with this.

2. Treatment of blood loss.

(a) A blood sample is taken for blood grouping and cross-matching of blood (if this is necessary).

(b) Reassurance. The patient requires constant reassurance by calm and sensitive medical and nursing staff, for the anxiety resulting from haemorrhage can be great.

(c) Rest and sedation. If shocked, the patient is nursed flat with one pillow but is allowed to sit up once his condition is stable.

(d) Blood transfusion. This is instituted if necessary, the rate and amount of transfusion being determined by the pulse rate, blood pressure, central venous pressure and haemoglobin. In severe cases two drips or transfusion under pressure may be required.

3. Diagnosis of cause of bleeding.

(a) History. This may provide a clear indication of the cause of bleeding.

(b) Gastroscopy. This should be performed as soon as convenient and if possible, when the patient's condition is stable. This should be within 12 (at most 24) hours of admission. Sometimes it has to be done as an emergency where severe haemorrhage is continuing or likely to recur. The stomach may have to be washed out with cold saline to obtain an adequate view. The cause of bleeding is seen in the majority of cases.

(c) Barium meal. This is done if gastroscopy fails to demonstrate the cause.

4. Arrest of bleeding. In many cases bleeding stops spontaneously. The younger the patient the more likely this is to happen. If severe bleeding continues or recurs within 24 hours, active steps to stop it have to be taken.

(a) Gastric cooling. Instillation of ice-cold saline via a tube or gastric balloon is sometimes used.

(b) Laser coagulation. This is an effective way of stopping bleeding

in selected cases. It is not readily available in many hospitals.
(c) Surgery. This is a definitive way of stopping the bleeding or preventing further severe bleeding. Occasionally it has to be done urgently as a life-saving procedure.
(d) Antacids and cimetidine are often prescribed but there is no evidence that they stop the bleeding.
(e) Antifibrinolytic inhibitors may be prescribed. Biggs et al (1976) have reduced the mortality from bleeding peptic ulcer using tranexamic acid.

OTHER CAUSES OF GASTROINTESTINAL HAEMORRHAGE

Peptic ulceration is the cause of gastrointestinal haemorrhage in over 80 per cent of the patients. The other main sites of haemorrhage are indicated in Figure 35.3.

The principles of management are similar to those described above.

Investigations which aid diagnosis include:
Gastroscopy
Sigmoidoscopy
Barium enema
Barium meal and small bowel meal
Colonoscopy
Angiography—coeliac axis, superior mesenteric and inferior mesenteric. This should be done during active bleeding to demonstrate its site.

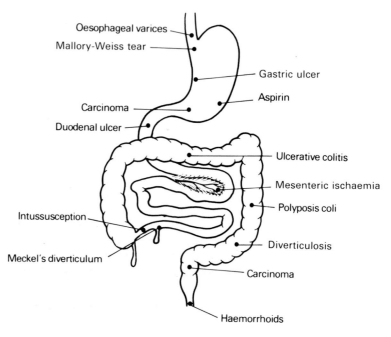

Fig. 35.3 Common causes of haemorrhage into gastrointestinal tract.

PYLORIC OBSTRUCTION (STENOSIS)

The outlet of the stomach may be obstructed by:

1. Congenital hypertrophy of the muscle (congenital pyloric stenosis).
2. Simple ulceration proximal or distal to the pylorus. An active ulcer may cause obstruction by virtue of its size or by surrounding inflammation and oedema, while a healed ulcer may cause obstruction by scarring.
3. A carcinoma in the pyloric antrum.

Whatever the cause, obstruction to the pylorus prevents food from leaving the stomach easily—solid food is retained and stagnates. As the condition becomes more severe fluid is slow to leave the stomach.

Because the stomach is nearly always full the patient has no appetite, feels distended in the epigastrium, vomits large quantities of foul material, loses weight and is constipated. Vomiting results in fluid and electrolyte depletion. On examination the patient's skin is dry and wrinkled, there is evidence of gross loss of weight and peristalsis may be visible. A hypertrophied pyloric sphincter may be palpated in the ten-day-old infant and an epigastric mass from carcinoma may be detectable in the adult suffering from carcinoma of the stomach. A barium meal will reveal delay in the emptying time of the stomach. Satisfactory gastroscopy is difficult because of the gastric residue, but can be performed after gastric lavage.

Management

Whatever the cause:

1. Fluid and electrolytes are replaced by intravenous infusion.
2. The stomach is emptied of its contents by a nasogastric tube and kept empty by frequent aspiration. If the contents are very foul a stomach washout, using a solution of sodium bicarbonate, is performed.
3. Intravenous nutrition is used with benefit in adult patients for 7 to 10 days prior to definitive treatment.
4. Definitive treatment depends on the cause but is surgical. This may be division of the pyloric sphincter (Ramstedt's operation) in the infant, vagotomy and a drainage operation in a benign pyloric stenosis, or a partial gastrectomy for carcinoma of the stomach.

GASTRIC STENOSIS (HOUR-GLASS STOMACH)

Occasionally a gastric ulcer is associated with such scarring that a stricture develops in the body of the stomach (hour-glass deformity). This causes a clinical picture similar to pyloric obstruction. It has to be dealt with in a similar manner, the definitive treatment being gastrectomy.

NEW GROWTHS OF THE STOMACH

Simple growths are rare, the commonest being a leiomyoma—a benign tumour of smooth muscle. Malignant growths are the third commonest cause of death from malignant disease and are relatively painless until far advanced. Their incidence in patients of blood group A is commoner than in the general population.

While surgery offers the only hope of cure, the survival rates, even in early cases, are extremely low. It is one of the most unfavourable sites in the body in which to develop a neoplasm.

Symptoms and signs

The early symptoms are few and very general in type. A feeling of malaise, increasing fatigue, and slight loss of appetite are the most common. Later pain, vomiting, and anaemia may develop. Loss of weight is usually rapid, and occasionally there may be a small haematemesis. An acute presentation with a large haematemesis or a perforation may occur. A growth in the pyloric antrum may cause pyloric obstruction. An early diagnosis may be made by biopsy of a gastric ulcer which macroscopically looks benign.

On examination of the abdomen there are no physical signs in early cases, but later the malignant growth can be palpated as a hard mass in the epigastrium. The liver may be enlarged and irregular from the presence of secondary deposits.

Investigations

1. Radiographic examination after a barium meal shows the typical appearance of a filling defect, with mucosal destruction.

2. Gastroscopy and biopsy confirm the diagnosis made radiologically. Alternatively this may be the primary investigation.

3. Examination of the gastric aspirate may reveal malignant cells.

4. Gastric secretion tests usually reveal the absence of hydrochloric acid (achlorhydria), but when the growth causes pyloric obstruction total acidity from fermentation may be increased. In all cases the amount of free hydrochloric acid is reduced. Such a test is not usually necessary.

5. Occult blood is usually present in the faeces.

Treatment

Removal of the stomach (gastrectomy) is the only operation which offers any hope of cure. If the growth is inoperable but pyloric stenosis is present or impending, considerable relief may be achieved by the performance of a gastroenterostomy to by-pass the growth. Should the growth be inoperable, careful nursing can do much to render the remaining days of misery more tolerable. Analgesic and hypnotic drugs will relieve pain, and vitamins by injection will delay deterioration. Antiemetics such as perphenazine (5 mg) may be prescribed. The diet should be light and nutritious, and in particular it must be what the patient fancies from day to day.

ACUTE DILATATION OF THE STOMACH

In this condition the stomach loses its tone and may fill almost the whole abdomen. Several pints of fluid are exuded into the cavity of the organ from its own walls and from the duodenum. The condition is similar to paralytic ileus with which it is in fact often associated.

Causes

1. After operations on the stomach or upper abdomen.
2. Occasionally it follows severe injury especially fractures of the dorsolumbar spine treated in a plaster jacket.
3. Sometimes the condition arises without any obvious cause.

Symptoms and signs

Symptoms and signs are identical with those of paralytic ileus. Large volumes of fluid may be vomited and aspirated from the stomach.

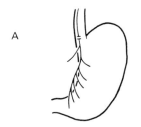

A

Treatment

The stomach must be emptied and rested, but the fluid balance must be maintained. These objects can be achieved by:
1. Nasogastric suction for at least 24 hours, or longer if necessary. Elevation of the foot of the bed and turning the patient on his left side may facilitate drainage of the stomach contents.
2. Intravenous fluids to maintain fluid and electrolyte balance.

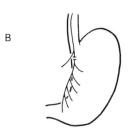

B

SURGERY OF THE STOMACH

1. Vagotomy. Division of the vagus nerves (vagotomy) denervates the stomach and significantly reduces gastric acid secretion. This is used in the treatment of duodenal ulcer and occasionally in the treatment of gastric ulcer. Division of the main trunks of the anterior and posterior vagus nerves is known as truncal vagotomy (Fig. 35.4A). If the vagi are divided below their hepatic and coeliac plexus branches, this is called selective vagotomy (Fig. 35.4B). It is rarely used now. If only the nerve fibres to the acid-secreting parietal cell mass are divided it is called proximal gastric vagotomy (or highly selective vagotomy, Fig. 35.4C).

C

Vagotomy also diminishes the activity of the stomach muscle so that defective gastric emptying tends to occur. For this reason a pyloroplasty or gastrojejunostomy is usually performed as a drainage procedure. This is not necessary after proximal gastric vagotomy because the innervated antrum tends to maintain normal gastric emptying.

2. Partial gastrectomy which may be performed for a gastric or a duodenal ulcer consists of removal of two thirds of the stomach. The stomach remnant is then sutured to the duodenum (Billroth I type, Fig. 35.5A) or to the jejunum (Billroth II or Polya type Fig. 35.5B). The Billroth I

Fig. 35.4 Types of vagotomy.
A. Total truncal vagotomy
B. Selective vagotomy
C. Proximal gastric vagotomy

Fig. 35.5 Gastrectomies.
A. Billroth I partial gastrectomy.
B. Polya partial gastrectomy.
C. Total gastrectomy with Roux-en-y oesophagojejunostomy.

reconstruction is usual in operations for gastric ulcer, the Billroth II form in cases of duodenal ulcer and antral carcinoma.

3. Total gastrectomy with anastomosis of the oesophagus to the jejunum (Fig. 35.5C) is performed in the rare case of a gastrin-secreting tumour of the pancreas, which may be too small to be located but causes persistent, recurrent, and often multiple peptic ulceration. The stomach is the target organ. More usually total gastrectomy is performed for carcinoma of the stomach.

Preoperative care

The preoperative care is similar to any major abdominal operation. Blood is crossmatched and, if necessary, anaemia is corrected. The risk of pulmonary complications is high following surgery in the upper abdomen so pre- and postoperative physiotherapy to the chest as well as the cessation of smoking is important. Fluid and electrolyte imbalance may require correction, especially in patients suffering from pyloric stenosis.

The stomach must be empty at the time of operation. Normally this occurs in 3 hours, and if emptying is not delayed it is unnecessary to pass a stomach tube. If pyloric stenosis is present, the stomach is emptied and washed out the evening before operation so that the patient is disturbed as little as possible the next morning. In severe pyloric stenosis gastric aspiration over several days is advisable.

A nasogastric tube is passed through the nose and left in position preoperatively. Some surgeons prefer to have the nasogastric tube passed by the anaesthetist while the patient is asleep, if its use is not necessary until after the operation. The end is left on open drainage or plugged with a spigot. Although the tube is usually passed through the nose some nurses and doctors who have had a gastrectomy performed have felt that intubation was rendered less intolerable by having it placed through the angle of the mouth.

Postoperative care

1. Care of the nasogastric tube. This tube, which was passed before or during the operation, is left in place afterwards and the stomach contents are aspirated hourly. The amount recovered is measured and recorded. The early aspirations consist of bright red blood which, in a few hours, changes to dark blood. In 24 hours the aspirate should be bile-stained. The amount aspirated diminishes until only a few millilitres of fluid are recovered, and the bowel sounds have returned. This indicates that the gastrointestinal tract has recovered its normal activity and that it is now safe to give fluid by mouth.

Thirty ml of sterile water are given. The stomach is aspirated an hour later. If it is emptying satisfacorily, the amount of fluid may be increased slowly to 90 ml each hour. The nasogastric tube is removed as soon as normal emptying of the stomach occurs. The diet is gradually built up with milk, eggs, strained soup etc. By the sixth day the patient is usually eating most foods.

Excessive aspirate may occur because the tube is too low and protruding through the stoma. It should be withdrawn so that it is in the body of the stomach. This position can be attained by with drawing the tube until no aspirate is recovered and then pushing it down again very cautiously 1 cm at a time until the stomach contents are again recovered.

Alternatives and modifications of nasogastric intubation

Some believe that a nasogastric tube is unnecessary and can be dispensed with. There is no doubt that, in the majority of cases, this is correct. In a significant minority, however, dilatation of the stomach occurs quietly and sometimes disastrously and this is preventable by an indwelling tube.

Morris Lee's two-way intubation tube is a double-barrelled tube, one barrel of which is much longer than the other. The longer one is manipulated into the jejunum (or duodenum) at the end of the operation and the nasal end is connected to a reservoir of fluid. This obviates the need for intravenous fluid. The shorter barrel is in the stomach and can be aspirated in the ordinary way. The underlying principle of its use is that the jejunum is often active and functioning while the stomach is still paralysed.

Kay has used a special tube from the cavity of the stomach to the abdominal wall to obviate the need for a nasogastric tube. It is a modified gastrostomy procedure.

2. The drainage tube. If a corrugated drain or tube has been inserted it should be removed on the 5th day, but if there has been a discharge of bile or intestinal contents this should be reported at once and the tube should not be removed.

3. General management. The maintenance of fluid and electrolyte balance is continued intravenously until the stomach is emptying and the diet is gradually built up. In most cases the patient is mobilised on the day following operation and fit for discharge from hospital in 8 to 10 days.

Complications

1. Haemorrhage. Small quantities of blood are usually aspirated from the stomach in the first 12 hours. Larger quantities of loss, however, require treatment. Morphia is administered and blood transfusion given. A nasogastric tube is usually in position and the stomach contents aspirated.

Treatment for haematemesis (p. 407) is instituted. If the bleeding persists the wound may have to be reopened and the bleeding point ligated.

2. Vomiting. Occasionally severe persistent vomiting occurs, due to the obstruction of the intestine which has been joined to the stomach. It may be necessary to re-operate when this complication is present. Acute dilatation of the stomach may follow gastric operations and the nasogastric tube must not be removed until the stomach has recovered its tone.

3. Staphylococcal diarrhoea, due to a pure growth of *Staphylococcus pyogenes,* may occur as a complication of any operation, but more than

50 per cent of cases are subsequent to gastrectomy. It should be stressed that:

(a) It may be epidemic.

(b) The patient is usually receiving broad-spectrum antibiotics.

(c) A nasogastric tube has been used.

Clinically the condition may simulate internal haemorrhage, coronary thrombosis or pulmonary embolism until the diarrhoea appears. There is a gross loss of fluid. In suspected cases a specimen of faeces is sent for immediate microscopic examination for Gram-positive cocci, to confirm the diagnosis. The culture is also performed for antibiotic sensitivity.

Treatment. Broad spectrum antibiotics are discontinued. Erythromycin (0.5g) four times daily is given intramuscularly but in severe cases 250 mg doses should be given by slow intravenous injection. Fucidin (500 mg) 6-hourly is also of value. Fluid loss is replaced by intravenous fluid. The patient is nursed in isolation.

4. Pulmonary complications may be prevented in many cases by deep breathing exercises and free movement in bed. Antibiotics are administered in established infection.

5. Peritonitis may occur from leakage at the anastomosis or from rupture of the duodenal stump (Fig. 35.6) The latter results in a duodenal fistula. (This can also occur from damage to the duodenum in the operations of right hemicolectomy or nephrectomy on the right side.) The drain will always discharge bile-stained fluid if the duodenum has ruptured. The commonest day for a rupture is the fourth or fifth postoperative day. It is impossible to resuture the ruptured duodenum because the ferments are already eating away its very substance. Therefore treatment consists of:

(a) Nothing by mouth.

(b) Gastric aspiration—continuously.

(c) Suction drainage through the stab wound.

(d) The parenteral administration of fluid to maintain the fluid balance.

(e) The administration of antibiotics.

Fig. 35.6 Rupture of the duodenal stump following gastrectomy is the commonest fatal complication. The escaping enzymes destroy so much of the wall that suture is impossible and the only hope lies in removing the enzymes by nasogastric tube and suction through the fistula.

6. Stomal ulcer. This is a more remote complication, heralded by recurrence of the original symptoms of indigestion.

A stomal ulcer is an ulcer at the line of junction (the stoma) between the stomach and the small intestine. Strict medical treatment is usually prescribed, but if this is not successful a more extensive removal of the stomach or vagotomy is performed.

A stomal ulcer may cause a gastrojejuno-colic fistula by perforation into the colon.

A recurrent duodenal ulcer can occur following vagotomy and drainage.

THE POST-GASTRECTOMY AND GASTRIC SURGERY SYNDROMES

1. The 'dumping' syndrome

A proportion of patients develop this syndrome after the main meal. The symptoms are of varying severity and include:

Dizziness

Sweating

Palpitation

Epigastric discomfort and feeling of fullness

Extreme weakness, and, on occasion, loss of consciousness.

These symptoms may appear half an hour to 3 hours after food, and may be relieved by lying down.

The patient is advised to avoid a large meal if any of the above symptoms appear. His diet must be revised to ensure adequate nutrition by means of small but more frequent meals.

The syndrome can also occur after vagotomy and drainage operations.

2. Bilious vomiting

This is due to the sudden discharge of bile from the proximal jejunum into the stomach via the gastro-jejunostomy.

3. Malnutrition

(a) Anaemia.

(b) Vitamin deficiency, particularly vitamin B.

(c) Gross loss of weight.

(d) Osteoporosis.

Treatment. Vitamin deficiency and anaemia can be treated medically by giving the appropriate vitamin preparation or iron. A gluten-free diet is sometimes of help.

4. Post-vagotomy diarrhoea

This is an occasional but very distressing sequel of vagotomy. The cause is unknown. If simple measures such as codeine phosphate fail, cholestyramine may be advised. For intractable cases a reversed jejunal segment may be created to slow down intestinal transit.

Advice on leaving hospital

It should be explained to the patient that at his operation the ulcer and a large portion of his stomach have been removed, or some other operation performed, but his tendency to form another ulcer remains.

The fundamental principles of early aftertreatment must be rest, relaxation, a calm attitude to life and its incidents, plenty of soft non-irritating food, taken at frequent intervals, and not lacking in any of the essentials of a good normal diet and no smoking.

The patient should be warned that initially he will probably only feel like eating small amounts at one time. He will need to be off work for 6 to 12 weeks. He should fairly quickly be able to get back on to a normal diet.

BIBLIOGRAPHY

Biggs J C, Hugh T B, Dodds A J 1976 Gut 17:729
British Medical Journal Editorial 1979 1:642

36

Diseases of the liver, the gall bladder and the pancreas

THE LIVER

Apart from being the site of synthesis of plasma proteins, glucose metabolism and the production of essential clotting factors, the liver also conjugates the breakdown product of haemoglobin, bilirubin, into an excretable form which leaves the liver by the biliary canaliculi in conjunction with the bile acids and salts. For its various metabolic activities the liver receives an abundant blood supply from the hepatic artery and the portal vein. The blood drains into the hepatic veins which join the inferior vena cava. The anatomical relationships of the liver, gall bladder and pancreas are illustrated in Figure 36.1.

INJURY

Injury to the liver usually takes the form of laceration, and is due to a

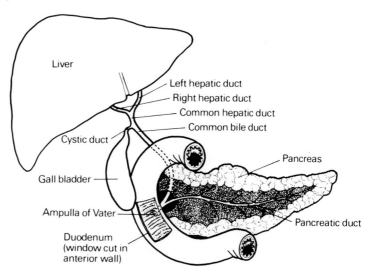

Fig. 36.1 The anatomy of the liver, the gall bladder and its duct and the pancreas.

crush injury of the abdomen in the majority of cases. Pain in the right hypochondrium, tenderness, and the signs of internal haemorrhage will be present. It is frequently associated with other abdominal injuries.

Treatment

The treatment consists of an exploratory laparotomy after blood replacement. If the tear is a minor one it may be sutured or simply left undisturbed. If the tear is a severe one the situation usually calls for a formal partial hepatic resection. The liver has remarkable powers of regeneration and may indeed regain its size following right hepatic lobectomy by the end of the third postoperative week.

INFLAMMATORY CONDITIONS

Viral hepatitis

Viral hepatitis comprises two microbiologically separate diseases serologically distinguishable from each other. Infective hepatitis is epidemic and believed to be transmitted by the faecal oral route, whereas serum viral hepatitis is transmitted by physical procedures and arises from:
    (i)   A pool of infected plasma or serum.
    (ii) A renal dialysis unit.
    (iii) Drug addiction.
    Serum hepatitis is associated with the serological entity Australian antigen (AuAg), much more commonly indicated as HB Ag, ie hepatitis B. It is acquired primarily within the walls of a hospital.
    All blood and serum products are potentially infected and the following precautions must, therefore, be taken:
    (a) All blood donors are tested for HB Ag.
    (b) All patients in dialysis units should be screened.
    (c) The sterilisation of syringes must be adequate.
    (d) Spilt blood should be disinfected with a hypochlorite solution or 10 per cent formalin.
    (e) Specimens of blood from suspected patients should carry a distinguishing mark.
    (f) All patients with liver disease, all those who have had previous blood transfusions and all drug addicts should be carefully screened.

Liver abscess

    1. *A solitary abscess* is usually a complication of amoebic dysentery. Surgical drainage of the abscess may be performed, but in most cases treatment consists of chloroquine or metronidazole with tetracycline for the secondary infection.
    2. *Multiple pyaemic abscesses* may occur as a complication of peritonitis. It is an extremely serious condition and chemotherapy alone offers the best prospects of cure. Multiple cholangiectatic abscesses may

develop from ascending infection within the bile ducts following obstruction of the common bile duct by a calculus or a growth. Chemotherapy and surgical relief of the obstruction are necessary.

Hydatid cyst of the liver

Hydatid disease is due to an infection caused by a parasite known as the *Taenia echinococcus*. The liver is one of the commonest sites for the infection. Surgical treatment consists of excision of the lining of the cyst and drainage of the cavity.

PORTAL HYPERTENSION

Cirrhosis of the liver may be caused by excessive alcohol intake, certain toxic agents and viral hepatitis. The liver substance heals by scar tissue and this may interfere with the normal flow of blood along the portal venous pathways contained within it. As a result there is back pressure on the portal venous system, this being most marked within the veins at the cardio-oesophageal junction. In time the veins become distended and tortuous, hence the term oesophageal varices. These thin walled veins may rupture thus giving rise to a massive upper gastrointestinal haemorrhage.

Shunting of the blood from the portal system into the systemic system by anastomosis of the portal vein to the inferior vena cava may be undertaken. This leads to a fall in the portal venous pressure. If a shunt is not feasible a direct attack on the bleeding by transthoracic ligation of the varices or endoscopic sclerotherapy may be undertaken.

NEOPLASMS OF THE LIVER

1. Primary carcinoma is uncommon in the Western world. It occurs more commonly in a cirrhotic liver than in a normal liver. The treatment is resection if possible.

2. Secondary carcinoma is almost invariably secondary to an intra-abdominal primary growth but is also quite common with neoplasms of the bronchus and breast. It may sometimes be temporarily controlled by intra-arterial cytotoxic agents.

INVESTIGATION OF THE LIVER

Liver function tests

Although these tests are nonspecific and often difficult to interpret they help to differentiate between obstructive jaundice which requires surgery and liver diseases which do not. Over three quarters of the liver may be destroyed before many of the tests show any abnormality. They attempt to provide information on:

Bile metabolism.
Plasma protein synthesis.
The liver enzymes.

Bile metabolism

Bilirubin is formed from haemoglobin in the cells of the reticulo-endo-thelial system (spleen, bone marrow, liver) where aged red cells are broken down. The bilirubin becomes attached to albumin in the plasma and is carried by the circulating blood through the liver. The bilirubin becomes conjugated (joined) to a substance called glucuronic acid in the liver and is passed by the bile ducts into the intestine. Here bacterial action converts it into stercobilinogen most of which is excreted in the faeces where, on exposure to air, it darkens to brown and is called stercobilin. Some of the stercobilinogen is reabsorbed from the intestine into the bloodstream and excreted in the urine as urobilin.

Urobilin in the urine. In complete obstructive jaundice there is no bilirubin in the intestines for the bacteria to convert to urobilinogen. Therefore there is no uruobilin to reabsorb into the bloodstream and none to pass into the urine. Tests for urobilin therefore are negative though the urine is dark due to a high content of bilirubin glucuronide.

Stercobilin in the faeces. The dark colour of the faeces depends on the amount of bilirubin entering the intestine. The stools are pale in obstructive jaundice.

Bile salts also appear in the urine in obstructive jaundice as they are drained back into the blood and excreted by the kidneys. Bile salts are detected by sprinkling flowers of sulphur on the surface of the urine in a test glass. If bile salts are present the sulphur sinks due to the lowering of surface tension.

Plasma proteins

Albumin and fibrinogen are synthesised in the liver. In severe liver disease therefore their level in the blood falls. The albumin may fall as low as 25 g per litre (normal 36–50 g per litre). The globulin level, however, remains unchanged, so the normal ratio of albumin to globulin (2:1) may be reversed. Globulin is not a single substance but a series of similar proteins called α (alpha), β (beta) and γ (gamma) globulins. When the liver is diseased the ratio of these globulins to one another in the plasma is altered. The thymol and zinc flocculation and turbidity tests are positive when these ratios are abnormal. Prothrombin is also synthesised within the liver, a process for which vitamin K is essential. If there is no bile in the intestine vitamin K cannot be absorbed and, therefore, in obstructive jaundice the prothrombin level is low. This requires correction before surgery can be carried out by the administration of vitamin K.

The liver enzymes

Serum alkaline phosphatase is removed from the blood by the liver and excreted in the bile. Normal values are about 35 to 105 International units per litre of serum. When the liver cells are diseased or the bile ducts blocked the level in the blood will rise. It should be noted that very high values·of serum alkaline phosphatase also occur in bone diseases when osteoblastic cells are overactive, e.g. rickets, Paget's disease, hyperparathyroidism, bone tumours.

Serum glutamate pyruvate transaminate (SGPT), 7 to 40 IU per litre, serum glutamate oxalacetate transaminase (SGOT), 7 to 40 IU per litre, and serum γ glutamyl transpeptidase (γ GT), 10 to 50 IU per litre, are enzymes whose levels are raised in conditions leading to damage of the liver cells such as viral hepatitis.

Liver puncture biopsy

Liver tissue may be obtained for histological examination either blindly by means of a Tru-cut or similar needle or by direct-vision needle biopsy using the laparoscope. It is helpful in the study of patients with liver disease when clinical signs and laboratory tests do not give a definite diagnosis. It is seldom indicated in jaundiced patients and is performed when sarcoidosis, Hodgkin's disease, or brucellosis are suspected.

Before the puncture is made the bleeding, clotting and prothrombin times are estimated and must be normal, liver function tests are performed, 2 units of blood are cross-matched and premedication with 15 mg morphia or 5 to 20 mg of diazepam is given. The patient lies on her back with a pillow under her right buttock, the right hand behind the head. The skin is cleansed, a local anaesthetic infiltrated and the liver biopsy needle is plunged into the liver. The biopsy specimen is placed in normal saline, labelled and sent to the pathologist. Postoperatively a watch should be kept for signs of internal haemorrhage.

Ultrasonography

This provides invaluable information about the size and consistency of the liver substance and is therefore, eminently suitable for the investigation of infiltrative disease of the liver, e.g. malignant secondary deposits.

Isotope scanning

This is similar to ultrasonography in its use but the information is more accurate.

Hepatic angiography

Occasionally arterial X-rays via the hepatic artery are used to investigate the liver. This artery is cannulated via the femoral.

CT scanning

This provides accurate and detailed information of the normality or otherwise of the liver.

Laparoscopy

Direct visualisation of the liver via a laparoscope can give valuable information concerning disease and on occasions avoid a laparotomy.

JAUNDICE

Jaundice is due to the retention of bile pigments in the tissues and in the blood. When the level of bilirubin within the blood rises (normal level is less than 15.4 μmol/litre) the patient becomes clinically jaundiced. The degree of jaundice may be measured by examination of the serum bilirubin. Whereas bilirubin is found in the urine in obstructive jaundice and in jaundice due to hepatitis, urobilin is absent in obstructive jaundice.

Jaundice may be classified by the site at which it is effectively caused, viz,:

Prehepatic. Haemolytic jaundice is a condition produced by the too rapid breaking up of the red blood corpuscles. It may be treated medically with cortisone or cured in some cases by removal of the spleen (p. 252).

Hepatic (diseases of the liver)
1. Viral jaundice has already been considered.
2. Cirrhosis.
3. Multiple secondary deposits.
4. Acute yellow atrophy.

Posthepatic (cholestatic jaundice). Due to obstruction of bile ducts:
1. Canalicular obstruction—chlorpromazine.
2. Bile ducts—stones carcinoma of the head of the pancreas.

Many of the above diseases are fully dealt with in medical textbooks. The important surgical form is due to obstruction of the common bile duct. This may result from:

(a) A stone impacted in the duct; or
(b) A carcinoma of the head of the pancreas obstructing the duct or a tumour growing in the common duct.
(c) Chronic pancreatitis (rarely).

Operative interference on a patient who is jaundiced can be dangerous. The blood has a lessened coagulability, due to the lack of vitamin K and consequently haemorrhage may be extremely difficult to control. Vitamin K is fat-soluble and therefore is not absorbed from the intestine in the absence of bile salts. For this reason vitamin K should be administered by intramuscular injection some days before and after operation. Large quantities of glucose are necessary to maintain the liver glycogen store and to help prevent further liver damage.

After operation a jaundiced patient requires special care, since not only is internal haemorrhage more likely to occur, but it may be more easily overlooked because *pallor cannot be observed*. The pulse volume and rate should be carefully watched (Fig. 36.2). As the condition improves, the colour of the stools is carefully noted each day, for they are a guide to the amount of bile reaching the intestine. When the patient is

Fig. 36.2 Postoperative hourly pulse chart—always important. Vital in jaundice, as pallor from haemorrhage is unobservable.

severely jaundiced the stools are almost white, and, as recovery occurs, tend to become more and more their normal colour. The urine is very dark in colour due to the presence of bile pigments.

There is an increased risk of renal failure. Mannitol after an intraven-ous fluid load, is used to prevent it (p. 428). An accurate record of urine output must be kept and any fall immediately reported. Wound healing is delayed and the susceptibility to infection is greater. Intolerable itching from retention of bile salts can be very distressing in persistent jaundice. Cholestyramine, which binds bile salts, is effective in relieving this symptom.

Jaundice in any form is very depressing mentally, and the nurse must make every allowance for irritability on the part of the patient. It is part of his disease.

THE GALL BLADDER

GALL-STONES

The most common disease of the gall bladder is caused by gall-stones formed by the precipitation of the constituents of bile. A gall-stone gives rise to symptoms when it moves. Movement may result in its obstructing the cystic duct with resultant acute cholecystitis, or the stone may migrate into the common bile duct causing obstruction to the main outflow of bile from the liver. There is a strong hereditary tendency in gall-stone formation. Ten per cent of gall-stones are pigment stones, 15 per cent are mainly composed of cholesterol, and 75 per cent are mixed in composition.

Fig. 36.3 Gall-bladder pain commences in the epigastrum and radiates to the back and shoulder.

Symptoms and signs of gall-stones

It has long been said that the most typical patient is a fat parous woman about the age of 40. This, however, is far from true. Gall-stones are equally common in the thin. They are certainly more common in the female than the male but they are by no means rare in men and are occasionally seen even in children.

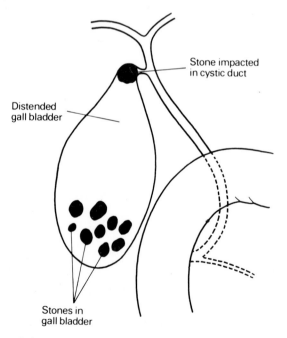

Fig. 36.4 Acute cholecystitis. A stone is impacted in the cystic duct. The gall-bladder, which contains numerous stones, is tense, distended and inflamed.

The patient may complain of recurrent bouts of flatulent dyspepsia precipitated by fatty goods. If a stone impacts in the neck of the gall bladder thus blocking the outflow the patient experiences severe upper abdominal pain originating in the epigastrium and then radiating around the flank to settle in the region of the right scapula (Fig. 36.3). The pain is usually colicky in type and is relieved by vomiting. This is the classical presentation of gall bladder colic.

If the pain persists and the abdomen is tender to palpation in the right hypochondrium it is very likely that the gall bladder has become acutely inflamed (acute cholecystitis), a diagnosis supported by elevated temperature and tachycardia (Fig. 36.4). Acute cholecystitis usually resolves on conservative therapy but occasionally may proceed to an empyema of the gall bladder.

Investigation of gall bladder disease

1. Direct radiographic examination of the abdomen reveals gall-stones only in 10 per cent of cases in which they are present because the majority of gall-stones are not radio-opaque. Therefore, only a positive X-ray will be of value.

2. Cholecystogram. The cholecystographic examination varies according to the opaque medium used and the technique employed.

The material, usually orablix, telepaque, or biloptin, is given by mouth the evening before. A radiograph is taken at 9 a.m. and if the gall bladder functions a fatty meal is then given and a further radiograph taken half an hour later. The patient will already have been prepared with the colon free from gas and faecal shadows. The material should be administered according to the makers' instructions, which should be closely followed. It is very important to be certain that the patient has not vomited the drug, as this renders the examination valueless. Filling defects, due to stones, will be seen within the gall bladder.

A diseased gall bladder will fail to concentrate the medium. As the medium is excreted by the liver and concentrated by the gall bladder the investigation is of little value in the presence of jaundice.

3. Cholangiogram (outlining of the common duct). This may be done:
(a) By the intravenous injection of biligrafin. Frequent radiographs are taken as the liver excretes the biligrafin.
(b) When the abdomen is open at operation or before a tube is removed from the common duct.

4. Ultrasonography. This is a valuable noninvasive investigation which is easy and quick to perform. The gall bladder and the bile ducts can be demonstrated. The presence of stones and dilation of the ducts can be seen.

5. Percutaneous transhepatic cholangiography is a useful procedure in obstructive lesions. It is usually done as an immediate preoperative investigation. The use of very thin needles makes it very safe.

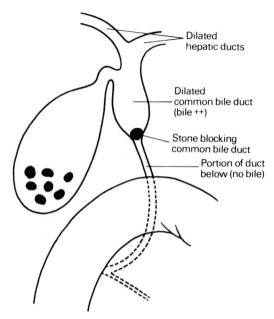

Fig. 36.5 Obstruction of the common bile duct by a stone. Note the duct above the stone and also dilatation of the hepatic ducts. This patient would be jaundiced.

Complications of gall stones

1. Acute cholecystitis.
2. Mucocele (filled with mucus) or empyema (filled with pus) of the gall bladder.
3. Common duct colic —stone in common bile duct.
4. Ascending cholangitis—infection secondary to stones in bile duct.
5. Obstructive jaundice (Fig. 36.5).
6. Acute pancreatitis.
7. Fistulous communication between the gall bladder and the duodenum with the possibility of the small bowel being obstructed by a gall stone (Fig. 33.4).
8. Carcinoma of the gall bladder.

Treatment

Acute cholecystitis and biliary colic. Most surgeons do not advise operation at the acute stage although this view is changing. The treatment usually prescribed is:

1. Rest in bed.
2. Pethidine (100 mg) by injection. Morphia is not recommended since it is said to produce spasm of the sphincter of Oddi which guards the common bile duct and pancreatic duct at the ampulla of Vater.
3. Antibiotics may be used.
4. Fluids (fat free) by mouth. An intravenous line can usually be avoided unless vomiting is severe.

Radical cure of gall-stones. Small radio-lucent gall-stones in a functioning gall bladder can be dissolved, in about 20 per cent of such cases, by the administration of chenodeoxycholic acid. Although it has been used clinically it is still not generally acceptable. The treatment is protracted and the stones may recur.

Removal of the gall bladder (cholecystectomy) removes the stones, the site of their formation, and a potential site for future problems. If excision of the organ technically is impossible, operation is confined to the removal of the stones and drainage of the gall bladder (cholecystostomy). Operative cholangiography is now performed routinely. If stones are present in the bile ducts they are removed and the common bile duct drained with a T-tube, the cross-limb of which is placed in the duct.

If the patient shows any of the features associated with the tendency to recurrent stone formation—the presence of biliary mud, papillary stenosis, intrahepatic stones or a grossly dilated common bile duct, an additional procedure to drain the duct may be undertaken. These include anastomosis of the duct to the duodenum or sphincteroplasty.

Care of the patient for gall-bladder operations

The usual preparation for any major abdominal operation is necessary. The main specific points concern the care of the drainage tubes. The nurse attending the patient in the theatre should take special care to note the exact position of each tube.

In all patients for cholecystectomy a nasogastric tube should be passed before the end of the operation. Patients after cholecystectomy tend to vomit a good deal of bile, and aspiration through a nasogastric tube for 24 hours eliminates this complication with its accompanying distress.

1. Drainage tube in the subhepatic pouch. The tube is inserted through a stab wound to drain the oozing of blood from the liver bed. It is also useful to reveal internal reactionary haemorrhage, and is usually removed after 48 hours. If there is any leakage of bile from the liver bed it also drains by this means.

2. Tube in the common duct. Bile flows along this tube, which is connected to a plastic bag. A T tube drain leading from the common duct to the outside (Fig. 36.6) will be inserted if the common bile duct has been explored. The volume of the bile excreted each day is measured and recorded and after 7 days a T tube cholangiogram is carried out. If this shows the bile duct to be patent the tube may be clamped for an hour or two. If the patient is pain free the tube may be withdrawn. The catgut sutures which previously secured it to the bile duct having by this time become friable and loose.

A specimen of bile may be sent for bacteriological examination. Where there has been severe cholangitis an antibiotic may be prescribed.

3. General care. The intravenous line commenced in the theatre can usually be removed on the second postoperative day and a normal diet is quickly resumed. If an anastomosis of the common bile duct to the duodenum has been performed the resumption of a normal diet should be more cautious.

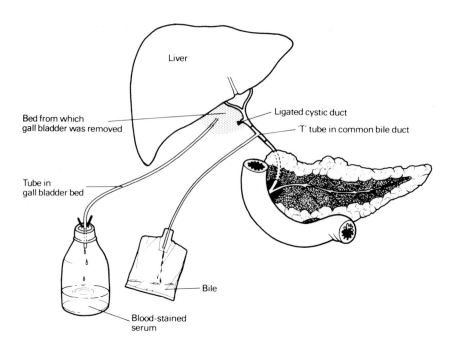

Fig. 36.6 The gall-bladder has been removed and its bed drained. The common bile duct was opened to remove a stone and closed around a 'T' tube which drains bile.

4. Jaundice. If the patient has been jaundiced or is jaundiced due to a stone in the common bile duct, vitamin K (10 mg) must be administered by injection preoperatively for three days and continued for several days after the operation. The jaundiced patient is liable to develop hepatorenal failure. This is now largely preventable by the administration of 500 ml of 10 per cent mannitol one hour before operation and this should be continued post-operatively. As mannitol produces a heavy diuresis, the fluid balance and electrolytes should be watched with great care.

Complications

1. Pulmonary complications are liable to occur especially at the base of the right lung. They may be prevented by adequate analgesia and breathing exercises.

2. Haemorrhage and bile leakage from the gall bladder bed—hence the importance of a subhepatic drainage tube.

3. Deep vein thrombosis and pulmonary embolism is more liable to occur in obese subjects. The incidence has probably decreased following the introduction of prophylactic subcutaneous heparin.

4. In the jaundiced patient there is always the danger of postoperative renal failure. This can be minimised by maintenance of a normal blood pressure during operation, careful pre- and postoperative intravenous fluid administration together with the administration of the osmotic diuretic mannitol during surgery.

5. Retained stone in the common bile duct. This will require further exploration, endoscopic division of the sphincter of Oddi, so that the

stone will pass into the duodenum or removal with a stone basket via the T-tube tract.

ASIATIC CHOLANGIO-HEPATITIS

Obstruction of the common bile duct by the liver fluke is quite common in the Far East. The smaller ducts in the liver are also involved and the patient presents with pain, Charcot's biliary fever and jaundice. As soon as he is fit the duct is emptied of stones and the liver fluke, but because of the presence of similar changes in the liver a wide opening in the lower end of the duct into the duodenum is effected so that inaccessible stones and flukes as well as pus can drain. The gall bladder is also removed.

CARCINOMA OF THE GALL BLADDER

The new growth usually occurs in a gallbladder which contains gall-stones. The rapid invasion of the liver by the growth renders most cases hopeless.

THE PANCREAS

The principal pancreatic diseases of surgical importance are acute and chronic pancreatitis and carcinoma. Rarely cysts, calculi, insulin and gastrin secreting tumours occur.

ACUTE AND RELAPSING PANCREATITIS

The great danger of this condition lies in the fact that the pancreatic juices, so potent in the digestion of fat and protein, digest the tissues with which they come in contact.

Although the exact cause remains unknown the following factors play a part in the aetiology:

(a) Gallstones.
(b) Alcohol.
(c) Viral infections such as mumps.
(d) Drugs such as steroids.
(e) Metabolic conditions—hyperparathyroidism and aminoacidurea.

Symptoms and signs

There is a sudden onset of epigastric pain which often spreads in a girdle-like fashion, frequently after a meal. The patient's general condition may remain good or he may show signs of shock, in varying degree. The face may be slightly cyanosed and the patient does not lie absolutely still as in the case of a perforated peptic ulcer, but tends to roll about. The temperature is subnormal in the first hours of the attack and the pulse rate is elevated. The abdomen is tender, but not rigid.

Investigation

1. The estimation of the serum amylase by the laboratory is of the greatest value. The normal value is 70 to 300 International units. In acute pancreatitis a reading of over 1000 units is usual. The test should be performed in the first 24 hours, and daily thereafter to monitor progress.

2. A white blood count may be elevated.

3. The serum electrolytes and blood urea should be estimated daily.

4. The blood sugar is estimated and urine tested for the presence of sugar. The pancreatitis may cause a temporary or permanent diabetic state.

5. Serum calcium is estimated. The serum calcium may fall due to its incorporation within areas of fat necrosis in the abdomen resulting from the action of pancreatic enzymes.

6. Peritoneal tap may be performed for diagnostic purposes. The fluid will show the presence of pancreatic enzymes.

7. Straight X-ray of the abdomen may show gall-stones or loops of dilated small bowel, secondary to the pancreatitis.

8. Ultrasonography. This will demonstrate gall-stones and may show pancreatic enlargement due to inflammation.

9. Cholecystography is performed when the attack has subsided if ultrasonography has not shown any abnormality.

Complications

1. Paralytic ileus.
2. Renal failure.
3. Respiratory failure.
4. Diabetes mellitus.
5. Obstructive jaundice.
6. Septicaemia.
7. Pancreatic or retroperitoneal abscess, which may require drainage.
8. Pseudocyst formation (a collection of fluid in the lesser sac) which may need to be drained into the stomach. One in 30 patients develop a pseudocyst within 6 weeks of an acute attack.
9. Recurrent pancreatitis.

Treatment

There is no specific treatment for acute pancreatitis, the management of the patient being entirely supportive in type.

1. Maintenance of fluid and electrolyte balance—loss of fluid into the retroperitoneal space maybe very great. Massive transfusions of whole blood and plasma protein fraction may be vital. A careful watch is necessary to maintain an adequate urinary output. Renal failure is a very real danger.

2. Alleviation of pain—this may be very severe and intractable. Codeine phosphate by injection is the best analgesic as it relaxes the sphincter of Oddi, but pethidine may also be required.

3. Suppression of pancreatic secretion by the use of continuous gastric suction to suppress the secretion mechanism is essential.

4. Calcium gluconate 10 ml 10 per cent solution i.v. may be required if hypocalcaemia occurs.

5. Antibiotics, and the use of anticholinergic agents to suppress pancreatic secretion are of unproven value. The use of aprotinin (an anti-enzyme) is not only unproven but extremely expensive. Surgical interference is rarely undertaken in the acute stage, except for complications.

6. Cholecystectomy is performed, if gall-stones are present, during the same admission once the acute episode has settled down.

CHRONIC PANCREATITIS

This is a condition in which the pancreas is slowly destroyed. It may follow acute pancreatitis but is a separate condition. Alcoholism is a prominent cause of chronic pancreatitis. It may present with:

Pain in the upper abdomen
Symptoms and signs of malabsorption
Jaundice
Diabetes

Investigations

Investigations include straight X-ray of the abdomen (which may show pancreatic calcification), cholecystography, ultrasonography, isotope scanning, sophisticated tests to determine the secretory capacity of the pancreas and chemical examination of the stools to measure malabsorption. Duodenoscopy and cannulation of the papilla of Vater and retrograde choledochopancreatography are formed to outline the pancreatic duct.

Treatment

Treatment is very unsatisfactory. Pancreatic enzymes orally and a high calorie, high protein diet may help. Continued alcoholism is the most important factor in predicting failure to improve. Surgical procedures undertaken for pain or persistent jaundice include division of the sphincter of Oddi, total or subtotal pancreatectomy and various operations for strictures in the pancreatic duct.

CARCINOMA OF THE PANCREAS

Symptoms and signs

Patients with carcinoma in the pancreas often have rather vague insidious symptoms for some time before they present to the doctor. Tumours in the head of the pancreas usually present with painless obstructive jaundice, those in the body and tail with persistent pain (often of a girdle-like distribution). Prior to such presentation the patient may have a general feeling of being unwell, some loss of appetite and weight, and vague epigastric or back pain.

Investigation

The diagnosis can sometimes be difficult to make. It depends upon some or all of the following tests.
1. Ultrasound scan of pancreas.
2. Isotope scan of pancreas.
3. Pancreatography via duodenoscope.
4. Cytology on duct aspirate, via duodenum.
5. Coeliac axis arteriography, to show pancreatic blood supply.
6. Percutaneous thin needle cholangiography, when patient is jaundiced
7. Laparotomy. This is often the way that the diagnosis is finally confirmed. Even then needle biopsy may be required to distinguish between neoplasm and inflammation.

Treatment

If the growth is mobile and has not spread anywhere it may be possible to remove it surgically. This is a long and technically difficult operation with a high mortality. If the patient is jaundiced he is prepared for operation in the way already described (p. 422). Anastomosis of the gall bladder to the jejunum (cholecystojejunostomy) or to the duodenum (cholecystoduodenostomy) relieves the jaundice. The prognosis in this disease is poor, the average life expectancy from diagnosis being about one year.

ISLET CELL TUMOUR OF PANCREAS

A tumour of the islet cell results in an excessive secretion of insulin. The patient suffers from recurrent hypoglycaemic attacks. Cure is effected by excision of the tumour.

GASTRIN-SECRETING TUMOUR

This tumour causes intractable duodenal and jejunal ulceration. The treatment is removal of the tumour if it can be located or total gastrectomy to remove the acid-producing organ being stimulated by the gastrin. Treatment with cimetidine is an alternative, to reduce gastric acid secretion.

BIBLIOGRAPHY

Williams K G, Dawson J L 1979 British Medical Journal 2-766

37

Diseases of the small intestine

Inflammation of the small intestine (enteritis) is common but, with the notable exception of Crohn's disease, usually recovers with medical treatment. Carcinoma, so prevalent in the gastrointestinal tract, is a rare finding in the small bowel. The dominant surgical lesion is intestinal obstruction which has been considered in Chapters 33 and 34. Its causes together with the special features of other particular conditions are reviewed here.

INJURY

Closed abdominal injury may result in a tear of the small intestine. The symptoms and signs are a combination of those of internal haemorrhage and peritonitis. After resuscitation laparotomy is undertaken and the intestine repaired.

MECKEL'S DIVERTICULUM

In the last 60 cm of the ileum a diverticulum of the bowel (Fig. 35.3) not unlike the appendix, may be present. It is a congenital abnormality. It varies in length from 5 to 50 cm and, like the appendix, it may become inflamed. The symptoms, signs, and treatment are similar to those of appendicitis. On other occasions it may be the cause of intestinal obstruction by ensnaring a loop of the intestine around a band of tissue connecting the diverticulum to the under surface of the umbilicus. The clinical features are those of intestinal obstruction. An important feature of the histology of Meckel's diverticulum is that it may contain ectopic epithelium such as gastric and pancreatic tissue. Ectopic gastric epithelium is apt to cause the adjacent epithelium to ulcerate and bleed. A bleeding Meckel's diverticulum is one of the causes of rectal bleeding in children. An ulcer may perforate. The diverticulum may twist on itself and become gangrenous, or intussuscept (see below).

CROHN'S DISEASE OR REGIONAL ENTERITIS

This is an inflammatory condition originally described in the terminal ileum. It is now accepted that it is a generalised disease involving any part of the gastrointestinal tract, the commonest sites being the terminal ileum and the colon. The cause is unknown. It may give rise to general ill health, abdominal pain and diarrhoea, or to symptoms similar to append-icitis, or to obstructive symptoms. Ninety per cent of all cases come to surgery eventually.

Obstruction, perforation or fistula formation are complications which occur. Skin ulceration and infection, iritis, arthropathy and peri-anal sepsis may also occur.

The diagnosis is made by radiology (barium enema, Ba meal and small bowel meal), endoscopy (sigmoidoscopy, colonoscopy, gastroscopy) and biopsy. It is sometimes difficult to distinguish it from ulcerative colitis. Corticosteroids and immuno-suppressive drugs such as azathioprine may be prescribed but are of doubtful long term value.

Acute obstruction usually subsides on treatment with nasogastric suction and intravenous fluids so that if operation is necessary it can be performed as an elective procedure. Resection is the usual procedure but the recurrence rate in other parts of the gastrointestinal tract is high as is the need for further operation. Yet most sufferers from the disease remain cheerful and hopeful that things will not get much worse from a condition which is virtually a life sentence.

INTESTINAL OBSTRUCTION

The main clinical features and treatment of acute intestinal obstruction, have already been considered in Chapter 34. Sometimes intestinal obstruction is incomplete (subacute). This may resolve but more often it progresses to complete destruction.

Causes

The bowel may be obstructed because:

1. Its lumen is blocked by a foreign body or a gall-stone.

2. Its wall is altered by disease such as Crohn's disease, new growths of various sorts, a stricture due or to an old tuberculous ulcer, drugs such as potassium chloride (in certain preparations), or to an intussusception.

3. The wall is constricted by something outside it; e.g. the neck of a hernial sac, adhesions (often from previous surgery), connective tissue bands. A loop of intestine may twist around itself (volvulus) or around an adhesion or band.

1. **Blockage by a foreign body.** One cause is a gall-stone. The fundus of the gall-bladder becomes adherent to the duodenum, and slowly a fistula between the two organs is formed (Fig. 33.4) A large gall-stone may pass through the fistula and become impacted in the narrowest portion of the small intestine, the ileum. If the stone is small it may pass without

difficulty. An impacted stone is removed after incision of the bowel and then the wall is re-sutured.

In some conditions of intestinal hurry, digestion has not time to occur and inadequately chewed food may block the lower ileum. This may result after gastrectomy or gastrojejunostomy. Swallowed foreign bodies such as marbles are occasionally the cause of blockage in the case of children.

2. The wall is altered by disease. Crohn's disease, which has already been discussed, is one cause. An important cause, particularly in infants under 12 months, is intussusception.

Intussusception. This is due to a small portion of the bowel becoming invaginated into the portion distal to it. As a result of peristalsis, the process is carried further until, as it were, the bowel, instead of being a single tube, now has three layers. The bowel is, in fact, telescoped into itself (Fig. 37.1).

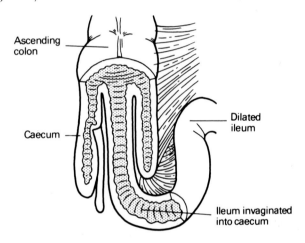

Ascending colon

Caecum

Dilated ileum

Ileum invaginated into caecum

Fig. 37.1 An intussusception.

Symptoms and signs. The child is usually a healthy male infant about 9 months old. His good health is probably the cause of excessive peristalsis driving one loop of bowel into the one below. The change of diet at the time may be a causal factor, and in the infant the Peyer's patches are enlarged so that they form a small tumour-like mass, disturbing the normal peristaltic wave. An alternative theory is that it is due to enlargement of Peyer's patches from an adenovirus which could account for its seasonal occurrence. The child screams with pain, which is typical of intestinal colic. The face becomes very pale when the colic is at its height and brightens in the intervals between the spasms. Vomiting is invariably present, and the passage of a small amount of bright red jelly-like blood clot per rectum is almost diagnostic. Careful examination of the abdomen reveals a sausage-like mass. Treatment consists of reduction of the bowel usually by operation, but retrograde pressure by barium enema may effect reduction. It should be given only under X-ray screening control. The nurse must watch especially for recurrence of symptoms on the first night after operation.

In the adult, intussusception occasionally occurs due to a neoplasm (usually polypoid) or a Meckel's diverticulum.

3. Lesions outside the bowel.

Causes

 Strangulated hernias

 Bands

 Adhesions.

Bands and adhesions may form as a result of previous operations or following inflammatory conditions such as generalised peritonitis, cholecystitis, appendicitis. As in all acute obstructions, urgent operation is essential to deal with the cause.

MESENTERIC THROMBOSIS

This condition presents with acute abdominal pain, circulatory collapse, the passage of blood from the rectum and abdominal tenderness. It is increasingly common as a manifestation of atherosclerosis. The mesenteric vessels are occluded by thrombosis or embolism. The main vessel or branch of it may be involved with gangrene of the segment of intestine supplied. The outlook is very poor however it is treated. Treatment includes resection, removal of the thrombus and anticoagulant therapy.

OPERATIONS ON THE SMALL INTESTINE

Enterolysis

This is the freeing of the intestine by division of bands or adhesions.

 Postoperatively the patient is treated with nasogastric suction and intravenous fluids until the paralytic ileus resolves. Where the adhesions have beem extensive or the intestine very dilated this may take several days.

Resection

A loop of bowel is removed. The continuity of the intestine is then restored by suture.

 This is usually performed for a gangrenous small intestine, for injury, or for neoplasm. Postoperatively the important points are aspiration of the stomach to relieve any distension above the anastomosis as well as parenteral fluid replacement. The relief of flatus by the passage of a flatus tube may ease discomfort.

Enteroanastomosis

This is the short-circuiting or bypassing of one portion of the bowel into another beyond a pathological lesion without removing the cause.

This is frequently performed for an obstruction which is not causing gangrene of the intestine, such as tuberculosis of the small intestine, severe adhesions, or Crohn's disease.

Enterostomy

This involves an opening of the intestine onto the abdominal wall.
1. For feeding purposes. This is performed:
   (a) Sometimes for inoperable cancer of the stomach.
   (b) Very occasionally for intractable gastric ulcer where the condition of the patient is too poor for radical operation, yet relief from medical treatment is very slight.
2. For ulcerative proctocolitis. The ileum is brought to the surface—an ileostomy (Ch. 38)—after removal of the colon and rectum. Very occasionally an ileostomy is performed to rest the colon without removing it.

Ileojejunal bypass

This has been performed for obesity. The immediate mortality is 5 per cent and the complications are many—wound dehisence, chest infection, pulmonary embolism, polyarthritis, electrolyte depletion and bypass enteritis. Weight loss is due not to malabsorption but to loss of appetite from a dilated bowel. The long-term results are poor.

Reversed loop in short gut syndrome

The short gut syndrome follows massive bowel resection in such conditions as mesenteric occlusion and internal strangulation. A loss greater than 75 per cent results in rapid intestinal transit, diarrhoea and malabsorption. If medical measures fail reversal of a 7.5-14.0 cm segment of the more distal small intestine is undertaken.

BIBLIOGRAPHY

Alexander-Williams J, Fielding J F, Cooke W T 1972 Gut 13: 973
Gazzard B G, Price H L, Libby G W, Dawson A M 1978 British Medical Journal 2: 1117

38

Stoma care

Stoma care commences when the decision to form a stoma has been taken. The successful management of a stoma (literally a mouth or opening) on the abdominal wall demands surgical and nursing skills, the cooperation of the patient as well as assistance from the pharmacist, the social worker, the housing authorities and maybe those responsible for refuse disposal. The support of the patient's family and the skill of the community nurse are essential. The indications for a stoma, the choice of stoma and the perioperative management are discussed in Chapters 39, 40 and 42.

Attempts have been made to make stomas continent surgically. The continent reservoir ileostomy has been designed but the complications associated with it have been too serious to commend it for general use. The magnetic ring implant (p. 448) in colostomies also has special complications.

TYPES OF STOMAS

1. Ileostomy. The terminal ileum is fashioned to project as a spout 5 centimetres long onto the skin of the abdominal wall (Figs. 38.1 and 38.2). The effluent is semi-fluid and corrosive.

2. Colostomy. The faecal discharge from an iliac colostomy is semi-solid but may be more fluid from a transverse colostomy.

3. Ileal conduit. A loop of ileum is isolated from the bowel, the upper part of the loop is closed and the ureters transplanted into the lumen. The lower end is brought out as a stoma. The small intestine is restored in continuity (Fig. 38.3). The loop of ileum acts as a urinary conduit.

4. Cutaneous ureterostomy. The ends of one or both ureters are attached to the skin surface.

PREOPERATIVE CARE AND COUNSELLING

There are three essential preoperative steps:

1. Acceptance by the patient. The patient is often very ill, which is

Fig. 38.1   Ileostomy showing coaption of skin to mucosa.

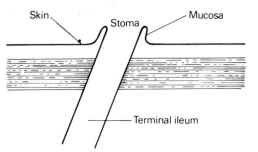

Fig. 38.2   Diagram showing the terminal ileum brought through the abdominal wall. The mucosa of the ileum is everted and sutured to the skin.

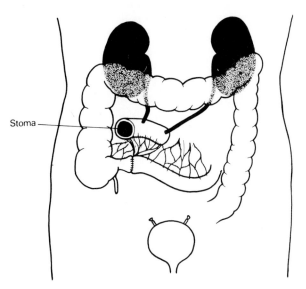

Fig. 38.3   Urinary conduit. The ureters are implanted into the isolated loop of the ileum. As shown the ileum is restored in continuity.

precisely the reason that major surgery terminating with an ileostomy is advised.

To the desperately ill patient with severe proctocolitis or severe intestinal obstruction any relief is welcome even if it involves the fashioning of a stoma. The patient suffering from a lesion such as carcinoma of the rectum, who feels comparatively well, finds a stoma difficult to accept.

The surgeon should preferably see the patient alone and satisfy himself that not only is consent obtained but that the patient understands to what he is consenting. His approach will depend to some extent on the personality of the patient and may vary according to the patient's age, intelligence, work and other relevant factors. The patient will be told that the stoma is a projecting moist and red spout of normal bowel. He must be reassured that he will be taught how to look after it, will not be discharged home until he is proficient in its care, and that afterwards he will have the support and care of the unit. He can be reassured that he need not worry about odours and other people will be unaware that he is wearing a bag. Nevertheless, the thought of a stoma is very distressing to most patients. Their fears about eating, the ability to work and to partake in normal activities should be allayed as far as possible.

The next person to discuss the problem with the patient is the stoma care nurse (stomatherapist). Her specialised knowledge and support in the hospital and in the future will inspire confidence. She may arrange a meeting with a patient of the same sex, who already has a similar stoma, who can encourage and help. The patient's relatives should also be involved at this stage.

2. Siting the stoma. This is marked on the abdominal wall a day or two before the operation by the surgeon and stoma care nurse together. The site chosen is usually midway between the umbilicus and the anterior superior spine but avoiding the patient's belt line. An appropriate appliance is fixed to the skin, avoiding scars, creases and boney prominences. The patient is examined lying in bed, sitting and standing to check that the site chosen is satisfactory. This can be further confirmed by leaving the appliance in place for 24 hours. The site is indelibly marked on the skin of the abdominal wall. This disc of skin is removed as the first step at operation before the abdominal wall is distorted by major incision. The siting for a temporary colostomy is not usually as important because it is done as an emergency and hopefully it will be closed before too long. The ongoing problems should not arise.

3. Allergy testing. The patient should be tested for allergy to the materials used in the appliance to avoid allergic reactions at a stage when they can be most inconvenient.

THE APPLIANCES

The problem facing the patient with a stoma, of whatever type, is that he has an opening which has no sphincter and which produces an effluent requiring collection and disposal. This requires a mechanism in which leakage is prevented, damage to the stoma and surrounding skin is avoided and odour prevented.

There is a wide choice of appliances available for all types of stomas. Continuous research is in progress to improve them. The final choice will be made by the patient, assisted by the stomatherapist. This can be decided only when the oedema and swelling of the stoma subside and the patient finds a technique of management at which he is efficient. He is in no way committed to use what has been applied in the immediate postoperative period. It is explained to the patient that the bag with which he comes back from the theatre is for the convenience of nursing observations and care and not for the patient's convenience. That will be considered later before he goes home.

The shape of the stoma may change as time progresses and it should be noted that while most are rounded some stomas are almost square.

The *two main types* of appliance are 'closed' and 'drainable'. The former are discarded when full, the latter can be emptied and retained. An appliance can be one-piece or two-piece (Fig. 38.4). The one piece consists of a bag and an attached adhesive square which sticks to the skin around the stoma. The two piece consists of a flange which adheres to the skin and a bag which can be removed from the face of the flange without disturbing the skin.

Fig. 38.4 Types of drainable stoma bags showing type of outlet and closures. Suitable post operatively or for an ileostomy.

The closed bag is usually used for a patient with a reasonably well formed stool while the drainable bag is used for a patient in whom frequent drainage of a loose or fluid stool is necessary (e.g. ileostomy, caecostomy or transverse colostomy). The urobags have a different kind of seal at the bottom to reduce the risk of leakage.

All stoma bags fitted at operation should be drainable and transparent so that the stoma can be inspected and the effluent drained with minimal disturbance to the patient. Later, opaque bags may be used to conceal sight of the effluent. A cover of cotton-polyester conveniently absorbs sweat from the skin. The bags are odourproof. Disposable bags are usually preferred. A belt may be worn with some appliances but with experience the patient may decide it is unnecessary. For those who engage in heavy work or sporting activities stronger non-disposable materials may be used and a belt may be necessary.

ILEOSTOMY

At the end of the operation a suitable appliance is fitted. The wound and the skin around the stoma may be protected by a sheet of stomahesive. However, most appliances now have protective squares incorporated into them thus ensuring minimal leakage onto the surrounding skin. As soon as possible the patient is taught to look after the stoma. The stoma is insensitive but delicate and easily traumatised. The surrounding skin has to be kept in good condition and will become sore if leakage occurs. The basic requirement is to maintain a perfect seal between the skin and the appliance, which may be changed as often as the patient feels it necessary but should not be left longer than 7 days.

Normally the rule for aseptic technique is 'from clean area into dirty area' but in the case of a stoma patient any soiling, due to a leaking bag etc., should be cleaned up and a fresh bag applied prior to any aseptic technique being carried out.

Postoperative care of the stoma

1. The abdominal dressing will have to be changed if it is soiled. The stoma bag should be changed before the midline dressing because the bag can stay on for several days whereas the dressing may need changing more frequently. This also allows the stoma bag to be undisturbed for several days should the surgical dressing encroach on the adhesive area of the bag. If the bag is put on after the dressing overlapping will occur leading to an inadequate seal and leakage.

2. The stitches. Some surgeons prefer to remove the stitches around a stoma after 5-6 days even if they are of catgut to avoid 'bumpy' healing, which predisposes to leakage. This is especially so in urinary stomas.

3. Baths. While still in hospital the patient can get into the bath with an appliance on if the wound is unhealed. Once it has healed a bath may be taken without the appliance. The skin will benefit from washing.

4. Skin soreness and leakage are discussed below.

Surgical complications at the stoma

1. Skin soreness is discussed below but, in addition to the causes mentioned, poor siting of the stoma may require revision.

2. Prolapse, recession or fistula formation, as well as obstruction may necessitate surgical refashioning of the stoma.

3. Bleeding is usually due to damage by the flange and will clear up as soon as the cause is recognised and corrected.

4. Recurrent disease does not occur in proctocolitis but may be the cause if the stoma was fashioned for Crohn's disease and further investigation is indicated.

5. Hernia formation adds to the difficulties of securing the appliance. It may be controlled with a suitable belt.

Changing the appliance

The final choice of the type of appliance will be made by the patient with the advice of the stoma nurse. Amongst the factors to be considered will be the general condition of the patient. For example an elderly person with arthritic hands and poor eyesight may find it difficult to manage an appliance and will require the simplest bag possible.

In a two piece appliance the bag is detached, the stoma wiped free of mucus or faecal material with a soft paper tissue and the new bag attached to the flange. When the whole appliance is changed, whether it is a one or two piece, the following equipment is necessary:

1. A new appliance.
2. Warm water.
3. White tissues.
4. Double sided plaster, stomahesive, Karaya washers or paste.
5. A pair of scissors.
6. A bowl lined with newspaper for discarded tissues and the appliance.
7. Deoderant.

Fig. 38.5 Ileostomy accessories:

Skin protection	Adhesives
Deodorants	Karaya paste
Bag covers	Flatus filter

Spenco flakes (render very fluid output more solid and lessen risk of leakage).

The new appliance is prepared and the old appliance removed by gently peeling it off. The stoma and the surrounding skin is wiped with soft tissue to remove old Karaya or faecal material. Adhesive material still adherent to the skin is best removed by the patient taking a bath rather than by using solvents. Otherwise the area is washed with warm water using no soap. The skin is thoroughly dried with tissues and adhesive is applied only when the skin is absolutely dry. The new appliance is fitted and the old appliance and soiled tissues wrapped in newspaper for disposal.

Leakage and skin soreness

This may occur because:
1. The skin was not completely dry.
2. The adhesive sheet was wrinkled.
3. The flange was not fitted correctly over the stoma or the hole in the appliance was not the correct size. This may also cause bleeding from injury to the spout of ileum. The stoma contracts for several weeks following the operation and it is essential to repeatedly check the size. Discs are provided by the manufacturers for this purpose.
4. The patient has increased in weight so the appliance is ill-fitting
5. Air from the bag has not been expelled.
6. The bag has been allowed to overfill or a bag which is too large has been used so that the flange is soaked in effluent.
7. The site of the stoma is poor.
8. Allergic reactions in the skin to the Karaya gum, the adhesive and other materials may occur. This is much less common with the use of modern hypoallergenic adhesives and materials.
9. Monilial infection of the mouth can extend to the skin around the stoma. Many patients have been on antibiotics which, as well as diarrhoea, may induce a monilial infection.

As soon as skin soreness appears every effort is made to discover and correct the cause. Assuming the preoperative allergy tests (p. 440) negative skin soreness is treated by application of stomahesive with Karaya gum to the excoriated skin so that it acts as a second skin on which the appliance can be placed. Various skin gels and barrier creams are also available. In severe reactions hydrocortisone cream may be prescribed. Stomahesive or other protective squares can be used on top to act as a surface on which to put the appliance. The cream content may prevent the bag sticking but there are barrier creams which will allow the adhesive to stick. Soreness sufficiently severe to require hydrocortisone while the patient is in hospital should have been investigated and corrected before it became so severe. It should be borne in mind that hydrocortisone is absorbed by the stoma.

If leakage is due to old scars, skin folds or creases around the stoma, these can be filled by a variety of pastes before fitting the appliance.

Other requirements of the patient

1. Access to the advice of a stomatherapist.

2. A bathroom in his home.

3. Ready access to a supply of new equipment.

4. A settled method of disposal of used appliances and wipes. The bag's contents can be emptied into the lavatory but the bag is wrapped in newspaper, placed in a plastic bag which is tied and disposed of in the dust bin. If this is not possible other arrangements are made with the authorities. They should not be burnt in an open fire as plastic gives off nasty acid fumes.

Fig. 38.6 Urinary ileal conduit with bag attached.

Fig. 38.7 Equipment for urostomy. Note the outlet on the bags, one of which shows night drainage tube attached.

ILEAL URINARY CONDUIT

The ureters are implanted into a free isolated loop of ileum (Fig. 38.3). The stoma, which looks identical with an ileostomy stoma, discharges urine and a little mucus but no faecal material (Fig. 38.6). The management of the appliance and the care of the stoma is identical to that of an ileostomy. Immediately after the operation a Foley catheter is inserted into the loop, the balloon inflated and the catheter brought out through the flange of the appliance into the collecting bag. Ureteric catheters may have been inserted and drain in the same way. Seven days later, if they have not been extricated previously, they are removed. A bag with a non-return valve should be used and at night a drainage bag with tubing can be attached if necessary (Fig. 38.7). Complications are similar to those of an ileostomy stoma but, in addition, the following may develop:

1. Obstruction of the stoma. It will be noticed that the urinary volume has diminished and the flow is slow. A gloved finger passed into the stoma is all that is usually necessary. A catheter may be inserted to drain the loop.

2. Urinary infection is a constant hazard. A specimen of urine is taken from the stoma with a sterile catheter for bacteriological examination—one from the bag is of no value. Mucus found in the urine from an ileal conduit is quite normal and not indicative of a urinary infection.

3. Phosphatic deposits and encrustation from infected urine may occur on the stoma. The urine is acidified with ascorbic or mandelic acid and the appropriate antibiotic administered. The patient is confined to bed and a wet dresssing of half strength vinegar dissolves the deposits and reduces the oedema in a few days. The bag needs to be a neat fit otherwise leakage will occur.

CUTANEOUS URETEROSTOMY

The ureters are stitched to the skin and urine collected by means of stick-on bags. The problems are much greater than those of an ileal conduit as leakage is more likely.

COLOSTOMY AND CAECOSTOMY

The formation of an 'artificial anus' entails bringing a portion of the large intestine to the surface of the abdominal wall so that its contents are diverted to the exterior.

This may take the form of either a colostomy or a caecostomy. Of the two, the colostomy is undoubtedly preferable because the faeces become more solid as they approach the rectum.

The faecal discharge from a caecostomy is thin and extremely irritant, so that, as a permanent arrangement, it is unsatisfactory. It is occasionally performed as an emergency measure in a patient who is so ill from obstruction of the distal bowel that exploration of the abdomen is impossible. After a low anastomosis in the distal bowel it may be performed as a temporary 'safety valve'.

A colostomy is performed either as a temporary or permanent measure for growths of the pelvic colon or rectum. It is almost invariable performed in cases of wounds of the rectum, so that the faecal flow is diverted from the wound. Congenital absence of the rectum or paraplegia in young adults is occasionally an indication.

CAECOSTOMY

A caecostomy is performed by the insertion of a tube into the caecum. The opening is usually valvular in type and frequently closes spontaneously after the tube has been removed.

The tube is connected to a drainage bag by the bedside so that the drainage is dependent and the discharge does not irritate the skin. After 24 hours when the caecostomy site is sealed off by inflammatory adhesions twice daily irrigation of 50 ml normal saline is commenced. As much as possible of the colonic contents as well as the irrigating fluid is withdrawn and drainage contines.

After 10 days, however, the tube drops out, and every effort must be made to prevent the skin from becoming inflamed and excoriated. Moist and petroleum jelly dressings tend to make the skin soggy. Stomahesive with a good seal will protect the skin.

A permanent caecostomy is almost unmanageable from the patient's point of view and if at all psssible it is avoided by anastomosis of the ileum to the transverse colon.

COLOSTOMY

The varieties of colostomy are illustrated in Fig. 38.8.

1. Loop colostomy. A loop of colon is brought to the surface of the abdominal wall and held in position by a thin rod or bridge passed through the mesocolon. The wound is then sutured. The colostomy is opened immediately.

2. Defunctioning colostomy. The loop is exteriorised and then divided so that there is no communication between the two orifices which are now separated by a bridge of skin. This provides complete rest to the distal colon.

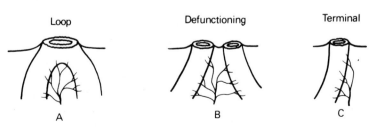

Fig. 38.8 Types of colostomy.

3. End or terminal colostomy. The colonic mucous membrane is sutured to the skin. Since this is usually performed only when all the distal bowel has been removed there is only one orifice and there is no possibility of subsequent closure. It is performed in conditions such as abdomino-perineal resection of the rectum. The patient should not be given any false hope that the colostomy can be removed.

A colostomy may be performed in the ascending, transverse or pelvic colon. The more distally it can be placed the better as the contents become more solid. A loop colostomy has a rod which is very slender and is brought out subcutaneously so that when the colon is opened and the mucosa sutured to the skin a colostomy appliance can be fitted immediately. The rod is removed about the tenth day.

As all colostomies are now opened at once, a colostomy bag is fitted at the end of the operation. Transparent drainable bags which can be emptied from the bottom without disturbing the seal are used. In the immediate postoperative period the effluent is usually very fluid and large in amount. Inspection of the colostomy is possible without disturbing the appliance. The stools become more solid after 4 or 5 days. The patient is now instructed in the use of a colostomy appliance. The choice is between a stick-on one-piece appliance which has to be changed every time the bag needs emptying and a two-piece appliance in which the bags are changed as necessary but the flange is changed only once or twice a week. The former may cause more skin irritation.

A magnet continent colostomy device. A magnetic ring may be implanted subcutaneously and the colon is drawn through it at the operation to make the colostomy. The stoma is treated on conventional lines for 3 to 6 weeks, when the magnetic cap is fitted. It is still under trial but is not without complications.

The orifices of a colostomy

A loop colostomy has two orifices (Fig. 38.9):
1. The active orifice through which faecal material is discharged and which leads proximally away from the growth.
2. The non-active orifice, which leads distally towards the growth. Usually only mucus is discharged from this opening.

The nurse should be able to recognise the active orifice, because it is through this opening that washouts are normally given. The active orifice in an iliac colostomy is usually the upper opening, the non-active one the lower. In a transverse colostomy the opening towards the right side of the abdomen is the active orifice and towards the left the non-active. A terminal colostomy has only an active orifice as the bowel below it (usually the rectum) has been removed. If the nurse is in any doubt, or the colostomy performed is not one with which she is familar, she should have no hesitation in asking the surgeon which is the active orifice.

A washout should be given through the non-active orifice:
1. Before a second stage operation for excision of the rectum or colon. (In this case the active orifice must, of course, also be washed out).

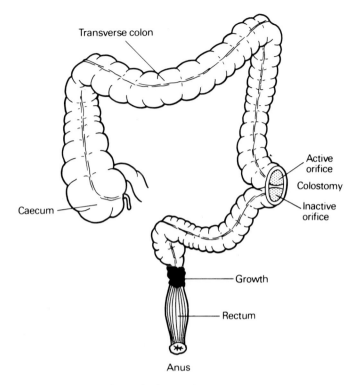

Fig. 38.9 Diagram of the orifices of a loop colostomy.

2. If the patient with a colostomy is troubled by excessive mucus or pus from a fungating growth.

Postoperative management of a colostomy

1. The rod or bridge is removed about the tenth postoperative day.

2. The sutures are removed about the fifth or sixth day if the wound has healed.

3. Regulation of the bowel. Normally the bowel will act without any special measures. If the bowel is obstinate a Dulcolax suppository may be inserted into the active opening of the colostomy and this usually produces a good result. Exceptionally, a washout through the colostomy may be given in the same way as rectal washouts are performed.

Once the bowel has been regulated, washouts and enemas are unnecessary. Some authorities find that about half their patients prefer washouts for control of the stoma. The appropriate apparatus has now made this procedure safe.

Diarrhoea may occur as a reaction to one or more components of the diet which must be traced and eliminated. Natural wheat bran is helpful in preventing diarrhoea. Diarrhoea may be checked by the administration of kaolin opiates, codeine or amphetamine sulphate. If it is persistent, however, it should be investigated.

4. Dressing. If full control of the stoma action has been achieved gauze or lint smeared with petroleum jelly is all that is necessary. A disposable plastic cap is worn attached with adhesive. The skin around the stoma should be washed with warm soapy water.

Complications of a colostomy

1. *Sepsis* in the wound.

2. *Prolapse of the bowel.* In this condition a loop of colon proximal to the colostomy intussuscepts and prolapses through the stoma. It is usually due to a technical error in selecting the wrong portion of the bowel at operation, although it is quite common in a loop transverse colostomy. The doctor will usually be able to reduce it in the ward.

3. *Retraction.* The loop may slip back into the abdomen, particularly if the mesentery is very short. Another cause for this complication is too early removal of the rod.

4. *Intestinal obstruction.* A loop of small bowel may become ensnared at the side of the colostomy. The symptoms are those of small bowel obstruction, and urgent laparotomy is indicated.

5. *Contracture of the colostomy orifice.* This is usually prevented by excision of an area of skin when performing the colostomy opening. Occasionally it may be necessary to dilate the opening by inserting a gloved finger or to refashion it surgically.

6. *Bleeding* may occur from injury to the junction of the colonic mucous membrane and the skin. The usual cause is a flange that is too small. This should be corrected. Sometimes small granulomatous patches develop. These can be cauterised with a silver nitrate stick. If there is no obvious local pathology to account for the bleeding reinvestigation of the colon is undertaken by the usual methods—radiography and endoscopy.

7. *Sore skin* is usually due to leakage, an ill fitting appliance or reaction to an ingredient in one of the appliance's components. In order to heal the skin the the cause must be established—then steps taken to remove or reduce it.

The size of the appliance may need altering—erosion can occur if the appliance rubs against the stoma whilst excoriation can occur if skin is exposed to the bag's contents. Faulty application e.g. stoma not central in gasket can result in both these conditions occurring together.

Appliances that have a precut gasket only offer a circular opening. Thus an elipse of skin will be exposed in the case of a double barrel colostomy. This area can be protected by the use of barrier cream or stomahesive which has been carefully cut to the correct shape. Leakage can be prevented by careful application of the bag using agents such as Karaya or stomahesive paste and Karaya powder to fill in gullies or flatten ridges as necessary.

Where reaction to a substance has occurred then contact with that substance must cease. A different appliance may be the answer, or the patient may prefer to keep their now familar appliance but introduce stomahesive and/or barrier cream. Castellani's paint has been found to be very effective in helping to heal a sore skin but, as it is spirit based, it will cause some considerable discomfort if the skin is broken—this effect can be resolved by diluting the solution with ordinary water.

Early detection and treatment of the problems outlined saves much time, effort and pain.

Instructions to the patient

There are 100 000 patients with a colostomy in Great Britain. Certain basic amenities are essential for the management of a colostomy. These include an indoor lavatory, a bath and hot water. Some patients with a colostomy should have top priority for housing. They also require more home help and modern cleaning and laundry methods. Some form of incineration is necessary for dressings. The laundry service for the incontinent should be used but, in most areas, it does not function at the weekend. The community services can be a tremendous help to the patient with a colostomy.

The patient should be taught how to attend to the colostomy. A colostomy is compatible with a useful and happy life but the initial training is most important. Routine washouts are unnecessary and can be harmful. There is a danger of colitis or perforation. With training the colostomy will function once or twice a day. Fruit and pips usually irritate the colostomy but what the patient can eat is largely a matter of intelligent investigation by himself. An agent which retains water and renders the stool soft but formed may be advisable. Agar or methyl cellulose in granules taken with water in the morning may be helpful.

The closure of a colostomy

When it is anticipated that a colostomy will ultimately be closed it is advisable to train the patient to perform sphincter exercises each day, so that there is no atrophy of the anal sphincter when it comes into action again.

The closure of a colostomy may be a dangerous operation unless the bowel is carefully prepared. It is essential to be certain that the bowel between the colostomy opening and the anus is not obstructed A barium enema is administered through the anus and the barium is allowed to run out of the colostomy opening. Radiographs will confirm the patency or otherwise of the segment of bowel.

Preoperative preparation

The main abdominal wound must be firmly and completely healed before the operation can be attempted. The lower bowel must be completely free of hard faecal material. Rectal washouts are given after the instillation of olive oil to soften the material. A further X-ray is taken to ensure no barium remains in the colon or rectum.

Postoperative treatment

Enemas must *not* be given for fear of perforating the sutured bowel, but a flatus tube or suppositories may be helpful.

A careful watch must be kept for the symptoms of peritonitis, due to a leak from the site of closure of the colon.

GENERAL ADVICE TO THE STOMA PATIENT

1. Diet. The patient can eat what he fancies and discovers what is unsuitable by trial and error. Digestion and absorption are largely unimpaired. Natural wheat bran helps to regulate the bowel. Many patients find onions, beans and peas keep the bowel very loose. The patient should drink as much fluid as before, alcohol is not forbidden but beer may need to be restricted because the large volume increases the quantity of the effluent.

2. Work and exercise. The majority of patients are able to return to their previous occupation and resume sporting activities. Most appliance manufacturers make activity pouches which can be worn when swimming, playing tennis, squash etc. Alternatively a plastic disc cup may be fitted over the stoma for such activities.

3. Drugs. Many drugs affect stoma function. Oral antibiotics may cause diarrhoea while the tricyclic antidepressants, by their anticholingenic action, cause constipation as will analgesics. A mild aperient may be required to counteract the constipation.

4. Washing the bag. A disposable bag can be washed out daily instead of being removed. A 50 ml syringe or a jug may be used to fill the bag with warm water. The bag is shaken and drained so that the patient is left with a clean bag.

5. Unsuitable lotions which may produce skin irritation include Savlon and Tinc Benz. Dettol should not be used to wash out a bag.

6. Rectal bowel action. Where the rectum has not been excised and is still in continuity with the bowel the patient will have an occasional bowel action. The patient who has had a total colectomy and ileostomy performed but in which the rectum has been closed from above should be warned that he may occasionally pass a little mucus.

7. Sexual advice. When all the wounds have healed normal sexual activities may be resumed and many ileostomists become parents.

8. Societies are self help groups formed by the patients themselves and groups include the Ileostomy, Colostomy and Urinary Conduit Associations. They will make domiciliary and hospital visits pre and post operatively and help mostly with day to day living whereas the medical staff are better able to give advice on appliances. By attending the meetings that are held the patients can obtain samples of new appliances without bothering their general practitioner.

BIBLIOGRAPHY

Care of Stoma Patient Conference 1975 Abbott Laboratories
Royal College of Nursing Stoma Care Forum 1979

39

Diseases of the caecum and the colon

The common diseases of the large intestine are inflammatory conditions, diverticular disease and new growths. The colon is one of the more favourable sites in the body in which to treat new growths.

INFLAMMATORY CONDITIONS OF THE COLON

Ulcerative proctocolitis

Non-specific ulceration of the colonic and rectal mucous membrane is a condition which is usually treated medically. The aid of the surgeon is sought when it is considered that the bowel is so diseased that excision is advisable. The usual operation is total procto-colectomy, but sometimes total colectomy is performed and the rectum retained. An artificial opening in the terminal ileum known as an ileostomy (Fig. 38.1) is fashioned. An alternative procedure if the rectum is retained is to anastomose the ileum to the rectum.

The patient may present with:

1. Acute fulminating disease which is a desperate emergency. Medical measures have failed, the patient is loaded with cortisone and is dying from a combination of gross toxic absorption, fluid and electrolyte depletion and haemorrhage. Total removal of the colon has to be undertaken as a lifesaving measure.

2. Relapsing proctocolitis although requiring the same extensive surgical ablation presents the opportunity to correct anaemia, fluid and electrolyte imbalance as well as vitamin deficiency. The problems arising from the formation of an ileostomy can be discussed with the patient.

At the end of the operation the main wound is sealed off and protected from the ileostomy. Postoperatively, resuscitation may be exacting, particularly following an operation for fulminating disease. The patient should be treated in an intensive care unit. The care of the stoma is an important procedure and has been discussed in detail in Chapter 38.

Antibiotic colitis

Diarrhoea is a fairly common sequel to antibiotic therapy. Occasionally it may herald the onset of:-

1. *Staphylococcal enterocolitis.* See p. 413.

2. *Pseudomembranous colitis* which may develop after antibiotic therapy and after surgical operation. Diarrhoea which is profuse but usually not bloodstained may occur during, or even a week or two after the antibiotic treatment is discontinued. The patient may be toxic, disorientated and collapsed. Sigmoidoscopy reveals the characteristic pseudo-membrane. The disease is caused by *Cl. difficile* which secretes a powerful necrotising toxin. The administration of vancomycin is usually curative.

Ischaemic colitis

This condition is due to arterial insufficiency in the colon. It presents with abdominal pain and diarrhoea (often blood-stained). It is usually diagnosed after investigation by a barium enema. The splenic flexure area is the portion most usually involved, and when the disease is localised to a short segment resection and end to end anastomosis may be performed.

Crohn's disease (see Chapter 37)

DIVERTICULAR DISEASE OF THE COLON

This is a condition of disorder of muscle function of the bowel. There is an increase in the tone of the longitudinal muscle and contraction of the circular muscle. The result is muscular hypertrophy. Diverticulum formation is a complication of this muscle abnormality and infection is a complication which may occur in a diverticulum. The corrugations of the bowel are very striking in a dissected specimen (Fig. 39.1). A diverticulum may perforate causing peritonitis or several diverticula may form a conglomerate inflamed mass, sometimes with abscess formation. The inflammatory mass may form a stricture and obstruct the bowel, and can be easily mistaken for a new growth. The inflammatory process may involve the bladder, and a fistula between the colon and the bladder is most commonly due to this condition (Fig. 33.4C). Diverticula can occur anywhere in the colon but by far the commonest site is the sigmoid colon.

Clinical features

The patient is usually past middle life, and, according to the course of the disease, the clinical features vary.

1. *Peritoneal symptoms* may be most prominent:
    (a) Pain, particularly in the left iliac fossa.
    (b) Constipation and some urgency of micturition.
    (c) Vomiting is usually present.
    (d) The temperature and pulse rate are elevated.
    (e) On examination a localised mass may be felt in the left iliac fossa.

Perforation of
diverticulum

Mouth of
diverticulum

Fig. 39.1 Segment of colon showing diverticular disease of the colon complicated by perforation.

2. Obstructive symptoms. A fibrous stricture may form. The symptoms are those of large bowel obstruction (p. 392).

Treatment

The majority of acute episodes subside with rest in bed and a low residue diet during the acute phase. As a long term measure high residue diet is advised to dilate the colon as much as possible.

If a palpable mass is present the Ochsner-Sherren regime (p. 383) is instituted. A perforation of the colon causes faecal peritonitis. After resuscitation laparotomy and peritoneal lavage are performed. The peritoneal cavity is drained. The affected segment of colon is resected either at the initial operation or at a later date. The bowel continuity is restored by a subsequent operation.

An elective resection of the colon with end to end anastomosis is indicated for fistula formation, recurrent abscess, haemorrhage and intractable disease.

HIRSCHSPRUNG'S DISEASE

This is a congenital lesion, probable genetic in origin, due to the absence of ganglion cells of the myenteric nerve plexuses (of Auerbach and Meissner) in the rectum and colon (Fig. 39.2). The bowel is paralysed, peristalsis does not occur and the contents of the gut cannot move. The normal bowel proximal to the paralysed section becomes very dis-

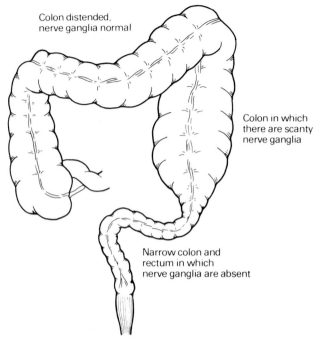

Colon distended,
nerve ganglia normal

Colon in which
there are scanty
nerve ganglia

Narrow colon and
rectum in which
nerve ganglia are absent

Fig. 39.2 Hirschsprung's disease

tended, with gas and faeces. The baby's abdomen is distended, he passes little or no meconium and soon vomits. If a little finger is passed into the rectum the colon may deflate and the baby be well for a few days before the symptoms recur.

Treatment

Treatment depends on the severity of the obstruction. Babies with only a short length of abnormal colon may be treated by the frequent passage of a soft rectal tube or small saline washouts. Diagnosis can then be confirmed by a radio-opaque enema and rectal biopsy. Babies with a long segment require an emergency laparotomy and a fashioning of a colostomy in the normal colon. Once the wound has healed and feeding established, the child can go home. There is no urgency to proceed to the next stage of treatment, which should be deferred until the baby weighs about 11.4 kg. He is then readmitted for the operation of rectosigmoidectomy.

NEW GROWTHS OF THE COLON AND CAECUM

Carcinoma of the large bowel causes 14 000 deaths each year in the United Kingdom. It is commoner in North-West Europe and North America. The areas in which there is a high incidence of the disease have a high standard of living. Several studies indicate a possible relationship between large bowel cancer and diet, either excess of fat or protein. The theory is that intestinal bacteria produce carcinogens from the dietary fat and from the bile steroids.

Familial polyposis of the colon is a condition in which carcinomatous change is inevitable and only a total proctocolectomy will save the patient. It should be undertaken before malignant change occurs and all members of the family must be examined regularly.

Malignant growths of the large bowel, usually carcinomas, are extremely common. They may occur anywhere, but the most common sites in order are the rectum, the pelvic colon, and the caecum. Although some growths, particularly in the caecum, are soft and proliferative, the majority grow around the bowel and eventually cause obstruction by forming a ring stricture (Fig. 39.3). This is particularly the case in the sigmoid colon and rectum.

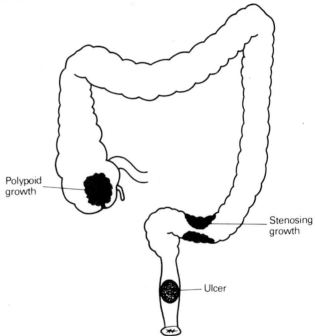

Polypoid growth

Stenosing growth

Ulcer

Fig. 39.3   The commonest sites and types of malignant growths in the large intestine.

Symptoms and signs

Increasing constipation in the most important symptom. At first, aperients give relief. Later the dose has to be increased, with a diminished effect, and finally the bowel action ceases. Many patients present with acute obstruction.

Pain is not prominent, and is usually described by the patient as being due to 'wind'. This is quite an accurate description, since his difficulty arises in his inability to pass flatus. The passage of small quantities of blood is an occasional complaint, but severe haemorrhage is uncommon.

Anaemia, particularly hypochromic in type, may be the presenting and only symptom of carcinoma of the caecum.

A lump in the right iliac fossa felt by the patient is unfortunately not an uncommon symptom in carcinoma of the right colon and caecum.

Other symptoms may occur. Increasing size of the abdomen is a frequent complaint, and is due to distension of the bowel. In later cases the distension is further increased by secondary deposits which cause ascites (free fluid in the peritoneal cavity).

Diarrhoea with mucus, particularly alternating with constipation, is not uncommon and is due to irritation of the bowel above the growth by retained faeces. Loss of weight appears slowly.

Examination of the abdomen may reveal a palpable mass or a distended large bowel. In early cases nothing abnormal can be made out on abdominal or rectal examination.

Investigations

Radiographic examination of the colon after the administration of a barium enema or barium meal may be performed. Exfoliative cytology (p. 221) may be undertaken.

Preparation of the patient for a barium enema. Preparation may be for 48 hours, or shorter preparation (an enema given the previous night, and a colonic washout next morning at least 2 hours before examination) may be satisfactory. Occasionally in the ambulant patients preparation by Dulcolax suppositories is satisfactory.

Sigmoidoscopy is of value for growths in the rectum and lower sigmoid colon up to 30 cm from the anus.

Fibreoptic colonoscopy (Fig. 39.4) enables the whole of the large

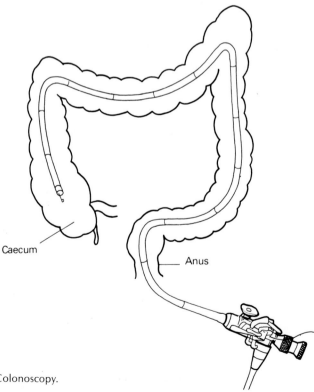

Caecum

Anus

Fig. 39.4 Colonoscopy.

intestine to be visualised. The examination is performed under sedation and is aided by image intensification X-ray control to check the position of the instrument. The examination may take up to an hour and should preferably be done after a barium enema study. In addition to diagnosis polyps can be removed with the diathermy snare without the patient having to undergo open surgery. A colonic anastomosis can be inspected to detect recurrence following resection for carcinoma. The colon should be clean and empty for a satisfactory examination.

Treatment

Treatment consists of a partial colectomy with anastomosts of the free ends of the bowel to restore continuity. The site and extent of the

Fig. 39.5 Colectomy: extent of resection of bowel and lymphatic field for carcinoma in various parts of the colon.

Irremovable tumour

Descending colon mobilised

Fig. 39.6   Colocolic anastomosis short-circuiting an irremovable tumour.

resection depends on the site of the growth (Fig. 39.5). A growth which cannot be removed is, where possible, short circuited (Fig. 39.6) to prevent the onset of intestinal obstruction. A defunctioning loop colostomy is performed above an obstructing irremovable tumour low in the bowel.

If the patient presents with acute large bowel obstruction, a colostomy, or sometimes a caecostomy, is performed as an emergency, and the obstructing growth removed at a later (second stage) operation. At a third operation the colostomy is closed.

THE CARE OF THE PATIENT FOR COLONIC OPERATIONS

Preoperative preparation

The preoperative preparation and care of a patient undergoing colonic surgery are as for any major abdominal procedure. Shortly before operation a nasogastric tube should be passed, and, for patients with disease in the sigmoid colon or rectum, a urinary catheter inserted.

There are two special aims in the preparation of these patients.

(a) *The relief of mild obstructive symptoms* if present so that a one stage procedure with restoration of continuity of the bowel can be undertaken. A light non-residue diet and repeated enemas and washouts over several days may be required to clear the bowel.

(b) *To prevent infection* at the anastomosis and in the abdominal wound. Colectomy involves cutting across and suturing the large intestine the lumen of which is normally teeming with bacteria. The single most effective procedure in eliminating infection is to ensure that the bowel is empty of faecal material at operation. This is achieved over 4 or 5 days. The diet is reduced to light non-residue and for the 2 days before operation only fluids are allowed by mouth. An aperient such as magnesium sulphate is administered regularly until the bowel is empty. The bowel is washed out morning and evening the day before operation and again on the morning of the operation until the effluent is clear. An hour immediately preoperatively a rectal tube is passed to recover any residual fluid. Care must be exercised with these procedures to avoid perforation of the diseased bowel.

Antibacterial substances may be administered orally for about 4 days preoperatively in an attempt to reduce the number of bacteria in the lumen of the gut. This carries the danger of propagating non-clostridial anaerobic organisms which may infect the anastomosis, causing leakage, and the abdominal wound, causing breakdown. The prevention of infection is better achieved by the administration in the immediate preoperative period of metronidazole (500 mg intravenously in 100 ml of saline) and a broad spectrum antibiotic such as gentamycin, tobramycin or a cephalosporin. These drugs are repeated 8 and 16 hours later.

The after care

The general postoperative care described in Chapter 4 is necessary. Enemas which may rupture the anastomosis should not be given but the passage of a flatus tube may help to relieve distension. This should not be used in low anastomoses. Some surgeons perform a three finger dilatation of the anus at the end of the operation for a similar purpose.

A low residue diet is consumed until the bowel has healed. Drains are removed when ordered, usually fourth or fifth day, and any signs suggestive of the development of a fistula, for example gas bubbles or a faecal discharge, reported at once.

Late complications include:

1. Bowel frequency is sometimes distressing after right hemicolectomy due to reduced water absorption. Isogel 5 ml t.d.s. or codeine phosphate 30-60 mg t.d.s. may help. In some cases lactose intolerance is the problem and a week's trial of excluding milk from the diet may be prescribed. When a considerable portion of the ileum has been removed as part of the operation bile salts may not be absorbed and watery diarrhoea may be produced. Cholestyramine 1-4 g may be advised.

2. Vitimas B_{12} deficiency. Vitimin B_{12} is absorbed from the lower ileum which is excised in a right hemicolectomy. After this operation a careful watch should be kept for the onset of macrocytic anaemia. Intramuscular Vitamin B_{12} may be required indefinitely.

40

Diseases of the rectum and the anus

The management of diseases of the rectum and anal canal demands considerable nursing skill. In many operative wounds healing is by secondary intention because primary suture is inappropriate or impossible.

EXAMINATION OF THE ANAL CANAL AND RECTUM

Such examination may include visual inspection of the anus and perianal region, digital rectal examination (called a PR, which stands for per rectum), proctoscopy, and sigmoidoscopy.

For all these procedures the patient is informed, privacy is ensured and the patient assisted to lie, if possible, in the left lateral position, with the knees well flexed and the buttocks near to the edge of the bed. The bedclothes are turned back to expose the buttocks and anal region and personal clothing is rearranged.

Rectal examination

This procedure is usually carried out by a doctor. A small tray is prepared containing:

Disposable glove (e.g. Dispos-A-Glove)
Lubricating jelly (e.g. KY)
Paper or gauze wipes
Paper bag (for disposal of used materials).

The person carrying out the examination puts on a Dispos-A-Glove, lubricates the tip of the index finger and anus and gently carries out the examination.

On completion of the examination, the anus is wiped with tissues and these, together with the used glove, are discarded into the paper bag. The patient is repositioned and made comfortable.

Proctoscopy and sigmoidoscopy

A proctoscope is approximately 10 cm long and is used for examining the

Fig. 40.1 Example of equipment used for proctoscopy and sigmoidoscopy.

anal canal. A sigmoidoscope is 30 cm long and is used for examining the rectum and lower sigmoid colon. Both examinations can be carried out in the outpatients department or in the ward. Occasionally it is necessary to perform the examination under general anaesthetic. A rectal examination should always precede a proctoscopy or sigmoidoscopy.

An example of some of the equipment needed is illustrated in Figure 40.1. It should include:

> Proctoscope
> Sigmoidoscope
> Light source and lead for each instrument
> Hand bellows for inflating lumen with air
> Suction apparatus and tubing
> Biopsy forceps
> Specimen jar for any biopsies taken
> Cottonwool balls, and carrier, for cleaning lumen
> Materials for rectal examination.

The instrument is well lubricated and inserted gently but firmly into the anus. The obturator is removed and the light lead attached. The eye-piece and bellows are attached, if the sigmoidoscope is being used. The nurse should stand where she can reassure the patient but also assist with the procedure if required. Suction or cottonwool balls may be required to clean the lumen before an adequate view is obtained. The instrument is advanced carefully always visualising the way ahead. Biopsies can be taken easily and painlessly from any abnormality seen, or from the rectal mucosa if needed. This is of great value in the diagnosis of rectal tumours, Crohn's disease and ulcerative proctocolitis. It is also of value in the confirmation of the presence of amyloid disease and Hirschprung's disease.

After the examination, disposable equipment and materials are discarded. Other equipment is removed, washed and soaked in antiseptic for at least 30 minutes.

BENIGN CONDITIONS OF THE ANUS AND PERIANAL REGION

Perianal abscess

Infection in the rectal or anal wall from an inflamed haemorrhoid or an abscess may spread into the perianal tissues or ischiorectal fossa (Fig. 40.2) or the infection may be blood borne.

Pain is often severe because the pus is under considerable tension. Pain on defaecation is usually present. The affected area is swollen, red, indurated and tender.

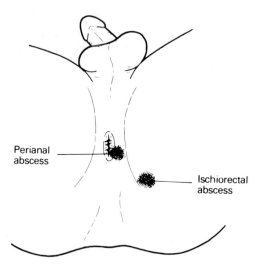

Fig. 40.2 Abscess formation around the anus.

Treatment

Very free drainage is necessary. This is achieved by surgical incision under general anaesthesia. As in all wounds around the anus, healing must occur from the depth of the abscess cavity. This is achieved by frequent salt baths and keeping the wound well open with a corner of a square of gauze soaked in eusol. If this is not carried out meticulously the skin heals over and one or more septic tracks are left in the depths of the wound with possible resultant fistula formation.

Fistula-in-ano

A fistula is a track lined with septic granulation tissue connecting two epithelial lined surfaces. The surfaces which the track connects in this region are the skin of the buttock and mucous membrane of the anal canal. The commonest cause is an ill-treated or neglected perianal abscess. Rarely multiple fistulae are present when the condition is tuberculous. Fistula-in-ano may be a complication of Crohn's disease.

A radiograph of the chest should be taken in all cases of fistula to exclude pulmonary tuberculosis, but this is rare nowadays. Disease higher in the bowel should be excluded by a careful history, and barium enema if necessary.

Symptoms and signs

A mucous or purulent discharge occurs around the anus. There is usually no pain until the opening becomes blocked and an abscess forms in the track behind.

Treatment

The two openings are found with a fine probe, and the track is excised. A wide raw area is left to granulate, and the same care is essential as in the case of an abscess to see that healing takes place slowly from the floor of the cavity. The specimen which has been excised is sent for pathological examination to exclude Crohn's disease, tuberculosis and new growth formation. The detailed preparation and aftercare are discussed later in this chapter.

Fissure-in-ano

This is the most painful of all anal conditions. Probably as a result of pressure from hard dry faecal material, a small crack (or fissure) appears in the posterior portion of the anal wall. There is severe pain on defaecation, which persists for several hours afterwards. The patient dreads another bowel action. The faeces, as a result, become still harder and drier. When the bowel has to act the pain is more severe than ever. A small skin tag, known as a 'sentinel pile', is usually present.

Treatment

In acute cases three-finger dilatation of the anus under an anaesthetic is sufficient to effect a cure. Dilation greater than three fingers may result in a tear of the anus. This requires admission for only half a day. If the fissure is thickened, excision of the crack and partial division of the internal sphincter is necessary.

Fig. 40.3 Pilonidal sinus.

Pilonidal sinus

This is a very common cause of recurrent abscess formation in the area between the tip of the coccyx and the anal margin (Fig. 40.3). Fine tracks lead from the skin into the tissues down to the coccyx.

Treatment

1. *Acute stage.* If an abscess forms incision is necesary. Any area seen to contain hair is laid open.

2. *Radical treatment* consists of wide excision of the area. A few millilitres of methylene blue may be injected into the track by means of a syringe and cannula, to outline the extent of the sinus. If the wound is clean it is closed by uniting the skin and obliterating the cavity by means of several deep nylon sutures tied over a roll of gauze. The wound is left undisturbed for 10 days. After this time it has healed. Alternatively the wound is left open to heal from the bottom by second intention. It is lightly packed with gauze or a silastic foam 'bung'. The patient is nursed lying on the side or in the prone position. The surgical treatment may be limited to opening up and laying open all visible tracks.

The hairy skin of the buttock should be shaved and kept shaved postoperatively. Special care is taken to remove any visible hair which may be seen in the granulating wound. The patient is advised to bath at least once daily, particularly following defaecation. He is also instructed to wipe the anus in a direction away from the sinus and not towards it. He should continue permanently with careful personal hygiene.

Recurrence following treatment is not uncommon.

Pruritus ani

Severe irritation and itching (pruritus) around the anus may occur from many causes. The commonest cause is threadworms. Other causes are a vaginal discharge, gross uncleanliness, haemorrhoids and diabetes. It may occur without any obvious cause. This is known as idiopathic pruritus ani.

Symptoms and signs

Severe irritation causes great distress, particularly at night in bed. The buttock area is covered with multiple scratch marks and the loss of sleep results in extreme weariness.

Treatment

The urine is tested for sugar because the condition may be caused by mild infection of the skin in diabetic subjects. Any obvious focus of irritation is treated. Warm baths of sodium bicarbonate and painting with 1 per cent gentian violet solution give considerable relief. Careful local hygiene is important. One of the many antipruritic or barrier creams may give relief. The injection of local anaesthetic into the affected are may be advised.

Haemorrhoids

Internal haemorrhoids contain an artery in the pedicle. The exact nature of a haemorrhoid is still a matter of doubt. They have been stated to be dilated veins, arteriovenous fistulas or merely, according to Thompson, displaced or prolapsed cushions of mucous membrane extruding from disruption of the supporting tissue. Great confusion has arisen from a lack of understanding of the terms 'internal' and 'external' haemorrhoids.

External haemorrhoids are small dilated veins covered by redundant folds of skin, and are situated on the anal margin. The only complication is a small haemorrhage into the skin folds. This causes severe pain which can be relieved by simple incision through which the haematoma is evacuated. No special preparation is necessary, and evacuation of the haematoma gives immediate relief. A simple gauze dressing is all that is necessary and it can be removed the next day. The patient has a bath and no further dressings are required.

Internal haemorrhoids. Internal, or true, haemorrhoids always originate inside the bowel (Fig. 40.4). There are three stages (degrees) of increasing severity:

1. Early in their development they are soft and bleed readily.
2. Later they become thickened and descend outside the sphincter on defaecation, but return spontaneously afterwards.
3. Still later they remain outside (prolapsed haemorrhoids).

Constipation and excessive straining at stool are thought to be important causes of haemorrhoids in a substantial proportion of patients. Burkitt has noted the rarity of haemorrhoids in rural Africans who consume a high residue diet which produces bulky stools. A patient with a history of passing hard stools or difficulty in defaecation should be advised to increase his intake of fluid and dietary fibre.

Fig. 40.4 The sites of the three primary haemorrhoids. With the patient in the lithotomy position these are 3, 7 and 11 o'clock.

Symptoms and signs

Bleeding is the earliest symptom, and severe anaemia may result if it is profuse. The blood is bright red and appears on defaecation. As they progress, irritation and distress during prolapse of the haemorrhoids are prominent complaints. Prolapse may occur suddenly or gradually. Sudden prolapse is extremely painful, and if the piles cannot be returned the patient is unable to walk. The anus and lower rectum may be examined visually by means of a proctoscope.

Treatment of prolapsed haemorrhoids

Treatment is directed to the relief of pain and the reduction of the inflammation locally. Rest in bed, preferably with the lower end of the bed raised and the patient lying on his side, is essential. Compresses of lead and opium or cold sodium sulphate are soothing as are warm baths. Morphia (15 mg) eight-hourly should be prescribed, and the diet should be confined to fluids. Anal dilatation may be advised and in many is effective even in painful prolapsed haemorrhoids.

Treatment by injections

Injections can be given only when the haemorrhoids are inside the anal canal. This is most effective for early bleeding haemorrhoids. Five per cent phenol in almond oil is injected by means of a haemorrhoid syringe submucosally. This is done through a proctoscope with the patient in the left lateral position or in the knee elbow position. Apart from a tiny amount of bleeding complications are unusual.

Anal dilatation

Lord believes that the primary defect is narrowing of the outlet of the anal canal. The anal sphincter is unable to dilate to whatever size is necessary to allow the stool to pass and faecal material has to be expressed. The rise in intraluminal pressure obstructs the venous return from the haemorrhoidal area. The haemorrhoidal plexus dilated with blood further obstructs the outlet. The aim of dilatation is to break this vicious circle.

1. Procedure. Dilatation of the anal sphincter up to eight fingers is undertaken under a general anaesthetic in an operating theatre. When dilatation has ironed out the constriction a sponge is placed in the anal canal to reduce the risk of haematoma formation. It is removed 1 hour later and the patient can go home.

2. Postoperative dilatation by the patient at home. The patient is instructed to pass a specially designed dilator 1½ inches long each day for 2 weeks after a hot bath before retiring, and on alternate days for the following month. It should be left in position for 1 minute. After this time the patient should pass the dilator only if there is any tightness.

Complications:
(a) Haematoma.
(b) Splitting. There is a danger of infection so the patient must be kept in hospital and antibiotics prescribed.
(c) Prolapse occurs occasionally and should be reduced.
(d) Incontinence. If it occurs it usually clears up in 2 weeks, but more recently some more persistent cases of sphincter dysfunction have been noticed and it would appear that for patients with a patulous anus dilatation is an unsuitable method of treatment.

Operative treatment

Haemorrhoidectomy is a very satisfactory operation and consists of ligation and excision of the three primary haemorrhoids. The preparation and after-treatment are considered on p. 470. Ligation with rubber bands is an alternative to formal operative ligation. It requires no anaesthetic and the patient is back at work next day. Discomfort is mild apart from transient mucus leakage. Complications are rare. In the presence of Crohn's disease the incidence of complications is high and if at all possible operative interference is best avoided.

Cryosurgery

The need for operation for haemorrhoids has diminished considerably since the introduction of Lord's dilatation. An alternative to surgical ligation is cryosurgery which necessitates hospitalisation for only 2 days.

Prolapse of the rectum

Conditions which predispose to rectal prolapse are chronic cough, constipation, phimosis, whooping cough, torn perineum from childbirth, occasionally threadworms, some neurological conditions, and senility. The essential aim of treatment in these conditions is to treat the cause.

Rectal prolapse may be:

1. *Incomplete.* In this form only the mucous membrane prolapses. This condition is usually seen in infants. In the adult it may be associated with haemorrhoids and is cured at the same operation. In infants, regulation of the bowels is usually all that is necessary. If the condition persists the buttocks are strapped together after the prolapse has been reduced, and the child is kept in bed.

2. *Complete prolapse* is a distressing condition associated with ageing, weight loss and decreasing muscle tone.

Treatment

If possible, the prolapse is replaced and the patient confined to bed. The foot of the bed should be elevated. If the patient's condition is satisfactory cure by operation may be undertaken. This consists of anchoring the rectum by an abdominal approach. In more feeble patients a suture of silver wire or nylon may be inserted around the anus to leave an aperture the size of the base of the operator's index finger. This is sufficient to allow a motion to pass a but small enough to prevent the mucosa prolapsing.

Simple stricture of the rectum

Simple stricture of the rectum may occur as a result of a gonococcal proctitis, ulcerative proctocolitis or as a complication of an operation for haemorrhoids or radiotherapy. Administration of an enema which is too hot may give rise to rectal stricture and it cannot be stressed too often that the temperature of all fluids used must be taken with a thermometer. Dilatation with special rectal bougies may be advised.

Proctitis

Inflammation of the rectum or anal canal unassociated with haemorrhoids or a new growth may be:

1. *Non-specific.* This is part of the condition of ulcerative proctocolitis (p. 451) in which the rectum is involved in about 70 per cent of cases.

2. *Specific.* Causes include bacillary and amoebic dysentery, gonococcal and tuberculous infection. The treatment is that of the cause.

SURGERY OF ANUS AND RECTUM (excluding removal of the rectum)

The anus and rectum, and the surrounding skin are teeming with vast numbers of pathogenic organisms. By any method of preparation it is impossible to have a sterile operating field. It is none the less important to render the area as free of organisms as possible, and operation in this area must be carried out under strict conditions of asepsis so that fresh forms of infection are not introduced. Because absolute asepsis is impossible, all wounds in this area require free drainage, and healing always occurs by secondary intention.

General preoperative treatment

1. The bowel. The bowel should be emptied before the operation. A mild aperient is given 2 nights before the operation, followed by an enema in the evening and a washout on the morning of the operation day. A rectal washout is given not later than 6 hours before the patient goes to the theatre.

Rectal washout. An enema saponis is given to ensure that the bowel is empty of faeces.

Equipment required (on a trolley):
Rectal tube or catheter
Connection tubing 0.6 m (2 ft) in length
Funnel
Small jug—1 litre
Large jug containing 4 l fluid (tap water) at 37.8°C(100°F)
Bucket
Incopad
Large polythene sheet
Disposable gloves
Lubricating jelly
Medical wipes/tissues.

The procedure is explained to the patient, and he is told that it may take 15 to 20 minutes. He is allowed to pass urine. He is placed in the left lateral position, with an Incopad under the buttocks. The polythene sheet is spread on the floor, and the bucket placed on it.

The small jug is filled with fluid. The funnel, connection tubing and catheter are assembled. The tip of the catheter is lubricated. Some fluid is run through to expel air, and then stopped. The patient is asked to take a deep breath, and the catheter is inserted about 6 cm (2½ in) into the rectum. The funnel is raised above the level of the buttocks and 300 ml (half pint) of fluid is run into the rectum. Before the funnel is empty it is inverted over the bucket and the fluid siphoned back. The process is repeated until the fluid returns clear, or the 4 litres of prepared fluid have been used.

Afterwards, the tube is withdrawn. The anal region is cleansed. If the patient desires, he is allowed to use a bedpan or commode. He is left comfortable in bed.

Used equipment is discarded. The fluid siphoned back and also that passed into the bedpan are measured and added together—the total amount thus returned is usually equal to the amount given.

After washing and drying her hands, the nurse reports on the amount of fluid given and returned, whether the final washout was returned clear, and any untoward effects experienced by the patient.

2. The perianal region. The skin around the anus, groin, and suprapubic area should be shaved and washed with soap. In painful conditions such as perianal abscess this is carried out after the patient has been anaesthetised.

3. The diet. During the 2 days before the operation the diet should be light, nutritious, and of the non-residue type.

The operation

The usual position for operation is the lithotomy position (Fig. 40.5). Sigmoidoscopy should always be performed to exclude any other disease in the anal canal, rectum or lower sigmoid colon.

Postoperative treatment

Pain. This is often severe, and repeated morphia injections are necessary. Hot baths are valuable for the relief of pain following an operation for haemorrhoids, and many patients like to spend several hours a day lying in a hot bath.

Haemorrhage may occur, and will be severe if the ligature of a haemorrhoid base has slipped. It must be reported at once and arrangments made for return to the theatre to secure the bleeding point. A rare but occasional complication is a secondary haemorrhage about the tenth day—this requires the administration of antibiotics, securing the bleeding point in the theatre and, if necessary, blood transfusion.

Fig. 40.5 Lithotomy position.

A tube covered with petroleum jelly may be left in the anal canal at the end of the operation for haemorrhoids, partly for the passage of flatus and partly lest haemorrhage should occur and not be revealed owing to the sphincter ani being in spasm.

The packs. The original packs in cases of fistula and abscess are usually removed at the end of 24 hours and replaced, after irrigation of the wound, by a light pack. In most cases flat packs are used, but one corner can be tucked into the wound to ensure that the skin edges are not allowed to fall inwards. A silastic foam 'bung' is a very good alternative dressing (see p. 106). Firm, deep packing with ribbon gauze is avoided.

A normal diet with an adequate fluid intake is allowed as soon as the patient desires it. The bulk of the stool is increased by giving bran or a hydrophilic laxative such as Isogel 10-20 ml/daily or Normacol 10-20 ml/daily. If the bowel has not moved by the third day two glycerine suppositories may be given or an olive oil enema, followed by a soap and water enema. A bath is taken after every bowel action.

Digital dilatation of the anus. Some surgeons consider this a particularly important after treatment following a haemorrhoid operation. It is commenced on the sixth day and performed daily for 2 days. Its purpose is to separate the 'sticky' surfaces so that stricture formation does not occur. However, if the patient is having a good bulky bowel action the same end is achieved.

Acute retention of urine. This is particularly liable to occur after a haemorrhoid operation, and after other perianal procedures. If the patient fails to pass urine with conservative methods of encouragement, then catheterisation must be undertaken (Ch. 43).

NEW GROWTHS OF THE RECTUM

Simple new growths are usually polypoid adenomas. The main symptoms are similar to those of haemorrhoids, and the treatment is excision.

Carcinoma of the rectum

Malignant new growths are very common.

Symptoms and signs

1. *Constipation.* Increasing constipation alternating with diarrhoea is not uncommon.

2. *Bleeding.* The blood is bright red in colour and is so important a symptom that it must not be attributed to haemorrhoids until carcinoma has been excluded. Pain in the rectum is a late symptom in most cases, but appears earlier in growths situated in the anal canal.

3. *Tenesmus.* With a polypoid growth of the rectum, the patient has a constant sensation of fullness associated with the desire to defaecate, which is not relieved by bowel action.

4. *Mucus and pus.* The discharge of mucus and pus may occur in a large fungating growth filling the rectum.

5. *Intestinal obstruction* may develop acutely if the lumen of the bowel has been narrowed by the growth.

6. *Sciatic pain* is sometimes the presenting symptom, and is due to infiltration of the sacral plexus by the growth.

7. *Digital examination* of the rectum will reveal a palpable growth.

8. *Sigmoidoscopic examination.* The higher reaches of the rectum and the lower colon may be examined by means of a sigmoidoscope and a portion of the growth taken for biopsy. The bowel should be emptied by a gentle aperient, followed by a Dulcolax suppository, 6 hours before examination. Some surgeons prefer no preparation at the first attempt.

Treatment

The standard operative procedure for most patients suffering from carcinoma is abdominoperineal excision of the rectum and terminal left iliac colostomy. The results are excellent. A more conservative procedure may be possible where the growth is situated in the upper third of the rectum. The sphincter is preserved, end to end anastomosis performed and a colostomy avoided. This is known as anterior resection of the rectum. Local excision only may occasionally be all that is necessary if the tumour is small; pathological examination shows removal to have been complete and histologically the tumour is well differentiated.

Pre-operative preparation

This is as for any major abdominal operation. The bowel and perianal area are prepared as described on p. 460 and p. 470. The site of a proposed colostomy must be marked on the abdominal wall. Blood (4 pints) should be cross-matched. Immediately preoperatively a nasogastric tube and a urinary catheter should be passed. Antibacterial substances are administered as for colectomy.

The operation

For abdominoperineal excision of the rectum two surgical teams combine, one operating in the abdomen and the other in the perineum at the same time. Resection of the rectum is always a severe operation. Blood transfusion is almost invariably required during operation. If an anterior resection is possible, a wash-out of the rectal stump with anticancerous agents may be undertaken in the theatre. This minimises the risk of implantation of cancer cells as well as diminishing the risk of recurrent tumour at the suture line. With the advent of modern stapling machines for anastomosing the bowel it is possible to perform an anterior resection and thus save the anal sphincter for some tumours in the mid-third of the rectum.

In women with malignant disease of the rectum some surgeons excise the posterior vaginal wall because the recto vaginal septum is the commonest site of recurrent disease. A year later it is impossible to tell whether the vaginal wall has been removed or not. As it is not sewn up the vagina remains normal in size and epithelialises.

The abdominal wound is closed and dressed according to the surgeon's preference. A colostomy bag is attached around the colostomy, preferably of the transparent type so that the stoma can be easily inspected. The perineal wound is usually sutured and drained with a wide-bore tube. If there is excessive haemorrhage or infection the perineal wound may be left open and packed.

Postoperative care

The patient is laid on his side and the head is kept low (on one pillow) until he recovers consciousness.

Blood transfusion is continued until the general condition is satisfactory.

Systemic antibiotic therapy is continued as after colectomy.

The colour of the stoma is checked regularly for the first 24 hours to ensure that it remains pink and viable. Any change should be reported.

The perineal drainage tube is connected to a low grade suction pump. The nature and quantity of fluid draining is carefully charted. Several hundred millilitres of sero-sanguinous fluid may drain in the first 24 hours. If the drainage is excessive, or fresh blood, it should be reported.

Nasogastric suction and intravenous fluids are continued until the paralytic ileus resolves and flatus is passed from the colostomy. Fluids should then be taken orally and the diet gradually increased.

The urinary catheter is maintained on closed drainage and urinary output carefully recorded. There may be some temporary disturbance of bladder function, both due to the change in anatomy after the operation and interference with the nerve supply to the bladder. The catheter is removed on about the fifth postoperative day.

The perineal drain can usually be removed about the third to fifth postoperative day when drainage has become minimal. If the perineal wound has been left open it requires daily irrigation with eusol or hydrogen peroxide and dressing as for an open wound. Considerable protein loss can occur from such a large open wound. A high protein diet should compensate for this. If a sutured perineal wound becomes infected it may require free drainage by removal of sutures and subsequent treatment as an open wound.

Abdominal sutures are removed on the tenth day, perineal sutures on the eighth.

The patient is instructed in the management of the colostomy.

Prognosis

The outlook for rectal tumours which have not spread beyond the bowel wall is, in general, good. However, many of these patients have symptoms for a long time before they seek medical help. The tumour spreads through the bowel wall to surrounding tissues, into the lymphatic system, and via the blood stream to the liver. Even in such cases it is worth, if possible, removing the primary tumour because the local symptoms are so unpleasant.

41
Hernia

DEFINITION

A hernia is a pouch of lining membrane protruding itself through a weak point in the covering structures. The most common site of a hernia is the abdominal wall. The term, however, includes a weakness at any point, for example, a defect of the skull results in what is known as a hernia cerebri.

SITE OF HERNIA

The weak points in the musculature of the abdomen are the canals through which certain structures normally run and scars. The hernias which occur at these sites (Fig.41.1) are named accordingly:

Fig. 41.1 The sites of some hernias on the abdominal wall.

1. Inguinal.
2. Femoral.
3 Umbilical (in the adult usually paraumbilical).
4. Epigastric.
5. Incisional through a scar (known as ventral if arising on the anterior abdominal wall).
6. Obturator.
7. Hiatus hernia (Chapter 32).
8. A rarer type of hernia is the diaphragmatic. The abdominal contents herniate into the chest.

The constituents of an abdominal hernia are:
   (a) The sac. This is the protruding pouch of peritoneum.
   (b) The contents. The most frequent are loops of the small intestine and the great omentum. They slip in and out, provided the hernia is not strangulated or obstructed. Long-standing friction results in adhesion of the contents to the sac. Almost any abdominal organ except the pancreas may be found in a hernial sac.
   (c) The coverings include all the tissues superficial to the hernia and consist of the stretched muscles and aponeuroses, the fascia, and the skin.

THE CAUSE OF HERNIA

A hernia may be congenital or acquired.

The commonest hernia in an infant is an umbilical hernia, from the failure of the umbilicus to seal off satisfactorily. The majority of small congenital umbilical hernias in infants cure themselves and reassurance of the parents is the only treatment necessary. In the larger ones a simple operation is necessary if they do not close spontaneously. In gross cases the whole of the intestines are outside the abdomen, a condition known as exomphalos. The condition requires urgent operation. Combined with an undescended testicle, congenital inguinal hernia is not uncommon in male children.

Hernias are frequently acquired as a result of tearing of the muscles due to strenuous work or play.

SYMPTOMS AND SIGNS OF UNCOMPLICATED HERNIA

Small hernias are noticed by the patient only after coughing or standing up. A swelling, with a slight dragging ache, is the commonest complaint. The skin over a large hernia may be in folds which tend to become eczematous as a result of friction

On examination there is an abnormal swelling with an expansile impulse on coughing. The swelling usually disappears, or can be reduced, on lying down.

COMPLICATIONS OF A HERNIA

1. Irreducibility of the contents occurs in long-standing hernias.

2. Strangulation The blood supply to the contents of the hernia (usually a loop of bowel or piece of omentum) is cut off, and, in addition to the local pain, the symptoms and signs of intestinal obstruction may be present (p. 391). There is no impulse on coughing, and the hernia is irreducible and tender. Unrelieved, the strangulated loop of bowel becomes gangrenous.

3. Progression. Increase in size is usual.

4. Intertrigo of the skin, i.e. abrasion due to two folds of skin rubbing together.

TREATMENT

Operative repair is the treatment of choice in most hernias. Many uncomplicated inguinal hernias are suitable for 'day' surgery. The patients can get up next day at home. The sac is excised after the contents have been reduced into the abdomen and the weakness repaired by suture of the muscles or by the introduction of special suture material if the muscles are weak. The patient is kept in bed for only one day, but in large recurrent hernias 3 to 4 days in bed are advisable. He is advised against very heavy lifting for 3 months. There are special cases, however, when this ideal course of treatment is not possible:

1. In the presence of special aggravating factors recurrence of the hernia is inevitable so these must be treated before operation on the hernia is contemplated. They are:

(a) Enlargement of the prostate.

(b) A urethral stricture.

(c) Constipation.

(d) A persistent cough.

2. The patient is temporarily unfit for operation

(a) In an infant the operation for hernia is undertaken at 3 months or even earlier.

(b) During pregnancy, provided the hernia is reducible, operation is best deferred until after parturition.

(c) After a severe illness such as pneumonia.

(d) Chronic bronchitis with an acute exacerbation.

3. The patient is unfit for operation

(a) Severe cardiac or pulmonary disease.

(b) Extreme age.

In all these conditions a truss may be advised, provided the hernia can be reduced and is not a femoral hernia. No truss so far designed will control a femoral hernia.

In babies an umbilical hernia is reduced by supporting with strapping. This is the only type of hernia support which may 'cure' the hernia, because obliteration of the umbilicus is a physiological process and adequate support may enable it to proceed to completion.

Special advice to a patient wearing a truss

Careful washing and powdering of the skin are necessary. The pad must be maintained in good repair, and if a spring is used in the truss it must be renewed before it becomes too weak.

The patient must be instructed to apply his truss while he is lying down in bed after the hernia has been reduced.

THE CARE OF THE PATIENT FOR A HERNIA OPERATION

Careful shaving of the suprapubic area and cleansing of the skin are essential. Slight cuts from shaving are very likely to give rise to infection, which will ruin the operation.

Abdominal exercises are commenced on the day following the operation. Retention of the urine may occur and must be relieved. Abdominal distension must be prevented by passing a flatus tube.

If the patient is very fat and the hernia is large it is usually wise to prescribe measures to reduce his weight before the operation.

Some patients have two very large inguinal hernias, and it is frequently decided to operate on them one at a time as the sudden reduction of the contents of two large hernias into the abdomen may give rise to cardiorespiratory embarrassment.

Certain terms connected with hernia operations give rise to some difficulty:

1. *Herniotomy* means opening of the sac.

2. *Herniorrhaphy* refers to the repair of the defect in the musculature.

3. *Hernioplasty* is a heniorrhaphy in which extra material, such as monofilament nylon or implants of Teflon are introduced for wide deficiencies.

Recurrence, which for inguinal hernias is in the order of 5 to 10 per cent, is due to faulty technique (failure to remove the sac), infection, straining, coughing and heavy lifting.

42

Diseases of the kidney and ureter

STRUCTURE AND FUNCTION

The kidneys are situated on the posterior abdominal wall behind the peritoneal cavity. The right kidney lies below the liver and behind the second part of the duodenum, while the left kidney, which is higher than the right, is situated behind and below the spleen. There are two major calices in each kidney which empty into the renal pelvis which has a capacity of 5 to 8 ml. The ureter, which joins the renal pelvis to the bladder, is about 25 cm long and its muscular coat provides the vermicular (peristaltic) movement. The ureter enters through the bladder muscle on an oblique course and terminates at the base of the trigone. In the female the ureter is only 0.5 cm from the cervix of the uterus.

The surgical significance of these facts is:

1. The surgery on the kidney and ureter is performed behind the peritoneal cavity whenever possible to avoid contaminating the latter with urine. If the peritoneum has been opened inadvertently at operation or if the approach has been transperitoneal a careful watch has to be kept for signs of peritonitis (Ch.34).
2. The oblique entry of the ureter through a tunnel in the bladder musculature prevents the reflux of urine from the bladder. It does not prevent the ascent of bacteria from the bladder into the ureter and thence to the kidney.
3. The proximity of the ureters to the cervix of the uterus enables a cervical growth to spread and obstruct the ureters.

The kidneys have a rich blood supply from the aorta through the renal arteries and the level is a critical one in resection of an abdominal aneurysm (Ch.24). The renal veins drain directly into the inferior vena cava so that a renal tumour may spread rapidly to the lung.

The main functions of the kidney are the control of water and electrolyte balance, the excretion of nitrogenous waste products and the elimination of drugs.

The kidney may be damaged and ultimately destroyed by failure of its blood supply, prolonged hypotension, toxins, bacterial infection, a mismatched blood transfusion, a new growth or any lesion obstructing the flow of urine down the ureter or the lower urinary tract.

INVESTIGATIONS OF THE URINARY TRACT

The repeated collection of specimens of blood and urine, intravenous urography involving abdominal compression in a darkened X-ray room, catheterisation and cystoscopic examination before a definitive operation is undertaken are a demanding ordeal for any patient. Unfortunately the only certain method of assessing progress or cure afterwards is a repetition of some or all of these procedures. These patients evoke special sympathy. The purpose as well as the details should be explained to the patient and, as far as possible, discomfort elimated.

The objects of investigation

1. To determine the precise anatomy. One kidney may be absent, the ureter may be reduplicated or some other anomaly may be present.
2. To assess renal function, bladder evacuation or exclude reflux into the ureter.
3. To localise the site and extent of disease.

1. Collection of specimens

Urine for routine examination is collected in a clean urinal or bedpan. Observations of colour, smell, deposits, specific gravity and pH are made. Tests for abnormalities (glucose, ketones, albumin, bile and blood) are carried out in the ward.

If bacteriological examination is required, a midstream specimen of urine (MSSU) is collected. Prior to this the genital area is cleansed with soap and water. The male patient is instructed to retract the foreskin and to pass a little urine into the urinal, to interrupt the stream and pass a little urine into a sterile container, and then to complete micturition into the urinal. The female patient is instructed to hold the labia apart, pass a little urine into the toilet or pan, to interrupt the stream and pass a specimen of urine into a sterile container or receiver and then to complete micturition into the toilet. She usually requires nursing assistance. The container is then sealed, labelled and sent to the laboratory without delay.

If the patient has an indwelling catheter a fresh specimen is obtained by spigoting the catheter for 20–30 minutes and then releasing the spigot and collecting the urine in the sterile container.

2. Examination of the urine

Urine specimens should reach the laboratory as soon as possible after being obtained—never more than 2 hours. This will include a search for the prescence of red blood corpuscles, pus, cancer cells, and organisms, as well as abnormal chemical constituents such as albumin and sugar. Measurement of urine output and specific gravity may be of help in assessing renal function.

3. Residual urine

The presence of residual urine is a most valuable sign of prostatic enlargement. It can usually be estimated by an intravenous urogram which, on the 'postmicturition' film, will show an outline of the residual urine. Occasionally it is necessary to measure the volume of residual urine. The correct method of doing this is as follows:

(a) The patient is requested to empty his bladder completely by his own efforts. The normal bladder is empty at the end of micturition and if a catheter is passed no urine will be obtained.

(b) If, after the patient has emptied his bladder to the best of his ability, a catheter is passed and urine is obtained, this is known as 'residual urine'. The volume should be measured and charted.

4. Blood urea

The normal is 2.50-6.67 mmol per litre. A more accurate test, because it is uninfluenced by diet or the state of hydration, is the serum creatinine, normal value 53-106 μmol per litre.

5. X-ray examination

Straight, or direct, X-ray examination of kidneys, ureters and bladder will, in 90 per cent of cases of stone, reveal their presence.

An intravenous urogram will reveal most abnormalities of the kidneys and, in addition, is a valuable test of renal function. A damaged kidney will not secrete the dye in sufficient strength to give a radiographic shadow.

In preparation for X-ray examination of the renal tract, the bowels should be emptied by the administration of vegetable aperient on each of the two previous nights. The passage of a flatus tube will reduce gas shadows, which so frequently interfere with a good film of the kidneys. The bladder is emptied.

On the morning of the examination no fluid or food is given. Films are taken at 5, 10, and 30 minutes, or longer, after the intravenous injection of 20 ml of 50 per cent solution of a medium containing an iodine compound. A small amount of leakage outside the vein in the arm is very painful, and if it should occur a hot fomentation is applied. The risk of idiosyncrasy to iodine should be anticipated by always having at hand 100 mg of hydrocortisone and a solution of dextrose for immediate intravenous injection.

Many patients complain of pain from the abdominal compression used in the examination to demonstrate the ureters more adequately.

6. Cystography

The bladder may be visualised when the dye injected for a urogram reaches the bladder, or alternatively a more adequate picture of the bladder may be obtained by passing a catheter and filling the bladder with dye. An X-ray taken when the patient is micturating—micturating cystourethrogram—will reveal whether there is reflux of urine into the ureters from the bladder.

7. Cystoscopy

This is visual examination of the interior of the bladder.

Preparation of a patient for cystoscopy

(a) The suprapubic area need not be shaved in the male unless the examination is likely to be followed by open operation.

(b) The patient should be encouraged to drink freely so that the secretion of urine can be observed from each ureteric orifice. There is no objection to the patient consuming plenty of fluid up to 3 hours before the anaesthetic unless the anaesthetist gives further instructions.

(c) The patient should empty the bladder before examination. The residual urine can then be measured when the cystoscope is passed.

(d) In the male, phimosis is sometimes present, and a dorsal slit may be necessary before the cystoscope is passed.

(e) Radiographs and notes must be available in the theatre.

(f) For every cystoscopic examination urethral dilators should be sterilised and at hand in case the condition should turn out to be complicated by a urethral stricture.

8. Ureteric catheterisation and retrograde pyelography

A ureteric catheter may be passed up the ureter of either kidney via the cystoscope to collect a specimen of urine secreted by that kidney. To ensure that the label on the specimen is correct it should be written out at once and care must be taken of the specimen, since damage or loss necessitates a repetition of the whole procedure.

If a retrograde pyelogram is to be performed the catheter is left in position and the patient is taken to the X-ray department, unless a special cystoscopy room equipped with X-ray apparatus is available. The radio-opaque medium is injected into the ureteric catheter with a syringe and the kidney and ureter X-rayed.

Instructions may be given for the catheter to be left in position until it falls out spontaneously. This procedure is frequently of value in aiding the patient to pass a small stone from the kidney or ureter. Two millilitres of sterile liquid paraffin may be injected into the catheter two-hourly for 12 hours to aid the passage of a stone. All specimens of urine which are voided must be retained for straining and examination in case a stone has been passed.

9. Ultrasonography

Ultrasonography is a noninvasive investigation easy to perform and repeat. Valuable information concerning the size and consistency of the kidney can be obtained.

10. Renal angiography

The renal arteries can be cannulated via the femoral artery and aorta. Injection of a radio-opaque medium demonstrates the kidneys. It helps to distinguish a cyst from a neoplasm and identifies abnormalities of the renal vessels.

11. Radioisotope studies

Radioisotope studies of the kidney may be undertaken to determine further information about renal blood flow, function, and drainage of the kidney. A radioactive isotope is injected intravenously and the kidneys scanned at varying intervals thereafter.

12. Renal biopsy

This may occasionally be performed, either percutaneously with a needle or by open operation.

13. Ureteroscopy

An instrument is now available which can be passed via the urethra and bladder into the ureter. The ureter can then be examined directly.

14. Nephroscopy

It is also possible to pass a telescope directly into the kidney percutaneously. This has as yet limited availability and use.

SYMPTOMS AND SIGNS OF URINARY DISEASE

Pain

1. **Renal pain.** This may be of two varieties:
   (a) A fixed dull aching in the loin. Lesions which distend the kidney frequently give rise to pain of this type. If the outer surface of the kidney is inflamed, as is commonly the case in pyonephrosis, adherence of the organ to the muscles in the loin may give rise to a very severe pain.
   (b) Renal colic or, more strictly, ureteric colic. The pain commences in the loin and radiates to the testicle in the male or the vulva in the female. It is severe and violent (Fig. 42.1). The expression of a small stone or clot frequently results in this type of pain.

Fig. 42.1 Ureteric colic radiates from the loin to the groin.

2. Bladder pain. Bladder pain may be felt as a suprapubic discomfort, but more commonly is felt as a burning pain in the urethra at the end of micturition.

Haematuria

The passage of blood in the urine is known as haematuria. Haemorrhage arising in the bladder usually results in the passage of bright red blood, more marked at the end of micturition. Bleeding originating in the kidney is more intimately mixed with the urine, and the urine passed is usually described as 'smokey'. In addition to gross bleeding, the presence of small quantities of blood may be discovered only by microscopic examination of the urine.

Causes

1. **Renal:**
   (a) Injury to the kidney.
   (b) Haemorrhage into a cyst of a congential cystic kidney.
   (c) Hydronephrosis.
   (d) Acute nephritis.
   (e) A stone.
   (f) Tuberculosis.
   (g) A neoplasm, e.g. innocent—angioma; malignant—hyperneph-roma, or nephroblastoma.
2. **Extrarenal:**
   (a) Hypertension.
   (b) Anticoagulants in excess.
   (c) The sulphonamide drugs.
   (d) Certain blood diseases.
3. **The bladder:**
   (a) Foreign body.
   (b) Severe cystitis.
   (c) A stone.
   (d) Neoplasms.
   (e) An enlarged prostate.
4. **Urethra:**
   (a) Trauma.
   (b) A stone.
   (c) Urethritis.

Following operation on any portion of the urinary tract haematuria is common and aggravated if clot formation occurs.

Increased frequency of micturition

Under nervous strain increased frequency of micturition is not an uncommon symptom. Irritation of the mucous membrane of the trigone of the bladder by infection, a stone or a growth are the usual urological causes. In tuberculosis of the urinary tract the mucous membrane is not only damaged but contraction of the bladder may result in unbearable frequency. Increased frequency is a prominent symptom of overflow retention (p. 503).

Difficulty in micturition (dysuria)

Difficulty with micturition is usually due to an enlarged prostate or to urethral stricture in the male. In the female it may be due to a painful urethral caruncle, a retroverted gravid uterus, or an impacted pelvic tumour.

Strangury

Strangury is the desire to pass urine when only a few drops are present in the bladder and is unrelieved by micturition. This symptom is fairly commonly associated with ureteric colic.

Scalding

Scalding, or pain on micturition, is usually due to infection.

Retention

Retention is the inability to pass urine.

Oliguria

Oliguria means that the urinary output is diminished—usually less than 300 ml in 24 hours.

Anuria

This is a condition in which no urine is formed by the kidneys or if glomerular filtrate is formed it is totally reabsorbed so the patient passes no urine, and on catheterisation none is recovered from the bladder. It may be due to a stone or other lesion blocking the ureter of the only kidney which the patient possesses.

Other causes are:

Acute tubular necrosis.

Shock. The urinary output is diminished, but as the patient responds to treatment kidney frunction is resumed.

Nephrotoxic drugs such as gentamicin.

The sulphonamide drugs. The crystallisation of the sulphonamide drugs in the renal tubules is liable to occur if the patient does not drink sufficient fluid when taking the drugs.

Incontinence

Incontinence is the patient's inability to control emptying of the bladder. It may be:

1. True incontinence

The sphincter is damaged, or the nerves eliminated so that coordinated micturition is impossible.

Incontinence is a cause of much suffering. The patient is always wet and damage to the skin occurs very rapidly. Many silently accept their misery from a sense of shame. Until recent times incontinence has been regarded as a disease to be treated instead of looking at continence as the result to be achieved whenever possible. Acute illness, injury or immobility may result in incontinence and will pass as soon as the patient recovers strength. Impacted faeces in the rectum may cause acute retention with overflow incontinence. These forms may be treated by catheterisation and the catheter is removed as soon as the underlying precipitating factor is cured or corrected.

Following cerebrovascular accidents the nervous control to inhibit micturition is diminished but not entirely destroyed. This results in urge incontinence and is aggravated by emotional stress. The most important need is to be able to empty the bladder without delay so that a bedside commode is essential by night as is physical proximity (a few yards on a level surface) to a lavatory by day. In addition habit training to establish a regular frequency pattern of bladder emptying is necessary. An alarm with a flashing light to remind the patient and staff unobtrusively for the need for a further visit to the lavatory is described by Rowe.

When habit training fails there is a variety of equipment available which includes disposable Incopads and napkins. Marsupial pants invented by Dr F.L. Williams hold an absorbent pad in a waterproof pouch on the outside of the garment. They are made of one way water repellent fabric which remains dry while allowing urine to pass through into the disposable pad. Because the pad is on the outside there is no need to remove the pants when the pad is changed.

Catheterisation with drainage into a bag or other device is a last resort.

2. False or paradoxical incontinence

The patient suffering from prostatic obstruction (Fig. 42.2) may develop acute retention with the result that a litre or more of urine may accumulate in the bladder. After a certain point 60 or 90 ml may overflow. The condition is really one of retention, and the incontinence is only a complication of this condition. Retention with overflow is a common description of this condition. This condition may also occur in women with an incarcerated gravid uterus.

3. Stress incontinence

Stress incontinence is a condition, usually seen in women, in which coughing, sneezing, laughing, or any condition which increases intra-abdominal pressure results in some escape of urine from the bladder. It occurs because the supports of the sphincter have been damaged, usually due to injuries sustained during childbirth, and some element of cystocele is present.

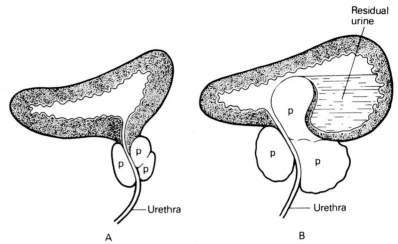

Fig. 42.2   A. Normal bladder after micturition.
B. Bladder obstructed by an enlarged prostate (p on the diagram).

DISEASES OF THE KIDNEYS AND URETERS

CONGENITAL ABNORMALITIES

Congential abnormalities of the urinary tract are legion. The commonest are:

Polycystic disease of the kidneys
Horse-shoe kidney
Absence of one kidney
Ectopic kidney.

1. Polcystic kidney (congenital cystic kidney). This is an inherited condition. It is probably due to failure of complete fusion of the cortex of the kidney with the medulla. Clinically, the disease is usually seen about the age of 40. Both kidneys are enlarged and irregular. The patient's symptoms are those of incipient renal failure from which, at a later date, he will die unless a renal transplant is successful. Non-inherited multicystic disease of the kidneys also occurs.

2. Horseshoe kidney. The kidneys are joined together across the midline, usually at their lower poles. The importance of the condition lies in the necessity for recognising it prior to operation. A horseshoe kidney is liable to all the diseases which may occur in an anatomically normal organ.

3. Absence of one kidney. This may occur as a result of failure to develop. Such knowledge is vital in cases of disease of the only kidney which is present.

4. Ectopic kidney. The kidney may be situated in the pelvis instead of in its usual position in the loin.

INJURIES TO THE KIDNEYS

Injuries to the kidney may occur as a result of a fall, a kick, or a road accident. The injury to the kidney may be anything from a bruise to a severe rupture, or damage to the renal vessels. If the peritoneum in front of the organ is torn, peritonitis may occur.

Clinical features

Loin pain and haematuria are present. Following a severe rupture of the kidney there is obvious haematuria, swelling, and pain in the loin combined with the general symptoms and signs of internal haemorrhage. An IVU should always be performed, mainly to check that the other kidney is present and normal.

Treatment

In occasional severe cases exploration of the kidney is necessary. In most cases healing occurs if the patient rests in bed. All urine voided is kept and the time of evacuation marked on the label so that the amount of blood in each specimen can be compared with that of the previous specimen.

HYDRONEPHROSIS

Hydronephrosis (pyelectasis) is a condition in which the renal pelvis is distended due to partial obstruction, usually at the pelvic-ureteric junction. The parenchyma of the kidney becomes compressed. In extreme cases it is no more than a thin sac and the number of functioning renal units may be very small indeed.

This condition develops as a result of intermittent obstruction to the outflow of urine. Complete obstruction results in atrophy of the kidney.

The obstruction is sometimes caused by failure of neuro-muscular coordination in the upper ureter, but most cases are secondary to some other condition. If the primary cause is unilateral, one kidney is affected. If the cause is bilateral, both kidneys may be affected. The ureter may also be dilated depending on the site of obstruction. The term pyelectasis is gradually replacing hydronephrosis in common usage and the affection of the ureter inaccurately described as dilatation is known as ureterectasis.

Conditions causing unilateral hydronephrosis

1. A stone in the urete·
2. The pressure of tumours on the ureter.
3. Kinking of the ureter from bands or aberrant blood vessels (extra vessels to the kidney in addition to the normal renal ones).
4. Neuro-muscular inco-ordination at the junction of the renal pelvis with the ureter. This may become bilateral.

Conditions causing bilateral hydronephrosis

1. Prostatic obstruction.
2. Urethral stricture and congenital urethral valves.
3. Phimosis.
4. Carcinoma of the cervix uteri.
5. Bilateral renal or ureteric calculi
6. Retroperitoneal fibrosis.

Complications

1. Renal failure (in bilateral cases).
2. Infection (pyonephrosis).

Treatment

Treatment of most cases will be that of the primary cause.

In severe unilateral cases a plastic operation on the pelvi-ureteric junction or nephrectomy may be necessary.

INFECTIONS OF THE KIDNEY

Pyelonephritis

Pyelonephritis is an infection of the renal pelvis and of the solid or parenchymatous portion of the kidney, often with small abscesses which destroy its substance.

Acute pyelonephritis unless treated seriously and with great care may lead to chronic pyelonephritis. The casual organisms are *Escherichia coli* or any of the common pyogenic organisms.

Pyelonephritis may occur in pregnancy and is predisposed to by progestin causing interference with the muscular contraction of the ureter rather than the effect of pressure of the uterus.

Clinical features

1. Pain in the loin and in the lower abdomen. The pain may resemble that of acute appendicitis. In addition there is usually frequency of micturition with scalding pain.
2. Pyrexia of the order of 39° C (103°F) is usually present. A rigor may be the presenting symptom.
3. Vomiting and the signs of a general febrile condition may be marked. On examination there is tenderness on the affected side in the region of the kidney. The urine contains pus and organisms.

Treatment

The causal organism is isolated and its sensitivity determined. While this is in progress the reaction of the urine to litmus must be determined. If it is acid an alkaline mixture is given, e.g. mist. potassium citrate. Antibacterial therapy is commenced and when the laboratory sensitivities are to hand any change of preparation which is indicated is made. Three litres of fluid must be taken daily. The dosage of antibacterial substances is based on an intake of 3 l of water.

When the acute stage has subsided full investigation of the urinary tract is carried out to determine any causal condition for the inflammation. The urine should be repeatedly examined for organisms when there has been apparent cure, otherwise chronic pyelonephritis may occur.

Chronic pyelonephritis is often slow to respond to treatment. Many cases in adults have had their origin in repeated urinary infection in infancy and childhood. Children who have had more than one attack of urinary infection should be investigated. Many will be found to have congenital anomalies of the renal tract. Some have neurological disturbances of the bladder leading to urinary retention and infection, while others will have anomalies of the junction of the ureter and bladder which allow reflux to occur up the ureters when the bladder contracts. This reflux can be minimised by instructing the patient in the art of double micturition—the child micturates, waits for a few minutes until the ureters drain into the bladder and then empties the bladder again. Reflux can be cured by a plastic operation in which a new valvular mechanism is constructed at the junction of the ureter and bladder.

Pyonephrosis

Pyonephrosis is a condition of inflammation of the kidney in which the renal pelvis is full of pus. It is often a hydronephrotic kidney which has become infected in which case the kidney is little more than a bag of pus. The patient complains of severe pain in the loin, which is swollen and tender. Rigors may be present and the temperature is often elevated to 39°C (103°F).

Treatment

Drainage of the abscess by nephrostomy or removal of the kidney will be necessary. Nursing treatment is similar to that of acute pyelonephritis.

Perinephric abscess

A perinephric abscess is an infection beneath the fatty capsule surrounding the kidney. The infection may arise as a result of the rupture of a small abscess in the kidney, but more usually it is blood-borne from a boil, carbuncle, or septic finger.

Symptoms and signs

The patient who has recently recovered from a staphylococcal infection runs a temperature for which no obvious cause can be found. There may be a dull ache in the loin. Later, the pain increases in severity and the loin becomes swollen and bulging.

Treatment

Incision of the abscess and drainage is usually required. The drainage tube will be left in position for at least a week, and in most cases a little longer. Antibiotics are usually unnecessary. Disease of the kidney may have to be dealt with subsequently.

Tuberculosis of the kidney

The kidney may be infected with tubercle bacilli from the blood stream or from a tuberculous lesion in some other portion of the genito-urinary tract. Unchecked, the disease is disseminated into the ureters, the bladder, and the opposite kidney.

Symptoms and signs

1. Frequency of micturition is the outstanding symptom.
2. Pain may be present in the loin, or true ureteric colic and haematuria may occur, due to small portions of granulation tissue passing down the ureter.
3. Painless haematuria.
4. The symptoms and signs of tuberculosis may be present elsewhere.

Investigation

Intravenous urogram may reveal distortion of the renal pelvis, and the typical cystoscopic appearance is a 'golf' hole appearance of the ureteric orifice.

Urine. The urine is acid in reaction, contains pus and is sterile on routine culture. Tubercle bacilli may be found on examination of the urine, early morning specimens being sent on three successive days, or only after culture on special media.

Treatment

Antituberculosis chemotherapy (Ch.9) is commenced. If resolution is not complete on chemotherapy, partial or total nephrectomy may be undertaken provided the disease is now limited to one kidney.

URINARY STONES

Kidney stones

Many stones are secondary to infection (recurrent pyelonephritis) or stasis in the urinary tract. Parathyroid overactivity is the cause in about 5 per cent of patients. Due to the concentration of the urine, the condition is said to be commoner in tropical climates. Patients who excrete abundant calcium in the urine, for example those with bone destruction from metastatic disease or those with bone decalcification due to chronic illness such as poliomyelitis or tuberculous arthritis of the spine, are more likely to form a stone. Excessive intake of calcium and vitamin D increases the likelihood of stone formation. Some patients who take excessive amounts of alkalies and milk for the treatment of dyspepsia absorb excess calcium. Others are hypersensitive to vitamin D (e.g. patients with sarcoidosis). Hypercalcuria is often idiopapathic (i.e. cause unknown). In the majority of patients with calcium-containing stones no definite cause for their formation is found. Some metabolic abnormalities (e.g. gout) give rise to the formation of specific types of stone.

Fig. 42.3 Stones in the upper urinary tract.

Types of stone

Renal stones may be:
1. Solitary.
2. Multiple.
They may be composed of:
(a) Oxalates (of calcium).
(b) Phosphates (of calcium).
(c) Uric acid.
(d) Urates.
(e) Cystine.
(f) Xanthine.

Symptoms and signs

Small stones give rise to prominent symptoms. They may pass from the kidney into the ureter. A large stone may form quietly, but cause greater damage to the kidney.

1. Pain. Typical ureteric colic is extremely painful. The pain in the loin is sharp and biting and radiates with greater severity to the testicle in the male or to the labia in the female. The patient writhes about in pain and may vomit.

2. Strangury. There is a great urge to pass urine every few minutes, but only a drop or two is voided.

3. Haematuria. The urine may be tinted with blood or there may be frank haemorrhage.

A small stone may be passed by the patient as a termination of the violent pain with considerable relief. When large fixed stones are present the pain is a more constant dull ache in the loin. Occasional bouts of pyrexia occur as a result of infection.

Investigations

Straight X-rays of the urinary tract and IVU are done to assess the site and size of any stones. Occasionally retrograde pyelography is necessary.

A search for a cause of stone formation is made. Calcium levels in fasting blood and 24 hour collections of urine are estimated. The blood and urine are examined for other abnormal constituents which may contribute to stone formation.

Urine must be cultured to detect any infection.

Treatment

1. Treatment of the acute attack. This consists of rest in bed and the relief of pain by the injection of pethidine.

2. In the quiescent stage. Antispasmodics are prescribed and the patient is advised to walk about. The indications for surgical removal of a stone are severe persistent symptoms, persistent or progressive back pressure on the kidney, and persistent urinary infection. The passage of a ureteric catheter may aid the passage of the stone, or at the ureteric orifice it may be removed endoscopically with a device such as Dormier's basket. If the stone fails to pass, its removal from the kidney (nephroli-thotomy) or ureter (ureterolithotomy) will be undertaken, and if the damage to the kidney has been severe, removal of the organ may be necessary.

3. Dissolution is possible by using an irrigating procedure but while cystine, phosphate and uric acid stones can be dissolved the commonest type of stone composed of calcium oxalate is refractory. Percutaneous nephrostomy using a catheter large enough for irrigation avoids the need for open surgery. It is a method to complement rather than compete with surgical removal and may be appropriate for patients unfit for surgery or a patient who has undergone several previous operations for renal stones.

4. Prevention of further stones. The patient should be advised to drink at least 3 litres of fluid a day to help prevent further stone formation. If a specific cause has been found this should be treated appropriately.

Ureteric stones

If the stone fails to pass spontaneously, or to pass after the passage of a ureteric catheter, it may have to be removed by operation.

Retroperitoneal fibrosis

Retroperitoneal fibrosis is a rare condition, sometimes caused by drugs like methysergide or some analgesics taken in excessive amounts. It may cause obstruction to the ureters or the inferior vena cava. Steroids may be used in treatment. Surgical relief of the obstruction is often necessary.

NEW GROWTHS OF THE KIDNEY

Simple tumours, although they do occur, are not very common. Malignant new growths are the nephroblastoma (Wilms' tumour) which is seen in infants and the hypernephroma (carcinoma of the kidney) of the adult. Both tumours are extremely malignant, and blood-borne metastases to other organs are early and extensive.

Carcinoma of the renal pelvis occurs sometimes in association with carcinoma of the ureter or bladder.

Symptoms and signs

Painless haematuria is the commonest symptom. Pain in the region of the affected kidney may be the presenting symptom. An enlarged kidney may be felt.

Investigation

The diagnosis is made by the use of some or all of:
    (a) Intravenous urogram (IVU)
    (b) Ultrasound scan of kidney
    (c) Renal angiography
    (d) Chest X-ray—to detect metastases
    (e) Skeleton X-ray—to detect metastases
    (f) Isotope bone scan—to detect metastases

Treatment

Removal of the kidney is the treatment of choice, but the end results are poor, since spread by the blood stream, particularly to the bones, occurs at an early stage in the disease. Radiotherapy may be given postoperatively and chemotherapy using actinomycin is also used.

RENAL FAILURE

Failure of the kidneys to clear the blood of waste products may be due to inadequate blood flow, damage to the kidneys or obstruction to the outflow of urine from the renal pelvis, from the ureters or from the lower urinary tract. It may occur suddenly or it may be the result of long-standing and progressive destructive disease. Uncontrolled, the patient will die.

Renal failure, whatever the cause, is aggravated by:
1. Incorrect fluid balance which causes waterlogging in the tissues.
2. Infection which causes tissue breakdown.
3. Ingestion of protein.
4. Excessive breakdown of protein such as occurs in starvation.
5. Potassium imbalance.

ACUTE RENAL FAILURE

Causes

1. Prerenal hypotension, which will recover as shock is treated.
2. Renal tubular obstruction by:
    (a) Mismatched blood transfusion. The tubules are obstructed by agglutinated (clumped) red blood cells.
    (b) Myohaemoglobin produced in muscles which have been severely crushed (the crush syndrome).
    (c) Precipitation of drugs such as crystals of sulphonamides.
    (d) Bile pigments, particularly when associated with a fall in blood pressure such as following operations on patients with obstructive jaundice (the hepatorenal syndrome).
3. Tubular necrosis.
    (a) Following operation and concealed accidental haemorrhage.
    (b) Certain metallic poisons.
    (c) From acute pyelonephritis.
    (d) Bacteraemic shock.
4. Post-renal or obstructive, for example a stone or other lesion blocking the ureter of the only functioning kidney which the patient possesses.

Clinical picture

The patient may remain well for several days. The striking feature is oliguria (300 ml or less), leading to complete anuria. The blood urea and the serum potassium rise each day. After about 6 to 10 days vomiting, breathlessness and increasing acidosis are evident. Before death, twitching and convulsions may occur.

Management

For low blood pressure the appropriate treatment to correct and overcome it is instituted. An obstructive lesion is relieved.

If the patient is anuric the most important nursing features are:

1. To stop all fluids until a satisfactory regime is instituted.
2. To stop all antibiotics and drugs because many of them are not now being excreted and cumulative effects are liable to arise.
3. All foods should be forbidden.

The patient may be kept alive for a very long time and the longer the time he is kept alive the greater is the chance that the kidneys may recover or regenerate provided the correct treatment is undertaken. Basically this consists of the fluid intake being limited to the amount lost by sweating and respiration. This amounts to 1 litre a day, but the body produces 500 ml of water which accumulates. Therefore the total amount of fluid which can be given to the anuric patient is 500 ml. To prevent the breakdown of body protein a high carbohydrate diet is essential and must contain about 2000 calories and should be mineral-free. The fluid and carbohydrates are best combined in a solution in 500 ml of Hycal (a flavoured liquid dextrose concentrate) which provides 2100 calories. This can be administered by drinking or by a nasogastric tube into the stomach. If the patient is unable to tolerate either method 500 ml of 50 per cent dextrose is administered every 24 hours by a polythene catheter into the inferior vena cava.

Because the patient's diet is lacking in vitamins they can be administered as a supplement.

When a diuresis occurs a volume of fluid equal to the amount of urine secreted plus 500 ml is given as potassium-rich fruit juice. The precise amount of fluid and its nature should be determined over 24 hours following blood and urine electrolyte estimations at least once daily.

In all cases of oliguria or anuria of sudden onset, mannitol 50 g in 500 ml of 5 per cent dextrose, is given in 30 minutes. If there is a response by diuresis, intravenous fluid and mannitol up to 100 g daily are given. A careful watch on the serum sodium is kept as mannitol tends to depress it. If there is no response to mannitol, structural damage has occurred and a modified Bull's regime is instituted. If this fails, peritoneal dialysis may be undertaken.

CHRONIC RENAL FAILURE

Causes

1. Chronic nephritis.
2. Polycystic disease of the kidneys.
3. Kidneys destroyed by calculi.
4. Hypertensive kidney disease.
5. Diabetic nephropathy.
6. Bilateral hydronephrosis.

The onset of disease is gradual, the patient is anaemic, the skin dry and retinitis is usually present. Vomiting, nausea and terminal intermittent respiration occur. The treatment is a low protein diet and dialysis. A renal transplant may be undertaken.

Dialysis

1. Peritoneal dialysis. Dialysis means the transfer of solutes across a semipermeable membrane. Substances in solution pass from areas of high concentration to areas of low concentration by diffusion.

During peritoneal dialysis, fluid of a known concentration is introduced into the peritoneal cavity. Blood vessels and the fluid in the cavity are separated by peritoneum which acts as a semipermeable membrane. The concentration of certain solutes in the dialysing fluid is lower than that in the blood and, therefore, salts for excretion diffuse into the peritoneal cavity.

Dialysing fluids contain a mixture of the normal plasma electrolytes in a 1.36 per cent solution of dextrose. A hypertonic solution (6.36 per cent dextrose) may be used to withdraw fluid. Heparin and antibiotics may be added as prescribed by the doctor.

The danger of infection makes sterility during any part of the process essential, and a bacterial filter is fitted to the inflow tube. Prior to the procedure the bladder must be emptied as there is a possibility of perforation of a distended bladder. The abdomen is shaved and cleaned with an antiseptic. A local anaesthetic is given. A catheter is then inserted into the peritoneal cavity and connected by tubing to two bags of dialysing fluid. The fluid is allowed to flow rapidly into the peritoneal cavity (1-2 litres in 10-15 minutes), it remains there for 20-30 minutes and is then allowed to drain.

It is essential that accurate fluid balance records are maintained as the amount of fluid introduced and that drained should correspond approximately. Patients should be weighed daily and observations of temperature, pulse and blood pressure maintained. Blood for urea and electrolyte estimations and dialysis fluid for culture and sensitivity are sent daily to the laboratory.

2. Haemodialysis. The artificial or mechanical kidney is basically a semipermeable membrane of Cellophane.

    (a) On one side of the membrane is a bath of fluid. The composition of the fluid is such that the substances which it is desired to attract into the bath are absent or of lower concentration than in the blood.

    (b) On the other side is the patient's blood.

The process is one of dialysis. The essential ions are kept in the blood by maintaining an identical concentration in the bath. The substances which it is particularly desirable to attract from the blood, in cases in which this is used, are urea and potassium (K^+).

The patient is connected to the machine by canalising an artery and vein. The blood passes along one side of the Cellophane and is returned to the previously filled reservoir of venous blood before being returned to the body by a vein.

The machine requires the undivided attention of a team— including a biochemist.

Renal transplantation

Renal transplantation has been discussed in Chapter 26.

Anabolic hormones

Breakdown of protein tissue (catabolism) increases the amount of nitrogenous and potassium products in the blood. Synthesis or building up of lean tissue is know as anabolism. Occasionally these anabolic hormones (Deca-Durabolin is one) are of value, particularly in:

(1) Some cases of acute renal failure, by depressing the formation of nitrogenous and potassium end products.
(2) To counter the protein breakdown (catabolic) phase following acute illness, trauma, or major surgical interference.

THE CARE OF PATIENTS FOR OPERATION ON THE KIDNEY

Operations on the kidney consist of:

1. Nephrolithotomy, that is, removal of a stone.
2. Nephrostomy. (Insertion of a tube into the kidney to drain pus or urine.)
3. Nephrectomy. (Partial or total removal of the kidney.)
4. Pyeloplasty to correct hydronephrosis.

Preoperative care

The general preparation of a patient for major surgery is appropriate. Infection in the kidney should be reduced as far as possible by the administration of antibacterial drugs according to the results of the sensitivity tests on organisms grown from the urine. The urinary function must be at the highest possible level. The blood urea reading is a fairly satisfactory rough guide. In most cases a figure of under 6.5 mmol per litre is desirable. The haemoglobin should be normal and 2 units of blood crossmatched.

The loin, back, abdomen, and chest are shaved in the usual way. A large cross is made on the loin or leg with a skin pencil by the doctor to indicate the side of the operation. Preoperative drugs are given as prescribed and the bladder is emptied. The bowel is emptied with suppositories the night before surgery.

Radiographs and notes must be brought to the theatre and arrangements are made for an X-ray to be taken on the theatre table during the operation if this proves to be necessary. In cases of stone the patient is X-rayed immediately before going to the theatre as the stones are sometimes passed 'silently' or change their position in the urinary tract while awaiting operation.

The operation

Most cases will be operated on lying on the side with the diseased side uppermost, the lower leg flexed, the upper leg straight, and the trunk secured to the table by a strap and maintained by sandbags or rubber cushions (Fig.42.4). A drain is usually inserted down to the kidney or kidney bed.

Fig. 42.4 Usual position for operations on the kidney.

Postoperative care

On return to bed the patient should be laid on the affected side. Later, he should be propped up to encourage drainage from the kidney down the ureter to the bladder. A careful watch must be kept for haemorrhage from the wound and in the urine. Some blood staining of the urine is inevitable for a day or two postoperatively except of course when the kidney has been totally removed.

The signs and symptoms of renal failure must be carefully watched for, and, in addition, the supervention of chest complications. Urinary antiseptics must be continued.

Pain must be relieved by analgesics.

The amount of urine, the presence of blood, or the onset of retention must be carefully noted. A fluid balance chart is essential.

Some degree of sepsis is almost inevitable if the kidney has been infected. The sutures are removed when the wound has healed, usually the 8th to 10th day. Paralytic ileus sometimes occurs following surgery in the retroperitoneal space. This should be treated as previously described (p. 386).

The drain left in the perinephric space is usually removed on the 3rd day, but if a tube has been inserted into the renal pelvis it is left until it loosens itself—about the 10th day. It should be connected to a drainage bag outside the bed. A primary leak of urine may occur from the drain site. This usually stops spontaneously.

The period in bed varies from 2 to 3 days in most cases.

OPERATIONS ON THE URETER

The preparation and aftertreatment are similar to that of an operation on the kidney. The only special points of importance are:

1. Skin preparation. The whole abdomen should be prepared on both sides, as well as the usual kidney area, since a ureteric stone may be removed through a lower midline incision.

2. X-ray immediately before the operation is essential and the patient must not be allowed to stand up or walk about after it has been taken. A stone which was in one portion of the ureter may have changed its position since the previous X-ray.

3. The drain. The wound often seeps urine for several days, and special care is necessary to control infection in the urine and in the wound.

URINARY DIVERSION

Transplantation of the ureters

The ureters may be transplanted into:

1. The pelvic colon, the patient passing urine by the rectum. This operation carries the risk of ascending urinary infection and also of excessive reabsorption of chloride ions from the rectal mucosa. Before operation the rectal sphincter should be examined for continence.

2. An isolated loop of ileum. This avoids the complications of colonic transplants but involves an ileostomy draining urine.

3. The skin of the abdominal wall (ureterostomy). They may be brought to the skin separately or together. Occasionally this is considered the only satisfactory way of diverting the urine.

Such operations may be performed for carcinoma of the bladder, after severe crush injuries, or for a severely contracted tuberculous bladder. An occasional indication is an ectopic bladder, a condition in which the pubic bones fail to fuse and the bladder mucous membrane lies on the abdominal wall, dribbling urine continuosly from the exposed ureteric orifices.

A common indication in children for transplantation of the ureters into an ileal loop is a paralýsed bladder with a myelomeningocele. The operation may be necessary because of incontinence or to prevent renal deterioration in the chronically infected neurogenic bladder. Transplantation into an ileal loop rather than the colon has the advantage of less electrolyte disturbance but is also necessary because the anal sphincters are paralysed. The main disadvantage is the need of a urinal bag.

Preoperative preparation

The mental preparation of the patient who is to undergo ureteric transplant either to the pelvic colon or into an isolated loop of ileum is extremely important. The change in habit following surgery must be fully explained to the patient.

Electrolyte balance and kidney function are corrected as far as possible. The bowel is further prepared by enemas and colonic washouts.

Postoperative care

The care is that of any patient returning to the ward following major surgery.

Points applicable to ureteric transplant to the pelvic colon:

1. Rectal tube in situ. Continuous drainage into a Bardic or Aldon bag should be set up. This tube is inserted while the patient is in theatre and should be watched very carefully postoperatively to ensure that drainage is constant. Should drainage be negligible this should be immediately reported to the medical staff.
2. A nasogastric tube is aspirated hourly as required.
3. Intravenous fluids should be given and correct fluid balance is very important.
4. Sedation.
5. There may be a urethral catheter in situ but this is only acting as a drain. There may also be a wound drain.
6. Aperients and enemas postoperatively are withheld as for any other type of intestinal surgery.
7. Dietary modifications may be necessary depending on electrolyte and blood urea levels both in the postoperative and convalescent stages. Table salt is avoided and sodium bicarbonate 1 g and potassium bicarbonate 1 g daily are given to counteract acidosis and hyperchloraemia.

Points applicable to ureteric transplant to ileal loop:

1. Catheter usually left in ileal loop. This is managed as rectal tube above.

2. Other points of management are similar to above. Dietary restriction is usually unnecessary.

3. The care of and problems arising from an ileal conduit have been discussed in Chapter 38.

43

Diseases of the bladder, and the male genital organs

The normal urinary bladder has a capacity of about 360 ml.

The symptoms and signs of disease of the urinary tract have been described in Chapter 42. Many of these occur as a result of diseases of the bladder and urethra.

INVESTIGATIONS OF THE BLADDER AND URETHRA

Many of the investigations described in Chapter 42 are used in diseases of the bladder and urethra. In addition the following may be useful in certain circumstances.

Urodynamic studies

This is a general term for tests designed to measure the muscle activity in the bladder and urethra as well as the rate at which the patient can pass urine.

A fine tube is passed into the bladder under aseptic conditions. With specialised equipment, recordings are made of the pressure within the bladder and urethra. The rate at which the patient can pass urine is also measured. These facts help to differentiate the various causes of abnormalities of micturition.

Urethroscopy

This is the visual examination of the inside of the urethra using an instrument with a telescope which looks straight ahead.

Urethrography

This is a radiological examination of the urethra, in the male, in which radio-opaque dye is introduced via the external urethral meatus. It is sometimes used in the investigation of urethral trauma or urethral strictures.

ACUTE RETENTION OF URINE

The patient is unable to pass urine and usually complains of severe pain.

Causes

1. *Reflex.* Postoperative retention is quite common. Following operations on the rectum and anus difficulty with micturition, if not actual retention, often occurs.

2. *Organic nervous diseases.* These are often slow in onset with no pain. Lesions of the central nervous system may affect the bladder centre in the spinal cord.
   (a) Fractures of the spine with damage to the spinal cord.
   (b) Multiple sclerosis, and other diseases of the central nervous system.
   (c) Children with myelomeningocele.

3. *Mechanical causes*
   (a) Rupture of the urethra.
   (b) Prostatic obstruction—this is the commonest cause of acute retention.
   (c) Urethral stricture and urethritis.
   (d) A stone, a foreign body, or a growth obstructing the neck of the bladder or urethra.
   (e) A retroverted gravid uterus.
   (f) Phimosis.

Clinical presentation

1. *Sudden acute retention* may occur in men with no previous history of urological disorder. The causes include drunkenness and hysteria.

2. *Acute retention* as a culmination of previous dysuria, increasing frequency and voiding a decreasing volume of urine. The attack may be precipitated by cold or being unable to empty the bladder at a convenient moment.

   In both types the patient is in severe pain and a firm, distended bladder is easily palpable.

3. *Acute-on-chronic retention.* This is the most dangerous form. The patient has had long-standing urinary symptoms with a bladder which has not been emptying properly. He is not usually aware of this but his general health may have deteriorated because of back pressure on the kidneys and renal failure. There is usually no complaint of pain and a complete unawareness of the severity of his condition. The large atonic bladder is painless.

Treatment and nursing care

The patient must never be catheterised and sent home forthwith. He should always be admitted to hospital, and the following measures instituted:

1. Analgesics and rest. The patient is in pain and anxious. Analgesics may be prescribed but catheterisation provides the best pain relief.

2. Mechanical relief. Mechanical relief is given by:

(a) Urethral catheterisation is the usual method which is employed. It is a common and important surgical procedure and will be considered in detail.

(b) Suprapubic catheterisation, by puncture with a trocar and cannula, will usually be performed only when it is impossible to pass a catheter by the urethra.

3. The maintenance of the excretion of urine by the kidneys is stimulated by the administration of liberal quantities of fluids.

4. Investigation of the cause includes clinical examination, examination of the urine, the blood, and an intravenous urogram in some cases.

CATHETERISATION

Catheterisation can be mechanically simple, but on occasions it is extremely difficult or impossible. The management of the catheterised patient and the prevention of infection require great care and patience by medical and nursing staff.

Complications of catheterisation

The problems which arise from catheterisation may be summarised according to the part of the urinary tract which is affected.

1. The urethra

(a) Trauma. The catheter may tear the delicate lining of the urethra. This is more likely to occur the more frequently the catheter has to be passed. A water-soluble lubricant is used. The more rigid the catheter the greater the trauma.

Fig. 43.1 Foley's catheter showing balloon inflated.

(b) The wider the catheter the greater is the pressure against the cells of the lining wall. A large catheter is more traumatic, but a small catheter once passed is more readily blocked by blood clot or debris.

(c) Urethritis may develop from catheterisation and infect the bladder causing cystitis, and the kidney causing pyelonephritis.

2. **The penis**

  (a) Meatal stricture is liable to develop from the combined effects of a large catheter and infection.

  (b) Balanitis and meatal ulceration. If the prepuce cannot be retracted a dorsal slit will have to be performed to avoid balanitis. Strapping the catheter to the glans penis may cause irritation. It is preferable to use a self-retaining catheter (Fig.43.1).

3. **The bladder.** The bladder may be infected by:

  (a) Careless catheterisation including neglect of asepsis.

  (b) Infection creeping up the lumen of the catheter. In this connection, air bubbles are particularly important as a source of infection. Closed drainage using a valved bag prevents airborne infection.

4. The kidneys. The kidneys are particularly liable to be infected in cases where long-standing chronic retention of urine has caused hydronephrosis and incompetence of the ureteric orifice allowing regurgitation of urine back into the ureters.

5. The blood. Bacteraemia or septicaemia may be caused by catheterisation or removal of a catheter in a patient with a urinary tract infection or when infection has arisen as a result of catheterisation.

The catheter

Catheters are available in a large variety of sizes, design and material. They are supplied presterilised by gamma rays.

Size

In general the smaller the catheter the less the trauma to and irritation of the urethra. If clear urine is to be drained a small catheter will suffice but if blood or pus is expected, a larger one is necessary.

Design

Most catheters are straight. Some have a shaped tip to assist passage in difficult cases. Most are self-retaining with a terminal balloon for this purpose (Fig. 43.1). The balloon is inflated via a small side lumen while urine drains through the main lumen (commonly called a two-way catheter). If irrigation of the bladder is necessary, to clear pus or blood, a catheter with a third lumen through which fluid can be instilled is used (commonly called a three-way catheter). Catheters with a single lumen, for drainage of urine, are made but only used in a few special circumstances (one-way catheter).

Material

Modern materials from which catheters are made are relatively non-irritant. For long-term use those made from silastic or coated with, for example, Teflon are used. Most catheters are soft and flexible. Some, with shaped tips, are stiffer for ease of insertion. Stiffer plastic catheters are available. Some people consider them preferable if bladder washouts are necessary because they do not collapse when suction is applied.

The 'Portex' Gibbon catheter (Fig. 43.2), a fine plastic catheter, constituted a major advance both because it is easy and safe to pass and also because it causes minimal urethritis. However, it had no self-retaining mechanism. This has been modified to include a balloon.

Fig. 43.2 Gibbon catheter.

The technique of catheterisation

Catheterisation can be an extremely dangerous operation. Force must not be used and unless full asepsis is maintained the patient may lose his life.

Many of these patients are agitated, in pain and dirty, so that the initial treatment consists of administration of an analgesic and giving the patient a hot bath. He may pass urine into the bath, obviating the need for a catheter. The majority do not, so catheterisation has to be undertaken.

A good light, an assistant and all the equipment necessary, including a variety of catheters, should be available.

1. The genitalia are washed.
2. After masking, a full scrub-up is undertaken and sterile gloves are put on.
3. The genitalia are cleansed with 0.25 per cent chlorhexidine.
4. The patient is draped with sterile towels.

5. A whole tube of gel containing lignocaine 1 per cent and chlorhexidine 0.25 per cent is injected into the urethra. The tube is supplied
   presterilised with a nozzle for injection.
6. A penile clamp is attached to keep the gel in the urethra. About 3
   minutes is necessary to produce adequate analgesia and antisepsis.
7. A catheter is passed using a no-touch technique (Fig. 43.3).
8. If the catheter is to be left indwelling it should be connected at
   once to a drainage bag (Fig. 43.7) with a non-return valve and a tap
   at the base for emptying. A specimen of urine is taken as soon as
   the bladder is entered. Further specimens, if needed, are taken by
   inserting a needle low down in the connecting tube before it
   enters the bag, so that the closed drainage system is not broken.
   The connecting tube is attached to the inner side of the thigh with
   adhesive tape.

Fig. 43.3 Method of passing catheter.

Catheter care

The external urinary meatus and the catheter as it enters the urethra
should ideally be cleansed with 0.25 per cent chlorhexidine 4 hourly. This
is sometimes impractical but it should be done at least twice a day.
Chlorhexidine cream should be applied around the meatus. A small
sterile dressing or a small ring of sponge over the catheter should be
placed around the meatus. All this is to remove urethral discharge which
accumulates around the meatus and to prevent infection entering
alongside the catheter.

If the bag needs changing the catheter should be clamped while it is
done to prevent ascent of air bubbles. The need for care to prevent
infection is as great when changing the bag as when passing the catheter.

When removing a catheter the balloon is deflated and the catheter
carefully withdrawn.

Suprapubic cystotomy

This may be performed for acute retention of urine if it is impossible to
pass a urethral catheter or if there is gross infection of the urine.

A fine catheter is passed percutaneously in the lower abdomen
through a trocar into the bladder under local anaesthetic. A specially
designed set is used. Alternatively the procedure can be performed by
opening the bladder through an incision in the lower abdomen and
inserting a self-retaining catheter.

DISEASES OF THE BLADDER

RUPTURE OF THE BLADDER

A blow on the lower abdomen, especially if the bladder is full, is one
cause of rupture. Through the tear, urine seeps into the peritoneum
(intraperitoneal rupture). As a complication of a fracture of the pelvis the
bladder may also be ruptured, but the tear is usually extraperitoneal and
there is no danger of peritonitis.

Both injuries are severe. Untreated, the patient with an intraperitoneal rupture develops peritonitis, while the patient with an extraperitoneal rupture develops extensive fulminating cellulitis as a result of extravasation of urine over the tissues of the abdominal wall and the perineum.

Clinical features

1. The patient is usually in a state of shock.
2. The lower abdomen is tender and rigid.
3. No urine has been, or can be, passed. The patient should be discouraged from attempting to pass urine because it flows through the rupture.
4. Catheterisation (which should be performed in an operating theatre) recovers only a small quantity of bloodstained urine.

Treatment

Shock is treated and a laparotomy performed. The bladder is sutured and the peritoneal cavity may be drained if the rupture has been intraperitoneal.

A urethral catheter or occasionally a suprapubic catheter is inserted to keep the bladder empty during healing. A drain may be placed in the retropubic space if the rupture is extraperitoneal.

CYSTITIS

Cystitis is a condition in which the bladder mucosa is inflamed. Many patients, particularly women, attribute any symptom, such as dysuria or scalding pain on micturition, to 'cystitis'. In many instances pyelography and examination of mid-stream specimens of urine reveal no abnormality. Only an initial specimen of urine or a urethral swab will contain pus and organisms.

Acute cystitis may be part of a general urinary infection. Chronic cystitis is usually associated with obstruction to the outflow of urine. The presence of a foreign body, such as a stone passed from the kidney, or an abnormality of the bladder, e.g. a diverticulum or cystocele, predisposes to infection.

Infection may pass down the ureter from a diseased kidney and give rise to a similar type of infection in the bladder. The organisms may be pyogenic or tuberculous. Ascending infection from the urethra is a common cause of cystitis in the female.

Most infections arise by ascent of bowel organisms from the perineum—haematogenous infections are rare except in the neonatal period. Since the incidence of urinary infection is greater in females, it seems reasonable to suggest that the shortness of the female urethra facilitates the entry of organisms.

Urethral stricture and prostatic obstruction as well as spinal injuries, all of which interfere with the effective drainage of the bladder, predispose to infection.

Symptoms and signs

The principal symptoms are suprapubic pain, scalding pain on passing urine and frequency of micturition. Haematuria may be present if the inflammation is severe.

In some cases an underlying neoplasm gives rise to the symptoms of cystitis. Examination of the urine reveals the presence of pus, organisms, and possible red blood corpuscles.

Treatment

The most important factors in treatment are to encourage the patient to drink plenty of fluid and to empty the bladder completely. In acute cases the patient has to be in bed, and consume 3 litres of fluid daily. The reaction of the urine if acid is changed by giving mist. potassium citrate. Antibiotics are prescribed only after bacteriological examination and sensitivity tests. Personal hygiene and care of the general health are important in overcoming the condition. When the symptoms subside a full investigation, particularly to discover any cause of defective bladder emptying which can be remedied, is undertaken. If bladder neck obstruction is present in the female endoscopic resection will be necessary.

Bladder washouts (lavage) are not usually performed unless specially ordered. Fluid must not be forced into the bladder under pressure, and bladder washouts should be of the correct temperature: 37°C (100°F). Normally 180 to 210 ml of fluid are instilled, but if the patient complains of pain before this volume has been used no attempt should be made to force a further quantity into the bladder. The common solutions used are:

> Silver nitrate 1/15 000 to 1/5000.
> Acetic acid 0.5 per cent.
> Hibitane 1/5000, in pure aqueous solution—not the form in which it is sent for ward stock.
> Noxyflex 1 per cent for continuous irrigation, 2.5 per cent for instillation.

Bladder lavage (irrigation)

> Bladder washout (irrigation) may be ordered for:
> Chronic cystitis.
> Haematuria with clot formation as the presenting sign of disease.
> Haematuria following operation on the bladder or prostate.
> The fluid usually used is sterile saline 0.9 per cent, at room temperature.

1. Continuous lavage—or closed system. The irrigating fluid is suspended from a drip stand, passes down a giving set, and enters the bladder through one arm of a three-way catheter. Together with the urine it drains out of the bladder via the other arm of the catheter into a drainage bag (Fig. 43.7). The rate of the flow of the irrigating fluid is prescribed by the doctor, e.g. immediately after operation it may be free-flowing, or 1.5 litre in 1 hour.

Before putting up a fresh container of irrigating fluid the drainage bag is emptied via its tap into a jug, and the contents measured. The nurse washes and dries her hands. The litre of fluid is checked and put up, and the flow regulated as prescribed. The amount of irrigating fluid and of drainage is recorded on a chart. Whilst the irrigation is in progress, the nurse observes:

(a) that urine is being secreted
(b) that the fluid is flowing into the bladder at the prescribed rate
(c) that it is draining out of the bladder into the drainage bag
(d) whether any bleeding is increasing or decreasing
(e) the presence of any clots
(f) any distension of or discomfort in the bladder or abdomen
(g) the amount flowing in as compared with the amount draining out
(h) the condition of the suprapubic wound (if there is one) and its dressing.

The irrigation continues until the urine is clear—usually, for not less than 48 hours and often for 3 to 4 days. The drainage system is changed as necessary. When the continuous irrigation is to cease, the patient is informed and made ready by being given privacy and by having personal and bedclothing rearranged.

The flow of the irrigating fluid is stopped, the giving set disconnected and the catheter arm spigoted—sterility being maintained—leaving continuous drainage of urine via the catheter and drainage tubing and bag. A note is made on the fluid chart to this effect. i.e. irrigation ceased. The patient is repositioned, encouraged to drink fluids in abundance, and all intake and output carefully measured and recorded. Used equipment is disposed of in the soiled dressing bag.

If requested, 24 hours after discontinuation, a catheter specimen of urine is collected and sent to the laboratory.

2. Hand irrigation. A basic dressing trolley is prepared, with the addition of a 50 ml catheter-tip syringe, irrigating fluid, bowl, receiver, spigot.

The patient is informed of what is going to happen and his cooperation obtained. The trolley is taken to the bedside, privacy is ensured, and the patient is placed in a comfortable position with his legs apart.

Using the aseptic technique, the dressing packet is opened and prepared. Outer packs are opened and the contents are placed on the sterile field. Some irrigating fluid is poured into the bowl. A towel is placed under the catheter, the receiver is placed between the legs. The spigot is removed and discarded, or the drainage bag is disconnected and its end covered with a sterile swab.

Using gentle pressure on a syringe 30 ml of fluid is instilled and then sucked back, noting the amount, colour, presence of clots etc. It is repeated as necessary until no clots return.

A clean spigot is put in, or the drainage bag is reconnected. The receiver is removed.

N.B. If after instillation of the first 30 ml no fluid is drawn back, the medical officer is notified at once, no attempt being made to introduce more fluid at this stage.

The meatus and nearby catheter are swabbed. The patient is dried and made comfortable. The trolley and its contents are removed. A report /record is made of the result.

STONES IN THE BLADDER

Bladder stones develop as a result of infection.

The stone may form in the bladder or may enlarge in the bladder after being passed from the kidney. The main symptoms are pain, frequency of micturition by day, haematuria and strangury.

X-ray reveals the presence of the stone, which is removed by the introduction of a crushing instrument *per urethram,* or, if too large and very hard, by the suprapubic route. Very occasionally a stone is not opaque and can be diagnosed only on cystoscopic examination.

NEW GROWTHS OF THE BLADDER

The majority of new growths of the bladder arise in the lining transitional epithelium. They may be single or multiple. They vary in their appearance, histology and behaviour from being relatively benign to frankly malignant (e.g. Fig. 43.4). They tend to recur. For this reason a patient suffering from the disease must be cystoscoped at regular intervals for the remainder of his life.

Workers in certain industries, of which rubber manufacture is an example, have a higher incidence of this disease than others and therefore should be screened for disease by cytological examination of the urine at regular intervals.

Symptoms and signs

1. Painless haematuria is the most constant symptom. At the end of micturition almost pure blood may be passed.

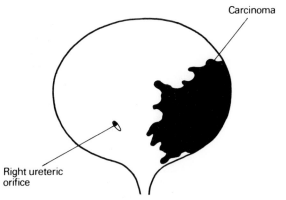

Fig. 43.4 Carcinoma bladder. The left ureteric orifice has been invaded and the left kidney will be non-functioning.

2. Increased frequency and scalding on micturition develop if secondary infection occurs.

3. Pain may be intolerable in the late stages of carcinoma, and frequently takes the form of severe sciatica from infiltration by the growth, of the sacral plexus.

4. Bimanual examination of the bladder, with a finger in the rectum and a hand on the abdominal wall, may reveal a swelling.

Investigations

1. Urine examination—for culture
    —for presence of blood
    —for cytology
2. Intravenous urogram
3. Cystoscopy and examination under anaesthetic

Treatment

1. Cystoscopy and endoscopic resection. The specimen is sent for histology. This is definitive treatment for tumours amenable to local removal.

2. Megavoltage radiotherapy. More extensive lesions may be treated by radiotherapy, either primarily or in addition to transurethral resection.

3. Cystodiathermy. This is used for the treatment of small recurrent tumours.

4. Total cystectomy with urinary diversion (Ch. 42). This is occasionally necessary for treatment of the tumour or for haemorrhage.

5. Cytotoxic drugs—into the bladder or systemically—are occasionally used.

6. Palliative. Continued haemorrhage is sometimes a problem. Instillation of silver nitrate or formol saline, or hydrostatic balloon distension of the bladder may be helpful.

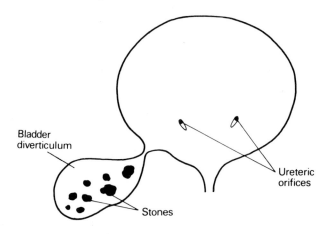

Bladder diverticulum

Ureteric orifices

Stones

DIVERTICULUM OF THE BLADDER

A diverticulum (Fig. 43.5) may occur in the bladder secondary to obstruction at the bladder neck or in the urethra or as a result of inherent weakness of the musculature of the bladder. The condition is frequently complicated by sepsis, stone formation, and the occurrence of a new growth.

The treatment is that of the causal condition combined, if necessary, with excision of the diverticulum.

DISEASES OF THE PROSTATE

The prostate is a gland about the size of a walnut, situated in the proximal portion of the male urethra.

PROSTATIC OBSTRUCTION

The commonest lesion is prostatic obstruction. This results in increasing urinary disturbance and if untreated damage to the kidneys. The bladder is never completely emptied, so that back pressure eventually causes hydronephrosis (Fig. 43.6). The patients are usually advanced in years, 60 or over being the usual age. Disturbance of the patient's general health may be very great.

Causes

1. Simple (benign) enlargement. This is the commonest type.

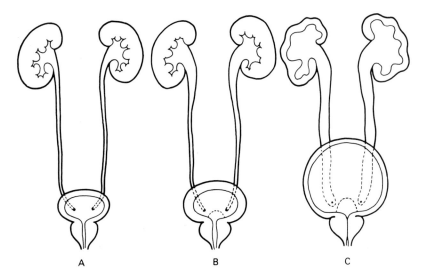

Fig. 43.6 The effects of prostatism. A. Normal. B. Moderate enlargement, hydronephrosis and hypertrophy of the bladder. C. Gross enlargement, extensive hydronephrosis and an atonic distended bladder.

2. *Prostatic fibrosis* in which the internal meatus is almost closed by narrowing.

3. *Carcinoma of the prostate.*

Symptoms and signs

1. *Increased frequency and difficulty of micturition* are prominent complaints. The patient's sleep is disturbed. The general health and well-being deteriorate from lack of sleep.

2. *Haematuria* may occur in some cases as a result of congestion.

3. *Pain and scalding on micturition* develop from infection of the residual urine.

4. *Acute retention of urine* may develop. About 1 in 10 patients present with acute retention. In a neglected case renal failure will set in, and the patient may be admitted to hospital in coma or in a semicomatosed state.

5. *Enlargement* of the gland may be felt on rectal examination.

Treatment

If at all possible prostatectomy in some form, or even in stages, is carried out. If the patient's condition is too poor then an indwelling catheter may be all that is possible and a Foley catheter, preferably made of inert silastic material, would seem to be the one of choice. Occasionally a permanent suprapubic catheter has to be left in place. The precise method of treatment will depend on:

1. *The nature of the obstruction*

2. *The effect it produces.* Most important are those on:
   (a) The kidneys.
   (b) The bladder.

Stone formation, infection or diverticulum formation may be extensive.

3. *General health of the patient.* Many patients have associated disease like myocardial insufficiency or chronic bronchitis. In such patients spinal or epidural anaesthesia can be used satisfactorily.

Choice of operations

Transurethral resection of prostate. Gland resected *per urethram* by resectoscope. No abdominal wound.

Retropubic (Millin). The prostate is removed by operation in the space between the back of the pubis and the bladder (which is not opened).

Transvesical (Wilson-Hey). The bladder is opened and the prostate enucleated.

Perineal approach, rarely used in the U.K.

The most satisfactory operation for prostatic obstruction is endoscopic resection. In expert hands 95 per cent of all enlargements can be dealt with by this method. There are no tubes beyond a urethral catheter. There is no wound in the abdominal wall, in the bladder or the prostatic capsule and the patient can usually be discharged on the fifth day passing urine satisfactorily.

Preoperative Care

1. General condition of patient. The fitness of the patient to undergo general, spinal or epidural anaesthesia must be assessed. Myocardial insufficiency, hypertension or chronic respiratory disease may require treatment preoperatively. Anaemia must be corrected, once the cause is ascertained.

Chest physiotherapy helps to diminish the risk of postoperative pulmonary complications.

2. Renal function

(a) A high oral fluid intake (in excess of 3 litres in 24 hours) should be encouraged in all patients. A jug of fluid should be available on the top of the patient's bedside locker and the nurse must encourage the patient to drink with unrelenting persistence. Sufficient fluid must be taken to keep the patient's tongue moist and a careful fluid balance chart must be kept.

(b) If the patient has a good urine output (in excess of 1.5 to 2 litres in 24 hours) and a normal blood urea, renal function is adequate.

(c) If there has been chronic retention, with back pressure on the kidneys, or urinary infection, the blood urea may be raised. In these circumstances a period of catheter drainage with a high fluid intake is necessary for 7 to 10 days to reduce the blood urea. This may not return completely to normal.

3. Urinary infection. Urine is cultured in the laboratory. If infection is present it must be treated with the appropriate antibiotic.

4. The pressure areas require meticulous care. Faulty junctions of the drainage apparatus result in a wet bed, and every effort must be made to keep the patient dry.

5. Two units of blood should be cross-matched for the operation.

6. A pubic shave should be performed.

7. Catheter removed. This should be done immediately preoperatively.

The operation

The number and arrangement of the drainage tubes will usually vary with the type of operation.

1. Endoscopic transurethral resection. As there is no wound the only drainage is through a three way Foley or similar self-retaining catheter. (Fig. 43.7).

2. Millin or Wilson-Hey prostatectomy. There is an abdominal wound. A drain is left in the retropubic space to drain the sutured incision in the prostatic capsule or bladder. A catheter similar to that used in endoscopic resection is used to drain the bladder.

Postoperative care

1. On return from the theatre. The patient is positioned recumbent in bed. The patient's general condition is checked, pulse and blood pressure measured and charted, the intravenous infusion checked to ensure that it is running satisfactorily and the bladder irrigation and

Fig. 43.7 Closed drainage of the bladder by a urethral catheter into an Aldon bag. The irrigating solution can be run through the other channel in the catheter.

drainage checked to make sure that it is running, a mental note being made of the degree of blood-staining of the effluent.

2. General condition. Continuing careful observation of the patient's general condition is very important especially in relation to the amount of bleeding. It should be noted whether the catheter drainage is becoming more or less blood-stained as time passes.

The pulse and blood are initially recorded every 15 minutes, then half hourly until stable. Any evidence of excessive or increased bleeding must be reported.

3. Intravenous infusion. This is maintained with the fluid ordered by the medical staff. Blood transfusion is often necessary.

4. Care of catheter. The details of managing continuous irrigation of the bladder and catheter care are as on pp. 507 and 509.

The irrigation is stopped when the catheter drainage is fairly clear (bleeding virtually stopped). The catheter is usually removed on the 2nd or 3rd postoperative day after transurethral resection or retropubic prostatectomy, as long as the urine is clear. After transvesical prostatectomy it is removed from the 5th to 7th day postoperatively.

5. *The drain.* This is removed about 48 or 72 hours postoperatively unless there is excessive drainage.

6. *General instructions.* A high oral fluid intake must be maintained. After removal of the catheter the patient is encouraged to pass urine regularly by the clock (½ to 1 hourly). The time interval is gradually extended so that after 2 or 3 days the patient passes urine as desired.

7. *Discharge home.* This is usually about 5 days after transurethral resection and 7 to 10 days after open prostatectomy. The patient must be instructed to drink plenty of fluid for 3 months and told that a little bleeding may occur from time to time initially.

Complications

1. *General complications.* This is an elderly group of patients in whom cardiovascular and respiratory complications are not uncommon. They must be treated appropriately. Deep venous thrombosis may also occur. It presents problems in management, for anticoagulants are contraindicated because of the likelihood of excessive bleeding.

2. *Haemorrhage.* Excessive haemorrhage may occur from the prostatic bed. Treatment includes blood transfusion, antifibrinolysins, and very occasionally surgical packing of the prostatic bed.

Secondary haemorrhage is an occasional complication about 8 days postoperatively and requires bladder washouts, free drainage and antibiotics.

3. *Clot retention.* The catheter may cease to drain because of blood clot in the bladder (this may be large amounts of clot or a small amount blocking the catheter). The patient complains of bladder pain and the bladder is palpable. The irrigation should be stopped until drainage is restarted. Milking the catheter, bladder washout and, on occasions, return to the theatre to clear the bladder may be necessary. Drainage bags are available which incorporate in their tubing a hand pump, allowing the catheter to be unblocked without breaking the closed drainage system.

4. *Infection.* Urinary infection may occur following prostatectomy. Bacteraemia or septicaemia may arise secondary to the urinary infection, especially after manipulation or removal of the catheter. Infection is suspected because of fever or rigors (occasionally bacteraemic shock) and confirmed by urine and/or blood culture. Appropriate antibiotics should be prescribed. Epididymo-orchitis may occur. This is usually a week or two after the operation.

5. *Suprapubic leakage.* This may occur after retropubic or transvesical prostatectomy, from the prostatic capsule or bladder wound. The catheter must be left in or re-inserted, only being removed when the fistula has been dry for 4 days.

6. *Incontinence.* Some patients have poor control of micturition after removal of the catheter. Treatment includes eradication of any infection, perineal exercises (stopping and starting the urinary stream), perineal

518 / Surgery for Nurses

faradism and the temporary use of a condom urinary drainage system.

7. *Late complications.* Urethral stricture sometimes occurs. The stream becomes thin and urine difficult to pass. It requires treatment by dilatation.

Dry ejaculation is often a sequel to prostatectomy because the bladder neck can no longer close. It requires no treatment except reassurance of the patient that all is well.

CARCINOMA OF THE PROSTATE GLAND

Carcinoma of the prostate is not uncommon. An established carcinoma of the prostate is usually too fixed to be removed. Occasionally a focus of malignancy is discovered on pathological examination of an enlarged prostate which has been removed for what was believed to be simple enlargement.

The symptoms and signs are similar to those of simple enlargement, but pain is more prominent in the perineum and bones. Spread of the growth to the bones occurs in this disease and the serum acid phosphatase may be elevated.

Investigations include estimation of the serum acid phosphatase, skeletal X-ray, isotope bone scan, occasionally lymphangiography, and needle biopsy as well as the usual tests to assess renal function.

Treatment

It may be decided to take no further steps in treatment beyond observation when a localised focus of malignancy has been discovered in a gland believed to be clinically simple.

In patients with symptoms, treatments available include:
(a) *Transurethral resection,* to overcome obstruction and to obtain tissue for histology. Open operation is contraindicated.
(b) *Radiotherapy,* either as treatment for the primary tumour or as palliative treatment for bone metastases.
(c) *Oestrogens.* A large number of preparations is available. They relieve symptoms but carry a significant risk of cardiovascular complications (including cerebrovascular accidents, myocardial infarction, thrombosis) as well as causing gynaecomastia. Antiandrogens and cytotoxic agents are also used.
(d) *Orchidectomy.* This sometimes gives good symptomatic relief but is not very acceptable to the patient.
(e) *Palliative surgery.* Hypophysectomy often relieves intractable bone pain. Laminectomy may be necessary to relieve spinal cord compression due to metastases.

PROSTATIC CALCULI

Prostatic calculi may occur as a result of infection or small abscess formation and of themselves, require no treatment. They are often found and removed incidentally during prostatectomy.

THE PENIS AND URETHRA

CIRCUMCISION

This operation is performed for phimosis (Fig. 43.8), paraphimosis (tight retracted foreskin which will not reduce), recurrent balanitis and religious reasons. If balanitis (infection under the prepuce) is present the prepuce is slit on its dorsal surface, since circumcision in the presence of infection is likely to be followed by extensive skin sloughing. In the infant circumcision is a very minor procedure, but in the adult it is a more severe undertaking.

Many infants are referred to clinics for advice on circumcision but only in a few is it necessary. The baby's prepuce is naturally tight and it may not retract easily until he is 3 or 4 years old. A common cause of reference is the ulcerated foreskin associated with ammoniacal dermatitis (napkin rash). For this condition, circumcision is strongly contra-indicated and will remove nature's protection for the glans and external urinary meatus and so allow ammonia to burn the glans. This will produce stenosis which is a complication of a meatal ulcer. Ammoniacal dermatitis is caused by bacteria from faeces fermenting the urea in wet napkins, with the production of ammonia. The treatment is to allow the child to be without a napkin as much as possible.

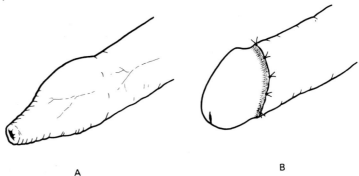

A   B

Fig. 43.8   A. Phimosis. B. Circumcision.

Complications of circumcision

1. Haemorrhage.
2. Infection.
3. Urethritis, particularly damage to the external urinary meatus.
4. Meatal ulcer.

Balanitis

This requires repeated saline baths, antiseptic dressings such as eusol, and the provision of free drainage by dorsal slit if necessary.

Carcinoma of penis

Carcinoma of the penis occurs occasionally, and treatment necessitates removal of the organ and the lymphatic glands in the groin.

The wounds

After the extensive dissection which is necessary to remove the glands in both groins it is usually difficult to secure healing of the wounds. The skin flaps are thin and lymph accumulates beneath. Firm pressure dressings are most important. Lymph which accumulates may be aspirated, with every care taken to avoid infection. Less effective is continuous suction.

Pin-hole meatus

This condition causes urinary obstruction. The treatment is enlargement of the meatus by meatotomy.

RUPTURE OF THE URETHRA

Rupture of the urethra is a serious injury sometimes caused by a fall astride a spike or the sharp edge of a kerbstone. Frequently it is associated with a fracture of the pelvis.

Clinical features

1. Bleeding occurs from the urethral orifice.
2. There is retention of urine.
3. Pain and swelling may be present in the perineum or around the part of the urethra injured.

Treatment

The patient is advised not to pass urine, because it would only flow into the tissues and add to the dangers. Morphia (15 mg) is prescribed to relieve the pain of retention until he can be taken to the theatre.

Opinion is divided as to the best emergency treatment of ruptured urethra. It depends partly on the site of rupture, associated soft tissue and other injuries, and whether the rupture is partial or complete. The possible treatments are:

(a) Exploration and repair of the rupture.
(b) Suprapubic catheterisation followed by repair of urethra, if necessary, at about 10 days.
(c) Urethral catheterisation, leaving catheter 10 to 14 days to allow rupture to heal.

Urethral stricture may occur as a complication of rupture. It will require treatment by dilatation or urethroplasty.

URETHRAL STRICTURE

The vast majority of urethral strictures used to be due to gonorrhoea but, with the easy cure of this disease by antibiotics, instrumentation and injury are now probably the commonest causes. The urinary stream gradually diminishes until the patient is almost unable to pass urine. Back pressure, if long standing, results in hydronephrosis of the kidneys and hypertrophy of the bladder. Periurethral abscess is an occasional complication.

The treatment consists of repeated dilatation with bougies. This is done under general or local anaesthetic. Alternatively urethrotomy (division of the stricture with a knife through a urethroscope) or urethroplasty may be performed. Following urethral dilatation rigors are liable to develop, due to bacteraemic shock. For this reason urethral dilatation is one of the few procedures in which a broad-spectrum antibiotic may be given prophylactically.

DISEASES OF THE TESTICLE, THE SPERMATIC CORD AND ITS COVERINGS

THE TESTICLE

Undescended testis

The testes develop near the kidneys *in utero,* and at birth both testicles are in the scrotum. The maldescent is frequently associated with a hernia and gives rise to symptoms only if recurrent nipping of the testicle occurs at the external abdominal ring.

Treatment

The testicle should be brought down by operation before the age of 4 years. Hormones are sometimes prescribed to encourage normal descent and development but their value is very doubtful.

The nurse must take care of any special stitch used to secure the testicle in position. The operating surgeon will give precise instructions about the postoperative care of the stiches and their date of removal. Often the testicle is placed in a subcutaneous pouch in the scrotum with no special stitch.

Acute epididymo-orchitis

Inflammation of the testis and epididymis is known as epididymo-orchitis.

Aetiology

In adolescents the commonest cause is its occurrence as a complication of mumps. In the adult the commonest organism is the *E.coli.* The gonococus is the second commonest cause of infection.

Symptoms

The testicle is tender and swollen and the scrotal skin may be oedematous. In many cases the condition is associated with a urinary infection, and increased frequency and scalding of micturition may be present.

Treatment

The patient should be confined to bed and the scrotum supported on a sling of broad strapping attached to the thighs. Urinary antiseptics or antibiotics, are prescribed. The urine should be examined for bacteria, or other abnormal constituents, and antibiotic sensitivities established.

Resolution is usual and drainage is rarely necessary. The acute stage subsides rapidly, but complete resolution takes two or three months, and recurrent attacks are not uncommon.

Ligation of the vas deferens may be advisable for recurrent attacks.

Chronic epididymo-orchitis

Causes

1. Tuberculosis.
2. Syphilis.

Tuberculous epididymitis may be part of a tuberculous infection of the urinary tract, or it may occur as a solitary lesion in the genito-urinary tract.

Treatment. Antituberculous chemotherapy (p. 79) is commenced. In refractory cases the epididymis may be excised.

Syphilis. A gumma gives rise to a large painless swelling of the testicle. At puberty a congenital syphilitic may develop epididymo-orchitis. The treatment is that of syphilis.

Torsion of the testis

Torsion of the testis gives rise to severe pain and acute swelling. Immediate operation is desirable and, because the same condition may occur on the other side, the opposite testicle should also be fixed in the scrotum.

Hydrocele

Fig. 43.9 Right hydrocele. The left side of the scrotum is normal.

A hydrocele is a collection of serous fluid in the tunica vaginalis or sac surrounding the testicle (Fig. 43.9). The condition may be secondary to disease of the testicle, but usually develops without any obvious cause.

Treatment

Aspiration by means of a needle and syringe inserted into the hydrocele under local anaesthesia may be performed.

The only preparation necessary is the cleansing of the skin with antiseptic. A torch is essential to transilluminate the swelling so that the surgeon can select an area of skin between the large veins and thereby obviate the formation of a haematoma. The puncture hole in the skin is covered by collodion gauze dressings.

Tapping is only a palliative measure and the sac refills, so that the procedure will have to be repeated fairly frequently.

Radical cure. This is effected by excision of the sac or by turning the sac inside out.

A drain will be inserted in the scrotum for 48 hours, and the scrotum must be supported on strapping across the thighs for ten days after the operation. This is most important if a massive haematocele is to be avoided.

Haematocele

A haematocele is a collection of blood around the testicle. The condition is sometimes due to trauma and sometimes to a new growth. Aspiration or open drainage may be necessary.

New growths of the testicle

New growths are not common but can be very malignant. There are a variety of histological types which behave somewhat differently from each other. The primary lesion may spread via the lymphatics to the para-aortic nodes and via the blood stream to bone.

Treatment

The testicle is removed and megavoltage therapy is prescribed for the abdominal glands.

THE SPERMATIC CORD

Funiculitis or inflammation of the spermatic cord may occur as a complication of epididymo-orchitis. The treatment is similar to that of infection of the testicle.

Vas

Venous plexuses

Testis

Fig. 43.10 Varicocele.

Variocele (Fig. 43.10)

Varicocele is a condition of varicosity of the veins in the spermatic cord, and occurs almost invariably on the left side. A slight dragging pain or, more usually, routine medical examination calls attention to the condition.

Treatment

The vast majority of cases require no treatment at all. A suspensory bandage is advised if the patient complains of pain. Operation may be undertaken and consists of excising the dilated veins. This is necessary if the patient is subfertile.

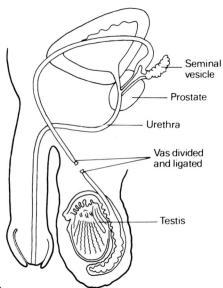

Fig. 43.11 Vasectomy.

Vasectomy (Fig. 43.11)

Vasectomy is division of the vas deferens. It may be undertaken:
1. As a method of family planning.
2. For recurrent epididymo-orchitis.

The surgeon must satisfy himself that the patient understands the nature of the operation, the difficulties of reversal and have the consent of the patient's wife. Before all these criteria are satisfied there is much to be said for a doctor specially interested in marriage counselling interviewing the couple before a decision is taken.

The operation is performed under local or general anaesthetic without the necessity for hospital admission.

The vas is divided through a small incision at the upper end of the scrotum on each side. Minor sepsis in the wound and a haematoma (which may require aspiration) are occasional complications. Semen examinations are essential until they show absence of spermatozoa. Until two negative tests are obtained one month apart vasectomy is not a safe method of contraception.

THE SCROTUM

A sebaceous cyst is probably the commonest lesion of the scrotal skin and is excised in the usual way.

Carcinoma of the scrotal skin is now extremely rare.

BIBLIOGRAPHY

British Medical Journal Editorial 1978 1:61
Dretler S P, Pfister R C, Newhouse J H 1979 New England Journal of Medicine 300:341
Roe P F 1977 Age and Ageing 6: 238-239

44

Injuries and diseases of the central nervous system

The central nervous system consists of the **brain** and the **spinal cord.**

STRUCTURE

THE BRAIN

The brain lies within the bony skull which provides it with some protection against injury. The largest part of the brain is made up of the two **cerebral hemispheres,** each with a surface folded into small crests (**gyri**) and grooves (**sulci**). Each hemisphere is divided into four lobes: The **frontal lobe**, lying anteriorly, is separated by the **central sulcus** from the **parietal lobe**, with the **occipital lobe** behind. The **temporal lobe** beneath the frontal and parietal lobes is separated by a deep groove, **the Sylvian fissure.**

The cerebral hemispheres

The surface of the cerebral hemispheres, the **cerebral cortex**, contains millions of nerve cells which give it a greyish pink colour (**grey matter**). Just beneath the cortex lies the **white matter** which consists of nerve fibres supported by a framework of connective tissue (**neuroglia**). Deep within each hemisphere, embedded in white matter are clusters of grey matter known as the **basal ganglia**, the **thalamus**, and the **hypothalamus**.

The brainstem

The **brainstem**, a single midline structure mostly made up of nerve fibres, extends from beneath the cerebral hemispheres to the spinal cord (Fig. 44.1). It is subdivided into:
  1. The **midbrain**
  2. The **pons**
  3. The **medulla oblongata**.
The **cerebellum**, comprising two laterally placed hemispheres and a

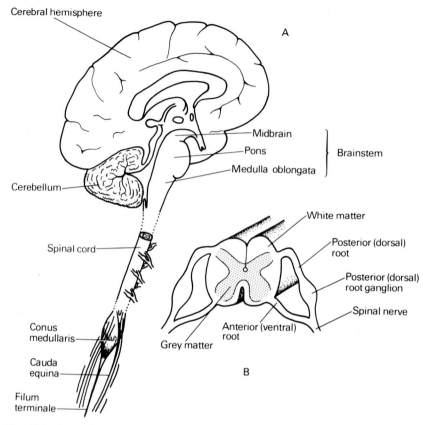

Fig. 44.1 A. Median section of the brain, showing the relationship of the cerebral hemispheres and cerebellum to the brainstem. The spinal cord is continuous with the medulla and ends in a bulbous swelling, the conus medullaris. B. The spinal cord in cross-section.

midline **vermis** lies on the back of the brainstem. The **cranial nerves**, excepting the first pair, enter or emerge from the front of the brainstem.

The blood supply

The brain derives its blood supply from the two **internal carotid** and two **vertebral arteries** in the neck. On the undersurface of the brain, branches join each other to form a ring, the **circle of Willis** (Fig. 44.2). From here major blood vessels (the anterior, middle, and posterior cerebral arteries) leave to supply well-defined parts of the cerebral hemispheres.

The meninges

The brain and the spinal cord are completely surrounded by three membranes—the **meninges**.

The dura mater, the outer membrane, is tough and fibrous. It is plastered to the inside of the skull, but also extends into the cranial cavity as folds separating the components of the brain. A midline fold, the **falx cerebri**, extending from the front of the head to the back separates the

Fig. 44.2 The base of the brain, showing the cranial nerves and major arteries. *Inset*: the circle of Willis.

two cerebral hemispheres, while a horizontal sheet (the **tentorium cerebelli**) slips between the cerebral hemispheres above and the cerebellum below. The brainstem descends through a gap in the tentorium, the **tentorial hiatus**.

The arachnoid mater lies beneath the dura and is a much thinner membrane.

The pia mater is very fine and closely applied to the brain itself. The arachnoid and the pia are separated by the **subarachnoid space**.

The ventricles

The brain is hollow, each cerebral hemisphere containing a large cavity, the **lateral ventricle**, filled with colourless watery **cerebrospinal fluid** produced by fronds of vascular tissue, the **choroid plexuses**.

The lateral ventricles join a **third ventricle** in the midline, and from here cerebrospinal fluid passes down the midbrain in a narrow **aqueduct of Sylvius** to reach the **fourth ventricle** (Fig. 44.3). Through three small

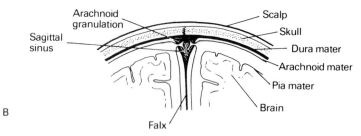

Fig. 44.3 A. The circulation of the cerebrospinal fluid.
B. Cross-section through the superior sagittal sinus. Cerebrospinal fluid drains from the subarachnoid space into the sagittal sinus through the arachnoid granulations.

openings in the roof of this ventricle, the fluid escapes to the subarachnoid space, bathing the outside of the brain. It circulates to the top of the head where it is finally absorbed into the **superior sagittal sinus**, a venous channel lying within the falx and draining into the internal jugular veins.

THE SPINAL CORD

The spinal cord is continuous with the medulla oblongata and extends down the spinal canal to the level of the lower border of the first lumbar vertebra. It consists of a central core of grey matter surrounded by a shell of white matter. At regular intervals along its length, the spinal cord gives off paired **anterior** and **posterior nerve roots** which join to form **spinal nerves**. These leave the spinal canal segmentally between adjacent vertebrae, and at the lower end are quite long resembling a horse's tail (the **cauda equina**). A gentle expansion, the **conus medullaris**, marks the end of the spinal cord which is attached to the coccyx by a fine fibrous strand, the **filum terminale**. The subarachnoid space extends down to the sacrum.

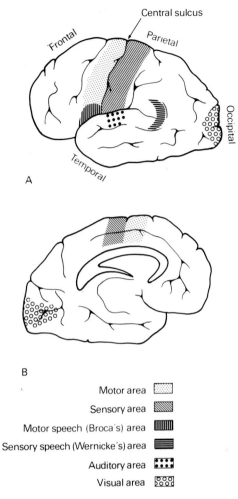

Fig. 44.4 Localisation of function in the left cerebral hemisphere
A. lateral aspect
B. medial aspect.

FUNCTION

The left cerebral hemisphere controls the right side of the body and vice versa. Furthermore in each hemisphere there are relatively discrete areas which appear to have specific functions (Fig. 44.4). Thus the gyrus just in front of the central sulcus (the **motor cortex**) has a predominance of cells which, when stimulated, induce movement on the opposite side. The gyrus behind the central sulcus (the **sensory cortex**) subserves general bodily sensation. The **visual cortex** lies in the occipital lobe.

Other aspects of brain function are represented in one hemisphere only. In right-handed people, speech (which involves both comprehension and expression) is organised in the left cerebral hemisphere, as is the ability to read, write, and do arithmetic.

The basal ganglia appear to be involved in the organisation of involuntary movements associated with change in posture and with emotional reactions. The thalamus, on the other hand, is principally a relay station through which nerve impulses are transmitted to and from the hemisphere. The hypothalamus takes part in the control and regulation of the visceral and metabolic activities of the body. The cerebellum has a controlling influence on posture and coordinates muscle tone to allow smooth voluntary movements.

At the cellular level, when a nerve cell (**neurone**) is stimulated, it gives off a small electrical discharge which travels along its length. It seems that the influence of one nerve cell over another is dependent on chemical transmitter substances. These are released when a neurone is excited, and may have a stimulating or inhibiting effect on adjacent nerve cells. There therefore exists a mechanism whereby electrical activity can be passed up and down the central nervous system through relays of nerve cells. In this way the brain receives information from the outside world (as well as from within the body), is able to make sense of it, and coordinates any action that may be appropriate.

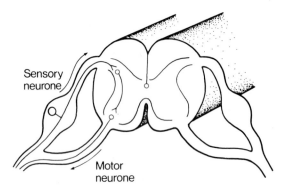

Fig. 44.5 The reflex arc.

The reflex arc (Fig. 44.5) is the simplest example of this mechanism. Taking a pinprick as an example, this stimulus excites a sensory nerve which reaches the spinal cord through a posterior nerve root. From here, further neurones are excited and a chain reaction follows up to the brain where the pain is appreciated. Meanwhile, within the spinal cord, other neurones directly stimulate a motor nerve leaving the cord through an anterior nerve root. Stimulation of this nerve causes muscle contraction, and the limb is smartly removed from the source of pain. All this, of course, happens in a fraction of a second, indeed before one becomes consciously aware of the pain.

THE NURSE, THE PATIENT, AND THE RELATIVE

ARRIVAL

Admission to a neurosurgical ward is a worrying time for the patient and his relatives. Much of the anxiety is generated from ignorance. The belief that neurosurgery comprises operations on patients helpless and hopeless is still widespread, and the fear of having one's faculties disturbed by surgery is understandable. The truth of the matter is that the neurosurgeon today is concerned with the management of a large number of eminently treatable conditions, and he aims to restore affected patients to a full and active life. Naturally he is also involved in serious and life-threatening conditions such as major head injuries and inoperable tumours, and he has his share of disappointment, frustration, and sadness.

First impressions are important, and a friendly welcome shown to a new arrival and his relatives does much to reassure a patient. He may be tired and hungry after a long journey. He may be worried by seeing other patients on the ward who are confused, restless, or perhaps have some difficulty with speech. People with bandaged heads provide an unfamiliar and sometimes distressing sight.

While the nurse is completing the various admission forms and settling the patient in bed, it is courteous to tell him the names of the ward sister and medical staff. Relatives require reassurance as much as patients, particularly when the patient is unconscious or has been admitted without their knowledge after an accident. They are frequently able to provide much of the patient's history and can amplify a referral letter from another hospital.

EXAMINATION

The houseman will wish to speak with the patient and his relatives as soon as possible after their arrival. He will build up a history of the patient's complaint which will help to establish the diagnosis. If the patient has been admitted unconscious from an accident and there are no eye-witnesses, the ambulancemen may have useful information.

After taking the history, a doctor will wish to examine the patient. Most of the examination will be conducted with the patient on his bed, but abnormalities of posture and gait will require room to stand and walk. The doctor will need the following equipment in the examination tray:

1. Scents for testing the sense of smell, e.g. oil of cloves, camphor, coffee, asafoetida.
2. Ophthalmoscope.
3. Torch.
4. Charts for testing visual acuity.
5. Solutions for testing the sense of taste, e.g. sweet—sugar, sour—citric acid, bitter—quinine, salty—salt.
6. Auroscope.
7. Tape measure, to assess muscle wasting or head circumference.
8. Patellar hammer.
9. Test tubes containing hot and cold water to assess temperature sensation.
10. Pins and cotton wool to assess pinprick and light touch sensation.
11. Tuning fork.

12. A pair of geometrical dividers to estimate two-point discrimination.
13. Some small familiar objects, e.g. keys, a spoon, a pen, to assess any speech disturbance (nominal dysphasia) and stereognosis.

By the time the examination is complete, the doctor should have a good idea of the diagnosis, but he will usually want to support his bedside assessment with appropriate investigations.

INVESTIGATION

Urinalysis

Chemical analysis, a cell count, and culture for organisms are performed on the urine of all patients. Further tests, such as specific gravity, urinary osmolarity and electrolytes, are performed should the need arise.

Blood tests

Every patient has blood taken for a full blood picture, ESR, electrolytes and urea, and grouping. Liver function tests, plasma proteins, calcium and phosphorus, and serological tests for syphilis may be indicated.

Lumbar puncture

Indications

1. **Diagnostic**. To establish the presence of blood or pus in the cerebrospinal fluid.
2. **Therapeutic**. To inject appropriate antibiotics in the treatment of meningitis.
3. **Anaesthetic**. For spinal anaesthesia.

Technique

A lumbar puncture may be performed with the patient sitting upright or lying on a bed in the left lateral position. Reassurance of the patient by the attending nurse is very important to the speedy successful performance of the puncture.

The skin over the back from the rib margin to the buttocks is first cleaned with antiseptic. Local anaesthetic is injected along the proposed course of the lumbar puncture needle, usually between the spinous processes of the 3/4 or 4/5 lumbar vertebrae. With the patient's spine well flexed to open the space between the vertebrae, the needle is inserted into the spinal subarachnoid space. The pressure of the cerebrospinal fluid is measured with a manometer. If the nurse now compresses the jugular veins in the neck, she will increase the intracranial pressure which registers as a rise on the manometer (Queckenstedt's test). Release produces a fall. Failure of the fluid to rise and fall freely in this test implies obstruction to its flow, perhaps by a spinal tumour. The cerebrospinal fluid is collected in three specimen bottles, and sent to the laboratory for cell count, culture, and protein, glucose and chloride estimation.

The cerebrospinal fluid is normally clear and colourless. If the puncture has been traumatic, the fluid will be bloodstained, but clears rapidly in successive specimen bottles. Fluid that is uniformly bloodstained in all three bottles confirms a subarachnoid haemorrhage. In meningitis, the fluid has a cloudy, even milky appearance.

At the end of the procedure, the needle is withdrawn and the puncture site is sealed and covered with a dressing. Drainage of cerebrospinal fluid lowers the intracranial pressure and post-lumbar puncture headache is occasionally a problem avoided by nursing the patient flat for 6 hours. If headache is severe, the foot of the bed should be raised.

It is important to avoid lumbar puncture when there is suspicion of raised intracranial pressure. Removal of fluid in this situation may induce 'coning' (see Head Injuries) with fatal results.

Fields of vision

This involves the formal charting of blind spots in the centre or at the edge of the visual field. Disturbance of normal function at different points along the visual pathway from the eyeballs to the occipital cortex produces certain well-defined visual field defects.

Electroencephalography (EEG)

This investigation records the electrical activity of the brain. It may prove helpful in localising irritative lesions.

Isotope brain scan

Many intracranial lesions cause a breakdown of the blood brain barrier allowing leakage of substances from the bloodstream into the brain substance. Because of this, they may be revealed by scanning the head with a gamma camera after the intravenous injection of a radioactive isotope, technetium

Radiographic examination

Plain X-rays

A chest X-ray is performed on all patients, and may reveal a primary lung cancer or secondary deposits from a tumour elsewhere. Skull X-rays may show evidence of raised intracranial pressure, thickening or erosion of bone, a calcified tumour, or displacement of a calcified pineal gland. The majority of skull fractures can be seen on X-ray. Cervical spine X-rays should be performed on patients with all but the most trivial head injuries.

Contrast studies

1. Air encephalogram. Air injected into the subarachnoid space by lumbar puncture rises into the head and provides silhouette pictures of the ventricles and the surface of the brain. Headache, sometimes severe, usually follows this investigation which has been largely superseded by less invasive procedures.

2. Ventriculogram. This involves the injection of air or carbon dioxide directly into the lateral ventricle through a burrhole (or anterior fontanelle in an infant). Again a silhouette picture of the ventricular system is obtained. Injection of Myodil or water-soluble metrizamide provides positive contrast studies.

3. Angiogram. The injection of iodine-containing contrast into the bloodstream outlines the cerebral blood vessels. The injection is made directly into the carotid and vertebral arteries, or more usually a catheter is passed from the femoral artery in the groin up the aorta to the great vessels in the neck. The procedure is usually performed under sedation.

Recent developments enable angiography to be performed following the injection of contrast into a vein rather than an artery (*digital intravenous subtraction angiography*). By avoiding arterial puncture, this technique is safer than conventional angiography, and since no sedation is required, the procedure, if necessary, can be performed on an outpatient basis.

4. Myelogram. Myodil or a water-soluble contrast medium is injected into the spinal subarachnoid space by lumbar puncture or occasionally a puncture in the neck. The contrast outlines the spinal cord, the roots of the cauda equina, and the spinal theca.

Computerised tomography (CT)

This non-invasive technique, available in neurosurgical centres, is quite painless, and merely demands that the patient should keep still during investigation which is completed in a few minutes. The head is scanned by a narrow beam of X-rays as a series of horizontal or vertical cross-sectional slices of pre-selected thickness.

Detectors mounted opposite the X-ray tube measure the rays after the beam has passed through the head. The machine gradually works its way around the head, and the information obtained is processed and reassembled as an image displayed on a television monitor. Intracranial structures are identified according to whether they are of high or low density compared with normal brain tissue.

Appearances may be enhanced by the intravenous injection of iodine-containing contrast. Contrast enhancement seems to depend on local blood flow (the more vascular a lesion, the greater the enhancement), and whether there has been a breakdown of the blood-brain barrier, allowing pooling of the dye.

Scanning may be carried out after the injection of water-soluble contrast into the subarachnoid space. This technique (*CT metrizamide cisternography*) is particularly useful in outlining tumours beneath the brain, while serial scanning may provide information on the circulation and reabsorption of cerebrospinal fluid.

High resolution scanning can portray lesions approximately 3 mm in diameter.

Magnetic resonance imaging (MRI)

-This technique, still very much in its infancy, relies on the tendency of nuclei with an odd number of protons or neutrons to align themselves when exposed to a strong magnetic field. The behaviour of the hydrogen nucleus (with its single proton) is fundamental in this respect. If a radiofrequency pulse is now applied, the alignment can be disturbed in such a way that when the pulse ceases, the original alignment with the magnetic field is restored and simultaneously energy is released as a radiofrequency signal. The properties of this signal are processed by computer to create an image.

There are no known hazards to this form of scanning which has considerable potential and may come to replace computerised tomography.

Intracranial pressure monitoring

In recent years, interest has grown in the direct monitoring of intracranial pressure. The pressure is conveyed from inside the head along a column of fluid to a transducer which allows the information to be presented on a chart or as a digital display. Pressure may be measured in the ventricles, the subarachnoid space, or outside the dura. Rising pressure can be detected before there is any change in a patient's physical signs.

OBSERVATION

Careful observation of patients with neurological conditions is of central importance to patient welfare. Clinical deterioration may develop rapidly; if not appreciated early and dealt with promptly, the outcome may prove fatal. The nurse's responsibility in this respect is therefore considerable, and if she has any particular concern about a patient, she should share this immediately with the sister or nurse in charge.

The observations required of a nurse comprise a simple neurological assessment and a note of the vital signs (Fig. 44.6).

Neurological assessment

1. Level of consciousness. This is really the level of responsiveness. It is the most important observation a nurse can make, and a little care in its recording is well worthwhile.

One of the difficulties in documenting the level of responsiveness is that different words have different meanings for different people. The Glasgow Coma Scale was developed in an effort to overcome this problem. It avoids terms like 'coma' and 'stupor' and instead defines the patient's response to external stimuli in three ways: (1) the circumstances in which he opens his eyes, (2) his best verbal response, and (3) his best motor response (Fig. 44.6). The options defined on the Scale are easily understood making observations between nurses consistent and reliable · (see Head injuries).

Fig. 44.6 A CNS observation chart, showing the features of cerebral compression in a patient whose head injury was complicated by an extradural haematoma.

The level of consciousness should be recorded at the time of admission so that a baseline is drawn to appreciate subsequent changes. Increasing intracranial pressure from any cause produces progressive deterioration in a patient's conscious level.

2. Pupillary changes. The size and reaction of the pupils to light must be recorded. In the early stages of cerebral compression, distortion of the brainstem may irritate the third (oculomotor) nerve and produce pupillary constriction, although this observation may easily be missed. With increasing compression, the third nerve fails to function, and the pupil dilates and becomes less responsive to light. If the cerebral compression is the result of a unilateral space-occupying lesion, then the pupil on this side is the first to become paralysed. The opposite pupil soon follows a similar pattern until ultimately both pupils are fully dilated and unresponsive to light (Fig. 44.7).

Pupil inequality by itself, as an isolated finding, is quite meaningless. The important point is the *progression* of pupillary signs combined with the overall assessment of the patient.

3. Limb movement. A unilateral weakness of the arm and leg (**hemiparesis**) or weakness of both legs (**paraparesis**) is easily demonstrated in a conscious and cooperative person. But if a patient cannot obey commands, a note should be made of any asymmetry of spontaneous movements of the limbs implying an underlying weakness. Likewise the response to painful stimuli may be different on the two sides of the body. Was this present on admission or is it a new finding?

Fig. 44.7 Unequal pupils in cerebral compression. The right pupil is dilated and does not react to light.

Vital signs

1. Pulse rate. Cerebral compression characteristically produces a slow bounding pulse.

2. Blood pressure. Raised intracranial pressure would normally drive blood out of the brain, so to ensure its adequate perfusion and nutrition, there is a compensatory rise in the blood pressure.

3. Respiratory rate. Usually the respiratory rate slows and breathing becomes deeper in the presence of cerebral compression.

4. Temperature. Blood in the subarachnoid space produces a moderate pyrexia. Temperatures in excess of 40°C may occur where there is damage to the hypothalamus or midbrain.

The frequency of these observations is decided by the doctor in charge. It should be emphasised that we seek to record the patient's progress with carefully documented observations; isolated findings are of little value.

As the nurse becomes familiar with the technique of recording a patient's signs, she will acquire further useful information which may never appear on a chart. Thus she will be able to tell a doctor about inappropriate behaviour, any speech problem, any tendency to ignore one side of the body, difficulty with coughing or swallowing, incontinence, fits, and many other observations which may prove helpful in the patient's management.

PREOPERATIVE NURSING CARE

All patients have some fear of surgery, and a neurosurgical operation is particularly worrying for those aware of their surroundings. There is anxiety about possibly not waking from the anaesthetic, or sustaining irreparable brain damage.

A patient is frequently reluctant to share these fears. He may also be worried about threatened unemployment, the care of his family, financial responsibilities, and religious beliefs. He may have understood very little of what he had been told by his doctors. All these problems snowball in many patients' minds, and a kind reassuring nurse who has time to talk can do more than anyone to help a patient approach his operation with calmness and greater understanding. The conduct of the nursing and medical staff does much to inspire (or undermine) a patient's confidence.

It is important that relatives should be kept abreast of a patient's progress. They at least must be told the diagnosis and prognosis as far as they are known. Relatives of patients recently rendered unconscious for one reason or another are often bewildered and frightened, and may place blind trust in nursing and medical staff in a desperate attempt to reverse events. They need comfort and reassurance, with the facts explained as simply as possible.

Unless an operation is an emergency, it is worthwhile spending a little time beforehand trying to improve the patient's physical condition. Smoking should be discouraged and any chest infection treated vigorously with physiotherapy and antibiotics. Debilitated patients may require rehydration and perhaps feeding by a nasogastric tube or intravenous line. Attention to pressure areas is of the greatest importance and repeated incontinence may make catheterisation desirable.

Consent for an operation is obtained by a doctor, who should at the same time explain the proposed operation in simple terms and outline any possible risks. The nurse may later be able to go over any points which are still unclear. She will introduce the anaesthetist the day before surgery, and explain the need for preoperative fasting. Reassurance of rapid regrowth of hair does much to make the shaving more tolerable for women, and the loss may be disguised with a scarf or wig. The patient should be told that he will come round from his anaesthetic with his head bandaged and an intravenous line in his arm.

POSTOPERATIVE NURSING CARE

Of supreme importance in the postoperative period is an open airway. The anaesthetist will only remove an endotracheal tube when he is satisfied that the patient can look after his own airway. He may wish to check the patient's blood gases, and is likely to give oxygen by face mask.

The patient recovering from an anaesthetic is at great risk of airway obstruction from secretions, vomit, and his tongue falling backwards. For this reason, he should be nursed semiprone (Fig. 44.8) or on his side, but never on his back. Regular suction of the mouth and throat removes secretions and stimulates the cough reflex which helps to keep the airway clear.

As soon as a patient enters the recovery ward after his operation, his condition must be recorded on the observation chart. Failure to regain consciousness and any new abnormal signs must be noted and reported at once.

A note is made of the operative findings, and details concerning drains, catheters, intravenous fluids, and drugs are recorded, together with any special remarks from the surgeon or anaesthetist. When the patient's conscious level has improved sufficiently to allow safe transfer, he is returned to his ward.

Thereafter his neurological condition continues to be observed carefully. Occasionally patients are confused and restless, particularly at night time. They may require the protection of cot sides and their hands may need to be bandaged to prevent injury. Restlessness may indicate a full bladder requiring catheterisation.

Fig. 44.8 The semiprone position.

Analgesia rarely needs to be strong after operations on the head, but should be given in adequate doses after spinal surgery. Intravenous lines are taken down once the patient is drinking normally and not feeling nauseated. Drains are usually removed 24 to 48 hours after the operation. At the same time, the patient may be encouraged to sit out of bed for a short period. The physiotherapist has a very important contribution to make throughout the patient's admission, but never more so than in the postoperative period. She will help with the care of the chest, and with the gradual remobilisation of the patient. Removal of sutures, from the head on the fifth and from the back on the tenth postoperative day, is always an important milestone for the patient.

Relatives should be kept informed of a patient's postoperative progress. They will discuss the final diagnosis with the doctor and the ongoing management. Foreseeable problems should be explained and solutions implemented where possible.

THE CARE OF THE UNCONSCIOUS PATIENT

There is a similarity between the unconscious patient and a newborn child. Neither can indicate his needs or desires, and the nurse does well to realise her patient is totally dependant on her.

The airway. The importance of a clear airway cannot be overstressed. If it is compromised, the resulting rise in the blood carbon dioxide and fall in the blood oxygen encourage swelling of the brain and a rise in intracranial pressure which may prove fatal. The patient should be nursed in the semi-prone position so that secretions and vomit will drain out of the mouth and the tongue cannot fall back. Regular removal of secretions by suction backed up with physiotherapy provides reasonable insurance against disaster. An oropharyngeal airway is useful to allow access to the mouth even when the jaws are clenched.

If there is any doubt at all about the airway, the safest procedure is to insert a cuffed endotracheal tube. This is mandatory, of course, if the patient is to be electively ventilated. If it seems as though a patient is going to require an endotracheal tube for more than a few days, he should undergo a tracheostomy since prolonged intubation encourages erosion or stenosis of the trachea.

The position. A pillow under the chest prevents a patient in the semi-prone position from rolling onto his face. Another pillow between the knees with the upper leg drawn up keeps the patient stable. There is no need for a pillow under the head (Fig. 44.8).

Nursing observations. The importance of careful observation has already been underlined (p. 535). The chart must record:
1. The level of consciousness.
2. The size and reaction of the pupils to light.
3. Limb movements.
4. The pulse, blood pressure, respiratory rate, and axillary or rectal temperature.
5. The frequency and nature of any fits.

Skin care. The patient should be turned every 2 hours to relieve pressure areas and prevent the development of sores.

Limb care. Two hourly passive movement of all the limbs helps to improve the circulation and may prevent contractures.

Nutrition. The unconscious patient may be fed very satisfactorily through a nasogastric tube. An adult usually requires 2.5 litres of fluid in 24 hours, but a pyrexia or hot environment may increase this figure. There are numerous proprietary feeds currently available which provide a balanced diet of proteins, fats and carbohydrates with vitamin supplements. Occasionally a patient may require intravenous feeding.

Mouth care. Regular toilet is very important in preventing infection of the mouth and salivary glands. Swabs of glycerine of thymol and ordinary toothpaste on a toothbrush suffice. Cracked lips need a lip-salve.

Bladder and bowel care. Urinary incontinence is best managed by catheterisation although, in the male patient, Paul's tubing may be strapped to the penis. The alternative is the frequent changing of sheets. Wet sheets encourage the rapid appearance of pressure sores.

Retention of faeces will require the assistance of suppositories and enemas. Diarrhoea is sometimes a problem with patients on synthetic feeds.

Eye care. The unconscious patient may not blink and the eyes should be kept moist with methyl cellulose drops. Dried secretions and lashes should be removed by irrigation with saline. The cornea should be protected by keeping the eyes closed with gauze pads soaked in saline. Infection usually responds to chloramphenicol ointment.

Other points. The hair should be kept clean and groomed. The nails should be clean and clipped. Pyjamas and nightdresses need to be changed. Most important of all, the patient needs to be spoken to with words of comfort and encouragement.

DEPARTURE

When a patient is considered fit for transfer, he will either be discharged home or returned to his referring hospital to continue convalescence. At times he may be a little reluctant to venture out of the unit he has come to trust over the previous few days. He should be reassured that his surgeons will continue to keep in touch with him on an outpatient basis, and if there are any specific problems, his family doctor can refer him back at any time. Instructions on any medication must be clearly understood, and an adequate amount supplied.

HEAD INJURIES

Head injuries are exceedingly common, and the majority are so trivial as never to be seen in hospital. Nevertheless there are over 150 000 hospital admissions for head injury each year, and most of these are treated in general surgical wards. Only a small minority require transfer to neurosurgical centres for specialised care and treatment of complications.

Injuries to the scalp

The scalp has a rich blood supply, and a wound will bleed profusely. Pressure on the wound with a firm bandage or the fingertips will usually control the haemorrhage, but a patient may be severely shocked from blood loss before he can reach medical help.

Injuries to the skull

Fractures of the skull may be simple (closed) or compound (open), single or multiple. They may affect the vault, or the base, or both:

(a) **Fractures of the vault** may be fissured (a simple crack) or depressed (where a fragment of bone is driven into the head).

(b) **Fractures of the base** may damage the cranial nerves with resulting impairment of function. Thus there may be weakness (**paresis**) or complete paralysis of muscles supplied by the cranial nerves (e.g. ocular muscles, facial muscles), and impairment or loss of sensation (e.g. smell, sight, hearing).

Anterior cranial fossa fractures may cause haemorrhage from the nose (**epistaxis**), leakage of cerebrospinal fluid down the nose (**CSF rhinorrhoea**), and a **subconjunctival haemorrhage** in the eye. This bright red haemorrhage characteristically has no posterior border for it results from blood tracking forwards from behind.

A middle cranial fossa fracture is suggested by bleeding and escape of cerebrospinal fluid from the external auditory meatus (**otorrhoea**), and the appearance of a dark bruise behind the ear (**Battle's sign**) a day or two after the injury.

Injuries to the brain

The brain is a soft organ with the consistency of porridge, enclosed in a rigid skull. Damage to the brain in a head injury may be local at the site of impact, and/or distant on the opposite side. If the moving head strikes an unyielding object, such as a road, movement of the skull ceases abruptly but the brain undergoes a slower deceleration and so becomes compressed at the site of impact. There follows a recoil movement of the brain which then strikes the opposite side of the skull thereby sustaining a second injury (**contrecoup** phenomenon).

Damage to the brain may be obvious to the naked eye (**contusion** and **laceration**), or only microscopic (**diffuse neuronal damage**). The severity of the lesion does not necessarily correlate with the patient's clinical condition; patients may be fully conscious and orientated with contused or lacerated brain, yet there may be prolonged unconsciousness with no macroscopic injury.

Further damage may be inflicted on the brain as a result of the initial injury. Swelling from **oedema** is a normal sequel to damage to any part of the body, and is part of the inflammatory response. Such swelling leads to raised intracranial pressure because of the unyielding nature of the skull. Pressure may be further raised by **intracranial haemorrhage** from vessels torn at the time of injury. Both oedema and haemorrhage can lead to serious cerebral compression. Because of this high pressure state the brain tends to be thrust down (i.e. herniate) through the opening at the base of the skull (the foramen magnum) compressing vital centres of the brain controlling the heart and respiration. This herniation is known as **coning** and may occur rapidly, demanding prompt treatment if the patient is to survive. If the signs of cerebral compression are to be picked up at the earliest possible moment, patients with head injuries require careful and continual observation by the nurse.

ASSESSMENT OF HEAD INJURIES

This relies on recording the sequence of events following a head injury. The time and details of the injury are important. Was the patient unconscious from the outset? When did the patient reach hospital? What was his condition on arrival? Are there any other injuries?

Nursing observations, described on p. 535, are begun immediately, and continued throughout the patient's stay in hospital. All patients who have lost consciousness from their injury are admitted to ensure that any complications that might arise are quickly discovered and promptly treated. The vast majority of patients admitted to hospital are conscious on arrival and make an uneventful recovery, returning home after 24 hours. Very frequently patients cannot remember events immediately preceding the accident (**retrograde amnesia**) or following the accident (**post-traumatic amnesia**). An estimate of these periods of amnesia should be made; the severity of the head injury appears to correlate with the duration of post-traumatic amnesia.

TREATMENT OF HEAD INJURIES

We have seen that the majority of patients admitted to hospital with a minor concussion make a rapid and complete recovery and are discharged after 24 hours. Patients who have sustained a major head injury provide a much greater challenge.

Resuscitation

The first necessity in the treatment of a major head injury is to ensure that the airway is preserved. Blood, secretions and vomit should be removed from the mouth and throat and the patient placed in the semiprone position. It may be necessary, after a rapid clinical examination, to paralyse the patient with muscle relaxants, and insert an endotracheal tube. Simultaneously an intravenous line is set up to replace lost fluids. Blood is taken for a full blood picture, blood gases, and grouping and cross-matching. The patient's head injury and neurological deficit are assessed, and a search made for any other injuries. Profuse haemorrhage from the scalp may be controlled with local pressure or an artery forceps. The nurse detailed to the patient records her observations.

X-rays

Once the patient's condition is stable, it is safe to move him to the X-ray department. Skull X-rays may reveal a fracture, intracranial air, and perhaps a shift of the pineal gland away from the midline. The paranasal and mastoid air sinuses may be opacified with blood. X-rays of the cervical spine may show an associated fracture or subluxation. A chest X-ray should be always be done for it may reveal rib fractures, a pneumothorax or haemothorax, or pneumonitis from aspiration of vomit. It will also show the position of the endotracheal tube if this has been inserted.

Further management

Further management depends largely on the conditon of the patient:

If he has now regained consciousness

   1. Closed head injury. It is legitimate to admit him to the ward for continued observation.
   2. Open head injury:
   (a) Leakage of cerebrospinal fluid from the nose or ear usually indicates a compound skull fracture. The fluid should be allowed to drain freely, and the patient should be instructed not to sniff or blow his nose if there is a rhinorrhoea. Prophylactic antibiotics are prescribed against the development of meningitis or a brain abscess. CSF rhinorrhoea and otorrhoea usually cease spontaneously, but if persistent, repair of the dural tear with a fascial graft may be necessary.
   (b) If there is a *scalp wound*, the scalp must be shaved to provide a good exposure. After infiltration of local anaesthetic and preliminary toilet, the wound is carefully examined with a finger to see if it communicates with a deeper injury. If the edges are ragged, they are excised. The wound is then sutured. The patient's immunity to tetanus should be checked and brought up-to-date if necessary. Scalp defects may require rotation of large skin flaps and split-skin grafting.
   (c) A compound depressed skull fracture requires elevation and usually removal of the indriven fragments. If the dura is torn, this should be repaired, if necessary with a fascial graft. A large postoperative skull defect can later be corrected by the insertion of a metal plate (**cranioplasty**).

If he remains unconscious or his condition deteriorates

The great concern here is whether or not the patient is suffering cerebral compression from a surgically treatable cause (viz. an extradural or subdural haemorrhage, Fig. 44.9). The simplest means of establishing this is by burrhole exploration of both sides of the head. The side of the fracture, or if there is pupillary inequality, the side of the larger pupil, is examined first. If a surface collection is found, then a **craniectomy** (removal of bone) or a **craniotomy** (cutting a bone flap) may be performed to remove the clot and stop the bleeding. If there is easy access to

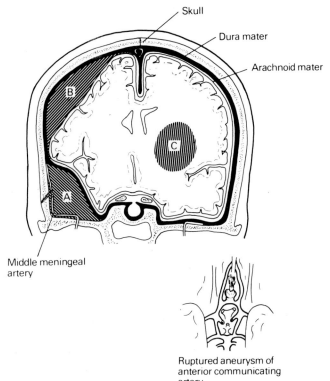

Fig. 44.9   Intracranial haemorrhage
     A. Extradural haematoma
     B. Subdural haematoma
     C. Intracerebral haematoma
Extradural, subdural and intracerebral haematomas are all space-occupying, unlike a subarachnoid haemorrhage.
Inset: A ruptured aneurysm of the anterior communicating artery.

a CT scanner, then a haematoma can usually be excluded without recourse to surgery.

In the majority of patients there is no surface clot but the brain is swollen. Measures to counteract this include:

(a) Intravenous mannitol (10 or 20 per cent)
(b) Intravenous frusemide
(c) Intravenous hypertonic urea (90 g in 200 ml of invert sugar)
(d) Elective hyperventilation.

Intravenous dexamethasone is very frequently given, sometimes in high dosage, but there is little evidence that it has a useful part to play in the treatment of head injuries.

The facility exists in some centres to monitor the intracranial pressure. This records the patient's response to treatment and may help in forming a prognosis.

The important role of the nurse in the ongoing management has already been described (see The care of the unconscious patient, p. 540).

Assuming consciousness is regained, the patient now embarks on a carefully planned programme of rehabilitation. The physiotherapist, occupational therapist, speech therapist, and medical social worker all have very important parts to play if the patient is to make full use of his abilities and return to a useful life.

COMPLICATIONS OF HEAD INJURIES

1. Complications of the unconscious state

(a) Early. Airway obstruction by vomit, blood or secretions; shock from other injuries.

(b) Late. Infection of the lungs and urinary tract; pressure sores; eight loss.

2. Intracranial haemorrhage (see Fig. 44.9)

    (a) Extradural
    (b) Subdural
        (i)   Acute—first 48 hours
        (ii) Subacute—2nd to 14th day
        (iii) Chronic—after 14th day
    (c) Subarachnoid
    (d) Intracerebral

3. Infection

    (a) Meningitis
    (b) Abscess

4. CSF leak

From:
    (a) Nose (rhinorrhoea)
    (b) Ear (otorrhoea)

5. Epilepsy

    (a) Early onset—during the first week after head injury
    (b) Late onset—after the first week

PROGNOSIS OF HEAD INJURIES

It is impossible to predict the extent of recovery from a major head injury with any great accuracy. Children in particular frequently recover well from major head injuries which would permanently and severely incapacitate an adult. As a rule, the improvement in a patient's condition is most obvious during the early weeks of convalescence, but progress may continue for as long as two years after the injury.

The Glasgow Coma Scale can be used as a means of scoring a patient's level of responsiveness between a minimum of three and a maximum of 15 points (see Fig. 44.10). In general terms, the higher the patient's score on admission, the better the prognosis. Conversely mortality exceeds 50 per cent when the score on admission is seven points or less. Likewise

Assessment	Response	Score
Eyes open	Spontaneously	4
	To sound	3
	To pain	2
	Never	1
Best verbal response	Orientated	5
	Confused	4
	Inappropriate words	3
	Incomprehensible sounds	2
	None	1
Best motor response	Obeys commands	6
	Localises pain	5
	Flexion — withdrawal	4
	Flexion — abnormal flexion	3
	Extension	2
	None	1

Fig. 44.10 The Glasgow Coma Scale and system of scoring. Note the scale in Figure 44.6 does not subdivide flexion to pain as the best motor response. The patient's score of 12 points on admission fell to 8 before she was taken to theatres but recovered to 11 points out of a maximum of 14 on return to the ward.

severe hypotension on admission (systolic blood pressure less than 70 mm Hg) carries a poor prognosis.

RESIDUAL DISABILITY

1. Physical disability

This occurs from damage to:
- (a) Cerebral hemispheres
  - (i) Dysphasia
  - (ii) Hemiparesis
- (b) Cranial nerves
  - (i) Anosmia
  - (ii) Visual field defects
  - (iii) Squints
  - (iv) Facial weakness
  - (v) Deafness and vertigo

2. Mental disability

There may be alteration of personality, and impairment of intellect and memory. Headache, dizziness, fatigue, irritability, and pain at the site of injury are common features of the normal recovery process following a head injury. When properly managed, they are short-lived, but they may persist for weeks or months (**post-concussional syndrome**).

DISEASES OF THE BRAIN

The neurosurgeon is commonly concerned with the management of patients with intracranial tumours, aneurysms and vascular malformations, hydrocephalus, and abscesses. Much of his work deals with spinal pathology—tumours, degenerative disease of the spine including prolapsed intervertebral discs, and vascular anomalies. He may also be asked for help in the management of intractable pain, epilepsy, and unwanted movements, e.g. in Parkinson's disease.

Intracranial tumours

The minority of these tumours are benign, e.g. meningioma. Those that are malignant may be primary (gliomas), or secondary (the result of metastatic spread from elsewhere).

Such tumours usually present with symptoms and signs of raised intracranial pressure:
1. Headache, often severe and frequently occurring in the early morning.
2. Vomiting, unrelated to food.
3. Increasing drowsiness.
4. Papilloedema (swelling of the optic disc in the eye).

In addition there may be localising signs, e.g. dysphasia, hemiparesis, visual field defects, according to the site of the tumour. Sometimes the patient presents with fits.

Many benign tumours can be completely removed and the patient cured. Surgical treatment for malignant tumours is less rewarding. Depending on its site and the patient's neurological deficit, a primary malignant tumour may be removed as far as the naked eye can see (macroscopic removal) or a palliative decompression may be all that can be offered. There may be a case for just obtaining histological confirmation of the tumour by burrhole biopsy. Whichever approach is adopted, it is usual for surgery to be followed by a course of radiotherapy.

Cerebral metastases, when multiple, are not amenable to surgical treatment, but occasionally a solitary secondary deposit can be removed with considerable relief of a patient's symptoms.

Aneurysms and vascular malformations

Subarachnoid haemorrhage, characterised by the sudden onset of very severe headache frequently accompanied by vomiting and loss of consciousness, is most commonly caused by rupture of an intracranial aneurysm (Fig. 44.9 inset). The condition carries a high mortality rate; many patients never reach hospital alive, and of those that do, 50 per cent will die within 8 weeks if left untreated. Death may be due to a further major haemorrhage, raised intracranial pressure from the mass effect of bleeding into the brain (forming an intracerebral haematoma), or vasospasm. Spasm of the arteries may be localised or diffuse. When severe, it compromises the flow of blood to the brain causing infarction. It is thought to result from the irritative effect of a blood component on the vessels but the details are poorly understood and there is no reliable treatment.

The minority of patients who recover well from their haemorrhage are candidates for angiography to localise the source of their bleeding. Subsequent surgery is aimed at reducing the likelihood of further, perhaps fatal, haemorrhage. The approach may be:

1. *Direct*, by protecting the aneurysm with a clip or by wrapping it with muslin or muscle, or

2. *Indirect*, by clipping or tying the parent vessel to reduce the pulse pressure of the blood to which the aneurysm is exposed.

Nowadays surgery is performed under the microscope, and improved surgical and anaesthetic techniques allow aneurysms to be approached which were previously considered inoperable.

Medical treatment, comprising bed rest and antifibrinolytic therapy, is reserved for patients too old or too ill for surgery, or who suffer from a serious co-existing medical condition which makes them a poor risk. Antifibrinolytic drugs aim to preserve the blood clot sealing the hole in the aneurysm while the normal healing process of repair is underway. A patient may still bleed again despite these drugs, which have their own side-effects, and their use in aneurysmal haemorrhage remains controversial.

Subarachnoid haemorrhage may also result from an arteriovenous malformation, but the haemorrhage is usually less severe and carries a lower mortality. Generalised or focal epilepsy is a more common presenting symptom while migrainous headache occurs less frequently. There may be an audible bruit, and diagnosis is confirmed by angiography. Where feasible, treatment is by surgical excision.

Hydrocephalus

Hydrocephalus describes an accumulation of cerebrospinal fluid (CSF) in the brain with consequent dilatation of the ventricular system. It usually results from an obstruction to the normal circulation of the fluid. The obstruction may lie inside the brain (e.g. aqueduct stenosis), when the hydrocephalus is described as internal or non-communicating, or outside the brain (e.g. from meningeal adhesions), when the hydrocephalus is external or communicating.

Congenital hydrocephalus is more common than acquired, and is almost always non-communicating. There may be other associated malformations of the brain. Because the bone plates of a baby's skull are mobile, the accumulation of CSF causes the head to enlarge. The fontanelles and scalp veins become prominent, the face seems relatively small, the eyes appear downcast ('sunset eyes'), and percussion of the head yields a crackpot note.

Hydrocephalus may be acquired from impaired circulation of CSF by a tumour or following meningitis or an intracranial haemorrhage. It is frequently communicating. Hydrocephalus acquired after fusion of the skull bones leads to symptoms of raised intracranial pressure (p. 548).

Treatment

Treatment is directed towards bypassing the obstruction to the circula-

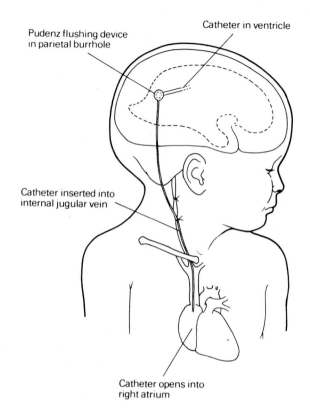

Fig. 44.11   Pudenz-Heyer ventriculo-atrial shunt.

tion of cerebrospinal fluid. Most commonly, the fluid is diverted into the bloodstream (ventriculo-atrial shunt) or peritoneal cavity (ventriculo-peritoneal shunt), where it is rapidly reabsorbed. A catheter is inserted through a burrhole into a lateral ventricle of the brain and passed subcutaneously behind the ear to the neck. If the fluid is to be diverted into the bloodstream, the lower end of this catheter is passed down the internal jugular vein and superior vena cava to the right atrium (Fig. 44.11). Otherwise the catheter is threaded subcutaneously to the epigas-

Fig. 44.12   The Pudenz-Heyer shunt system.

tric region where the abdomen is opened to gain access to the peritoneal cavity. Retrograde flow of blood or cerebrospinal fluid up the shunt is prevented by a valve system, e.g. the Pudenz valve (Fig. 44.12), which also provides a means of testing the patency of the shunt; an incompressible valve implies a distal obstruction, while a proximal obstruction is suggested by a valve that fails to refill after emptying.

Occasionally hydrocephalus may be treated by:

1. A direct attack on the site of the block.
2. Removal of a choroid plexus papilloma producing excessive CSF.
3. Short-circuiting a block by passing a catheter from the lateral ventricle to the cisterna magna (Torkildsen's ventriculocisternostomy).
4. A thecoperitoneal shunt (from lumbar theca to peritoneal cavity).

Cerebral abscess

A cerebral abscess is usually caused by staphylococci or streptococci. It may result from direct extension of infection from the middle ear or paranasal air sinuses, from infected head injuries, or occasionally it may arise from blood-borne infection from distant sources, e.g. bronchiectasis and pneumonia.

There is usually a history of preceding infection. A mild pyrexia may be accompanied by signs of meningeal irritation—neck stiffness and resistance to passive extension of the knee with the hip joint flexed (Kernig's sign). There may be signs of raised intracranial pressure with focal disturbance of function, e.g. dysphasia, hemiparesis, visual field defects. Fits may be a feature. Diagnosis is by computerised tomography of the brain.

Treatment

Treatment consists of drainage of the abscess by aspiration through a brain needle. Aggressive treatment with systemic antibiotics should be started before the results of culture of the pus and sensitivities are known; the regime may subsequently need to be modified. With the potent antibiotics presently available, it is probably no longer necessary to inject antibiotics into the abscess cavity. The patient's progress is monitored clinically and by serial scanning; the abscess may require repeated aspiration. At a later date it may be appropriate to excise the abscess remnant.

Computerised tomography and improvements in culture technique (particularly of anaerobic organisms) have markedly reduced the mortality rate of this dangerous condition.

INJURIES OF THE SPINE AND SPINAL CORD

THE SPINE

Cervical

The cervical spine may be injured by excessive flexion, extension, lateral flexion, or rotation. Flexion injuries tend to produce wedge compression fractures which are stable and unlikely to injure the spinal cord. Rarely there may be posterior prolapse of an intervertebral disc. Flexion-rotation injuries may cause subluxation (unstable), dislocation, or fracture dislocation (very unstable with likelihood of spinal cord injury). Hyperextension may produce a subluxation unstable in extension, with possible cord injury.

Thoracic and lumbar

Most fractures result from excessive flexion of the spine, producing stable wedge compression of the vertebral bodies without threat to the cord. Less commonly, flexion combined with a rotation force produces a dislocation or fracture-dislocation that is very unstable and usually injures the cord or cauda equina.

Treatment

Reduction is unnecessary in stable fractures. A collar for the neck and gradual remobilisation for the back are all that is needed. Subluxations and dislocations first require controlled reduction by traction, if necessary by open operation, followed by immobilisation in a plaster collar or jacket. There may be a case for fusing the spine with a bone graft thereby allowing the patient to mobilise more quickly.

THE SPINAL CORD

The cord or cauda equina are damaged in only a small proportion of spinal injuries. Injury in the thoracic and thoraco-lumbar region is most common.

Complete transection of the cord is usual in thoracic injuries and may occur in the neck. There is a complete flaccid paralysis, sensory loss, and suppression of sphincter control below the site of injury. This state of **spinal shock** fades over days or weeks as the paralysis becomes spastic and visceral reflexes return uncontrolled by higher centres.

The neurological deficit may be patchy in incomplete transection of the cord. Severe injury to the cauda equina causes a permanently flaccid paraplegia and sensory loss, with no return of the visceral reflexes, unless the nerve fibres recover their function.

Treatment

The fracture. Bony displacement in the cervical spine should be reduced. If there is evidence of a disc prolapse on emergency myelography, this demands removal. Paraplegia from thoracic injuries is deemed to be the result of complete transection of the cord, and nothing is gained from attempts at reduction. In the thoraco-lumbar and lumbar regions, where the neurological injury is likely to be incomplete, immediate reduction and internal fixation should be considered.

Nursing care. The patient is nursed on his back and on his side, being turned every 2 hours. The skin requires special attention and a sheepskin under the patient reduces the risk of pressure sores. The limbs require full passive exercise and massage to encourage the circulation and prevent contractures. Breathing exercises reduce the risk of developing hypostatic pneumonia. An indwelling catheter drains the bladder. Within about 3 months of complete transection, the bladder begins to empty as a reflex as soon as it has reached capacity—the **automatic bladder.** Injury to the sacral segments of the cord or the cauda equina interrupts this reflex arc, and emptying of the bladder is dependent upon a local reflex in the bladder wall itself. This **autonomous bladder** can be encouraged to empty by abdominal compression or straining.

The patients are fully aware of their neurological deficit, and encouragement and confidence in their ability are the corner-stones of their rehabilitation. Patients with complete cord transections learn to lead a useful life from a wheel chair, while many of those with injuries to the cauda equina are able to get about with elbow crutches or walking sticks. The contribution of the physiotherapist during this difficult time cannot be overstressed.

DISEASES OF THE SPINE AND SPINAL CORD

CONGENITAL DISEASES

Spina bifida

1. Spina bifida occulta
2. Meningocoele
3. Myelomeningocoele

These conditions are due to incomplete closure of the vertebral canal, particularly in the lower portion of the spine.

1. Spina bifida occulta is a condition in which the bony arch of the spinal canal is deficient. In mild cases there are no symptoms or signs, and the condition is diagnosed as an accidental finding on X-rays. Sometimes there is a sacral pit, and the overlying skin may be covered with a soft tuft

Fig. 44.13 Lumbar meningocoele.

of hair. There may be partial paralysis of the feet due to tethering of the nerves of the cauda equina. Club foot deformities may occur.

An operation may have to be undertaken to release tethered nerves, and deformity of the feet may require correction.

2. Meningocoele (Fig. 44.13). Here the meninges bulge on to the skin, so that there is a large bluish cyst which becomes more tense as the baby coughs or cries. The spinal cord itself is not involved. The condition is evident at birth.

Unless the greatest care is taken, the meninges may rupture, with the escape of cerebrospinal fluid. There is then a risk of infection, and meningitis may prove fatal.

Treatment. If the skin overlying the meningocoele is healthy, there is no urgency to operate. It is essential that the skin be very carefully protected—maceration from wet napkins must be avoided. Wool or lint may be used to pad the swelling which should be washed, dried and powdered at each napkin change. If the covering is very thin, or has ruptured, a decision must be made whether or not to close the defect. The operation involves excision of the membranes and repair of the back by mobilising fascia and skin.

Most of these children will grow up to be normal adults after closure of the defect, although some will have minor neurological defects in the legs or difficulty with the anal or bladder sphincters.

3. Myelomeningocoele. This is a condition in which nervous tissue bulges through the bony defect and the spinal cord is exposed on the surface as a flat ribbon. It is usually associated with some paralysis below the level of the lesion. Paralysis may be minor or in the most severe cases complete paraplegia may exist. In addition, there may be deformities of the lower limbs, deformities of the vertebral column, dribbling incontinence, and hydrocephalus.

Treatment. The decision on whether or not to repair a myelomeningocoele is often difficult but should be made as early as possible. The baby should be handled gently to avoid rupture of the delicate sac. A moist saline pad should be placed over the lesion and lightly bandaged in position.

If it is agreed to close the defect, a specimen of the mother's blood as well as details of the pregnancy and labour should be sent with the baby on transfer to a neurosurgical unit for operation. Surgery aims at mobilising and burying the exposed cord which is then covered with fascia and skin. Postoperatively the baby is nursed on his side in an incubator, being changed from side to side every two hours, or alternatively partly suspended face downwards in elastic slings passed under the abdomen. Babies are nursed with the head low for the first few days to minimise leakage of cerebrospinal fluid from the wound. The baby should he handled as little as possible and should be fed in the incubator. There is a high risk that he will go on to develop hydrocephalus which will require the insertion of a shunt.

As these children grow, they impose an increasing strain on the family. Help from various social service organisations and the educational authority is usually invaluable.

ACQUIRED DISEASES

Tumours

(a) Tumours of the vertebral column.

Primary tumours, e.g. myeloma are unusual.

Secondary tumours are very much more common, and have usually spread from the lung, breast, thyroid or prostate. Vertebral erosion and collapse lead to cord compression.

(b) Tumours of the spinal cord and meninges.

Primary tumours of the spinal cord, e.g. ependymoma, are not common.

Secondary tumours are exceedingly rare.

Tumours arising from the root sheaths (**neurofibromas**) and the meninges (**meningiomas**) are relatively common and benign. Malignant tumours are rare.

Clinical features

Tumours of the spine and spinal cord present with symptoms and signs of cord compression:

1. At the level of compression: a lower motor neurone lesion with flaccid weakness and wasting, depressed tendon reflexes, and local sensory root irritation producing pain and hyperalgesia.
2. Below the level of compression: an upper motor neurone lesion with spastic weakness, increased tendon reflexes, and sensory impairment.
3. Loss of bladder and bowel control, and sexual function in men.

Treatment

For tumours of the vertebral column, decompressive laminectomy may be indicated in an effort to prevent increasing paraparesis and preserve sensation and bladder function. Surgery may be followed by radiotherapy. Tumours of the spinal cord are usually irremovable; histological confirmation is obtained by biopsy, and treatment is by subsequent radiotherapy. Neurofibromas and meningiomas can frequently be removed intact and the patient cured.

Laminectomy is comfortably performed with the patient in the sloping crouch position (Fig. 44.14). Like the Moslem praying position, it keeps pressure off the abdomen and so reduces bleeding from venous congestion. Much of the patient's weight is taken on the buttocks so there is no venous stasis from compression of the legs. Furthermore the surgeon can sit at the foot of the table and still have an excellent view.

Nursing care is similar to that described for injuries of the spine.

Degenerative disease of the spine

Degenerative changes in an intervertebral disc may encourage herniation (prolapsed intervertebral disc) or stimulate new bone formation and hypertrophy of ligaments (spondylosis).

Fig. 44.14 The sloping crouch position for laminectomy.

Cervical spondylosis is the commonest cause of pain in the neck and upper limbs in middle and later life. New bone formation (osteophytes) may encroach on an intervertebral foramen, compressing a spinal nerve and producing lower motor neurone symptoms and signs, and perhaps some sensory impairment. Narrowing of the spinal canal may lead to cord compression with spastic weakness, increased tendon reflexes, and possible sensory impairment. If symptoms are rapidly progressive, a cervical discectomy (with or without fusion) or decompressive laminectomy may be indicated.

Degenerative disc disease of the **thoracic spine** is comparatively rare, but early recognition and treatment is important if permanent paraplegia and loss of sphincter control are to be avoided. The disc is reached by a posterolateral approach.

In the **lumbar region,** roots of the cauda equina may be compressed by stenosis of the spinal canal, but more commonly by a prolapsed intervertebral disc. The patient complains of lumbar backache with pain radiating through the buttock, down the back of the thigh and outer side of the calf to the outer border of the foot (sciatica). There is often a history of injury to the back. Pain is characteristically worsened by movement and straining, and eased by rest. A central disc prolapse may produce pain in both legs precipitated by exercise and relieved by rest (intermittent claudication of the cauda equina). Examination reveals a rigid lumbar spine, resistance to passive straight-leg raising, wasting and weakness of the leg, impaired sensation, and depressed tendon reflexes. Treatment is initially conservative with bed rest on a firm mattress and analgesics. Traction to both legs is occasionally helpful, or the patient may be supplied with a corset or plaster jacket.

If pain persists despite an adequate trial of conservative treatment, operative removal of the prolapsed disc may be indicated. After subsidence of the acute attack, the patient should be advised to:

1. Avoid heavy lifting.
2. Sleep on a firm bed.
3. Avoid sitting in too low a chair and rising too suddenly.
4. Perform spinal exercises daily and swim if at all possible.

A change of occupation may be necessary.

Infections

Extradural abscess. This is usually the result of spread of infection, often trivial, from elsewhere in the body. The patient has a fever and complains of severe back pain. Neurological signs rapidly develop. Surgical drainage is urgent if permanent damage to the spinal cord is to be avoided.

Tuberculous osteitis (Pott's disease). This condition is now rare in the U.K. A blood-borne infection, it most commonly affects the thoracolumbar spine. The spine is rigid, and local back pain may be referred to the abdomen or chest, mimicking appendicitis or pleuritic pain. There may be vertebral collapse classically producing a kyphosis. Neurological signs may appear as the disease progresses and are due to cord compression; there may be a complete paraplegia. A local abscess may form, and rarely pus may track down beneath the psoas fascia to point in the groin (psoas abscess). Antituberculous therapy (rifampicin, ethambutol, INAH, pyridoxine, perhaps streptomycin and PAS) and a good diet should be combined with complete rest of the spine, if necessary in a plaster bed. Abscesses require drainage through an anterolateral approach, and subsequent spinal fusion may be indicated. Paralysed limbs require the care outlined under Injuries of the Spinal Cord.

BIBLIOGRAPHY

Hickey J 1981 The clinical practice of neurological and neurosurgical nursing, J B Lippincott Company, Philadelphia

45

The peripheral nerves

The peripheral nervous system comprises the **cranial nerves** related to the brain stem, and the **peripheral nerves** related to the spinal cord.

INJURIES TO THE PERIPHERAL NERVES

There are three types of injury:
1. **Neurotmesis**—interruption of the axon and its myelin sheath.
2. **Axonotmesis**—interruption of the axon with preservation of the myelin sheath.
3. **Neuropraxia**—axon and myelin sheath preserved.

Eventual recovery of function can be expected with neuropraxia and axonotmesis, but some degree of permanent functional loss is inevitable with neurotmesis. Complete division produces:
1. *Motor changes*, i.e. immediate loss of power and later wasting of the muscles supplied by the nerve.
2. *Sensory changes.* All sensation is lost in the area of skin supplied by the nerve.
3. *Trophic changes.* By this is meant the curious undernourished appearance which the skin develops. At first white, dry and scaly, the skin later becomes shiny and bluish, and painless ulceration may occur.

Partial division produces an incomplete disability.

Prevention

The nurse must take every precaution to avoid injury to the nerves. This just requires a little thought in the general nursing care. Important examples are:
(1) The arms of an unconscious patient must never be allowed to hang over the edge of the bed or operating table as this may compress the radial nerve causing a wrist drop.
(b) Intramuscular injections in the buttock should be given in the upper outer quadrant, well away from the sciatic nerve.

(c) Skin traction on a Thomas's splint or abduction frame must avoid the neck of the fibula. Compression of the adjacent lateral popliteal nerve may produce a foot drop.

Treatment

The vast majority of nerve injuries are not operated upon until the surgeon is certain that division has occurred. In many instances he will advise waiting to see if spontaneous recovery takes place.

In all cases he will require that the paralysed and/or anaesthetic area be kept in good condition to make full use of any recovery that may take place. The following general principles are fundamental:

Paralysed muscles must not be overstretched. For example, a drop wrist should be held in a cock-up splint, and a drop foot should be splinted at a right angle. Massage is valuable in encouraging the local circulation. Passive exercises help to avoid contractures. Electrical (galvanic) stimulation is useful in maintaining circulation and movement.

Insensitive skin requires special care. Insensitive fingers are easily burnt quite painlessly by cigarettes. The patient must be warned of the danger, and it may be wise to cover the fingers or hand with a kid glove to increase the margin of safety. Hot-water bottles, bed cradles, radiant heat lamps, and other ward furniture may all constitute similar hazards.

TUMOURS

Tumours may arise in the nerve cells themselves or in the nerve sheaths. Multiple tumours of the nerve sheath are characteristic of neurofibromatosis (Von Recklinghausen's disease—Fig. 45.1).

Tumours present as a tender lump that can be felt beneath the skin, or there may be intermittent pain radiating to the periphery of the nerve associated with impaired motor or sensory function.

Treatment is excision where possible.

Fig. 45.1 Neurofibromatosis.

NEURALGIA

This describes paroxysmal pain along the course of a nerve. Examples are trigeminal and glossopharyngeal neuralgia, postherpetic neuralgia, and phantom limb pain.

Surgical treatment aims at intercepting the sensory pathway. Numerous procedures are described but relief is by no means guaranteed.

LESIONS OF INDIVIDUAL NERVES

THE CRANIAL NERVES

Number	Name	Function	Lesion
I	Olfactory	Mediates the sense of smell	Commonest cranial nerve to be damaged in head injuries. Avulsion causes loss of the sense of smell (anosmia).
II	Optic	Mediates sight	Injury or compression produces partial or complete blindness.
III	Oculomotor	Controls constriction of the pupil, movement of the lens, and inward, upward and downward movement of the eyeball	Injury or compression produces a dilated pupil and a divergent squint.
IV	Trochlear	Controls downward and outward movement of the eyeball	Injury or compression produces an inability to look downwards and outwards. Rarely occurs as an isolated finding.
VI	Abducens	Controls outward movement of the eyeball	Injury or compression produces a convergent squint.
V	Trigeminal	Mediates facial sensation. Controls muscles of mastication	Impaired function may result from injury or compression. The cause of trigeminal neuralgia is unknown.
VII	Facial	Controls muscles of facial expression	Injury or compression produces a lower motor neurone facial weakness (Fig. 45.2). The cause of Bell's palsy is unknown.
VIII	Vestibulo-cochlear	Mediates balance and hearing	Injury or compression produces deafness and imbalance.
IX	Glosso-pharyngeal	Mediates sensation from the back of the tongue and throat	Rarely injured. Compression may produce difficulty in swallowing.
X	Vagus	Controls palate and vocal cord movement, heart rate, and movement and secretions in the gastrointestinal tract	Compression may produce difficulty in speaking, swallowing and coughing. Vagotomy reduces gastric acid secretion (Chapter 35).
XI	Accessory	Innervates sternomastoid and trapezius muscles	Damage interferes with head, neck and shoulder girdle movements.
XII	Hypoglossal	Innervates the tongue	Damage produces wasting and weakness.

Fig. 45.2 A lower motor neurone facial weakness affecting the right side of the face.

THE PERIPHERAL NERVES

1. *Axillary nerve.* May be injured in trauma around the shoulder joint, resulting in wasting of the deltoid muscle and weakness of shoulder abduction.

2. *Radial nerve.* May be injured in fractures of the humerus, causing a wrist drop from paralysis of the extensor muscles (Fig. 45.3A).

3. *Ulnar nerve.* Injury or compression at the elbow leads to wasting and weakness of some of the forearm muscles and small muscles of the hand. In addition, sensation may be impaired over the inner one-and-a-half fingers and medial border of the hand (Fig. 45.3B).

4. *Median nerve.* Injury causes wasting and weakness of the small muscles of the thumb, and sensory loss over the lateral aspect of the hand and outer three-and-a-half digits (Fig. 45.3C).

5. *Sciatic nerve.* This may be injured by trauma or by the nurse with misplaced injections into the buttock. Infiltration of the nerve roots by primary or secondary tumours in the pelvis may cause sciatica. There is weakness of the foot and impaired sensation over the foot and lower leg.

6. *Lateral popliteal nerve.* Compression at the head of the fibula produces a foot drop and impaired sensation between the big and second toes.

7. *Femoral nerve.* Weakness of the quadriceps femoris and pain and parasthesiae over the front of the thigh may occur as femoral neuritis complicating diabetes melitus. Occasionally the cause is a retroperitoneal tumour. A similar clinical picture may result from prolapse of the L3/4 intervertebral disc, when surgery may be indicated.

A

B

C

Fig. 45.3 Peripheral nerve palsies
A. Radial nerve palsy—wrist drop.
B. Ulnar nerve palsy—claw hand. Note the wasting of small muscles between extensor tendons to digits.
C. Median nerve palsy. Note the wasting of the small muscles of the thumb (thenar eminence).

46
Diseases of bone

Diseases of bones and joints cannot be properly understood without a sound knowledge of the anatomy, and a study of Figure 46.1 would be well worth while before reading further.

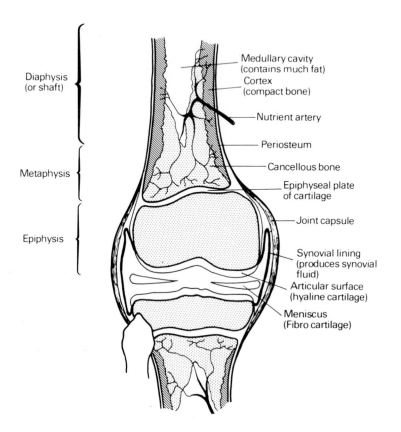

Fig. 46.1 Knee joint to show anatomy of typical bone and synovial joint.

CLASSIFICATION OF BONE DISEASE

Diseases of bones can best be classified as follows:
1. Congenital
2. Traumatic
3. Infective
4. Metabolic
5. Neoplastic

CONGENITAL DISEASES OF BONE

Babies may be born with mild or severe failure of development of the bones and in some cases bones which are normally present may be completely absent. This is best seen in the tragic results of thalidomide therapy where the complete absence of one or more limbs was not unusual. Lesser degrees of deformity such as a congenitally short femur or a congenitally short radius (producing a radial club hand known as Madelung's deformity) are also occasionally seen. A rare condition which leads to severe disability is that known as congenital pseudarthrosis of the tibia where the junction between the upper two thirds and lower third of the tibia fails to develop properly and gives rise to a false joint in the middle of the bone. These children may need years of treatment before they are able to walk on the tibia without splintage. Another type of congenital abnormality is the group in which hamartomata form. These are areas in the bone which do not develop in the normal way and may give rise to bone cysts or areas of fibrous dysplasia in the bone. These most commonly occur in the metaphysis or the epiphysis of the bone.

TRAUMATIC LESIONS OF BONE

These have been covered in Chapter 21.

INFECTIVE DISEASES OF BONE

Bone may be infected by the ordinary pus forming bacteria giving rise to the condition known as osteomyelitis, which may be acute or chronic. Other infecting agents are the tuberculosis bacillus and the organisms which affect the bowel such as those causing brucellosis, typhoid and dysentery. The usual mode in which the bacteria gain access to the bone is through the blood stream and this is known as haematogenous spread. Bones can however be infected directly from compound wounds into the bone.

Acute osteomyelitis

This is a common condition in young children and must be suspected

Fig. 46.2 X-ray of femur affected by chronic osteomyelitis, Involucrum shown by continuous line. Sequestrum shown by dotted line.

whenever an ill child with a high temperature presents and diagnosis is not immediately obvious.

It is worthwhile considering symptoms and signs of this condition in parallel with the pathology of the disease. The initial infection gains access to the bone via the blood stream, having entered the circulation from some other septic focus in the body, such as a boil or a sore throat. The bacteria settle in the bone in the metaphysis where the blood vessels are branching into finer and finer arterioles and capillaries. If the body's defences do not contain the bacterial infection then the bacteria begin to multiply and a small abscess develops in the bone close to the cortex. As is usual with abscesses oedema soon develops around the abscess and the pressure in the bone is increased. At this stage the child is feverish with no particular localising signs. There are certainly no changes on X-ray at this stage. As the bone abscess spreads so the infected oedema passes through the tiny channels in the cortex of the bone and starts to elevate the periosteal lining from the outer aspect of the cortex. At this stage the child might begin to complain of some localised pain in the affected area and as the disease progresses so there might develop clinical tenderness on palpation of the site of bony infection. If this remains untreated the bone from which the periosteum has been elevated will die because its blood supply has been damaged. The abscess may then enlarge through the soft tissues and eventually discharge through the skin giving rise to a discharging sinus. At this stage the acute disease has become a chronic infection. A small or large area of bone may be deprived of its blood supply and die. Dead bone eventually becomes separated from live bone and it is then known as a sequestrum. The infective process and the presence of dead bone excites the living bone to produce new bone to repair the damage and it is not unusual for the new bone formed completely to surround the various dead pieces of bone rather like an envelope surrounds a letter. It is for this reason that the new bone formed is known as an involucrum (Fig. 46.2).

Treatment of osteomyelitis

The treatment of acute osteomyelitis is aimed at preventing the spread of the abscess and bone death. One of the ways of combating infection is the use of antibiotics. In these modern days many bacteria are resistant to commonly used antibiotics and it is always helpful to find out which particular organism is causing the infection. Blood cultures are therefore essential in any child with a high temperature and an undiagnosed condition, as these will often tell the surgeon which organism is causing the infection. If the organism is not known it is quite common to use a combination of antibiotics such as Fucidin and Erythromycin to cover as wide a spectrum of bacteria as possible. The limb should also be rested in a splint.

If the signs of infection begin to settle with the child's affected limb splinted then surgery may not be necessary. However, if the infection remains clinically active and the child's temperature high, and if the site of infection can be accurately localised then some surgeons will operate on the bone to relieve the tension in it by drilling the bone and allowing the pus to escape.

The initial treatment therefore is rest and antibiotics and the second treatment which may be necessary is surgical drainage, just as in any other surgical infection elsewhere in the body.

Once the disease has reached the chronic stage with the formation of sinuses and sequestrae it is necessary to remove the dead sequestrae by surgical operation before the chronic osteomyelitis will heal up.

Tuberculous osteitis

This once very common disease is now much less common. Tuberculosis is still however seen occasionally and one of its favourite sites is the spine. Tuberculous infection does not progress as quickly as does pyogenic infection and the physical signs are not so dramatic. Generalised constitutional debility is often present together with localised pain or discomfort. The abscess which is formed does not excite the body's defence mechanism to such an extent so that there is little local hyperaemia and therefore little localised warmth. This is why a tuberculous abscess is often known as a cold abscess (Ch. 9). However the damage it can do is considerable and if the abscess bursts from the vertebral body through into the spinal canal it can cause paraplegia,—the so called Pott's paraplegia.

The treatment of tuberculous osteitis whether in the spine or elsewhere is complete rest of the affected part and the exhibition of antituberculous drugs such as Pasinah and Rifampicin. Streptomycin is little used these days because of its dangerous side-effects upon the ear and its tendency to produce a severe fibrotic reaction.

In earlier days patients with tuberculous osteitis were often kept in hospital for many years until the infection became quiescent but nowadays most surgeons would treat the lesion initially with rest and chemotherapy but would be much more ready to perform a surgical excision of the affected area if the disease failed to settle fairly quickly.

Other infections of bones

Infections of bone by other organisms are treated by means of suitable antibiotics or chemotherapy which kill the bacteria or prevent them from multiplying. In the case of those organisms which normally infect gut it is often difficult to isolate the bacteria themselves but fortunately there are various blood tests which can be done which will give the surgeon considerable help in making the diagnosis. These tests estimate the amount of the natural body defence protein which is mobilised to agglutinate the infecting organisms so that antibrucella, antityphoid or antidysenteric titres are often helpful in reaching a diagnosis. Once the diagnosis has been made then the appropriate treatment can be ordered.

METABOLIC DISEASES OF BONE

Bone, like any other tissue, is living and therefore the normal biochemical processes of living tissues go on within the bone. Thus bone is constantly being remodelled, the blood stream brings new chemicals to the cells and takes away used ones. These chemicals may be organic (proteins and carbohydrates) or inorganic (calcium and phosphorus). It is estimated that the calcium content of the human body is completely changed every seven years. It is not surprising therefore that occasionally things go wrong with the living processes (metabolism) in bone.

Parathyroid disease

One of the ductless glands that controls the calcium and phosphorus metabolism of the body is the group of glands known as the parathyroids. These small glands are situated on the posterior surface of the thyroid gland and produce parathormone. If an excess of parathormone is produced, e.g. should an adenoma of the parathyroid gland develop, then the calcium in the bones is rapidly mobilised and is lost to the body through the kidneys. This may give rise to an acutely painful illness where the bone becomes extremely thin and weak and there is a danger of formation of kidney stone. The treatment is to remove the offending parathyroid tumour. A more chronic parathyroid disease may give rise to the formation of multiple cysts in the bone, a condition known as osteitis fibrosa cystica.

Fig. 46.3 Rickets.

Rickets and osteomalacia

Another of the chemical agents responsible for the control of the calcium metabolism is vitamin D and an absence of vitamin D in a growing child will give rise to a condition known as rickets. Rickets can also be caused by a failure to take in an adequate amount of calcium through the gut or by an excessive amount of calcium being excreted through the kidneys. Rickets can therefore be caused by inadequate calcium in the diet, by an insufficient vitamin D intake or by an excessive excretion of calcium by the kidneys (renal rickets). Whatever the cause the bones do not develop properly, they become soft, there is swelling of the epiphyses and widening of the epiphysial plates of cartilage and the shafts of the bones will bend (Fig. 46.3).

The treatment of rickets requires correction of the basic metabolic defect and if bone deformity has occurred this will need correction either by manipulations and plaster or by osteotomies to straighten the bones. Once the epiphyses have fused and bone becomes adult then deficiency of vitamin D or calcium gives rise to softening of the bone which in adults is known as osteomalacia. The treatment is the same as for rickets. These two diseases are becoming more common in temperate climates as more dark skinned people emigrate from their own sunny warm countries. This is because sunlight is essential to the formation of vitamin D within the body when the diet is deficient in this vitamin.

Paget's disease

Fig. 46.4 The skull of a patient with Paget's disease.

Paget's disease of the bone is an affliction of the elderly and is very common indeed. The causation of the disease is unknown but it is well known that a great increase in the blood supply of the bone occurs and a great increase in the rate of calcium changeover within the bone also occurs. This gives rise to considerable new bone formation so that the bones become thicker, but because of the lack of calcium they also become softer. Sufferers slowly develop the bowed legs and the enlarging skull which are typical of the disease (Fig. 46.4). Pathological fractures in this condition are common. Because of the increased blood channels within the bone the action of the heart is put under strain and congestive cardiac failure may occur. Sarcomatous change is much more common in Pagety bone than in normal bone.

Gout

Gout is an abnormality of metabolism which causes the deposition of sodium urate crystals within the ends of the bone and within the joint linings. These crystals may become so large that they burst through the skin overlying the bone giving rise to what is known as a tophus. An acute attack of gout can be one of the most painful experiences in life but fortunately it can be treated easily and effectively by means of anti-inflammatory agents and can be prevented by means of special drugs to increase the excretion of uric acid.

NEOPLASTIC DISEASES OF BONE

Tumours of bone may be benign or malignant. If malignant they may be:
1. Primary.
2. Secondary.

As will be seen from the diagram at the beginning of this chapter, bone is composed of a number of tissues including bone itself, cartilage, blood vessels, nerves and fibrous tissues, e.g. the periosteum. Primary tumours may develop in any or in a combination of these tissues, whereas secondary tumours, deposited in bone via the blood stream from primary cancer in other organs, will have the same characteristics as the primary growth from which they were derived.

Benign tumours of bone

These are quite common and usually require no treatment unless they are interfering with joint movements or causing pressure symptoms on neighbouring organs. Such tumours may be osteomas (pure tumours of bone tissue), chondromas (pure tumours of cartilage tissue), or fibromas (pure tumours of fibrous tissue) or they may be mixed, e.g. osteochondroma which has some bone tissue and some cartilage tissue within the growth.

Fig. 46.5 Drawing of a femur cut longitudinally to show the spread of osteogenic sarcoma within the bone.

Malignant tumours of bone

The primary malignant tumours of bone are largely diseases of younger people and the most malignant of all unfortunately affect children before growth has ceased. Because the bone is not a glandular tissue malignant disease of the bone is not known as carcinoma but as a sarcoma. Again the malignant tissue may arise in any of the components of bone.

The most common primary malignant tumour of bone in children is osteogenic sarcoma which arises from the cells which are actively producing bone. Such tumours give rise to new bone formation which is often laid down in a radial manner giving the so-called 'sunray appearance', on X-ray. These tumours are highly malignant and give rise to pain and swelling. They metastasise rapidly via the blood stream to the lungs and are usually fatal within a very short period (Fig. 46.5).

Modern methods of treatment are however giving rise to hope that better results may be obtained in the future. If the tumour is accessible it is excised, often by means of amputation, and the surgical treatment is followed up by serial treatments with a mixture of cytotoxic drugs to try and control the secondary spread of the tumour.

Another rare tumour which is distressing in its rapidly fatal course is the so called Ewing's tumour which is thought to arise from the endothelial cells of the blood vessels in the bone. This tumour is more usually treated by local excision followed again by serial cytotoxic therapy and radiotherapy. Other primary malignant tumours such as chondrosarcoma and fibrosarcoma in bone usually arise in a later age group and are not so rapidly fatal, and in fact there are many instances of 20 years survival after such lesions have been treated.

Secondary tumours of bone

Secondary deposits may be laid down in bone from cancers elsewhere in the body. By far the most common primary tumour to give rise to secondary bone deposits is cancer of the breast and secondary deposits of breast cancer in bone are the commonest bone tumour that is seen. However secondary deposits may also present in bone from carcinoma of the bronchus, the prostate, the kidney, the thyroid and the uterus. They are often only diagnosed when a pathological fracture occurs through them but are sometimes diagnosed by X-ray after the patient complains of persistent pain.

Cancer of the breast and the prostate are sometimes 'hormone dependent' and secondary deposits from such cancers are often treated by exhibiting hormones to the patient. Thus a secondary cancer from the prostate may be treated by performing an orchidectomy and treating the patient with stilboestrol. In most circumstances secondary bone tumours are treated by means of radiotherapy and occasionally by cytotoxic drugs.

47

Diseases of joints, muscle and tendons

ANATOMY OF JOINTS

Joints may be freely mobile, in which case there is a cavity between the bone ends which is lined by a synovial membrane producing fluid to lubricate the movement of the joints (see Figure 46.1). Such joints may be of several mechanical types: the ball and socket joints seen in the very mobile joints such as the hip and the shoulder; hinged joints moving freely in one plane only such as the elbow and the knee; pivoting joints such as that between the head of the radius and the lower end of the humerus, which allow rotation of one bone on the other; or gliding joints such as the joints between the small bones of the wrist (the carpus) or the foot (tarsus.) The less mobile joints are those in which the bone ends are joined by fibrous tissue or cartilage and this situation is seen in the discs between the vertebral bodies, or the fibrocartilage between the two pubic bones at the front of the pelvis. The ribs have synovial joints between their posterior ends and the vertebral column but have flexible areas between the front ends of the ribs and the costal cartilages joining the ribs to the sternum anteriorly.

CLASSIFICATION OF JOINT DISEASE

Diseases of joints may be classified into the following four groups:
1. Congenital.
2. Inflammatory.
3. Traumatic.
4. Degenerative.

CONGENITAL JOINT LESIONS

Congenital dislocation of hips

The most important condition to consider under this heading is congenital dislocation of the hips. The causation of this condition is not fully understood but a very important factor in its production is the position of the baby's legs whilst in the womb. Extended breech deliveries, where the legs are acutely flexed with the knees lying straight up the front of the trunk, give rise to congenital dislocation of the hips much more commonly than do the normal vertex deliveries. The neonatal paediatrician will test new born babies' hips for stability within the first few hours of birth and if there is any suggestion that the hips may be unstable the babies are usually nursed in double nappies to keep the legs abducted so that the head of the femur is positioned securely within the acetabulum. If the hip instability persists then special splints may be used to keep the legs in the abducted position at the hip joints. By the use of this treatment a large percentage of dislocated hips are stable by the time the baby starts standing and walking. However if the hips remain dislocated by the time the child is of standing age then treatment must be instituted to reduce

Fig. 47.1 An X-ray showing congenital dislocation of the right hip.

Fig. 47.2 The same patient as Fig. 47.1 after operative reduction and stabilisation by osteotomy of the pelvis immediately above the acetabular roof. The osteotomy is held open by a wedge of bone fixed by a Kirschner wire. A gonad shield is in place to protect the ovaries from irradiation during the X-ray.

the hip and keep it reduced until the acetabulum is fully developed. This may require nursing on special abduction frames with traction on the legs followed by a period in a plaster of Paris spica. Should this treatment fail to keep the hips well in position then surgical treatment may be necessary in the first years of life in order to stabilise the head of the femur within the acetabulum (Figs. 47.1 and 47.2).

An open reduction of the dislocated hip may be necessary and this is sometimes combined with osteotomies of the pelvis on that side to tilt the acetabular roof well over the head of the femur. This position is then maintained until the bone and soft tissues have healed after a period in a plaster spica. At a later date (3 months) a derotation osteotomy of the femur should be performed.

INFLAMMATORY LESIONS OF JOINTS

Inflammatory lesions may be caused by infecting organisms such as bacteria or they may be caused by non-infective conditions such as rheumatoid arthritis.

1. INFECTIVE JOINT DISEASE

Infection gives rise to a hot, swollen and acutely painful joint which the patient will protect by muscle spasm, and will avoid moving at all costs because of the pain. As in acute osteomyelitis the temperature will be raised and in fact infective arthritis is often caused by osteomyelitis close to the joint.

An important cause of acute infective arthritis in new born babies is infection reaching the joint through an infected umbilical cord. In older patients the infection reaches the joint through the blood stream or by direct infection from a compound wound of the joint. The treatment is to rest the joint completely, to isolate the causative organism and to treat the infection with the appropriate antibiotic. More often than not operative drainage of the joint becomes necessary just as in osteomyelitis or in any other severely infected surgical lesion.

As in the case of fractures the muscles which control the affected joint must be kept as strong as possible by regular static exercises (i.e. exercises without moving the joint).

Tuberculous infection of joints is less common than it used to be but it still occurs. The treatment of such joints follows exactly the same principles, i.e. rest, muscle exercises, appropriate chemotherapy and occasionally surgical drainage.

2. NON-INFECTIVE INFLAMMATORY CONDITIONS OF JOINTS

Rheumatoid arthritis

This disease is one of the most widespread and crippling in the world. It consists of inflammatory synovitis in which the inflamed synovium spreads over the joint surface and eats its way into the articular cartilage thus causing great pain and deformity. It may affect the patients at any age although it is more common in early middle age.

Its cause is unknown but, for some reason, the body defence mechanisms fail to recognise protein molecules produced by the body, and attack these proteins with antibodies at certain sites. This causes the release of toxic products which damage the affected tissues. The synovium is one of the major targets of such a reaction but rheumatoid arthritis also affects the walls of blood vessels, the lungs and the eyes, so that a patient with a severe form of rheumatoid arthritis may become extremely ill.

Treatment of rheumatoid arthritis

Many different types of anti-inflammatory drugs have been produced in order to treat this painful condition and it is wise to start treatment with the simpler drugs such as salicylates and to progress to the more complicated drugs with their larger proportion of side-effects only if the condition fails to respond to simple treatment, including splintage where necessary and physiotherapy.

A course of gold injections is sometimes given as it has been found that the injection of heavy metals is sometimes helpful. Systemic steroid treatment is also sometimes prescribed in the event that no other drug seems to be having any effect. However the serious side effects of long term steroid therapy must always be borne in mind. More recently drugs such as penicillamine and immuno-suppressive drugs have been tried with good effect in some patients. The surgical treatment of rheumatoid arthritis consists of one of several methods:

(a) Injections of radioactive substances such as radioactive gold or yttrium into the larger joints has recently been shown to be very effective.

(b) Excision of the affected synovium. This operation (synovectomy) is practised quite frequently when an accessible joint is persistently painful and swollen.

(c) Excision of the whole joint and replacement with an artificial joint is practiced more and more when the disease has destroyed the affected joint.

Other conditions resembling rheumatoid arthritis

'Rheumatism' is a lay term for a very large number of diseases which may cause inflammatory synovitis of joints. Such conditions as psoriasis, gout, pseudogout (inflammation of joints caused by crystals other than uric acid) and joint inflammations associated with various bowel diseases are some examples. A particular condition which may present in a similar way to rheumatoid arthritis is ankylosing spondylitis. This is a condition which affects the spine mainly but can also affect other joints in the body. It is characterised by pain and increasing stiffness so that eventually the spine may become completely rigid—the so-called poker back.

Fig. 47.3 Position of table for menisectomy or exploration of the knee joint.

(i) The tourniquet position, high up on the fleshy part of the thigh to diminish pressure on the large nerves to the lower leg.

(ii) The calf is several inches away from the bottom leaf of the operating table.

(iii) The knee joint is lifted by a sand-bag under the lower thigh and the surgeon can flex and extend the joint during surgery if necessary.

TRAUMATIC LESIONS OF JOINTS

Acute dislocations and compound joint injuries have been dealt with in Chapter 21. Internal derangements of joints may be caused by trauma such as the very common torn meniscus in knee joints.

Torn cartilage (meniscus) in knee

This is almost always caused by acute rotation strains usually during sporting activities and the two classical symptoms of this condition are locking of the joint and giving way of the joint. If symptoms occur frequently then arthroscopic examination of the knee is necessary to confirm the diagnosis. It is sometimes possible to remove the offending meniscus arthroscopically, but if this proves difficult then a full arthrotomy is required as shown in Figure 47.3.

Recurrent dislocations

A damaged joint may become so unstable that it dislocates on frequent occasions during normal movement. This happens particularly to the freely mobile shoulder joint and also to the patella.

A shoulder joint which dislocates recurrently requires surgical stabilisation and several operations have been devised to prevent further recurrence.

In the same way a patella which dislocates frequently is a considerable disability and again requires surgical stabilisation. One of the methods is to transfer the attachment of the patellar tendon from its central point on the upper tibia to a position more medially placed on the upper shaft of the tibia.

Slipped upper femoral epiphysis (Fig. 47.4)

Before the epiphysial plate of cartilage between the head of the femur

Fig. 47.4 X-rays showing fixation of bilateral slipped upper femoral epiphyses.

and the neck of the femur has become ossified there is considerable mechanical strain upon it because of the amount of weight it bears and because of its rather vertically placed position. The head of the femur sometimes slips upon the epiphysial plate and a deformity occurs in the hip joint. This condition is more likely to happen in fat children with poorly developed sexual characteristics. Should a slip occur then the treatment is to reduce the slip by slow gentle traction and then fix the head to the neck of the femur by means of pins passed up the femoral neck.

Perthe's disease

This is a condition occurring in children between the ages of six to ten which results in softening of the epiphysis of the head of the femur. It gives rise to a painful limp and the treatment is to rest the child in bed on traction until the pain diminishes. The pathological process in the head of the femur takes 2 to 3 years to complete its cycle, and it is important that the head of the femur should be well contained within the acetabulum during this period.

Treatment is only necessary if the head of the femur is partly outside the acetabulum. In this case treatment consists either of an operation to position the head of the femur in the acetabulum or else the child is kept in a special type of splint which achieves the same object.

The pathological process in Perthe's disease is known as osteochondritis and this process occurs in many other parts of the body during the growing period, such as the knee, elbow and ankle.

Prolapsed intervertebral disc

An intervertebral disc is a form of joint between the bodies of the vertebrae and consists of an outer tough elastic annulus fibrosus and an inner semi-fluid nucleus pulposus. When the annulus fibrosus is ruptured by trauma the central nucleus can bulge out through the weakened spot. This can often be shown by a myelogram. If this traumatic bulge presses upon one of the lumbar nerve roots it gives rise to sciatica. The treatment of this condition is dealt with in Chapter 44. An alternative operative position to that shown in Chapter 44 is illustrated in Figure 47.5. This is also used for operations on the spine.

DEGENERATIVE DISEASES OF JOINTS

Like any mechanical joint the joints of the body wear away with increased use and increased age. Therefore heavy people who lead active lives are more liable to develop arthritic changes than are slightly built persons who take a less active part in life. Again, like any mechanical joint, a human joint which has been damaged by disease or injury when the patient is young will wear away more quickly than a normal joint so that degenerative changes also occur in patients who have had fractures into

Fig. 47.5 Position on table for spinal operations.
  (i) The body is in a comfortable, relaxed position as spinal surgery may take several hours.
  (ii) The pelvis is supported by sand-bags and the chest by a pillow so that there is no pressure on the abdomen. This means that there is no pressure on the vena cava so that the spinal veins do not become engorged with blood.
  (iii) One (or two) arms are easily accessible for I.V. drips, B.P. measurement or for injections by the anaesthetist.
  (iv) This position can be used for operations on the cervical spine, the thoracic and lumbar spine or the sacrum.
  (v) Note the special head-rest attachment on the table.

joints, patients who have had diseased joints, e.g. rheumatoid arthritis or septic arthritis, and in patients who have had cartilages removed, Perthe's disease or slipped epiphysis. Degenerative changes in joints give rise to friction instead of the usual smooth movement and this causes pain, synovial inflammation and swelling together with a tendency for the bone to become irregular in shape and to give rise to irregular out-growths from the side of the joint known as osteophytes. These changes occur not only in synovial joints but also in the less flexible joints such as the intervertebral discs and the sacroiliac joints. They may give rise to quite severe deformities of the joints such as those seen in hallux valgus.

Treatment of degenerative joint disease

Nonoperative treatment consists of resting the joint, reducing the weight of the patient—and this is a most important aspect as a reduction in weight obviously will reduce the stress upon the joint—various forms of physiotherapy and occasionally appropriate splinting. However as a rule surgical treatment usually becomes necessary and such treatment usually is one of three types of operation:
  1. arthrodesis
  2. arthroplasty
  3. osteotomy.

1. Arthrodesis

Arthrodesis consists of the excision of the joint surfaces and the apposition of the raw bony ends so that the bones join together and the joint no longer exists. This has the effect of relieving the pain permanently and providing a stable mechanical structure. It has however the great disadvantage of permanently restricting mobility of that part of the body. This may not be very important in such areas as the spine but it becomes increasingly important in the mobile limbs. Arthrodesis is therefore used mainly in the spinal column to treat degenerative arthritis, in the toes to treat deformities and occasionally in the hip and the knee in the younger patient. When the joint is arthrodesed it requires to be immobilised in the same way as a fracture until the bone is soundly fused.

2. Arthroplasty

Arthroplasty means repair of a joint. A joint may be rendered mobile and painless merely by excising the joint and allowing the space between the bones to fill with blood clot which becomes organised into fibrous tissue. This is the principle behind such common procedures as Keller's operation, where the proximal two thirds of the proximal phalanx of the big toes is removed, or the less common practice, Girdlestone's operation, where the head and neck of the femur are excised leaving the hip joint as a rather elastic flail joint. Such arthroplasties are known as excision arthroplasties and the postoperative care consists of a period of immobilisation until the blood clot is organised followed by mobilisation exercises and encouragement of normal activities as far as possible.

In more recent years surgeons have concentrated not only on excising the affected joints but on replacing them with prosthetic materials. These materials, be they metal, plastic or silicone rubber, are either impacted into the bone or are secured to the bone by means of an acrylic resin cement. Practically all joints in the body can be replaced except those in the spinal column, but the indications for such operations are mostly to be found in the ball and socket hip joint. The hip joint can be replaced by a metal socket and a metal ball, the former being screwed into the ileum

Fig. 47.6 X-ray showing osteoarthritis of right hip joint.

Fig. 47.7 The same patient as in Fig. 47.6 showing that the hip has been replaced with a Charnley total hip prosthesis.

and the latter impacted into the femur (Ring). The metal components may be secured to the bone by cement (McKee) but the more commonly used hip arthroplasty now is that where a metal femoral prosthesis articulates with a polyethylene acetabular component both of them being secured to the bone by cement (Charnley and other types, Figures 47.6 and 47.7).

Whichever method is used great care is placed upon preoperative skin preparation, the eradication of any septic focus within the body and antibiotic cover for the operation. Many surgeons prefer to perform such major joint replacement surgery in a hyper-sterile theatre so that orthopaedic surgeons often appear like spacemen operating in plastic tents. All these precautions are designed to reduce the risk of infection to a minimum as infection deeply placed within the body in relation to foreign material will give rise to persistent sepsis and loosening of the prosthesis which will then have to be removed.

Postoperatively the antibiotic cover is continued for several days, the patients are prevented from sitting or walking for several days and precautions are taken to reduce the other great danger in operation, i.e. pulmonary embolus from thrombosis of the deep veins in the leg or the pelvis. Many regimes are adopted to prevent this complication such as the use of plasma expanders, (e.g. Dextran 40) mechanical massage for the calves, small doses of anticoagulants, small doses of aspirin, platelet antistickiness drugs such as plaquenil, and active foot and ankle exercises by the physiotherapist. The patient is usually able to be discharged from hospital walking between sticks about a fortnight after the operation. Other joints which are commonly replaced are the metacarpo-phalangeal joints of the fingers and for this operation very flexible silicon rubber prostheses are used. A large variety of artificial knee joints has been produced, the one most widely used being the total condylar knee prosthesis. Shoulder joints, elbow joints and ankle joints are also occasionally replaced where necessary.

Fig. 47.8   X-ray showing treatment of an osteoarthritic right hip in a younger patient by inter-trochanteric osteotomy.

3. Osteotomy

Division of a bone close to a joint either above it or below it produces relief of pain. The reason for this is poorly understood but part of the answer must lie in the relief of mechanical strains upon the joint and part of the answer in the division of nerves running from the joint.

An osteotomy of the upper tibia is an extremely useful operation to halt the progress of degenerative disease in a knee which has developed either valgus or a varus deformity. The limb requires immobilisation in plaster for a few weeks until the bone is joined after which rehabilitation is begun. Osteotomy of the upper femur between the lesser and greater trochanters (the so-called intertrochanteric osteotomy) has been used for many years to relieve the pain of osteoarthritis of the hips and it is still used by many surgeons in the treatment of the younger patient with an osteoarthritic hip (Fig. 47.8). If the operation of osteotomy fails to produce the desired effect then arthroplasty can still be carried out whereas if arthroplasty has been the first choice, followed by complications, then there is no other operation to fall back upon. Osteotomy is also quite frequently used in younger patients for deformity and early degenerative changes in the big toe joint. It should not be forgotten that the big toe joint is an extremely important joint in the body as it is one of the major weight bearing joints.

MISCELLANEOUS

There are many conditions which are not strictly joint lesions but which occur in the peri-articular tissues.

Bursitis and tenosynovitis

Bursae are sacs of fluid placed in the tissues to lubricate movements of tendon or skin over bone and these bursae quite often become inflamed; a typical example is housemaids knee (Fig. 47.9). The tendons themselves are closely surrounded by filmy sheaths which are similar in structure to the synovial linings of joints. Inflammation of these sheaths is known as tenosynovitis and such an inflammation may cause thickening of the tough outer sheath enclosing the synovial sheath causing constriction of the tendon. Such a condition requires release of the tendon by incision of the thickened sheath.

Fig. 47.9   Pre-patellar bursitis (housemaid's knee).

DISEASES OF MUSCLES AND TENDONS

INJURIES

These injuries are discussed in this chapter because muscles and tendons are closely associated with bones and joints.

Muscles are frequently partially torn, in which case they bleed and large haematomas may develop in their sheaths, or they may be severely bruised by direct violence with a similar end result. The treatment is rest followed by restoration of function when the pain and swelling subside.

Tendons may rupture either through injury (e.g. Achilles tendon rupture in athletes) or because of disease (e.g. the extensor tendons of the fingers in rheumatoid arthritis). The usual treatment of these injuries is surgical repair of the ruptured tendons.

When the flexor tendons of the hand are accidentlly severed, primary suture is usually only undertaken by expert surgeons in special hand surgery centres. Most accident surgeons find they get better results by suturing only the skin as a first measure and then inserting a tendon graft to replace the severed tendon some weeks later. All patients who have had hand surgery require nursing with the hand elevated for the first few days to avoid postoperative swelling. This complication is the main cause of poor results.

There is a circular cuff of muscle tendons which surrounds the shoulder joint from the front to the back passing across the top of the joint. This is known as the rotator cuff and tears and inflammatory lesions of this are extremely common occurrences. They are best treated by local injection of hydrocortisone into the tender area and by various forms of physiotherapy. A similar condition occurs at the elbow, either on the medial or the lateral side but more usually laterally. This is an inflammatory lesion of the muscle origin from the bone and has acquired the colloquial name of tennis elbow.

MISCELLANEOUS

Dupuytren's contracture

This condition causes curling up of the fingers because of contracture of the tough tissue underlying the skin of the palm. It is an inherited condition and is progressive. The skin of the palm becomes infiltrated by the thickened palmar fascia and it becomes nodular and ridged (Fig. 47.10). The treatment of this condition is excision of the thickened tissue deep to the palmar skin.

Fig. 47.10 Dupuytren's contracture of the palm and left ring finger.

Ganglion

A ganglion is a tense, painful cyst arising from the synovial lining of a joint or tendon sheath. It is full of jelly-like material and can sometimes be burst and dispersed by direct pressure or a sharp blow. If not, excision is the usual treatment.

Poliomyelitis

Mention must be made of this condition although it is becoming increasingly uncommon in those countries where an active immunisation programme is under way. The disease is caused by a small virus which attacks the anterior horn cells in the spinal cord; hence its name. This causes inflammation, swelling and eventual destruction of the nerve cells affected so that the muscles supplied by these nerves become paralysed. The disease is characterised by a high fever, indistinguisable at first from fever caused by any other disease, but the diagnosis becomes clear once the paralysis develops after forty-eight hours or so. The disease may affect practically every muscle in the body or may be highly selective affecting a few muscles here and few there. In the more severe forms of the disease the patient will often require assisted respiration and indeed this may become necessary as a permanent measure. However more commonly the patient survives with his respiratory mechanism intact and is left with varying degrees of paralysis.

Surgical treatment of poliomyelitis

Surgical treatment is confined to stabilising unstable joints by various methods, by strengthening the action of various weak groups of muscles, by transferring the tendons of strong muscles to reinforce the action of the weaker ones and to correct deformities which may have been allowed to develop during the acute illness.

If a lower limb is paralysed whilst the patient is young then it does not grow so quickly as the unaffected opposite limb and because of this a difference in leg lengths may be one of the more disabling affects of an attack of poliomyelitis. Surgical treatment can help to lengthen the affected limb by means of slow and continuous traction on a divided bone over a period of 2 to 3 weeks or surgery may be directed towards preventing growth of the longer limb. This can be done by preventing growth at the epiphysial plates of cartilage. The operation is known as epiphysiodesis if bone is placed across the epiphysial plate or as epiphysial arrest if metal staples are placed across the epiphysial plate.

Ingrowing toenail

This painful condition should more properly be described as an overgrowth of the skin fold at one or the other, or both, sides of the great toenail. At all events a deep groove, or sulcus, develops between the nail and the skin which inevitably collects dirt and skin secretions, subsequently causing inflammation and often purulent infection (Fig. 47.11).

This chronic, painful condition can be prevented by correct cutting of the nail (straight across, not back into the corners), wearing well-fitting shoes and by careful attention to foot hygiene. It can sometimes by cured by skilled foot care, but often excision of the infected nailfold and part of the nail is necessary. Sometimes radical excision of the nail bed, preventing further growth of the nail, may be needed.

Fig. 47.11 An ingrowing toenail.

48

Diseases of the ear, the nose, and the throat

Diseases of the ear, the nose, and the throat are considered together because these structures are linked anatomically and are affected by the same pathological processes. Until recently, surgery in this area was aimed at eradicating the common infections but the emphasis has now moved towards reconstruction. Hearing can often be restored and function can be re-established even after major resections for malignancy.

THE EAR

SYMPTOMS OF EAR DISEASE

1. Deafness means that the patient has a hearing loss which may be mild or severe. If the cause of the deafness lies in the outer ear or the middle ear, it is said to be a conductive deafness. If the cause lies in the inner ear or the auditory nerve, it is a sensori-neural deafness. The most common cause of deafness in childhood is serous otitis media whereas in adults, presbycusis is most common. Presbycusis means the deafness of the elderly and it is a sensori-neural hearing loss caused by the degeneration of nervous tissue.

2. Pain. Earache or otalgia is a very common complaint. In children, the commonest cause is acute otitis media whereas in adults it is otitis externa. The pain may arise from the ear itself or from an adjacent site with a shared nerve supply. The commonest site for referred pain is the throat, where infections or, more rarely, malignant tumours are responsible.

3. Discharge. A discharge from the ear may be mucoid, purulent or bloody. It must be distinguished from the escape of wax which is a normal process. Commonly, the cause of a discharge is otitis externa or otitis media and in the latter event, a perforation will be present in the tympanic membrane.

4. Vertigo is a form of dizziness where the patient experiences a spinning sensation. It is a common symptom when the balance, or vestibular system of the inner ear is diseased. It is accompanied by nausea and vomiting and it is difficult to treat.

5. Tinnitus, or noise in the ear, is a very common complaint. Its quality varies from a high-pitched whistle to the clanging of bells or recognisable snatches of music. It is a distressing symptom and although it can sometimes be alleviated, it can seldom be cured.

DISEASES OF THE OUTER EAR

Bat ear

The pinna protrudes from the side of the head because the ridge of the antihelix has not formed. The child may be the object of derision and the antihelix can be reconstructed fairly easily through an incision on the back of the pinna.

Wax

Wax or cerumen is a normal substance produced in the external ear canal. It is made up of epithelial scales mixed with the secretions from special glands in the skin of the outer ear. In most people, the wax escapes as it is formed but in some, it remains in the ear canal, obstructing it and causing deafness. Olive oil or liquid paraffin ear drops will soften the impacted wax which is then removed by syringing.

It is important that the water in the syringe should be at body temperature so as not to stimulate the inner ear and cause dizziness. The jet of water is directed at the wall of the ear canal and the wax is washed out. A receiver is held beneath the ear and the patient's clothing is protected by a mackintosh sheet. The ear must be dried gently after the syringing and it should be examined by a doctor to exclude any damage to the tympanic membrane.

Foreign bodies

These are commonly found in the ears of children and the variety is immense. Sometimes they can be removed by a probe or syringeing but the child is often frightened and uncooperative and a general anaesthetic will be necessary. The ear must always be checked to exclude any underlying damage.

An insect in the ear is treated similarly.

Otitis externa

This is an inflammation of the outer ear which is lined by skin. The condition is usually bilateral and the symptoms start with itching. The patient scratches the ear which becomes infected, painful, and sometimes blocked by a thin muco-purulent discharge. Allergy, stress, and the presence of infected water may all play a part but the treatment is the same. Any precipitating cause is removed and a swab is taken for culture and sensitivity. The ear canal is cleaned gently, thoroughly, and frequently using a wisp of cotton wool on the tip of a suitable probe. Drops are then instilled directly or used to impregnate a small wick of ribbon gauze which is left in the ear for one or two days. The drops may be simple disinfectants or may be combinations of topical antibiotics (to kill the bacteria) and steroids (to reduce the inflammation). The condition tends to recur.

Boils

A boil, or furuncle, is found in the outer hair-bearing skin of the ear canal. It is very painful because the skin at this site is firmly tethered to the underlying cartilage. Like boils elsewhere, it is caused by the staphylococcus and the relevant antibiotic is only necessary when the symptoms are severe. Analgesics are necessary and the possibility of underlying diabetes must be excluded.

Tumours

Malignant tumours of the ear are commonest in the outer ear where both basal cell carcinoma and squamous carcinoma are found. The small lesion is treated with radiotherapy but the larger will need surgical excision.

MIDDLE EAR DISEASE

In order that sound may pass efficiently through the ossicles, the Eustachian tube must allow air to enter the middle ear from the nasopharynx. In children particularly, the tube becomes blocked and this obstruction is responsible for many conditions in the middle ear.

Serous (secretory) otitis media

When the Eustachian tube becomes blocked, the air trapped in the middle ear is absorbed into the surrounding tissues and is replaced by thin fluid. In time, small glands appear in the lining of the middle ear and the mucus which they secrete, explains the popular name of 'glue ears' which is given to this condition. It is seen most in those children where an immature musculature and repeated upper respiratory tract infections, predispose to tubal obstruction.

The child develops a hearing loss which may pass unnoticed. However, the parents may have noted that the child's school work has deteriorated or that he turns up the television. There may also be associated episodes of earache caused by a superadded infection of the fluid. An examination of the ear will reveal the presence of fluid behind the tympanic membrane and a simple whisper test or an audiogram will confirm the presence of a hearing loss.

If the condition is temporary or intermittent, nothing need be done since most children outgrow the condition. If it is more severe, an

Fig. 48.1 A grommet for insertion in secretory otitis media. Ten times the normal size.

alternative means of allowing air into the middle ear, must be found. A hole is made in the tympanic membrane (a myringotomy) and the hole is prevented from healing by inserting a small plastic tube (grommet, dottle or stopple) (Fig. 48.1). At the same time, any underlying cause (sinusitis or enlarged adenoids) is treated.

As long as the grommet remains in place and remains unblocked the hearing is normal. However, the grommet drops out after an average period of 6 months. When the condition is recurrent, larger tubes may be inserted to aerate the middle ear. The majority of patients with grommets in place can be allowed to go swimming although ear plugs are advisable. It is hoped that the patient will have outgrown the problem by then, but a grommet may need to be reinserted if fluid reaccumulates.

Acute otitis media

The middle ear is in continuity with the nasopharynx and is therefore very prone to infection from it. This is especially so in the presence of serous otitis media when a convenient culture medium is available for the invading bacteria. The middle ear mucosa becomes inflamed and the cavity fills with pus which escapes by bursting out through the tympanic membrane into the external ear.

The patient, who is usually a child with a cold, develops an earache of increasing severity which ceases when the membrane bursts. The perforation usually heals after 2 to 3 days but this should be checked after one month and the presence of an underlying serous otitis media excluded.

The patient should be confined to bed and given analgesics. A covered hot-water bottle applied to the ear is helpful and warm olive oil drops will soothe the inflamed membrane. If a patient is seen before the perforation occurs, penicillin should be given and should be continued for at least 5 days and until the inflammation has settled. A swab should be taken from the discharging ear and sent for culture and sensitivity. Complications may arise but these are now rare. The commonest was acute mastoiditis, a condition in which an abscess develops in the mastoid bone and bursts out behind the ear. It is now only seen in children whose natural defence mechanisms are not functioning normally.

Chronic otitis media

When a middle ear infection becomes persistent it is called chronic otitis media. Permanent damage is done to the tympanic membrane and to the ossicles and the patient may be very deaf with a large central perforation and a persistent discharge. The discharge is particularly likely to occur when the patient has a cold because infected secretions pass up the Eustachian tube.

An attempt is made to remove any source of infection in the nose or nasopharynx and the local discharge can be controlled by regular toilet and the instillation of ear drops. When the ear has been dry for several months it is suitable for a surgical repair of the perforation. A piece of fascia is taken from the surface of the temporalis muscle and the thin tissue is grafted over the perforation. The graft may be laid on the inner or the outer surface of the tympanic membrane and the operation is known as a myringoplasty (myrinx is Greek for the tympanic membrane). Similarly, any loss of ossicular continuity can be corrected by repositioning a damaged ossicle or by replacing it with a piece of bone or a prosthesis. This operation is called tympanoplasty. More recently it has become possible to remove the tympanic membrane and its attached ossicles, in one block from a cadaver. These homograft tissues can then be implanted into a suitable patient but the operation is technically very difficult.

Cholesteatoma

This is a cyst lined by squamous epithelium and filled with layers of epithelial scales. The cyst forms from an in-pouching of the upper segment of the tympanic membrane, into the middle ear cavity. Initially the epithelial scales escape into the external canal, but as the mouth of the pouch narrows, they are retained and accumulate. The cholesteatoma is unique in that it has the property of eroding most of the tissues which it encounters. The contents of the cyst become infected and the condition may be regarded as a form of chronic otitis media.

The extent of the damage is determined by the direction in which the cholesteatoma enlarges. Usually the ossicles are damaged, but an upward extension will produce a brain abscess or meningitis. Similarly, a medial extension may produce a facial paralysis or damage the inner ear.

The patient complains of deafness and an offensive scanty discharge. There may be evidence of a complication and an examination of the ear will reveal a marginal perforation with white epithelial scales protruding. The treatment of a cholesteatoma is surgical and some form of radical mastoidectomy is necessary for its removal.

There are two forms of mastoidectomy operation. In a simple or cortical mastoidectomy, a hole is drilled from the surface of the mastoid bone into the mastoid antrum and the localised disease is removed. The operation does not interfere with the middle ear and postoperatively, the external canal and tympanic membrane may appear normal. For a cholesteatoma, this operation alone would be unsuitable because the middle ear itself is involved. A simple mastoidectomy is done first and then the bony wall between the simple cavity and the external canal is removed. The remnants of the tympanic membrane and the ossicles are also removed and we are left with a large cavity which can be seen on postoperative examination. This is the radical mastoidectomy and the ear will be safe although the patient will still be deaf and may still have a discharge. There will also be good access for toilet.

Otosclerosis

In otosclerosis, abnormal bone grows across the margins of the oval window and on to the footplate of the stapes which can no longer vibrate. The condition is commoner in women; it begins in early adulthood and the deafness progressively worsens. The treatment is a choice between a hearing aid and surgery and the operation is known as a stapedectomy. The mobile part of the stapes is removed and hole is made in the fixed footplate. A piston (or a similar prosthesis) is placed in the hole and hooked around the incus to re-establish sound transmission. The inner ear is at risk during the operation and this must be clearly explained to the patient. Some dizziness almost always occurs temporarily and this is countered by a drug such as Stemetil.

DISEASES OF THE INNER EAR

Any disease affecting the inner ear causes damage to the delicate nerve endings responding for hearing and balance and the patient may complain of vertigo, deafness, or tinnitus. Surgery is rarely of any assistance but a hearing aid will help the deafness which is very common in old age.

Trauma, loud noises and some drugs may damage the inner ear and they should be avoided if possible. In Meniere's disease, there is an accumulation of endolymph in the inner ear and the patient suffers from episodes of severe vertigo. If the hearing is good, certain specialised operations can be attempted but the results are not often convincing. If the hearing is bad, the inner ear can be destroyed in an operation known as a total labyrinthectomy and the result is often very beneficial.

A tumour known as an acoustic neuroma may occur in the internal auditory canal and its symptoms will mimic those of inner ear disease. The ear, nose and throat surgeon carries out many investigations to distinguish between these in an attempt to diagnose a neuroma at an early stage.

DEAFNESS

Deafness is a disability which separates the sufferer from society. Communication becomes difficult and there is a tendency for the non-aggressive personality to become a recluse. Although hearing aids may help, they never provide normal hearing and they may aggravate the disability. When speaking to deaf people, especially the elderly, the speaker should face his companion and speak clearly and distinctly. It must be remembered that deafness varies for sounds of different pitch and the patient may hear some sounds normally. Shouting usually distorts speech even more and it often causes distress and acute discomfort.

If any child is suspected of deafness he should be regarded as being deaf until proved otherwise. If thought to be significantly deaf he should be given an aid as soon as possible.

Points of interest in ear surgery

Incisions for ear operations may lie behind, or in front of, the pinna.

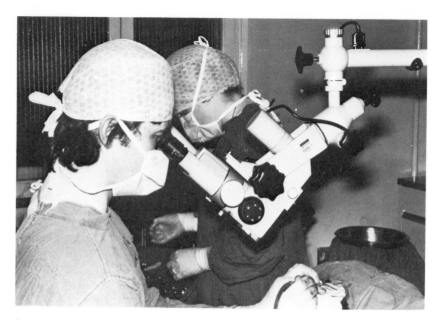

Fig. 48.2 An ear operation using the operating microscope.

Fig. 48.3 Instruments in ear surgery.
Left to right—Crocodile forceps Myringotomy knife Aural speculum Tilley's aural dressing forceps Jobson Horne probe.

Since the hair often encroaches on the operation site, it is usually necessary to shave a narrow band in order to allow the application of an adhesive sterile towel.

The examination of the ear is carried out with a head mirror, a head light or an electric auriscope. Since the middle ear structures are so small, a binocular operating microscope is employed for middle ear operations (Fig. 48.2). The instruments used in middle ear surgery are angled so that the manipulating hand does not obscure vision down the narrow external canal (Fig. 48.3).

DISEASES OF THE NOSE

SYMPTOMS OF NASAL DISEASE

1. Bleeding. The medical term for a nose bleed is epistaxis. The blood may escape through the nostrils or it may run backwards into the nasopharynx and throat.

2. Obstruction. This may be fluctuant or permanent and it is caused by mucosal congestion, a deviated septum or nasal polyps. The congestion may be infective or allergic. The patient with nasal obstruction, snores and mouth-breathes.

3. Discharge. This is usually watery in allergic conditions and purulent in infective conditions. A unilateral persistent discharge is caused by a foreign body (in children) or a tumour (in adults). A discharge which passes backwards into the throat is known as a postnasal drip.

4. Loss of the sense of smell. This is an under-rated disability and little understood. Since taste is mainly gained through the sense of smell, the patient is unable to appreciate his food.

NASAL LESIONS

Fractured nasal bones

The nasal bones are flattened or deviated to one side following trauma. If the patient is seen within 3 weeks, the deformity may be corrected under general anaesthesia. If treatment is sought much later, a rhinoplasty becomes necessary. In this operation, the skin of the nose is separated from the underlying nasal skeleton and the shape is corrected as desired.

Septal abscess

Trauma causes bleeding between the septal cartilage and the overlying muco-periosteum. This haematoma will cause nasal obstruction and unless it is drained it will form an abscess with subsequent destruction of the cartilage.

Deviated nasal septum

A significant deviation of the septum causes nasal obstruction and interferes with the drainage of the sinuses. It is corrected by one of the two following operations:

1. Sub-mucous resection (S.M.R.) of the nasal septum. The muco-periosteum is raised and the deviated portion of cartilage is removed.
2. Septoplasty. The offending cartilage is straightened and repositioned in the mid-line.

Epistaxis

A nose bleed presents in two ways. In the young patient, bleeding occurs from a superficial septal blood vessel lying just inside the nostril on a spot known as Little's area. Bleeding is initiated by the slightest trauma or infection and it is usually trivial. The first aid treatment is to grip the tip of the nose between thumb and forefinger and to exert firm pressure over the bleeding point for 3 minutes. If the epistaxes occur regularly, the offending vessel is cauterised under local or general anaesthesia and any underlying nasal infection is treated.

In the elderly patient, bleeding is often heavy and arises from larger vessels at the back of the nose. There is often a history of vascular disease and access to the responsible vessels is poor. The nose is packed with ribbon gauze impregnated in paraffin or a suitable disinfectant and this is left in place for one or two days. Pressure can also be exerted on the bleeding area by inflating a special balloon. A blood transfusion may be obligatory and the surgical ligation of the arteries supplying the nose sometimes becomes necessary.

It must be emphasised that an epistaxis is often a sign of some underlying systemic disease.

Infection

The common cold or coryza is the commonest nasal infection. It is an acute viral rhinitis which presents with sneezing, mucosal congestion and a mucoid discharge. After 2 days, a secondary infection by various bacteria results in a purulent discharge and the condition settles within 1 week without any treatment.

Allergic rhinitis

An inflammatory congestion of the nasal mucosa can be caused by an allergy as well as by an infection. The symptoms, although similar, present in varying patterns. In hay fever, the nasal mucosa is allergic to grass pollen and the symptoms of sneezing, obstruction and a watery discharge are only present during the early summer months. With perennial rhinitis, the symptoms are present throughout the year and numerous allergens, such as feathers and house dust, may be responsible.

If possible, the allergen should be identified and avoided, and in some cases a course of desensitisation injections is helpful. Anti-histamine drugs suppress the symptoms but produce unwanted drowsiness as a side-effect. Many patients respond well to steroid nasal sprays such as Beconase, but these should be prescribed with care.

Nasal polyps

Allergic rhinitis is sometimes associated with the appearance of polyps in the upper part of the nose. Localised areas of mucosa become swollen and droop downwards into the nasal cavity to give the appearance of skinned grapes. They cause nasal obstruction and there is no treatment apart from surgical removal which is carried out under local or general anaesthesia. Nasal polyps are harmless but they tend to recur because the underlying problem has not been cured.

Fig. 48.4 Instruments for nasal surgery
Nasal speculum
An adenoid curette
Trocar and cannular for sinus wash outs.

Vasomotor rhinitis

When the nasal mucosa becomes swollen and congested without any evidence of infection or allergy, the condition is known as vasomotor rhinitis. It is caused by an alteration in the behaviour of blood vessels supplying the mucosa and it is sometimes believed to have a psychological basis. The main symptom is nasal obstruction and it is difficult to treat.

Decongestant nasal sprays or drops are not advocated since they aggravate the condition when used persistently. When the mucosa overlying the inferior turbinate bone is particularly swollen, it may be reduced in volume by the application of surface cautery or sub-mucosal diathermy. A polluted or centrally-heated environment makes the condition worse and the patient should be encouraged to take a healthy diet, plenty of fresh air and exercise.

THE ADENOID

This is the name given to the pad of lymphoid tissue which lies on the roof of the nasopharynx behind the nose. In the past, it has been held responsible for a variety of symptoms in children but its role as a scapegoat has recently become much diminished. The adenoid is normally enlarged between the ages of four and seven and on rare occasions it may be so large as to obstruct the nasal passages and affect the opening of the Eustachian tube. The adenoid gradually atrophies after the age of eight.

The removal of the adenoid is still carried out for nasal obstruction and in the treatment of serous otitis media although its role in these conditions has not been proven. The operation of adenoidectomy is done with the mouth held open by a special gag and with the patient in the supine position. The adenoid curette (Fig. 48.4) is guided behind the soft palate and the pad of lymphoid tissue is scraped out. Care must be taken not to damage any other structures during this blind procedure. Since the main complication is haemorrhage, it is imperative that the patient is carefully observed during the postoperative period.

Points of special interest

The nose is examined by raising the tip and shining a light inside. The view may be improved by retracting the margins of the nostril with a nasal speculum. The back of the nose is examined by placing a small mirror through the mouth and behind the soft palate. When a light is directed at the mirror, the reflection of the nasopharynx and posterior nose is seen. Nasal operations occur at the upper end of the respiratory tract and special emphasis is therefore placed on the protection of the lower airway. As in the ear, the instruments are angled to permit better vision and a headlight is employed to concentrate light at the site of operation.

Postoperatively, the nose is almost always blocked by oedema, and the obstruction is eased by nasal douches using warm sterile saline. The patient inevitably mouth-breathes and regular mouth-washes prevent the resulting dryness.

THE SINUSES

There are four sets of air sinuses on each side of the skull; the maxillary sinus (or antrum), the frontal sinuses, the ethmoid sinuses and the sphenoid sinuses. They are placed around the nose and are therefore called paranasal sinuses. Each sinus is an air-filled space in the skull and each drains into the nose by a small opening, the ostium. The largest sinus is the maxillary antrum which lies in the cheek bone and it is this which is most often infected. If all the sinuses are infected, the condition is known as pan-sinusitis. Sphenoid sinusitis is very rare.

Maxillary sinusitis

When the nose is infected by the common cold, the lining of the maxillary antrum is involved in the same way. As long as the ciliated epithelium, which lines the antrum, remains healthy and as long as the ostium stays open, there is no problem. Once the ostium blocks, mucus and pus accumulate in the antrum and the patient is said to have acute maxillary sinusitis.

The patient is pyrexial and ill and there is a throbbing pain over the affected cheek which is also very tender to pressure. The nose is often blocked and examination will show the presence of pus which is swabbed and sent for culture. The patient is kept in bed and given suitable analgesics and the symptoms usually settle on antibiotics, penicillin being the treatment of choice.

In some patients, the infection becomes chronic and the lining mucosa becomes thickened, polypoid and partially destroyed. The patient has a blocked nose and a postnasal drip. The antrum is no longer able to drain via the ostium and surgical treatment is necessary.

The first step is to carry out an antral washout. A trocar and cannula (Fig. 48.4) is introduced into the antrum via the nostril and the thin layer of bone below the inferior turbinate. The trocar is removed and a syringe is applied to the cannula which is flushed out with saline. The accumulated pus is removed and the ostium is unblocked. This procedure may need to be repeated but if it is inadequate, it will be necessary to construct a permanent drainage opening below the inferior turbinate. This is known as an intranasal antrostomy and it gives the antral mucosa the opportunity to return to normal. If the situation is irreversible, the infected mucosa is removed through an opening constructed in the front of the antrum beneath the upper lip. This is known as a Caldwell-Luc operation and it allows good access to the antrum.

Ethmoiditis

There are several small ethmoid sinuses which lie between the orbit and the upper nose. They are often involved by chronic infection in conjunction with the antrum. Acute ethmoiditis is unusual and it is only seen in children. Oedema of the soft tissues around the eye is seen and it is treated with penicillin. If an abscess forms it may need to be drained.

Frontal sinusitis

An acute infection of the frontal sinus is dangerous because it is so near to the brain. The patient should therefore be admitted to hospital and given systemic penicillin. A nasal swab is taken for culture and if the condition does not settle, the sinus is drained through the roof of the orbit. Chronic frontal sinusitis is difficult to eradicate and it tends to recur in spite of surgical treatment.

Tumours

Malignant tumours can reach a considerable size in the maxillary antrum before they produce symptoms. The symptoms, when they appear, depend upon the direction of spread. Problems may arise with the eye, the teeth or the nose and there may be a swelling of the cheek. It must be emphasised however, that the commonest cause of a swollen cheek is an infected tooth of the upper jaw. The treatment is by radiotherapy, surgery or a combination of the two. Surgery may involve the removal of an eye and considerable cosmetic deformity results. The prognosis for malignant tumours in this area is poor.

THE THROAT

The trachea and the oesophagus meet at the hypopharynx which continues upwards into the oropharynx. At its junction with the pharynx,

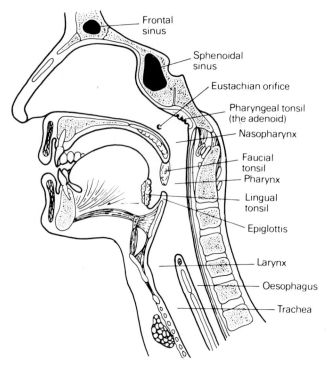

Fig. 48.5 The pharynx, the larynx and trachea.

the structure of the trachea has become modified to form the larynx. These three structures the larynx, the hypopharynx and the oropharynx, together with adjacent tissue, constitute the throat (see Fig. 48.5).

SYMPTOMS AND SIGNS OF THROAT DISEASE

Dysphagia or difficulty in swallowing is a serious symptom if it persists for longer than a few days. Together with pain, it is commonly found in tonsillitis but a more serious cause is a malignant tumour or an impacted foreign body.

Pain usually presents on swallowing and it often radiates to the ear.

Hoarseness. This means that there is a roughness of the voice, caused by some factor which prevents the smooth approximation of the vocal cords. Infections are the commonest cause but an early tumour of the vocal cords should always be suspected.

Cough. This is an explosive release of air through the vocal cords and it suggests the presence of an irritation in the larynx or trachea.

Stridor or noisy breathing. It may be present during inspiration, expiration or both. It implies that there is a narrowing of the respiratory tract.

EXAMINATION OF THE THROAT

The throat is examined by indirect or direct laryngoscopy. An indirect laryngoscopy is done by pressing a warmed mirror against the soft palate and observing the reflection of the larynx and hypopharynx. It can be difficult to do this when the patient has a sensitive throat and a direct laryngoscopy becomes necessary. This involves the insertion of an illuminated metal tube into the pharynx under general anaesthesia. The larynx is then examined directly through the tube. A narrower and longer tube is employed for an oesophagoscopy. The need for direct laryngoscopy under general anaesthesia has recently decreased because of the use of flexible fibreoptic laryngoscopes and oesophagoscopes.

DISEASES OF THE THROAT

Infections are very common especially in childhood when serious, especially when the larynx is involved. In adults, malignant tumours are relatively common and major surgery may be necessary.

Tonsillitis

When the surface of the tonsil and the oropharynx becomes inflamed, the patient has pharyngitis. He has a sore throat but he is not ill. When the deep tissues of the tonsil are acutely infected, the patient has acute tonsillitis. He has a sore throat but he is also ill and runs a high temperature. The infecting organism is commonly a virus but secondary bacterial infection occurs especially with the streptococcus. Whatever the infecting organism, the clinical features are the same and the examination findings vary with the stage of the illness. The tonsils are usually large, red and covered with patches of purulent debris which have been extruded from the tonsillar crypts. The upper cervical and sub-mandibular lymph glands are often enlarged and tender. In the very small child there may be no sign apart from a refusal to take food.

The condition is commonest in childhood between the ages of five and eight but it does occur in young adults who have not gained immunity. The patient is ill for 2 or 3 days and gradually improves over the next 5 days.

Treatment consists of rest in bed and isolation of the patient. He is encouraged to drink, and swallowing is made easier by the administration of an analgesic such as aspirin. Antibiotics are not usually necessary because most episodes are viral in origin and the natural course of the condition is short. In the more severe attack or where a complication is feared, an antibiotic is advisable and penicillin is probably best.

If the acute attacks recur five or six times a year and there is a significant interference with schooling or work, a tonsillectomy should be considered. If the child is around the age of seven or eight when first seen, it is worthwhile postponing surgery for 1 year because most gain immunity around this age. A simple enlargement of the tonsils is not an indication for their removal. It must be appreciated that tonsillitis and other upper respiratory tract infections are so common around the age of five that infrequent attacks must be considered as part of the normal process of growing up.

Fig. 48.6 Position after tonsillectomy. Pillows are placed behind the mattress on one side.

The operation is carried out under general anaesthesia and the tonsil is dissected from the underlying pharyngeal tissue. The adenoids are no longer removed routinely at the same time and the operation is never done while the tonsil is inflamed.

Postoperatively the patient should be nursed on the side with the head down so as not to inhale blood or a tonsil fragment (Fig. 48.6). The main complication is haemorrhage and its early recognition is essential. Observations are made on the respiration, colour, pulse and blood pressure and any excessive swallowing should be reported to the surgeon who will examine the patient. If bleeding occurs, the patient is returned to the theatre for ligation of the bleeding point.

The following day the patient is encouraged to eat and drink and an analgesic such as soluble aspirin is given before each meal. The throat is very sore and the pain may radiate to the ear. Children are normally kept in for about 3 days and adults for a day or so longer. Secondary bleeding may occur about 1 week after the operation but this is due to infection and it responds well to penicillin.

Peritonsillar abscess (quinsy)

Rarely in adults, the tonsillitis does not settle and the infection spreads on one side, into the adjacent pharyngeal wall and soft palate. A unilateral abscess forms and the swelling pushes the tonsil up to, or even across, the mid-line. The patient cannot open his jaws and the saliva which he cannot swallow, dribbles from the mouth.

The traditional treatment of this peritonsillar abscess is to incise it and the patient is given a course of penicillin. The tonsils are removed 6 weeks later to prevent a recurrence. Recently there has been a tendency to remove the tonsils when the patient presents with the quinsy.

Most patients sent up to hospital with a suspected quinsy are usually found to have a persistent bilateral tonsillitis as part of the picture of glandular fever.

THE LARYNX

Acute laryngitis

The larynx may be involved in any acute upper respiratory tract infection. In adults, this causes hoarseness and the best treatment is to rest the voice. In children, however, the larynx is smaller and any additional narrowing by inflammatory oedema interferes with the airway. Initially the child has stridor (croup) but severe respiratory obstruction can result. Admission to hospital, humidity in an oxygen tent, naso-tracheal intubation or a tracheostomy may all become necessary if the symptoms are severe.

Chronic laryngitis

The patient is persistently hoarse in this condition and a tumour may be suspected. The vocal cords are red and thickened and the patient often follows an occupation which demands an over-use of the voice in a smoky environment. Treatment is notoriously difficult because the patient may need to lose his job in order to achieve the essential voice-rest.

Vocal nodules are small swellings which occur on the vocal cords and are thought by some to be a form of chronic laryngitis. They cause hoarseness and if large, they can be removed by direct laryngoscopy.

Tumours of the larynx

Benign. Laryngeal papillomata are small viral warts which grow in the larynx of the small child. They produce hoarseness, stridor and respiratory obstruction and they are removed by suction diathermy, cryosurgery or more recently by the laser. A tracheostomy is done if the symptoms are severe but the papillomata eventually disappear when immunity is gained by the host.

Malignant. A patient suffering from a laryngeal tumour presents with hoarseness. In the early stages he may be treated by radiotherapy with preservation of the voice and a good prognosis. In the later stages and for those tumours which recur after radiotherapy, a laryngectomy is carried out.

The larynx produces speech and prevents the entry of food into the trachea. Both these functions are lost after a laryngectomy. After the removal of the larynx one is left with the cut end of the trachea and a defect in the pharynx. The latter is sutured up while the trachea is brought out through the middle of the neck and sutured to the skin.

Postoperative care of the laryngectomy

1. The care of a tracheostomy has been discussed in Chapter 16.

2. A laryngectomy is a major procedure because the patient loses his main organ of communication. He can no longer ask for attention and initially he requires the constant presence of a nurse. Many patients are not accustomed to writing and they become intensely anxious, frustrated and depressed. Great demands are therefore made upon the patience and sympathy of the attendant nurse. The patient is provided with a pencil and pad and a bell is placed within easy reach. A selection of word-cards is also useful (Fig. 16.2). In time many patients learn a new form of speech whereby air is swallowed and regurgitated to produce a vibration in some suitable piece of tissue. This is a similar mechanism to that of the 'belch'. The degree of clarity achieved by this technique, varies with the motivation of the patient.

3. Feeding is initially achieved through a naso-gastric tube while the pharyngeal defect is healing. An adequate liquidised diet is given and a close eye is kept on the patient's weight and upon his fluid output.

Basic nursing care is at a high premium because the patient is often elderly and in poor physical condition. However, the rewards are great because the patient is sometimes totally rehabilitated.

Tumours of the pharynx

These tumours present with dysphagia or with a gland in the neck. Radiotherapy is often the first treatment of choice but many come to need surgery. Pharyngeal tumours often involve the adjacent larynx and so an adequate excision includes the larynx as well as the pharynx. It is no longer possible to suture the defect in the pharynx as after a laryngectomy and a method has to be found to bridge the gap. This continuity is provided by the transference of a section of gut or by employing grafted tubes of skin. The employment of myocutaneous flaps has improved the results of these repairs. This flap is an 'island' of skin and underlying muscle from the shoulder or chest wall with its blood supply intact. The patient commonly develops fistulae and stenosis at the site of the operation and the postoperative period is a protracted one. A block-dissection of the lymph glands in the neck is commonly done with a pharyngo-laryngectomy.

The postoperative care is the same as that after a laryngectomy although the problems are worse because of the bleeding difficulties. Much effort is needed in preventing the patient from becoming depressed.

Tumours in the mouth and oropharynx are now often removed by the laser.

49
Diseases of the eye

Ophthalmology, a knowledge of the art of healing eye diseases, first became a specialty in its own right at about the middle of the 19th century after which, particularly in Vienna, considerable advances were made in the understanding and treatment of eye disease. Hospitals specialising exclusively in eye disorders developed in this country and others, but there has now been for a time a welcome and useful trend towards the integration of eye units into general hospitals.

Ophthalmalogical practice tends to be dominated by the treatment of blindness due to cataracts and glaucoma in old patients and other conditions in the ageing eye, and in the young, squints and congenital abnormalities, which often have a genetic basis. Infections and traumatic cases occur at all ages. Examination of the eye gives an important input to general medical and neurological examination.

THE EYE UNIT

The eye unit comprises the outpatients department, the ward, (which has facilities for surgical day-stay patients), and the operating theatre.

The ophthalmic outpatient department is gaining importance as the hub of the management of ophthalmic patients, undertaking treatment of an expanding range of eye conditions with an increasing requirement for a suitable suite of dark rooms etc.

The ophthalmic ward is likely to contain fewer beds in future, with a reduction in the length of stay of patients. A resultant greater nursing activity per bed will be somewhat offset by the reduction in the overall number of beds. Mobility of the patients will continue to be a useful goal.

The ophthalmic theatre is generally likely to be situated in a suite of other theatres sharing recovery room facilities. A surgical microscope and many other types of ophthalmic surgical equipment will be available.

The delicacy of ophthalmic surgical instruments, problems in their cleaning and their liability to damage must be stressed.

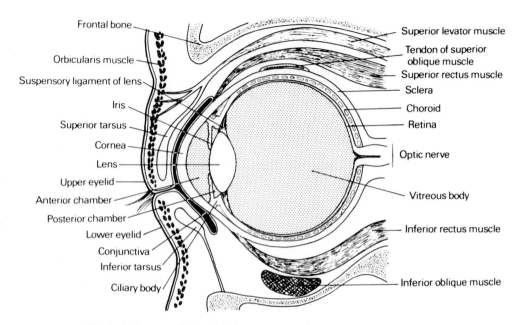

Fig. 49.1 Section of the orbit showing internal structure of the eye.

ANATOMY AND PHYSIOLOGY OF THE EYE

A basic understanding of ophthalmology requires a knowledge of the anatomy and physiology of the eye, as well as optics.

Figure 49.1 shows a section of the eye within its orbit. The eyeball should be regarded as an optical organ whose function is to place an image on to the retina. **Rods** are light sensitive retinal cells which are responsible for peripheral and night vision; **cones** provide central and detailed vision. As far as embryonic development is concerned, the retina belongs to the brain and within its layers a considerable processing of the image, which at this stage is inverted, occurs before a coded visual message is passed on through the visual pathways to the visual cortex resting within the occipital bone, and further on to areas of the brain where visual memory is stored, the actual seeing area of the brain.

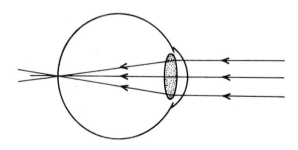

Fig. 49.2 Diagram to illustrate normal eye—emmetropia

Optics and the eye's refractive errors

The refractive properties of the eye place images accurately on to the retina in most people (see Fig. 49.2), a state which is called **emmetropia.**

In **accommodation** the crystalline lens becomes fatter due to a slackening of the suspensory ligament of the lens, due to contraction of the sphincteric ciliary muscle. This enables the eye to focus and view near objects. It is only when the age of 50 years is approached that the lens becomes hard and less able to change its shape, making reading glasses necessary. A state of **presbyopia** is now established. Most people will only ever need reading glasses but as old age approaches the strength of these glasses will need to be increased as accommodative power diminishes further.

Hypermetropia is a refractive error and means long sight. The eye is adapted to viewing distant objects (see Fig. 49.3) generally because it is too small. Glasses with a convex lens are required to place the image on the retina. Hypermetropia may not manifest itself until later life since accommodation can compensate for a time. The early prescription of reading glasses may then become necessary.

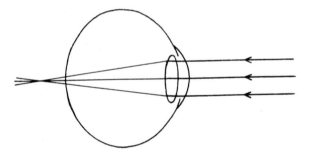

Fig. 49.3 Diagram to illustrate hypermetropia (long sight).

Myopia means short sight. Focussing of near objects is generally possible even in middle and old age but since images of distant objects form in front of the retina, the eye is generally too large (Fig. 49.4). A concave lens in the patient's glasses of a suitable strength will then place the image back on to the retina.

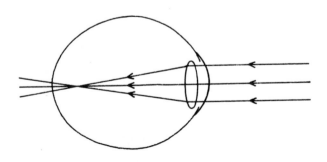

Fig. 49.4 Diagram to illustrate myopia (short sight).

Astigmatism indicates that the refractive power of the eye varies in different planes and a blurred image results. Regular astigmatism can be corrected by suitably ground lenses.

Such refractive errors can be measured by retinoscopy and an appropriate strength of glasses is then prescribed.

Contact lenses rest on the front of the eye and are most popular among the short sighted. There are optical advantages for the highly myopic in contact lenses since the field of vision is unimpaired by spectacle frames. Contact lenses are of advantage in some medical and surgical ophthalmological conditions.

EXAMINATION OF THE EYE

This is in general best undertaken in the ophthalmic outpatient department whenever possible. Traditionally a suitable dark room is available on the eye ward but this should be for the use of inpatients only since

there are objections to the access of casualties and outpatients to a surgical area.

An accurate history is first taken including notes of any previously diagnosed general medical conditions. Examination of the eye starts with the eyelids and surrounding skin, and any disorders of movement of the eyes or the pupil are noted. A dense cataract may be seen. The visual acuity is recorded in all cases generally by Snellen's test type (Fig. 49.5) at 6 metres (20 feet) or half that distance when the letters are viewed through a mirror. Further examination requires a whole variety of instruments, some of which are cumbersome, hence the need for their mobility on castors, and adequate space.

Fig.49.5 Snellen's test type—internally illuminated, four sided, rotating drum test type. (Hamlyn (Instruments) Ltd)

Ophthalmoscopes permit a view of the retina which will often need to be facilitated by dilatation of the pupil. In binocular ophthalmoscopy, so vital in retinal detachments, the patient generally lies on a couch. By means of a **retinoscope,** refractive errors (see above) are measured so that appropriate glasses can be prescribed.

Slit lamp microscopes provide a detailed examination of the eye in a thin optical section so that individual layers can be observed in microscopic detail. Thus corneal conditions can be assessed, sometimes aided by fluorescin eye drops, and the anterior chamber searched for inflammatory cells. Attachments to the slit lamp microscope permit measurement of the intra-ocular pressure i.e. tonometry by applanation in glaucoma. Diagnostic contact lenses are used to observe the angle of the anterior chamber by means of a gonioscope, an important test in glaucoma, or provide a view of the retina (3 mirror lens).

Visual field examination by a variety of methods, i.e. perimetry or central fields by the Bjerrum screen, is an important part of the follow-up of glaucoma patients and the diagnosis of intracranial tumours. A suitably quiet and lighted room is required.

Disorders of the lacrimal drainage apparatus may require a lacrimal sac washout in a suitable treatment room.

Assessment of colour vision is required as part of eye examination to assess suitability for various types of employment.

BASIC NURSING OF EYE CONDITIONS

The following general principles are of special importance in the nursing of patients suffering from disease of the eye.

1. Attention to minute detail is essential.

2. An aseptic or no-touch technique should be maintained when carrying out treatment.

3. The terms guttae (gutt.) and oculentum (oc.) are extensively used and indicate eye drops and eye ointment respectively. The use of 'cream' indicating oc. is to be discouraged since a cosmetic or culinary meaning might be understood.

4. Since there is a danger that the dropper tip of drop bottles may touch eyelids or eyelashes which harbour bacterial and other contaminants, they have largely been replaced by single dose containers, e.g. 'minims' or 'opulets', which must only be opened immediately before use and then discarded, to avoid cross infection.

5. All drops should be carefully checked as the instillation of wrong drops may lead to a disaster. Drops which dilate the pupil may be particularly dangerous in certain patients as they can produce acute glaucoma with a serious risk of damage to the vision. It is therefore most important that the name be carefully read.

6. In general, where there is a purulent discharge the eye is not covered, in order to allow the discharge to escape.

7. Where there has been an abrasion or wound of the eye, or a foreign body has been removed from the cornea, then the eyelids may be kept

closed by means of a pad and bandage fixed firmly over the eye. This will offer the patient much relief. Further protection may be given in postoperative patients following intraocular surgery, including cataract extractions, by using a strong shield (cartella) which fits over the pad. By abutting on the bone above and below, protection of the eye against an accidental knock, for instance from the patient's hand when he is sleeping, is provided.

8. The majority of patients require covering of the affected eye only. In certain circumstances, however, padding of both eyes is necessary, for example often before and after retinal detachment operations.

9. A patient with both eyes padded needs to be treated with the same care and consideration as a blind person.

10. Care of a case of excision of the eye. Immediately postoperatively, a firm pad and bandage are required to reduce swelling and bruising. Subsequently the socket will require the instillation of drops or ointment of a suitable antibiotic until healing has occurred. A plastic shell is worn for 3 to 4 weeks to prevent shrinkage and to shape the socket until an artificial eye is worn. In most cases, a better cosmetic result is obtained by replacing the excised eye with an implant which forms a movable base for an anteriorly placed prosthesis.

OCULAR INJURIES

All parts of the eye and bony orbital walls are liable to injuries. It follows that even apparently trivial eye injuries should be referred to a properly equipped eye department or room in the accident and emergency department specially adapted for eye examination. Visual acuity is always recorded from each eye separately, with glasses if normally worn using Snellen's Test Type (Fig. 49.5).

A history is always necessary. Important clues, for example to the presence of a metallic intra-ocular foreign body when flying metal fragments may have injured the eye, would otherwise be missed. Such injuries may have originated, for example, from a hammer striking the end of a chisel. In suspected cases an X-ray is necessary.

Corneal abrasions will be revealed by fluorescin staining.

Foreign bodies may lie superficially in the cornea or conjunctiva. Their detection often requires magnification and an adequately bright light source. Most of those seen in a casualty department will be metallic, embedded in the superficial layers of the cornea, and require expert removal by a sharp needle on the slit lamp microscope with prior topical anaesthesia using guttae amethocaine 1 per cent. Subtarsal foreign bodies are only found by eversion of the upper or lower eyelids and are usually removed by means of a small moist swab on a stick.

A metallic intra-ocular foreign body (see above) leads later to blindness when, as in most instances, it is made of iron, so an X-ray of the orbits in suspected cases is essential. Removal is by a powerful electro-magnet.

Lacerations of the eyelids, especially their margins, require expert surgical closure in the eye department. There may be a perforation of the cornea or sclera due to sharp objects e.g. glass fragments in road traffic accidents. An irregularly shaped and eccentrically situated pupil is an important sign that a full thickness wound of the cornea has resulted, with loss of aqueous humour from the anterior chamber. An emergency operation is then necessary to close the wound, and the ophthalmologist will need to assess the patient for other injuries to the eye.

Blunt injuries to the eye, some of which result from ball games, result in a variety of injuries to different parts of the eye. Hence a **hyphaema** may result in which a level of blood is seen in the lower part of the anterior chamber. A **traumatic cataract** may have resulted from a sort of 'concussion' of the eye. **Vitreous and retinal haemorrhages** as well as **retinal tears** leading to **retinal detachment** may also occur.

Injury to the bony walls of the orbit results from severe blunt injuries. In a blow-out fracture of the maxilla, orbital contents are forced into the maxillary antrum. The optic nerve may be severely damaged by fractures of the orbit at its apex.

Chemical burns of a variety of types are seen. Alkalies, e.g lime, are in general the most severe. Irrigation of the conjunctival sac with copious amounts of fluid, generally tap water, is urgently necessary after spillage of chemical into the eyes. Careful scrutiny of the upper and lower conjunctival fornices after eversion of the eyelids is necessary so that adherent particles of lime can be removed with a moist swab.

Exposure of the eyeball due to inadequate closure of the eyelids, made worse by absence of the blinking reflex in a variety of conditions, is a serious situation requiring the instillation of eye ointment, preferably albucid, and urgent referral to an ophthalmologist. The commoner causes are proptosis (or a forwards displacement of the eyeball) often due to thyroid disease, the unconscious patient, including general anaesthesia when the eyelids should be closed with adhesive tape, facial palsy, or a coloboma (= a notch of the upper eyelid, either traumatic or developmental in the newborn). A tarsorrhaphy (closure of the eyelids) is often necessary since severe corneal ulceration and loss of the eye may occur.

CONDITIONS OF THE EYELIDS

Coloboma

This is a developmental defect in the upper eyelid in the newborn and requires the urgent attention of an ophthalmologist. Otherwise the serious condition of exposure keratitis occurs.

Stye (hordeolum)

A stye is a staphylococcal infection of an eyelash follicle in which pus under pressure produces pain and the lax eyelid tissues allow great surrounding swelling (oedema).

Treatment

This is by local heat and antibiotic treatment. Spontaneous resolution is the rule.

Blepharitis

This is an inflammation of the lid margins, prone to recur after cessation of treatment.

Treatment

The crusts are removed with moist swabs of saline or weak sodium bicarbonate solution. Irrigation with the latter twice to three times a day using an eye bath over a 2 weeks' period generally offers relief for a time.

Meibomian cyst (Chalazion)

A swelling in the lid varying from lentil to large pea size results from accumulation of scavenger cells (macrophages) packed with oily material from a Meibomian gland. Normally the oil is secreted onto the lid margin and covers the surface of the tear film reducing evaporation of tears.

Treatment

Incision of the lesion and curettage, usually under local anaesthesia, is required in many cases although spontaneous resolution may occur.

Entropion

Entropion is a turning in of an eyelid. This causes the eyelashes to rub on the cornea, giving discomfort, but more seriously, corneal ulceration may be produced. Irritation in the eye or tight bandaging may produce spastic entropion. This is relieved by curing the primary condition or removing the bandage as appropriate. Common causes of entropion are changes in the lid due to age (senile), scarring or mechanical factors.

Treatment

Treatment is by surgery.

Ectropion

In this condition the eyelid turns outwards. The tears cannot reach the lacrimal punctum and the patient will be troubled by watering (epiphora). The exposed conjunctiva becomes inflamed and thickened, giving an unsightly appearance in more severely affected patients. A laxity of the eyelid in the old, facial palsy and contracture due to scar tissue are the commonest causes.

Treatment

Treatment is by surgery.

Ptosis

Ptosis or a drooping of the upper eyelid is due to swelling or weakness of the muscle which elevates the upper lid. The latter may arise from a failure in development, or acquired disease or injury affecting the muscle, the nerve-muscle junction (myasthenia gravis), or the nerve supply which is derived from the third cranial nerve and the sympathetic nervous system.

Tumours of the eyelids

A common malignant lesion is basal cell carcinoma (rodent ulcer) which is mostly suitable for local excision, with a skin graft if necessary; radiotherapy is only rarely recommended.

CONDITIONS OF THE CONJUNCTIVA AND CORNEA

Conjunctivitis and corneal ulcers

Symptoms and signs

This is characterised by a complaint of a gritty sensation in the affected eye and often intolerance to a smokey atmosphere. Photophobia may also be present. The eye appears red and, in cases uncomplicated by corneal involvement, the conjunctiva immediately surrounding the cornea will be unaffected. Pupillary size and reaction to light are normal.

If in addition corneal ulceration is present, vision is usually impaired. Patients usually complain of ocular pain and photophobia with a foreign body sensation. A localised area of the cornea is mostly involved which appears grey and may be more easily seen as a green area after fluorescin is applied to the conjunctival sac. A secondary iritis may occur in severe cases.

Responsible organisms are bacteria, e.g. staphylococci, pneumococci and sometimes the *Pseudomonas pyogenes*.

Viruses are commonly the cause, especially herpes simplex, with invasion of the conjunctival sac from cold sores and the characteristic dendritic corneal ulcer. Some adenoviruses cause affection of the local (pre-auricular) lymph nodes. Such viruses and other organisms sometimes cause epidemics of infection in patients attending outpatients or casualty departments, but the use of single dose packaging for eye drops (instructions must be strictly followed in their use) has resulted in increased safety for patients from such calamities. Fungi are also occasionally responsible for severe chronic corneal ulcers.

Treatment is by appropriate antibiotics and it is fortunate that antiviral agents are now available in herpes simplex infections. Secondary acute iritis will need treatment with mydriatics. A common end result is corneal scarring with resultant loss in vision. Perforation of the cornea with panophthalmitis and loss of the eye may sometimes result.

Allergic types of conjunctivitis, in which the cornea may also be involved, occur and chronic, sometimes severe, cases are described as 'spring catarrh'. These require different treatment including the cautious use of anti-inflammatory agents, e.g. corticosteroids.

Ophalmia neonatorum

This was formally due in many cases to the gonococcus, but conjunctivitis in the newborn is now much more commonly due to viruses, e.g. chlamydia, although bacteria, e.g. staphylococci, are sometimes responsible. The cornea is now usually spared from severe involvement. The occasional gonococcal conjunctivitis is still best treated with penicillin eye drops.

Trachoma

Trachoma is caused by a virus so large in size that it shares some characteristics with bacteria in so far as it can be seen with the ordinary microscope after staining. It responds slowly to suitable antibiotic treatment. Trachoma is endemic to many parts of the world, particularly the Middle East, Far East and South America, where a large part of the population is affected at some time. The effects are initially mild but later become severe during the prolonged course of the illness. Occasional cases are found in immigrants to Britain. In the acute stage a very red eye with discharge and large follicles in the conjunctiva lining the eyelids gives an appearance almost like sago grains. The upper part of the cornea is later affected and the lining of the lids (palpebral conjunctiva) becomes scarred, leading to entropion, and further damage is caused by the trauma of ingrowing eyelashes. Secondary infection may be a further cause of serious corneal damage so that trachoma is a leading cause of blindness in the world as a whole.

New growths

At birth, small dermoids may be present at the junction of the conjunctiva and cornea, and dermolipomas occur sometimes in the posterior parts of the conjunctiva. Naevi are benign pigmented growths like freckles. Malignant change in them is rare. The commonest site for epitheliomas is the junction of the cornea with the sclera.

Corneal grafts

In this operation part of the diseased cornea is replaced by healthy corneal tissue from the eye of a dead person. Mostly a penetrating or full-thickness graft is done, but sometimes a lamellar or partial thickness graft is sufficient. The operation requires particularly meticulous attention to detail in all those concerned: surgeon, nursing staff and anaesthetist. The recent availability of tissue typing provides increasingly compatible donor material. Improved clarity of the corneal graft is then possible.

AFFECTIONS OF THE IRIS

The uveal tract comprises the iris, ciliary body and the choroid.

Inflammation of the various parts is called uveitis. Clinical types are: **acute iritis** in which the iris and ciliary body are involved, **chronic cyclitis** and **choroiditis**—each has its characteristic causes. **Sympathetic ophthalmitis** follows perforating eyeball injuries and very rarely, ophthalmic operations.

Acute iritis

Acute iritis is characterised by a painful red eye with photophobia and blurred vision with adhesions between the small pupil and the crystalline lens behind it. Inflammatory cells are seen in the aqueous humour. It can often be associated with systemic illnesses, e.g. sarcoidosis as well as ankylosing spondylosis. Symptomatic relief is obtained by dilatation of the pupil with mydriatics including atropine eye drops. Secondary glaucoma can result.

Chronic cyclitis

Chronic cyclitis runs a chronic, usually mild course and its cause is usually obscure. Treatment has little effect on the condition.

Choroiditis

Choroiditis is usually due to an easily recognisable cause, e.g. toxoplasmosis or *Toxocara canis* larval infestations, either of which is probably contracted from domestic or other animals. Symptoms are blurred vision as the inevitable inflammatory reaction spreads into the vitreous humour. In many cases no treatment is necessary but careful follow-up by the clinician is required.

Melanomas of the uvea

The uvea contains abundant pigmented cells, and is the site of naevi or 'freckles' which can easily be seen on the iris or in the ocular fundus with an ophthalmoscope. Inevitably malignant melanomas also occur at these sites. Malignant melanomas of the choroid, the commonest intra-ocular tumour, as well as those of the iris and ciliary body, are mostly slow to enlarge but result in visual loss. Choroidal tumours are liable to result in spread outside the eye most commonly to the liver, but such spread is often not discovered until many years after the eye has been enucleated. Improved modern treatment by radiotherapy or even local excision can sometimes save the eye.

DISEASES OF THE RETINA

Detachment of the retina

Separation of the retina from the choroid results from an accumulation of fluid from the vitreous body which has passed through holes in the retina. The retina becomes separated from the choroid. These holes arise from a predisposition or weakness in the retina arising in some myopic eyes, after trauma, or following cataract operations. Partial loss of the field of vision in correspondence with the extent of detached retina usually progresses quite quickly and it is essential that the patient is admitted to the eye unit as soon as possible. Early symptoms which coincide with the retinal tear, i.e. the sudden appearance of 'floaters' in the vision, must be correctly interpreted with prompt examination by an ophthalmic surgeon.

Detachment of the retina due to tears or holes is called a simple retinal detachment and this is treated surgically. A careful search for all responsible holes is essential and a drawing made in the dark room using a binocular indirect ophthalmoscope. At operation all holes are localised and cryothermy applied to them. The holes are closed nowadays by the use of silastic sponge which achieves buckling of the sclera and choroid by overlay sutures to meet the retina, obliterating the space between the choroid and retina. It is essential for reattachment of the retina that the buckle or indentation is accurately placed. Silicone rubber is also used by insertion into suitably placed pockets which have been dissected in the sclera. Encircling bands are often used since they enhance the indentation. Before and after the operation, both eyes are usually padded to encourage absorption of the fluid which separates the retina from the choroid. Bed rest with appropriate positioning of the patient may also help to encourage absorption of the sub-retinal fluid. The patient is warned against stooping or bending after the operation. Laser or light coagulation treatment has no real value once the retina has detached, but can be used to seal holes before the retina detaches.

Retinal detachment may also occur secondary to local or general inflammatory or neoplastic disease.

Retinoblastoma

This is a malignant growth of the retina which occurs in young children, usually in the first months or years of life. The condition may necessitate excision of the eye, but irradiation from cobalt plaques and chemotherapy may enable the eye to be preserved with safety. The condition may be bilateral, particularly with the autosomal-dominantly inherited variety. Spontaneous retinoblastoma due to a somatic mutation usually affects one eye only.

Retrolental fibroplasia

Retrolental fibroplasia is a condition which sometimes occurs in premature babies treated with oxygen at high concentrations. It affects both eyes and is characterised by the formation of fibrous tissue behind the lens and detachment of the retina is often present.

Retinopathy

This is associated with several medical conditions.

Hypertension and arteriosclerosis. Severe changes appear in malignant hypertension. Oedema of the optic disc with retinal haemorrhages and exudates can be seen with the ophthalmoscope. Reduced visual acuity may result. In less severe hypertension or arteriosclerosis, the following changes occur:

The vessel walls become thicker than normal and 'nipping' of the veins by the arteries occurs at crossing points. Veins may be obstructed leading to multiple retinal haemorrhages and oedema in the area of the retina served by the vein. This is called retinal vein thrombosis. Arterial obstruction due to an embolus or to arteriosclerotic blockage of the blood flow in the ophthalmic artery may simply be due to 'hardening of the arteries'.

Diabetic. The individual features visible with the ophthalmoscope are usually quite characteristic. Tiny round (dot), or slightly larger (blot) haemorrhages can be seen in the retina. These arise at the site of microaneurysms in the capillaries. White hard exudates appear, particularly in the posterior fundus. In time many patients show a tendency to the formation of new blood vessels on the retina and optic disc producing vitreous haemorrhage and retinal detachment. Diabetic retinopathy is the commonest cause of blindness in young adults in Europe and North America. Proliferative diabetic retinopathy may now often be prevented or treated by extensive ablation of the retina using photocoagulation or laser applications.

AFFECTIONS OF THE LACRIMAL APPARATUS

The lacrimal gland secretes tears which form a layer over the conjunctival sac and cornea. The fluid drains out of the conjunctival sac, via the lacrimal puncta, into the canaliculi to the lacrimal sac and via the nasolacrimal duct into the inferior meatus of the nose. If there is blockage in any of these structures, then the tears are unable to drain away and they pour on to the cheek, resulting in epiphora. The stagnant tears may become secondarily infected. A lacrimal abscess, or a mucocele, may result. Blockage of tear flow inevitably results in conjunctivitis. Although treatment by topical antibiotic is necessary, the condition will recur and operation, i.e. a new drainage channel made into the nose (dacryocysto-rhinostomy), or in some cases removal of the infected sac altogether (dacryocystectomy), is often necessary. In small children, probing the tear duct may be sufficient.

GLAUCOMA

In this condition the pressure within the eye is elevated, usually due to insufficient escape of aqueous humour from the eye rather than its excessive production. Without adequate treatment, blindness results sooner or later. Where the rise of tension is associated with some known pathological event, such as anterior uveitis, a dislocated lens or an intra-ocular tumour, then the condition is known as secondary glaucoma.

Glaucoma in infants is called buphthalmos. This results from non-development at the outflow channels for the escape of aqueous humour from the eye. The term buphthalmos indicates an enlargment of the eye which is typical for the condition. Photophobia is also usually present in the infant. Detection and treatment by an ophthalmologist are vital.

Glaucoma in adults (usually the old)

If no other pathological condition is evident in the eye, glaucoma is classified as acute with a closed 'angle', or chronic with an open 'angle'. Some chronic cases arise from a gradual closure of the angle.

In **acute closed angle glaucoma** there is a sudden elevation of the intra-ocular pressure due to sudden closure of the outflow channels in the 'angle' made by the iris and the cornea, at the iris root. The patient complains of severe pain in the eye often with vomiting, and the vision becomes blurred. The acute attack is often preceded by intermittent angle closure when the patient may complain of 'rainbows' round light bulbs, an important warning signal. The pupil becomes dilated and the eye feels hard, with resultant corneal oedema. Immediate referral to the local eye unit is necessary where treatment with intensively applied pilocarpine eye drops, as well as Diamox administered by injection rather than orally, is started. Early operation is the rule since the affected eye quickly becomes blind. An iridectomy or drainage operation, which facilitates escape of aqueous from the eye, is necessary. The unaffected eye normally needs a prophylactic (preventive) iridectomy.

Chronic open angle glaucoma. The onset of this condition is gradual so that permanent and extensive damage to vision may already have occurred before the condition is diagnosed. The field of vision may be very restricted and blindness may result although externally the eye appears normal.

Treatment

Drugs which exert an effect on the autonomic nervous system are used. Hence, those with a parasympathetic effect, e.g. guttae pilocarpine and phospholine iodide, reduce the intra-ocular pressure. Some adrenaline preparations are also useful as are drugs which block sympathetic effects (beta blocking agents).

If the raised pressure in the eye is not adequately controlled, then surgery is advised. Follow-up requires a regular assessment of the visual fields and tonometry.

OTHER AFFECTIONS OF THE EYE

Strabismus (squint)

The majority of squints begin in childhood and often arise from a refractive error in one eye. Poor vision due to any pathological eye condition also results in a squint. The majority of squints are concomitant, i.e. the angle of squint is constant in all positions of gaze, but the squint may also have originated from a hypoplasia or developmental weakness of intra-ocular muscles. Neurological disease affecting the 3rd, 4th or 6th cranial nerves causes a paralytic squint. It is therefore vital that any serious underlying neurological cause should be detected and treated at an early stage.

Severe amblyopia (a lazy eye) results if a squint in a child is not treated promptly by spectacles and appropriate occlusion or patching of an eye. When vision has improved sufficiently, correction by surgery is indicated but this is not often undertaken before the age of 3½ or 4 years. Horizontal deviations, convergence more frequently than divergence, predominate.

The onset of squints in adults coincides with diplopia (double vision) and a paralytic cause predominates. The orthoptic department is essential to the management of squints.

Nystagmus

This is an oscillatory, rhythmical, involuntary movement of the eyes in any direction, mostly horizontal. Ocular causes are often hereditary, e.g. albinism or aniridia (absence of the iris), congenital cataract or retinal malfunction. Disease of the central nervous system, e.g. disseminated sclerosis, arteriosclerosis, and inner ear disease may also be responsible.

Cataract

The normal crystalline lens is a soft, clear structure. With age it becomes harder but generally remains clear. The development of lens opacification is the condition known as cataract.

A cataract may occur as a congenital condition, and infection of the mother with rubella in the early stages of pregnancy is one such cause. Iridocyclitis, retinal detachment or injury may be the primary cause. Diabetes and some other general medical conditions may hasten on a cataract. Most commonly, cataract arises as a senile condition.

As the cataract progresses, light is less able to enter the eye and the vision deteriorates.

Treatment

When the patient's life-style is significantly impaired, a cataract extraction has become necessary. A considerable change in the focussing of the eye then results so that in most patients thick convex spectacles are necessary to achieve useful vision with a resultant increase in image size.

Some patients, especially the older ones, find difficulty in getting used to their new glasses. The use of contact lenses or intra-ocular artificial lenses, which are inserted into the eye at the time of the cataract extraction in some suitable patients, restore a normal image size for the patient.

Care of the patient for cataract surgery

A preoperative assessment is made for general medical conditions especially diabetes, cardiovascular and respiratory disease. The eyes are carefully examined to exclude possible infection and some surgeons give broad spectrum antibiotic drops for at least 48 hours preoperatively. The operation is carried out under general or local anaesthetic. The former is increasingly preferred by modern ophthalmic surgeons.

Postoperative care of the patient

This has been simplified by the use of ophthalmic surgical microscopes and increased attention to detail in suturing the incision into the anterior chamber, with the availability of improved needles and sutures.

Prompt mobilisation with early discharge home of the patient, often 1–2 days after the operation, is now possible and highly desirable for the well-being of the patient. The operated eye should be covered with a shield at night in order to reduce the risk that the patient may knock his eye during sleep. Mydriatics and local antibiotic eye drops are instilled daily. Temporary glasses are often necessary for the operated eye and those with previously poor vision rapidly become accustomed to them.

Complications

1. Postoperative mania is not uncommon in elderly patients and may subside with sedatives, but often requires the uncovering of the eye.

2. Prolapse of the iris may occur, through a gap in the incision into the eye. It is liable to occur in restless patients. Further operation may then become necessary, consisting of the excision of the prolapsed portion and resuturing of the wound.

3. Intra-ocular infection is a very serious complication and can lead to the loss of the eye.

4. Chest complications may arise as in any operation performed on a patient of advancing years who, of necessity, has been immobilised and confined to bed.

5. Haemorrhage into the eye may result from sudden movement, stooping, clumsy application of eye drops, or squeezing of the eye after instillation.

Orbital cellulitis

The whole orbit may be involved in a severe infection which may require appropriate systemic antibiotic treatment.

50
Gynaecology

Gynaecology is defined as the study of diseases peculiar to women. Today gynaecology has changed because of alterations in social attitudes. For example, population control is of worldwide concern and the gynaecologist is not only involved with the teaching and practice of contraception but also with the problems which arise as a result of contraception.

The Abortion Act of 1967 has resulted in large numbers of women coming into gynaecological wards for termination of pregnancy and yet in the next bed there might be a woman being investigated for infertility.

The nurse must always be conscious of the patients' feelings. A friendly word and a sympathetic ear will do much to help these patients and allay fears.

ANATOMY

The vulva. The labia majora are two skin folds which bound the vulval cleft and meet anteriorly at the mons pubis.

The labia minora are two small skin folds lying between the labia majora. The labia minora enclose the vaginal vestibule and each divides anteriorly to form the prepuce of the clitoris.

The clitoris consists of erectile tissue.

The mons pubis is a cushion of fat lying in front of the pubic bone.

The hymen is a septum which partially closes the vaginal orifice.

Bartholin's glands lie within the substance of the posterior part of each labia majora, the ducts of which open on the inner side of the labia minora.

The urethral orifice lies between the clitoris anteriorly and the vaginal orifice posteriorly.

The perineum is the area between the vagina and anus.

The external genital organs are illustrated in Figure 50.1.

Internal genitalia. The internal genitalia comprise the vagina, uterus, Fallopian tubes and ovaries (Figs. 50.2 and 50.3).

The vagina is a muscular canal extending from the hymen below to the cervix of the uterus above. The cervix projects into the vaginal vault and divides it into four fornices, anterior, posterior and the two lateral fornices. Anterior to the vagina is the urethra and bladder, posterior there is the rectum and pouch of Douglas.

The uterus is a pear-shaped, hollow, muscular organ about 7.5 cm long, lying in the middle of the pelvic cavity supported by ligaments. It is covered by peritoneum, except laterally where the anterior and posterior peritoneal layers pass towards the lateral walls of the pelvis forming the broad ligaments. The Fallopian tubes and the blood and lymphatic vessels of the uterus are enclosed in the broad ligaments. The uterus is divided into the body and the cervix. The part of the body above the insertion of the Fallopian tubes is known as the fundus. The uterus is lined by the endometrium, which is composed of tubular glands of columnar epithelium. The cervix, which is the lower part of the uterus, is 2.5 cm in length and projects into the top of the vagina.

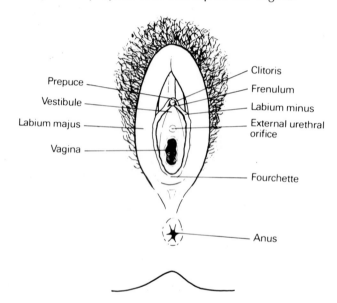

Fig. 50.1 Female external genital organs.

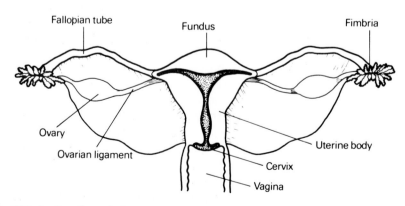

Fig. 50.2 Section through the uterus.

EXAMINATION OF PATIENT

A gynaecological examination consists of inspection and palpation of the abdomen. Examination of the breasts should also be routine. This is followed by inspection of the vulva and a bimanual examination, which may be carried out either in the left lateral or dorsal position depending on the preference of the gynaecologist.

The labia are separated and the vulva inspected. The fore-finger and middle finger are then inserted into the vagina and passed up the vagina into the anterior fornix; the other hand is placed on the patient's abdomen just above the symphysis pubis. It is then possible to palpate the body of the uterus between the two hands. The vaginal fingers are then placed in the lateral fornices, and the ovaries and tubes are similarly palpated. They are normally not felt, unless the patient is very thin.

The vagina and cervix are then visualised by inserting a vaginal speculum into the vagina. Any lesions of the cervix or vagina will then be seen, and it is at the time of visualising the cervix that a cervical smear should be taken. The equipment necessary for this procedure is illustrated in Figure 50.5. While the procedure itself is illustrated in Figure 50.6. Swabs are taken from the cervix, the vagina and the vulva when there are signs of inflammatory disease.

Other special investigations are estimation of the pituitary, the ovarian and the adrenal hormones when indicated. A midstream specimen of urine is also frequently indicated when there are urinary symptoms.

Fig. 50.5 Requirements for Papanicolaou cervical smear.
1 Sponge holder
2 Vaginal speculae (Sims and Cuscoe)
1 Ayre's spatula
1 Glass slide
1 laboratory form

Container for slide with alcohol ether
3 Wool balls
1 Disposable glove
Bag for discard
Tube of lubricant.

Fig. 50.6 Method of taking cervical smear.

DISORDERS OF MENSTRUATION

Amenorrhoea

Amenorrhoea is the absence of menstruation. Amenorrhoea may be true amenorrhoea or false amenorrhoea (cryptomenorrhoea).

   1. True amenorrhoea may be:

(a) *Physiological.* Before puberty and after the menopause, during pregnancy and lactation.

(b) *Pathological.*

   (i) Primary—when menstruation has never occurred. Primary amenorrhoea may have general causes such as severe chronic systemic disease i.e. tuberculosis, nephritis, heart disease, endocrine disorders or there may be local causes such as absence or underdevelopment of the uterus or ovaries including chromosomal abnormalities.

   (ii) Secondary—when menstruation has occurred for a time and has then ceased.

     Secondary amenorrhoea may have general causes such as a general systemic disease, including any severe illness; endocrine disorders; obesity and malnutrition; contraceptive pills; irradiation or removal of both ovaries; hysterectomy; psychological causes such as shock, grief, change of environment.

Treatment

Treatment of amenorrhoea consists in finding the cause and if possible treating it.

2. False amenorrhoea (cryptomenorrhoea) is where the patient has commenced her menses but there is no external bleeding. This is due to an imperforate hymen or imperfect canalisation of the vagina. The blood collects in the vagina forming a haematocolpos, and in neglected cases blood fills the uterus (haematometra) and even the tubes (haematosalpinges).

Abnormal bleeding

1. Menorrhagia. Excessive or prolonged blood loss at normal intervals.
2. Epimenorrhagia. The periods occur at frequent intervals and are excessively heavy or prolonged.
3. Epimenorrhoea. The periods occur at frequent intervals, but the loss is normal.
4. Metrorrhagia. Irregular and heavy bleeding, including bleeding between periods.
The above types of bleeding may be caused by:
  (a) Hormonal disorders, either an imbalance between oestrogen and progesterone or an excess of oestrogen.
  (b) Local disease, e.g. uterine growths such as fibroids or polyps, pelvic inflammatory disease.
Treatment. Find the cause and treat it.
5. Postmenopausal bleeding. This is bleeding from the genital tract that occurs after the menopause. The cause must always be diagnosed as it may be due to malignancy. Other causes are oestrogen hormonal therapy, urethral caruncle, vaginitis, polyps, ovarian tumours.
Treatment. Find the cause and treat it.

Dysmenorrhoea

Dysmenorrhoea is painful, incapacitating menstruation; there are two main types—primary and secondary dysmenorrhoea.
1. Primary. Occurs in girls and young women. It is a spasmodic pain in the pelvis, lower abdomen and back. Nausea, vomiting and fainting may occur. It commences at the beginning of a period and lasts 12–24 hours. It occurs only when the ovary is ovulating.
Treatment. Adequate analgesics and anti-prostaglandins, reassurance and encouragement to continue one's normal activities and, if this is unsuccessful, suppression of ovulation by hormones, the oral contraceptive pill being ideal. Hypnotherapy may also be useful. Dilatation of the cervix has fallen into disrepute because of the cervix becoming incompetent and causing habitual abortions.
2. Secondary. This is associated with pelvic disease, i.e. fibroids, inflammatory disease. There is a history of regular, painless menses for some years before the onset of dysmenorrhoea. The pain may commence before the menstrual flow.
Treatment. Find the cause and treat it.

DISORDERS ASSOCIATED WITH PREGNANCY

ABORTION

Definition

The termination of pregnancy before the 28th week, the foetus showing no signs of life.

It occurs spontaneously in 10-15 per cent of all pregnancies. It is caused by many factors: foetal abnormality, uterine abnormalities, hormonal disturbances, severe acute or chronic maternal disease.

Types of abortion

1. *Threatened abortion.* Vaginal bleeding occurs but the cervical canal remains closed and there are no painful uterine contractions and no part of the pregnancy sac is expelled. Treatment is by rest in bed and sedation. If progesterone deficiency can be demonstrated progestogens may be given. The pregnancy is subsequently shown to be continuing normally.

2. *Inevitable abortion.* There is severe bleeding with painful uterine contractions. The cervix dilates. Treatment is to evacuate the uterus by surgical operation. Blood transfusion may be required.

3. *Incomplete abortion.* There is severe bleeding with painful uterine contractions. The cervix dilates and part of the pregnancy sac is expelled. Treatment is surgical evacuation of the uterus. Blood transfusion may be required.

4. *Complete abortion.* This is the same as an incomplete abortion but the pregnancy sac has been expelled complete and, therefore, surgical evacuation of the uterus is not always required. Blood transfusion may be required.

5. *Missed abortion.* This is where the pregnancy dies but is not expelled from the uterus. The uterus should be encouraged to empty itself by administering either an oxytocic or prostaglandin infusion intravenously, or alternatively it may be removed by surgical evacuation if the size of the uterus is not too large.

6. *Habitual abortion* is where three or more successive abortions have occurred. This is usually associated with a uterine abnormality, i.e. congenital malformations, incompetent internal cervical os, or it may be due to hormonal imbalance. Investigate to discover the cause and treat it.

7. *Septic abortion.* Any type of abortion which is complicated by infection of the genital tract. The infection is controlled with the appropriate antibiotic followed by surgical evacuation of uterus.

8. *Therapeutic abortion.* The induction of abortion carried out for medical indications. The Abortion Act 1967 states that if, in the opinion of two registered medical practitioners, the continuation of the pregnancy is likely to endanger the life of the pregnant woman or involve risk to her mental or physical health or that of her existing family or if there is a substantial risk of foetal abnormality, then abortion may be carried out.

The uterus may be evacuated vaginally by aspiration curettage up to the 12th week; after the 12th week the uterus is usually emptied by medical means such as intra-amniotic prostaglandins and/or an intravenous prostaglandin infusion. An abdominal hysterotomy is sometimes performed.

ECTOPIC PREGNANCY

An ectopic pregnancy·is where the fertilised ovum becomes inplanted elsewhere than in the endometrium of the uterine body. It may occur in the ovary, peritoneal cavity or Fallopian tube. The commonest site is in the Fallopian tube (Fig. 50.7).

In a tubal pregnancy, as the ovum develops, either rupture of the tube or extrusion of the developing ovum into the peritoneal cavity occurs. Both processes are associated with abdominal pain, haemorrhage into the peritoneal cavity and shock.

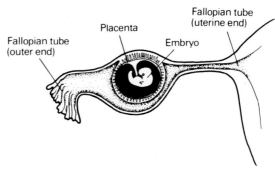

Fig. 50.7 Ectopic pregnancy in the Fallopian tube.

Symptoms and signs

There is usually a history of amenorrhoea and maybe early subjective symptoms of pregnancy. When tubal rupture or tubal abortion occurs there is lower abdominal pain and in half the cases there is some vaginal bleeding. The associated internal haemorrhage can cause referred pain to the shoulder tip and also can lead to pallor, shock, and collapse characterised by a rapid pulse and low blood pressure. On examination the abdomen is tender with some fullness and muscle guarding; free fluid may be demonstrated. Vaginal examination is often inconclusive because of extreme tenderness and pain on movement of the cervix.

Treatment

Resuscitation by blood transfusion followed by laparotomy and removal of the damaged tube. If the diagnosis is in doubt laparoscopy may be carried out before laparotomy.

HYDATIDIFORM MOLE

This condition is produced by degeneration of the chorion in early pregnancy; the foetus dies and disappears. The chorion is converted into a mass of small cysts often growing at a rapid rate.

It gives rise to severe morning sickness and symptoms of preeclampsia (raised blood pressure, oedema and proteinuria). Vaginal bleeding occurs and vesicles may be expelled. On examination the uterus is frequently larger than dates. Ultrasound scanning will show a charateristic 'picture' and no foetus will be demonstrated. Estimation of chorionic gonadotrophins will reveal a very high level and pregnancy tests will be positive in high dilution.

Treatment

The uterus is encouraged to abort the mole by either an oxytocic or prostaglandin infusion. Following abortion of the mole a curettage is performed under anaesthesia to remove any retained products.

A careful follow-up is imperative because of the risks of developing choriocarcinoma (p. 634). This should include routine clinical examinations and estimation of chorionic gonadotrophins for a minimum of two years.

INFERTILITY

Infertility is where a woman of reproductive age is unable to become pregnant. It may be primary infertility, where she has never been pregnant, or it may be secondary, when she has had a previous pregnancy.

It must be remembered that both the male and the female should be investigated.

Causes of infertility.

1. Male
   (a) Low sperm count (oligozoospermia).
   (b) Absent sperms (azoospermia).
   (c) Failure of ejaculation.
2. Female
   (a) Failure of ovulation. This might be due to pituitary failure causing lack of gonadotrophins, to ovarian failure, or to high prolactin levels.
   (b) Blocked or damaged Fallopian tubes.
   (c) Infections of the endometrium, especially an infection by tuberculosis.
   (d) Poor penetration of the cervical mucus by the sperms.
3. Coital problems. This can be due to apareunia, dyspareunia, infrequent coitus, or the incorrect calculation of the 'fertile' time.

Investigations

1. Male. Semen analysis is performed. A specimen of the seminal fluid is obtained and a sperm count is done, the motility of the sperms and the number of abnormal forms is noted.

2. Female

(a) Demonstration of ovulation by serial hormone studies, the examination of the endometrium in the 2nd half of the menstrual cycle, or by regular daily basal temperature recordings.

(b) Pituitary activity can be assessed by serial estimations of the follicular stimulating hormone (FSH) and the luteinising hormone (LH) levels in the blood. Serum prolactin levels are estimated.

(c) Tubal patency can be demonstrated by injecting a radio-opaque fluid through the cervix, it then passes through the uterus and tubes, an X-ray is taken and the uterus and tubes visualised and any spill of the fluid from the fimbrial ends of the tube denotes patency. This technique is known as hysterosalpingography. Tubal patency can also be demonstrated by laparoscopy and again injecting a dye through the cervix. If the tubes are patent dye can be seen spilling from the fimbrial ends of the tubes.

(d) Infections of the endometrium are recognised by performing a D and C. Part of the specimen of endometrium is sent for histology and part for special culture to recognise an infection e.g. by tuberculosis.

(e) A specimen of the cervical mucus is obtained approximately one hour following intercourse. It is then examined under a microscope and the depth of penetration of the sperms noted.

Treatment

1. Male. Sometimes a testicular biopsy is required to determine whether the testes are capable of forming sperms. If the capability is present the sperm count may be improved by treatment with clomiphene citrate. This is a synthetic drug which acts as a gonadtrophin.

2. Female. If there is a failure of ovulation and the ovaries are normal ovulation can be induced by either clomiphene citrate (Cyclofenil) or human gonadotrophins (Pergonal). These drugs must be carefully controlled because of the danger of multiple pregnancies.

Blocked tubes are treated by tubal surgery. The success rate is poor and even if successful can predispose to ectopic pregnancies. Some patients may be suitable for in vitro fertilisation, which can only be carried out in specialised units.

Infections of the endometrium are treated with the appropriate antibiotic.

Poor penetration of the cervical mucus by the sperms is now thought to be due to the woman developing antibodies against the sperms and treatment so far is unsuccessful.

High serum prolactin levels are treated by a course of bromocriptine.

Artificial insemination

Artificial insemination is done with the husband's seminal fluid (A.I.H.) where he is unable to achieve intercourse because of impotency. It is also done with a donor's seminal fluid (A.I.D.) where the husband has oligo or azoospermia, and the couple wish this form of treatment.

THE GENITAL TRACT

INFECTIONS OF THE GENITAL TRACT

1. Vulvovaginitis. Infections of the vulva are usually associated with infections of the vagina and they are considered together as vulvovaginitis. The signs and symptoms of vulvovaginitis are a vaginal discharge and irritation of the vulva (pruritus vulvae). The commonest causes of vulvovaginitis are listed below.

(a) *Trichomonas vaginalis,* a small unicellular organism, causes trichomoniasis. The woman can infect herself from the anal canal but it can also be spread by sexual intercourse; it is usually asymptomatic in the male.

It is characterised by a yellow discharge containing small bubbles of gas and the vaginal walls are reddened; there is vulval irritation.

Diagnosis is confirmed by examining a drop of the discharge under a microscope when the actual organisms can be seen.

Treatment is metronidazole tablets (Flagyl) 200 mg orally three times a day for 10 days or a higher dose for a shorter length of time. The partner should be treated also.

(b) *Candida albicans (Monilia)* causes a fungal infection (moniliasis, or thrush) and is especially common in diabetics. The discharge is thick and white and there is intense irritation. The diagnosis is confirmed by culture of a vaginal swab; the fungus can then be identified by microscopy.

Treatment is by nystatin pessaries, or other anti-fungal pessaries and cream. The partner should also be treated with anti-fungal cream.

(c) *Gonorrhoea.* This infection by the *Gonococcus* is again becoming more prevalent. It is a venereal disease and manifests itself by a vulvovaginitis; it can also cause infection of Bartholin's glands, cervicitis and urethritis. The discharge is yellow and there may be accompanying dysuria.

Diagnosis is by cervical and urethral smears which show the gonococci; these may be grown on culture.

A course of an appropriate antibiotic cures the infection.

(d) *Chlamydia.* This organism has now been shown to cause vulvovaginitis, cervicitis and salpingitis. A special culture medium is required. The treatment is erythromycin 500 mg q.i.d. for 10 days. The partner should also be treated.

(e) *Non-specific infections.* Many bacteria can cause vulvovaginitis, and diagnosis is made by culturing a vaginal swab, identifying the bacteria and giving the appropriate antibiotic.

If this occurs in elderly patients after the menopause it is called senile vaginitis, and is due to the reduction of oestrogen causing the vagina to contain less lactic acid and therefore, to be more easily infected. Treatment is by giving a short course of an oestrogen either orally or in pessary form.

2. Cervicitis. This is an acute infection of the cervix, commonly due to the gonococcus but can follow puerperal sepsis or even arise from a vulvovaginitis.

There is a purulent vaginal discharge and pus can be seen exuding through the external cervical os.

The organisms should be indentified from a swab and the appropriate antibiotic given.

3. Endometritis. This due to infection of the endometrium of the body of the uterus.

Acute endometritis usually occurs after abortion or childbirth. It causes a raised temperature and pulse rate, and a bloodstained purulent discharge. The treatment is to identify the bacteria by a swab and give the appropriate antibiotic.

Chronic endometritis may be due to tuberculosis and is diagnosed by endometrial biopsy. It can also occur where there is blockage of the cervical canal. The uterus distends with retained pus and forms a pyometra. The most frequent cause in an elderly patient is a carcinoma either of the body of the uterus or the cervix.

4. Salpingitis. This condition should be more correctly referred to as salpingo-oophoritis as both the tubes and ovaries are usually involved. It may be acute or chronic.

Acute salpingo-oophoritis. This may be gonococcal, may follow infection at childbirth or abortion, or may spread from an abdominal focus, e.g. the appendix.

The patient complains of severe lower abdominal pain, the temperature and pulse rise, tenderness and rigidity of the lower abdomen may be present. There may be a purulent vaginal discharge.

On examination the lower abdomen is found to be acutely tender; on pelvic examination movement of the cervix causes pain and palpation through the fornices is extremely painful. A leucocytosis develops.

Chronic salpingo-oophoritis. This can follow acute salpingo-oophoritis or it may be due to tuberculous infection. The patient presents with general ill-health, lower abdominal pain, menstrual irregularities, vaginal discharge, and infertility. The majority of cases resolve with antibiotic therapy or short-wave pelvic diathermy. In cases which do not resolve with treatment surgery is required for removal of the infected tubes. If the patient is over 40 years old then hysterectomy with removal of both tubes and ovaries is the best treatment.

Treatment

A cervical swab should be taken to identify the bacteria and then the appropriate antibiotic is given.

Complications

(a) Pyosalpinx—the tube becomes sealed and distended with pus.

(b) Tubo-ovarian abscess—a large abscess cavity forms involving both tube and ovary.

(c) Pelvic abscess.

(d) Narrowing of the tube due to adhesions and subsequently an ectopic pregnancy.

(e) Infertility due to blocked tubes.

DISPLACEMENT OF THE GENITAL TRACT

1. Prolapse

Uterovaginal prolapse is where the supports of the vagina and uterus are weakened so that the walls of the vagina bulge into the cavity of the vagina and may protrude through the vaginal introitus. The uterus may also descend down the vagina and emerge at the vaginal introitus.

The vaginal and uterine supports are weakened by child-bearing, and also after the menopause there is atrophy of these supports. There are various types of uterovaginal prolapse.

(a) *Cystocele.* This is prolapse of the anterior vaginal wall together with the base of the bladder.

(b) *Rectocele.* This is prolapse of the lower part of the posterior vaginal wall together with the rectum.

(c) *Enterocele.* This is prolapse of the upper part of the posterior vagina wall together with the pouch of Douglas.

(d) *Uterovaginal prolapse, first degree*—the uterus descends the vagina until the cervix reaches the introitus.

(e) *Uterovaginal prolapse, second degree*—the cervix protrudes outside the introitus.

(f) *Uterovaginal prolapse, third degree*—the whole uterine body lies outside the introitus; this is sometimes known as a procidentia.

Clinical features

(i) The patient may complain of a lump in the vagina or a feeling of 'something is coming down'.

(ii) Backache and a bearing-down sensation.

(iii)Disturbances of micturition, frequency and dysuria, stress incontinence.

(iv)Bleeding due to the protruding prolapse becoming ulcerated.

(v) Difficulty in defaecation.

Treatment

The treatment of choice is a surgical repair of the prolapse. This consists essentially of excising the redundant parts of the vaginal walls and tightening-up the supporting fascia and pelvic muscles.

(a) Cystocele. This is repaired by anterior colporrhaphy.

(b) Rectocele. This is repaired by combining a posterior colporrhaphy with reconstituting a new perineal body by an operation known as a perineorrhaphy; the operation is, therefore, known as posterior colpoperineorrhaphy.

(c) Enterocele. This is repaired at the same time as the posterior colpoperineorrhaphy.

(d) Uterovaginal prolapse. The minor degrees are repaired by anterior colporrhaphy and posterior colpoperineorrhaphy, and the Mackenrodt ligaments are tightened combined with amputation of the cervix; this is known as a Fothergill's operation, or a Manchester repair.

The major degrees are better treated by a vaginal hysterectomy followed by an anterior colporrhaphy and posterior colpoperineorrhaphy.

If patients are unfit or unwilling to have an operation a pliable ring pessary made from polythene or vinyl is squeezed and inserted into the vagina: when it opens out it takes up the slack in the vaginal walls. The patient is not cured but her symptoms are relieved; however, she must attend at approximately 3-monthly intervals for the vagina to be inspected for infection or ulceration and for the ring to be changed.

2. Retroversion and retroflexion

Backward displacement is usually a combination of retroversion and retroflexion (Fig. 50.8). The condition occurs normally in approximately 15 per cent of women and is usually symptomless.

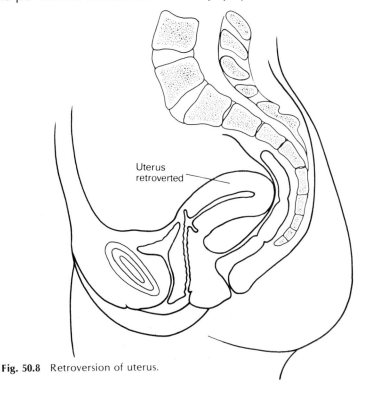

Uterus retroverted

Fig. 50.8 Retroversion of uterus.

It may first occur in the puerperium as the uterus involutes, or it may be drawn backwards by fibrosis from infection or endometriosis, or may be pushed backwards by tumours such as a fibroid or ovarian tumour.

It is now thought that the retroversion is symptomless and any existing symptoms, i.e. backache, menorrhagia, dysmenorrhoea, infertility and abortion, are symptoms of the associated condition.

If, however, the ovaries prolapse into the pouch of Douglas, dyspareunia can result and is an indication to perform one of the uterine suspension operations.

A Hodge pessary may be inserted to correct the retroversion, but it is usually only used to confirm that the symptoms the patient is complaining about are due to the retroversion.

TUMOURS

1. Vulval tumours

Benign

Bartholin's cyst is caused by blockage of the duct of Bartholin's gland and contains mucoid fluid (Fig. 50.9). It is treated by marsupialisation (incision into the cyst and suturing its lining to the skin leaving a permanent stoma).

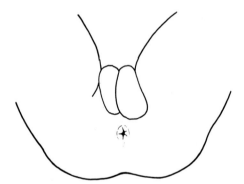

Fig. 50.9 Bartholin's cyst.

Fibromas, lipomas and papillomas. These should be excised.

Malignant

Squamous cell carcinoma of the vulva usually arises in women past the menopause and can be predisposed to by leucoplakia. It presents as an ulcer with everted edges. The inguinal lymph glands are involved in the course of the disease.

Treatment is by excision of the vulva and removal of the inguinal, femoral and iliac glands (radical vulvectomy). Radiotherapy may be used for recurrences, but the tumour is not usually radiosensitive.

2. Urethral tumours

Benign

Urethral caruncle. This is a small pedunculated swelling of the posterior lip of the urethral meatus; it is very tender, may cause dysuria and slight bleeding. It consists of adenomatous vascular tissue.

Treatment is by excision, frequently done by diathermy.

Malignant

Carcinoma of the urethra is very rare.

3. Vaginal tumours

Benign

Vaginal cysts. These are usually asymptomatic and found on routine examination. If causing symptoms they are excised.

Malignant

Primary carcinoma of the vagina is rare and is treated by radiotherapy. **Secondary carcinoma** may follow uterine carcinoma.

4. Uterine tumours

Benign tumours

Polyps can arise in the uterine cavity or cervical canal. They cause menorrhagia, intermenstrual bleeding, postcoital bleeding and post-menopausal bleeding.

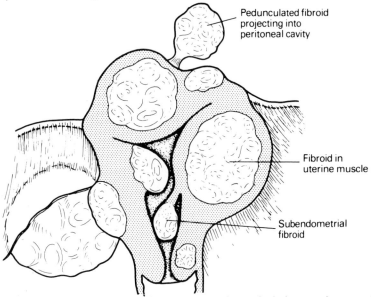

Pedunculated fibroid projecting into peritoneal cavity

Fibroid in uterine muscle

Subendometrial fibroid

Fig. 50.10 A fibroid uterus showing the various sites from which the growths may arise.

Treatment. The uterine cavity polyps are curetted away and the cervical ones removed by twisting them off.

Fibromyomas. These are more commonly known as fibroids (Fig. 50. 10). They occur usually after the age of 30 years and never arise for the first time after the menopause. They are more common in women who have not had children. Fibroids are more likely to arise in the body of the uterus than the cervix. They are composed of muscle and fibrous tissue, may be single or multiple and can be from a pinhead size to enormous size. They can lie under the peritoneal surface (subperitoneal) or protrude into the cavity (submucous) or be in the wall of the uterus (interstitial). They may also develop pedicles (pedunculated).

Fibroids may be symptomless, but the common symptoms are menorrhagia, and pressure symptoms due to their weight. Pain is due to complications such as degeneration of the fibroids or torsion of a pedunculated fibroid. Enlargement of the abdomen may be the only complaint.

Treatment. Small asymptomatic fibroids do not require any treatment. Myomectomy is performed if the woman is of child-bearing age and has no children or is desirous of further children. Abdominal hysterectomy is performed if the woman is past child-bearing age or has completed her family.

Malignant tumours

Carcinoma of the cervix (Fig. 50.11). This can arise at any age but is more common between the age of 40 and 50 years. However it is now

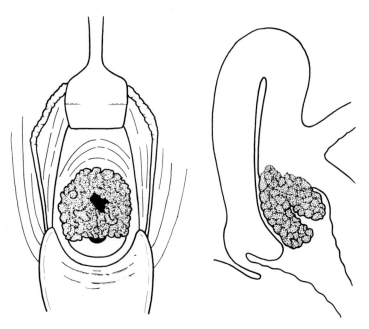

Fig. 50.11 Carcinoma of the cervix. A large carcinoma as seen through a vaginal speculum. Note that the bladder is already invaded by the growth.

occurring more frequently in younger patients. There is evidence to suggest that the causative factor is transmitted by coitus; it is more common in people who commence coitus early in life and have many sexual partners. As it is rare in Jews, it is also suggested that it may be related to coitus with uncircumcised partners. There are various stages of carcinoma of the cervix.

Stage O. This often known as either pre-invasive carcinoma or carcinoma in situ. This stage precedes the development of many cases of invasive carcinoma. It is asymptomatic and can only be discovered by a cervical smear followed by biopsies. Many cases do not progress to invasive carcinoma.

Stage I. Invasive carcinoma confined to cervix.

Stage IIa. Spread to vaginal vault.

Stage IIb. Spread to parametrium but cervix not fixed.

Stage III. Spread to lower two-thirds vagina or parametrial spread and cervix fixed.

Stage IV. Involvement of bladder and rectum or metastases outside the pelvis.

Symptoms

(i) A watery discharge which may be bloodstained and offensive.

(ii) Irregular vaginal bleeding.

(iii) Postcoital bleeding.

(iv) Pain; this is a late symptom signifying involvement of other organs.

(v) Incontinence of urine or faeces due to fistula formation.

Diagnosis. Cervical cytology by routine cervical smear in all women over 30 years at regular intervals yields about five positive smears per 1000. These are followed up by biopsy of the whole squamocolumnar junction (cone biopsy), or by colposcopy and a limited biopsy.

Treatment. If the biopsy shows the carcinoma to be pre-invasive and it is completely excised the case may be followed up by repeated smears, otherwise total hysterectomy is the treatment of choice. The more recent and developing form of treatment for pre-invasive lesions is to identify the lesion by staining with an iodine preparation, examining the cervix with a colp-microscope and destroying the lesion with a laser beam. This form of treatment is particularly valuable in the younger woman as it is much less destructive and will have less effect on a subsequent pregnancy and labour.

If the biopsy shows it to be invasive then the choice is between radiotherapy and surgery in operable cases, the results being much the same. Most gynaecologists these days favour radiotherapy.

If surgery is decided upon, Wertheim's hysterectomy is done. This is a total hysterectomy and bilateral salpingo-oophorectomy; the upper third of the vagina is removed and also the pelvic lymph glands.

Prognosis. The five-year survival rates are:

Stage I 75 per cent

Stage II 50 per cent

Stage III and IV 10 per cent

Carcinoma of the body of the uterus. Usually occurs in women past the menopause but can occur before. Occurs equally in women who have had children and those who have not. It is an important cause of post-menopausal bleeding.

Symptoms. Intermenstrual bleeding and postmenopausal bleeding. There may be some uterine enlargement.

Diagnosis is by diagnostic curettage of the uterus.

Treatment. Total hysterectomy and bilateral salpingo-oophorectomy and removal of a wide cuff of the vagina.

Some gynaecologists give pre-or postoperative radiotherapy to reduce the risks of recurrence at the vaginal vault. Progestogens are now given to most patients pre- and postoperatively for up to 2 years. Radiotherapy and progestogens can be used palliatively in inoperable cases.

Choriocarcinoma (chorion-epithelioma). This highly malignant tumour follows a hydatidiform mole. It is treated by total hysterectomy and bilateral salpingo-oophorectomy. Any metastases will respond to folic acid antagonists such as methotrexate. This may be combined with a cytotoxic drug.

5. Ovary

Ovarian tumours are often referred to as ovarian cysts but it must be remembered that many of them are solid tumours. They can arise in any age group. There are many different types of tumour arising from different types of tissue. They can be benign or highly malignant; they may even be a secondary tumour to a primary in the stomach, colon or breast.

Symptoms are few. Uncomplicated cysts are often symptomless; swelling of the abdomen may be the only complaint. Menstrual upset is rare. Pain can occur if complications such as torsion (Fig. 50.12), rupture or

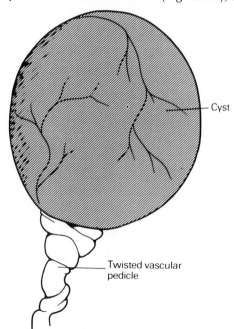

Cyst

Twisted vascular pedicle

Fig. 50.12 Torsion of an ovarian cyst.

infection arise or if the tumour is malignant. Pressure symptoms such as oedema of the legs or dyspnoea may occur.

Treatment. If benign, the tumour is resected leaving part of the ovary. Malignant tumours if operable are treated by total hysterectomy and bilateral salpingo-oophorectomy. If inoperable as much as possible of the tumour should be removed, and the patient should then be treated with cytotoxic drugs, e.g. cisplatin. Most tumours are not radiosensitive.

6. Fallopian tubes

Tumours of the Fallopian tubes both benign and malignant are extremely rare.

ENDOMETRIOSIS

This is a condition where endometrial tissue occurs in ectopic situations such as ovaries, myometrium and other pelvic organs. It is benign.

Symptoms. Endometriosis only occurs during reproductive life. It causes infertility, secondary dysmenorrhoea, menstrual upsets, and dyspareunia.

Endometriosis causes the formation of tender, bilateral masses involving the tubes and ovaries. These are known as 'chocolate cysts' as they contain a chocolate-like fluid. The uterus can become enlarged.

Treatment. In young women the affected tissue is excised attempting to conserve some ovarian tissue. Prolonged hormone therapy with danazol for up to 12 months causes the endometriosis to regress. In older patients total hysterectomy and bilateral salpingo-oophorectomy is performed. Danazol is usually given both pre- and postoperatively.

PREOPERATIVE AND POSTOPERATIVE CARE OF PATIENTS

Preoperative preparation

Prior to any operative procedure the patient must be suitably prepared. The patient is admitted to hospital 1 or 2 days before operation. Some minor procedures are now performed as day cases.

1. Routine observations are made on admission: temperature, pulse, blood pressure.
2. Urinalysis.
3. Vaginal swab if any evidence of infection.
4. General medical examination.
5. Haemoglobin checked, blood grouped and cross-matched if considered necessary.
6. Consent form signed. Husband's signature should be obtained in a younger patient if the operation will render her sterile. This is however not legally essential.
7. Patient's abdomen or perineum shaved for major operations.
8. Bowel preparation is important, enemas or suppositories are necessary in some cases.

9. A bath or bedbath is necessary the evening before operation and the morning of surgery.
10. Night sedatives are given to ensure that the patient has a good sleep before surgery.
11. Food is withheld for 6 hours before operation.

Postoperative care

(a) Minor cases

(i) Immediate postoperative care is the same as for any postoperative theatre case.
(ii) Minor cases are allowed up and about as soon as they are able to manage.
(iii) Vaginal blood loss is observed.

(b) Major cases

(i) Immediate postoperative care is as for any postoperative theatre case.
(ii) Observation of pulse, temperature, blood pressure, wound condition and vaginal loss are made and recorded.
(iii) Analgesics are given as prescribed.
(iv) Intravenous therapy may be ordered.
(v) Fluid intake and output is recorded.
(vi) The patient should be seen by the physiotherapist as soon as possible after surgery.
(vii) Early mobilisation is extremely important to prevent deep venous thrombosis.
(viii) Haemoglobin estimation is carried out on the second postoperative day.
(ix) Vaginal pack. Following major vaginal surgery there is frequently a vaginal pack inserted to prevent bleeding. This often causes difficulty in micturition and, therefore, a catheter is also inserted. The pack is usually removed in 24 hours and the catheter in 48 hours. Following the removal of the catheter the patient may be catheterised on a subsequent day to determine whether there is any residual urine following micturition. If there is, the catheter will be left in situ for a further 48-72 hours.
(x) On the seventh to 10th day abdominal sutures or clips are removed.
(xi) After major surgery patients are usually discharged from hospital on the 10th to 14th postoperative day and are subsequently seen in the follow-up clinic. They may be discharged earlier after more minor procedures.

GYNAECOLOGICAL OPERATIONS

D and C. This stands for dilation of the cervix and curettage of the uterus. This is usually done for diagnostic reasons, the curettings being examined histologically. Curettage can be therapeutic in cases such as incomplete abortion.

Abdominal hysterectomy. A total hysterectomy is where the complete uterus is removed. A subtotal hysterectomy is where only the body of the uterus is removed and the cervix left behind; this is not often carried out except where there are technical difficulties in removing the cervix.

Salpingo-oophorectomy is removal of one or both Fallopian tubes and ovaries. This may be carried out for ovarian or tubal disease; it is often combined with hysterectomy.

Ovarian cystectomy. This is removal of a benign ovarian cyst by shelling it out of its capsule and reconstructing the remains of the ovary into its normal shape.

Salpingostomy and reimplantation of tubes. These are performed in cases of infertility where tubal blockage has been demonstrated.

Wertheim's hysterectomy. This is performed for carcinoma of the cervix and is described under that heading.

Pelvic floor repair and vaginal hysterectomy. These are performed for prolapse and are described under that heading.

Simple vulvectomy and radical vulvectomy. These are performed for malignant tumours of the vulva.

Sterilisation is an operation carried out to prevent further pregnancies. Many methods are used but most are based on dividing the tube, separating and ligating the cut ends.

Laparoscopy. This is the insertion of a laparoscope through the abdominal wall to visualise the pelvic organs. It is principally a diagnostic procedure but sterilisation can also be performed in this way by diathermising the tubes or constricting the tubes with small rubber rings or metal clips.

Myomectomy. The removal of fibroids from the uterus and reconstruction of the uterus.

Shirodkhar's operation. This operation is the insertion of a purse-string suture around the cervix to prevent habitual abortions due to an incompetent internal cervical os.

Vacuum curettage. This is to terminate a pregnancy in the first 12 weeks.

Colposcopy. This is the insertion of an instrument into the vagina to visualise the cervix, frequently a microscope is attached and it is then known as colpo-microscopy.

Hysterotomy. This is the abdominal removal of a pregnancy, usually in the mid-trimester.

FAMILY PLANNING

A nurse should know something of the methods available and where expert help and advice can be obtained.

Male contraception

1. Coitus interruptus. This is withdrawal of the penis from the vagina immediately before ejaculation and is one of the oldest methods used. It is unsafe and psychological strain can be placed on both partners.

2. Condom or sheath. They are worn over the penis during intercourse to prevent the seminal fluid being deposited in the vagina. It is reasonably effective but may be made safer by the use of a spermicidal agent.

Female contraception

1. Rhythm method (safe period). This is the only method acceptable to some people. It is based on the fact that in a regular menstrual cycle ovulation occurs 13 to 15 days prior to the next period, and fertilisation is possible up to five days before or 2 days after ovulation: Allowing for an extra day at either end, intercourse should be avoided for these 12 days of the cycle. It is an unreliable form of contraception.

2. Occlusive caps (diaphragm, cervical cap). These are devices which cover the cervix and mechanically obstruct the entrance of spermatozoa. If used with a spermicidal cream or jelly it is a good form of contraception.

3. Chemical contraceptives. These are all chemical agents which kill spermatozoa. They are incorporated in jellies, creams, pessaries and aerosol foams. They are relatively ineffective when used alone but should be combined with a mechanical barrier, i.e. sheath or diaphragm.

4. Intrauterine contraceptive devices (IUCD). IUCDs are small plastic devices which are inserted into the uterine cavity. There are many designs, i.e. Lippes loop, Saf-T-Coil, etc. Some have copper wire round the stem. The copper is supposed to react with the cervical mucus and repel the sperms. The mode of actions of IUCDs is uncertain but it is now thought that conception takes place but the fertilised ovum cannot become implanted in the uterine cavity. They are not ideal as they may cause menstrual upsets, dysmenorrhoea, pelvic infections, or ectopic pregnancies. They can also perforate the uterus and enter the peritoneal cavity. Also pregnancies can occur with them in place and it is, therefore, recommended that they be used in conjunction with a spermicidal agent.

5. Oral contraception. Oral contraceptives are usually a combination of oestrogen and progesterone, or progesterone alone. The first are taken cyclically and the second continuously. They act in several ways. Ovulation is inhibited; the cervical mucus is rendered hostile to sperms which are, therefore, unable to penetrate the cervical mucus; and lastly the endometrium is not suitable for implantation of any fertilised ovum.

It is a reliable form of contraception and with the newer low dose pills the side effects are minimal. It is contraindicated in certain circumstances, i.e. known thrombotic disease, liver damage, etc.

Sterilisation

This is by tubal ligation in the female or ligation of the vas deferens in the male. It is a permanent method of contraception.

51
Iatrogenic disorders

The aim of all medical treatment is, if possible, to cure the patient and to relieve symptoms. Unfortunately the treatment itself sometimes gives rise to complications or specific disorders.

In some instances mishaps occur which could easily have been avoided. In other cases a condition arises which could not have been foreseen. In many cases the complications and risks of treatment are well recognised but are either unavoidable or considered a low price to pay compared with the benefits gained.

The conditons resulting from medical intervention are called iatrogenic disorders.

The following is a brief summary of such disorders.

They may be:

1. Physical injuries from surgical apparatus or a surgical environment.
2. Chemical injuries.
3. Drug toxicity and idiosyncrasy.
4. Direct operative complications.
5. The effects of surgical ablation.

It is incumbent upon all who are involved in the care of patients to avoid or minimise the occurrence of iatrogenic disorders.

PHYSICAL INJURIES

These are numerous and fairly obvious. They include:

Burns

These may occur from:

1. *Chemicals* used on the wrong tissue or in too concentrated a strength. There is no substitute for a personal check of the label on the container.

2. *Hot-water bottles.* These burns can be avoided by not using hot-water bottles. They are unnecessary.

3. *Surgical diathermy* incorrectly used. A high-frequency current

generates heat passing through the body but does not cause an electric shock. This has already been considered in detail (Ch. 10).

4. Radioactive material. Treatment by radiotherapy may give rise to burns of skin or deeper organs.

Explosions

See Chapter 10.

Foreign bodies

See Chapter 10.

A needle may break off in the tissues. A swab or instrument may be left in the body at operation. This is always avoidable by adherence to strict checking methods.

Pressure and traction

These injuries may arise from:

1. Tourniquets. Their use is rarely required for control of haemorrhage and if used to provide a bloodless operation field they must be removed by the person who applied them.

2. Plaster casts and splints. If too tight, plaster casts and splints act as tourniquets with the most devasting effects.

3. Pressure sores. These may occur from the roughened edges of a plaster. Even more important are sores in which the body weight is one factor. Others are loss of sensation, incontinence, excessive sweating, oedema and an impaired circulation.

4. Nerve paresis. This is particularly liable to occur if the brachial plexus is stretched or the radial nerve suffers pressure from lying on the edge of the table. The lateral popliteal nerve may be damaged by severe pressure or may be stretched from traction over the neck of the fibula. Drug injection into the radial or sciatic nerves may also cause paresis.

Confinement to bed

This may cause no special trouble, but it may initiate a chain reaction giving rise to conditions such as:

1. Thrombosis and embolism. The incidence of these is diminishing but not abolished by early postoperative ambulation and the measures mentioned in Chapter 18.

2. Diminished blood volume. This occurs from confinement to bed and, in general, patients should be up and about before operation or, if this is impossible, the blood volume should be restored preoperatively. If it is not, drugs used for the induction of anaesthesia which cause vasodilation may bring on early circulatory collapse. A small amount of bleeding will cause a similar effect.

3. Retention of urine. This is commonly due to some degree of prostatic obstruction, particularly in elderly men.

4. *Pressure sores and deformities,* such as drop foot.

5. *Faecal impaction.*

The surgical environment

The best surgical environment is that in which the access of infective organisms to wounds is prevented. This ideal is rarely achieved completely.

DRUGS AND THERAPEUTIC SUBSTANCES

A few general principles are important. They are:

1. Identification

This is fundamental. If a drug is to be injected the solution must be drawn into the syringe after the label has been read by two people one of whom is a qualified nurse or a doctor. The same care is essential with fluid for infusion. Mixtures dangerous for infusion should be coloured, for example, sodium citrate for use in the bladder.

Blood is particularly important. The most essential precaution is that the correct cross-matched bottle for the patient is the one being handled. Then it should be checked that:

(a) It is the correct group.

(b) The Rh typing is correct.

(c) That it is not out of date.

(d) A careful watch should be kept that the first 50-100 ml are causing no reaction.

2. Drug therapy in progress when surgery is necessary

This should be reviewed in the light of possible consequences. Particularly important are:

(a) **Anticoagulant therapy.** This must always be temporarily reversed by the intravenous administration of protamine sulphate for heparin, or of vitamin K in the case of warfarin.

(b) **Corticosteroid therapy.** This delays healing, but if the dosage is reduced too rapidly the original condition for which the patient is being treated may flare up in a fulminating form. Therefore before surgery corticosteroid therapy must be increased so that the response to injury (p. 295) can occur. Afterwards it is reduced gradually.

Drug reactions. There are many complications of steroid therapy which may be of surgical importance. The commonest are:

(i) Reactivation of quiescent pulmonary tuberculosis.

(ii) Bleeding from a peptic ulcer.

(iii) Development of fulminating infections, such as appendicitis, which progress silently.

(iv) The rapid development of cardiac failure.

Other complications include thrombosis, osteoporosis, psychosis, myopathies and skin reactions such as acne and hirsutism.

(c) The correct drug by the wrong route. This may cause great harm. Thiopentone, so effective intravenously, causes arterial thrombosis with gangrene of the hand if given into the brachial artery.

(d) The correct rate. This must be determined for any substance given intravenously.

Complications of drug therapy

Sensitivity in some individuals is almost inevitable; there is almost no drug to which some individual may not be sensitive. This may vary from a severe anaphylactic reaction to a mild skin rash.

Resistant organisms may develop.

Normally suppressed organisms may proliferate.

Anaemia and damage to the blood-forming tissues may occur. Chloramphenicol, the sulphonamides and most of the cytotoxic drugs used in malignant disease, as well as radiotherapy, are particularly notable.

Crystallisation in the kidney may occur from some sulphonamides associated with an inadequate fluid intake, particularly with an acid urine.

Damage to the nucleus of the VIIIth cranial nerve is almost always due to the aminoglycosides (streptomycin, neomycin).

Vitamin B deficiency is most liable to occur from alteration of the intestinal flora by the tetracycline group of antibiotics.

Jaundice may occur from blood plasma (infective) or drugs. Notable are:

Halothane—used in anaesthesia.
Methyldopa—used for hypertension.
Chlorpromazine—an anxiolytic drug.
Phenylbutazone—an anti-inflammatory agent.
Ampicillin ⎱ antibiotics.
Tetracycline ⎰

Intestinal ulceration with stricture formation may result from enteric-coated diuretic capsules containing potassium chloride.

Gastric erosions are common from the irritation of aspirin as well as phenylbutazone.

Coma and respiratory failure may be quite alarming following small doses of morphia in a sensitive patient.

Abdominal pain may be severe from excessive dosage of vitamin D, while constipation may result from ganglion-blocking drugs used in the treatment of hypertension.

Sclerosing peritonitis is a complication of practolol.

Retrolental fibroplasia may result from the administration of oxygen in excess of 35 per cent, to the newborn.

Gangrene may result from severe spasm produced by ergot.

Glaucoma is aggravated by atropine.

Citrate intoxication after massive blood transfusion. In addition to causing reduction of serum calcium stored blood contains excess of potassium ions.

DIRECT AND INDIRECT OPERATIVE COMPLICATIONS

These have been considered under specific diseases, but in general may be:

1. Direct damage from trauma.
2. Obstruction postoperatively.
3. Fluid leakage from the (i) blood vessels, (ii) the suture line in visceral anastomoses.
4. Metabolic changes from surgical intervention. Re-operation may be indicated for (a) fluid leakage (including haemorrhage) and (b) obstruction.
5. Infections.

OPERATIVE ABLATION

The effects which arise from operative ablation depend on the extent of the ablation, to what extent the functional reserves of the body are adequate and to what degree, if any, disability can be overcome or minimised by artificial means. Many of the physiological consequences which arise take time to manifest themselves. The longer the results of many ablations are studied, the more wide-reaching their effects are discovered to be.

Miscellaneous iatrogenic lesions

The obvious sequelae of amputation of the limbs or the breast need no special stress except the importance of ensuring that such mutilation is undertaken only for compelling indications.

Even where the functional reserve is adequate, as in the kidneys, the ovaries or the testes, a conservative attitude to removal is essential, since time may bring similar or more severe disease to the contralateral organ.

Ductless gland ablation can be largely overcome by administration of the appropriate hormone if its removal causes a deficiency. More difficult and more complicated are the effects of extirpation of large amounts of gastrointestinal tract.

Physiological and anatomical shortening of the digestive tract

The stomach. The greatest effects in proportion to the amount removed are seen after gastrectomy, partly due to anatomical and physiological exclusion of the duodenum. The main effects are:

1. Limited intake of food.
2. Anaemia.
3. Vitamin deficiency.
4. Intestinal hurry.
5. Defective absorption.
6. Enterocolitis (possibly from achlorhydria).

7. Other syndromes:
   (a) Face flushing.
   (b) Hypoglycaemia.
   (c) Bilious vomiting.
8. Osteoporosis.

The small intestine. Resection of large lengths of the small intestine results in loss of weight and some frequency of stools.

Intestinal hurry occurs in all conditions of physiological shortening of which gastrectomy is one of the most important examples.

The large intestine. This has a considerable functional reserve and more than half can be removed without any great effect.

The gall-bladder. Cholecystectomy results in dilute bile dribbling into the duodenum as it is formed. Most patients after cholecystectomy have no great disability although there may be a certain amount of windy discomfort and a bowel action which is freer than usual.

After removal of the gall bladder the patient should be able to eat a reasonable amount of fat but not excessive quantities. In the immediate postoperative phase fat should be liberally supplied to encourage biliary drainage and to avoid further colic from inspissated mucus or a tiny fragment of gravel which may form the nidus of a further stone.

The pancreas. Pancreatectomy, which is usually undertaken for neoplasm, causes:

1. Diabetes, control of which presents no great difficulty.
2. Steatorrhoea, diminished by giving pancreatic enzymes.
3. Diminished calcium absorption.
4. Fat and protein absorption is also disturbed.

Most operative procedures produce after-effects which are usually of a minor nature. The more seriously ill the patient beforehand the more ready he is to accept these discomforts, but where preoperative symptoms, especially pain, have been slight the less likely is the patient to be tolerant of postoperative symptoms. It is rightly said that the bad results of operations for peptic ulceration are more frequently the results of bad selection of patients than of bad surgery.

SOME BIOGRAPHICAL NOTES

Hippocrates (460-370 BC) is considered to be the father of modern medicine for he severed medicine from witchcraft and superstition and transformed it into a science based on observation. He travelled widely throughout Greece setting up teaching centres and left model clinical records for posterity (his descriptions of epilepsy and puerperal septi-caemia could be found in any modern textbook). His work was assisted by his emphasis on good nursing and a balanced diet. The Hippocratic oath is a tribute to the high ethical standards he brought to the profession.

Galen (AD 130-200). Prior to 1500, Galen was second only to Hippo-crates in medicine, and his theories, both correct and erroneous, were accepted without question. After serving the Roman Emperor Marcus Aurelius as personal physician, he retired to write and to study. He was the first experimental physiologist and discovered that the arteries contained blood and that contraction of muscle occurred independently of the nerve supply. Among his other important discoveries were his explanations of respiration and inflammation. His work on anatomy was less successful for he based all his findings on the dissection of animals. As a physician he placed great reliance on drugs, notably opium, sugar and alcohol. While some of his teaching misled, his collection of 80 books preserved much that was finest in ancient medicine throughout the Dark Ages.

Ambroise Pare (1510-1590). By his own skill and personality, Pare raised the status of surgery from a despised mechanical art to that of a major profession, using the new discoveries in anatomy to advance surgery. By the discovery that gunshot wounds were not poisonous and required soothing applications rather than boiling oil and by his advocacy of artificial limbs for wounded soldiers, he brought much relief to the surgery of the battlefield. To prevent bleeding after amputation, he replaced the indiscriminate use of a red hot cautery with a simple ligature. Among his other work was the invention of artery forceps, detailed discussion of the treatment of fractures and dislocations and the suggestion that syphilis was the cause of aneurysm. He established himself in a position of great authority as surgeon to four French kings, and riled the established physicians of the time by scorning such remedies as powdered mummy and a unicorn's head.

Andreas Vesalius (1514-1564). By freeing anatomy from many of Galen's errors, Vesalius laid the foundation on which many subsequent advances in medicine and surgery could take place. At the age of 23 he was Professor of Anatomy at Padua University and his great work, the *Fabrica*, published in 1543, corrected Galen on many points, completely destroying Galen's osteology and muscle anatomy. For instance, he found the lower jaw consisted of a single bone, that loss of the spleen was compatible with life, and he destroyed such fallacies as the double bile duct and the five-lobed liver. His work on the spinal cord showed the means by which the brain acts on the various muscles of the limbs and trunk. By 1555 he had laid the basis of Harvey's discovery of the circulation by denying the existence of interventricular pores and by noting the existence of valves in the vein without appreciating their significance. His later years were spent as physician to the Emperor Charles V.

St Vincent de Paul (1576-1660) was the founder of the Sisters of Charity. Destined for the Church he was sold into slavery on his capture by pirates. After his release he returned to Paris to fight against poverty, ignorance and infection. Initially 120 well-to-do ladies would visit the poor in teams of four but no nursing was undertaken until St Vincent widened the membership of the Order to include peasant women, known as Sisters of Charity, who were taught simple nursing procedures. The ladies and Sisters of Charity were then amalgamated and the first Nursing Order had been formed, performing heroically on the battlefields of seventeenth-century France. After St Vincent's death the Order waned because it failed to follow the advances in surgery and medicine, but at the time of the Crimean War the Sisters of Charity inspired Florence Nightingale to provide a similar standard of nursing of British soldiers in the Crimea.

William Harvey (1578-1657). It was as Lumelian lecturer that William Harvey delivered the following statement in 1616 which revolutionised the whole of medical science: 'The movement of the blood is constantly in a circle and is brought about by the beat of the heart'. With a sound knowledge of anatomy, Harvey saw that the valves in the veins would permit the blood to pass only to the heart while those in the great arteries permitted blood to flow only away from the heart. He then calculated that the quantity and velocity of the blood was such as made it physically impossible for the blood to do other than return by a venous route. His conclusions were published in his famous book *De Motu Cordis*. His *De Generatione Animalium*, published in 1651, was the first English work on embryology, also containing the first chapters in English on obstetrics. As a staunch Royalist, Harvey compared the heart to his king, Charles I 'the centre of all strength and power'.

John Hunter (1728-1793) was not only one of the foremost surgeons of all time but the most versatile of scientists. He raised surgery to a technical science firmly grounded in physiology and surgical pathology. To assist him in his work he founded a great menagerie of 13 000 specimens and it was his study of the capillary system of the deer which led to his treatment for aneurysm which is still in use today. Among his other discoveries were the arterial supply of the gravid uterus, the olfactory nerve in the nose and many features of the lymphatic system. As a surgical pathologist his descriptions of phlebitis, pyaemia and shock were revolutionary and his technical inventions, such as artificial feeding by a tube in the stomach and apparatus for forced respiration, were of the highest order. As a biologist his work led him to the principle that functional activities in the lower forms of life were simplifications of those in the higher. His love of science caused his death which was as a result of a mistaken inoculation of syphilis and gonorrhoea. A certain incoherence in writing was more than compensated for by his work as a teacher, as three famous doctors (Jenner, Abernethy and Astley Cooper) were his pupils.

Edward Jenner (1749-1823) was a country doctor in Berkeley, Gloucestershire, who noticed that those who had had cowpox (a mild form of pox contracted by milkmaids from cows) never became infected with smallpox. In May 1796 he conducted a crucial experiment by vaccinating an 8-year-old boy with pus from the hand of a dairymaid infected with cowpox. The boy failed to develop smallpox following inoculation eight weeks later. Cowpox was technically known as vaccinia so it was inevitable that Jenner's process became known as vaccination. Not only was one of the most terrible diseases banished from this country but a principle had been established which eventually led to the immunisation of man against many infectious diseases.

James Blundell (1790-1877) was the pioneer in the field of blood transfusion. He discovered the value of transfusion by injection of the blood of a dog into the circulation of another dog but discovered that a dog would die if injected with the blood of a sheep. This established the incompatibility of the blood of different species and prevented the practice of injecting animal blood into human beings. By further experiment he showed that a smaller quantity of blood than the amount lost would resuscitate an animal. The first transfusion of human blood took place on 12 December 1818 on a patient who was fatally ill. His first successful recovery was for a postpartum haemorrhage for which the patient received 8 oz of blood, recorded in the *Lancet* of 1829. Blundell showed, contrary to existing belief, that the blood was not injured by its passage through instruments and that a few air bubbles in the circulation were quite harmless. The problem of coagulation proved difficult and later led to his invention of a special apparatus enabling the blood to be transferred from donor to recipient with minimal physical interference.

Theodor Fliedner (1800-1864) was a Lutheran clergyman responsible for the experiment which began nursing reform. In 1826 he founded an association to help discharged prisoners and relieve the sick poor of his parish. This association led in 1836 to the development of a new hospital which was founded at Kaiserswerth, where Fliedner trained women called deaconesses to help him in his work. It was the first nursing experiment to exist independently of a religious order. The deaconesses were examined in medicine and pharmacy but, unlike the nursing training of Florence Nightingale, this was more on the lines of a comprehensive social service including training in cooking, laundering and gardening. Kaiserswerth was the first school of nursing and left a lasting impression with its spirit of dedicated service. At the time of Fliedner's death 1600 deaconesses were nursing as far apart as Turkey and the U.S.A.

William Thomas Norton (1819-1868) was a dental partner of Horace Wells (1815-48), whose career was ruined when he gave an unsuccessful public demonstration using nitrous oxide to anaesthetise a patient. A Boston chemist recommended to Morton the use of sulphuric ether and the first successful public demonstration was given at the Massachusetts General Hospital on 16 October 1846 when an operation for a vascular tumour was successfully performed. Morton ruined his reputation by attempting to patent the drug and made no further contribution to the subject.

James Simpson (1811-1870). In Edinburgh, the Professor of Midwifery, James Simpson, found ether unsatisfactory in midwifery and used a new drug, chloroform. His first experiment was upon himself and, on recovering consciousness, rightly remarked, 'This is far stronger than ether'. The drug was first administered on a child for an operation for osteomyelitis on 15 November 1847. More powerful and pleasant than ether, chloroform became the standard anaesthetic drug in Britain for the next 50 years and the new medical science of anaesthetics was born with far-reaching effects for the development of surgery.

Florence Nightingale (1820-1910) was the first outstanding figure in the history of nursing. Before she went to the Crimea nursing did not exist as a profession of high ethical and technical standards. She was able to overcome the social barriers which prevented women entering nursing. In 1854 she was able to go to the Crimea where, amid the filth of the hospitals in Scutari, she courageously fought her own battle for cleanliness and care of the patients. She never ceased to fight for sanitary conditions in the army medical service, being influential in later Royal Commissions. Her *Notes on Nursing* and *Notes on Hospitals* emphasise the principles of personal and communal hygiene as well as administrative efficiency.

By 1860 a grateful nation had contributed £50 000 to the Nightingale Fund which was used to establish a nursing school at St Thomas's Hospital London. The great medical advantages of this period could only be of benefit to mankind with trained and educated nurses. Her most notable administrative reform was the removal of nurses from the supervision of the medical staff to that of the matron. She set a standard of nursing education which was a model for all subsequent English and Commonwealth schools. After choosing the probationers herself, she ensured that they would be instructed in the basic sciences by the medical staff and would receive practical instruction in the wards under the supervision of the sisters. In later years she pressed for many reforms in workhouse nursing and was responsible for the grant of a Royal Charter to the Royal British Nursing Association in 1893.

Louis Pasteur (1822-1895) is considered to be the founder of modern bacteriology for by extensive study of milk and beer he proved that organisms naturally present in the air are alive and can produce putrefaction, but on heating lose their power and are killed—a discovery fundamental to aseptic surgery. By injecting anthrax bacilli, greatly reduced in strength, into a sheep, he was able to immunise it against subsequent infection by the virulent bacillus. This, and similar experiments, led him to conclude that the origin or extinction of infectious disease in the past may have simply been due to the strengthening or weakening of its virulence by external conditions, and the principle was applied with success in the case of preventive vaccination against hydrophobia. In 1885 the Pasteur Institute was opened and Pasteur surrounded himself with brilliant pupils—among them:

Emile Roux, responsible for epoch-making work on the diphtheria antitoxin;

Yersin, who found a vaccination against plague, and

Calmette, who discovered preventive inoculation against snake bites.

Truly Pasteur was one of the pioneers of modern preventive inoculation.

Lord Lister (1827-1912) was the greatest surgical figure of modern times. As Professor of Surgery in Glasgow, he studied the work of Pasteur from which he deduced that infection in wounds was analogous to putrefaction in wine, and selected carbolic acid as a means of destroying the organisms in the wound. Thus Lister discovered the principle involving the prevention and cure of sepsis in wounds. He insisted that everything touching the wounds should be treated with antiseptic and sought constantly to improve his dressings, eventually deciding on a gauze containing the oxides of mercury and zinc. The effects of the new principle were shown by a dramatic drop in the mortality rate of amputations and compound fractures. Abdominal, cranial and chest surgery date from the invention of the antiseptic system which had made possible the surgery of the hollow cavities of the body. Lister's antiseptic principle was later developed into an aseptic system by Halsted and Spencer Wells.

Among Lister's other achievements were the invention of the sinus forceps, probe pointed scissors and the catgut ligature. He further showed that an uninfected clot if undisturbed can be organised into living tissue, and a piece of dead bone may be absorbed in an aseptic wound.

He was President of the Royal Society 1895-1900 and became the first medical peer in 1897.

Hugh Owen Thomas (1834-1891) spent his whole professional life in the poorer areas of nineteenth-century Liverpool, but no one did more to advance the treatment of bones and joints. In his day excision and amputation were the remedies for the chronic diseases of the joints but, instead, Thomas applied the principle of complete rest for the treatment of tuberculous joints and this prevented many amputations. To ensure that the diseased part was not compressed or the circulation of the blood impaired, Thomas invented his famous fracture splint, now known as the Thomas splint. His other inventions included a wrench for the reduction of fractures and an osteoclast to break deformed bones before resetting them. The effect of the Thomas splint was not seen until World War I when it was responsible for the reduction of the mortality rate of fracture of the femur from 80 per cent in 1916 to 7 per cent in 1918—only now was Thomas seen as a great pioneer. His work was continued by his nephew, Sir Robert Jones, who developed the modern methods of tendon transplantation and bone grafting.

Robert Koch (1843-1910). When he delivered his paper on the anthrax bacillus in 1876, Robert Koch had produced the greatest discovery in bacteriology for he had proved that an infectious disease can often be caused by a specific micro-organism. He also showed how to fix and stain bacteria. In 1882 he announced the discovery of the tubercle bacillus which made possible all subsequent work on the cure for tuberculosis. On his visits to India and Egypt as the head of the German cholera Commission of 1883 he discovered the cause of cholera—the *Vibrio cholerae*— and its transmission by water and food. His work on rinderpest, tropical malaria and bubonic plague was extremely valuable and for his services to medicine he was awarded the Nobel Prize in 1905.

Wilhelm Conrad Roentgen (1845-1923) was Professor of Physics at Wurzburg who, while working with a Crooke's tube, discovered that shadows were forming on a photographic plate. After careful experiment he found that, by making his tube light-proof, a greenish fluorescent light would be thrown on a platino-barium screen 9 feet away. These rays passed through substances ordinarily opaque, such as the soft parts of the body, revealing the bones. He read his paper to the Wurzburg Society and when Professor Kolliker submitted his own hand to be photographed all doubts were allayed, Kolliker suggesting the new rays, which had been called X-rays, be known as Roentgen rays.

Among the many honours he was to receive for this discovery were the Rumford Gold Medal of the Royal Society and the Nobel Prize.

Sir Alexander Fleming (1881-1955) was responsible for the greatest contribution to the science of medical treatment made in the first half of the twentieth century—the development of antibiotics. In 1928, on examining one of his culture plates in his laboratory at London University, he found that the growth of the mould was the same as on other culture plates but the microbes near the mould, instead of forming into a yellow opaque mould, had dissolved. He then placed various microbes near the mould with different effects—for instance the diphtheria microbe was among those destroyed whilst the typhoid and influenza microbes were not so affected. Thus an antibiotic had been discovered—something alive in the mould was killing other living microbes. Fleming called this substance penicillin and it has been responsible for inhibiting the growth of the causative organisms of many common infectious diseases. During the Second World War it was used to great effect in the treatment of war wounds and gas gangrene.

Fleming was knighted in 1944 and received the Nobel Prize in 1945.

TABLE OF APPROXIMATE NORMAL VALUES

There may be some variation between laboratories depending on the method of estimation employed. This is particularly true of enzymes.

Haematology

Haemoglobin—14.6 g/100 ml or 100 per cent
Red cells—5 million/mm³
White cells—
    Adults—4 to 10 000/mm³
    Infants—10 000 to 25 000/mm³
Differentiated white cell count—
    Polymorphs 40 to 75 per cent
    Lymphocytes 20 to 50 per cent
    Monocytes 1 to 6 per cent
    Eosinophils 1 to 6 per cent
    Basophils 1 per cent
Platelets—150 000 to 350 000/mm³
Bleeding time—1 to 5 minutes
Coagulation time (capillary)—2 to 8 minutes
Erythrocyte sedimentation rate (ESR)—
    Men 0 to 10 mm/hour
    Women 0 to 20 mm/hour
Blood viscosity—1.50 to 1.75cp(centipoise)

Blood chemistry

Electrolytes—
    Serum sodium (Na^+) 136-144 mmol/litre
    Serum potassium (K^+) 3.5-5.0 mmol/litre
    Serum chloride (Cl^-) 95–105 mmol/litre
Acid/Base balance—
    Plasma alkali reserve (or carbon dioxide combining power)—50 to 75 ml CO_2/100 ml plasma, often referred to as 50 to 75 volumes per cent or 20–30 mmol/l
    Arterial P_{CO_2}—35 to 45 mm Hg
    Standard bicarbonate 22–30 mmol/litre
    Base excess of blood—±2 mmol/l
pH of 7.35–7.42
Blood glucose (fasting)—3.0–5.0 mmol/litre
Blood urea—2.50–7.5 mmol/litre
Serum acid phosphatase—2.2–3.7 ng/100cm³
Serum alkaline phosphatase—35–105 International units/litre
Serum amylase—70–300 International units/litre
Serum bilirubin—5–17 μmol/litre
Serum calcium—2.25–2.62 mmol/litre
Serum cholesterol—3.35–6.46 mmol/litre
Serum creatinine—50–100 μmol/litre
Serum gamma glutamyl transpeptidase
    (γGT)—10–50 International units/litre
Serum glutamate oxalacetate transaminase
    (SGOT)—7–44 International units/litre

*Serum glutamate pyruvate transaminase
   (SGPT)*—7–40 International units/litre
Serum iron—12.5–32 μmol/litre
Serum lactic dehydrogenase (LDH)—90–500 International units/litre
Serum phosphate—0.81–1.4 mmol/litre
Serum proteins—
   Total—60–80g/litre
   Albumin—36–50g/litre
   Globulin— 20–30g/litre
 Serum thyroxine (free)—8.8–26 μmol/litre
Serum uric acid—0.12–0.40 mmol/litre

Cerebrospinal fluid

Protein—200–400 mmol/litre
Chloride—119–126 mmol/litre
Glucose— 2.2–4.2 mmol/litre
White cells— 0 to 5/mm³

Index